Clinical Genetics
in Nursing Practice

Third Edition

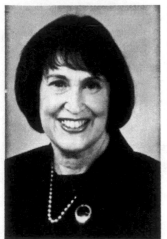

Felissa R. Lashley, RN, PhD, FAAN, FACMG (formerly Felissa L. Cohen), is Dean and Professor of the College of Nursing at Rutgers, The State University of New Jersey. Prior to that she was Dean and Professor of the School of Nursing at Southern Illinois University, Edwardsville and Clinical Professor of Pediatrics at the School of Medicine at Southern Illinois University, Springfield. Dr. Lashley received her BS at Adelphi College, her MA from New York University, and her doctorate in human genetics with a minor in biochemistry from Illinois State University. She is certified as a PhD Medical Geneticist by the American Board of Medical Genetics, the first nurse to be so certified, and is a founding fellow of the American College of Medical Genetics. She began her practice of genetic evaluation and counseling in 1973.

Dr. Lashley has authored more than 300 publications. Both prior editions of *Clinical Genetics in Nursing Practice* have received Book of the Year Awards from the *American Journal of Nursing*. Other books have also received *AJN* Book of the Year Awards including *The Person with AIDS: Nursing Perspectives* (Durham and Cohen, editors), *Women, Children, and HIV/AIDS* (Cohen and Durham, editors), and *Emerging Infectious Diseases: Trends and Issues* (Lashley and Durham, editors). *Tuberculosis: A Sourcebook for Nursing Practice* (Cohen and Durham, editors) received a Book of the Year Award from *Nurse Practitioner*. Dr. Lashley has received several million dollars in external research funding, and served as a member of the charter AIDS Research Review Committee, National Institute of Allergy and Infectious Disease, National Institutes of Health.

Dr. Lashley has been a distinguished lecturer for Sigma Theta Tau International and served as Associate Editor of *IMAGE: The Journal of Nursing Scholarship*. She is a fellow of the American Academy of Nursing. She currently serves as an editorial board member for *Biological Research in Nursing*. She received an Exxon Education Foundation Innovation Award for her article on integrating genetics into community college nursing curricula. She is a member of the International Society of Nurses in Genetics, and was a member of the steering committee of the National Coalition for Health Professional Education in Genetics, sponsored by the National Human Genome Research Institute, National Institutes of Health. She served as President of the HIV/AIDS Nursing Certifying Board. Dr. Lashley received the 2000 Nurse Researcher Award from the Association of Nurses in AIDS Care; the 2001 SAGE Award by the Illinois Nurse Leadership Institute for outstanding mentorship; and received the 2003 Distinguished Alumni Award from Illinois State University, and in 2005, was inducted into their College of Arts and Sciences Hall of Fame. She served as a member of the PKU Consensus Development Panel, National Institutes of Health. She serves as a board member at Robert Wood Johnson University Hospital in New Brunswick, New Jersey.

Clinical Genetics
in **Nursing Practice**
Third Edition

Felissa R. Lashley, RN, PhD, FAAN, FACMG

 Springer Publishing Company

To my own special loved ones—my F_1 generation: Peter, Heather, and Neal and their spouses, Julie, Chris, and Anne, but especially for my wonderful and awe-inspiring F_2 generation: Benjamin, Hannah, Jacob, Grace, and Lydia Cohen. I love you more than words can say. Thanks to my P_1 generation: Ruth and Jack Lashley for love and support through the years.

Springer Publishing Company, Inc.
11 West 42nd Street
New York, NY 10036

Acquisitions Editor: Ruth Chasek
Production Editor: Pamela Lankas
Cover design by Joanne Honigman

05 06 07 08 09 / 5 4 3 2

Library of Congress Cataloging-in-Publication Data

Lashley, Felissa R., 1941–
   Clinical genetics in nursing practice / Felissa R. Lashley. — 3rd ed.
      p. ; cm.
   Includes bibliographical references and index.
   ISBN 0-8261-2366-X
   1. Medical genetics. 2. Nursing.
   [DNLM: 1. Genetics, Medical—Nurses' Instruction. 2. Genetic Diseases,
Inborn—Nurses' Instruction. QZ 50 L343c 2005] I. Title.

RB155.L37 2005
616'.042'024613—dc22

                                                              2004028505

Printed in the United States of America by Integrated Book Technologies.

Contents

Introduction

I wrote the first edition of this book more than 20 years ago, and the discoveries in genetics since then have been phenomenal. The new knowledge and applications of human genetics to health and to society have made it even more necessary that nurses "think genetically" in their practice and, indeed in their lives. Genetic factors can be responsible in some way for both direct and indirect disease causation; for variation that determines predisposition, susceptibility, and resistance to disease and also for response to therapeutic management. Genetic disorders can be manifested initially at any period of the life cycle. In addition, improved detection, diagnosis, and treatment have resulted in the survival into adulthood of persons who formerly would have died in childhood and who now manifest common adult problems on a background of specific genetic disease. Genetic disorders have an impact not only on the affected individual but also on his/her family, friends, community, and society. Genetic variation is important in response to medications, common foods, chemicals that comprise pollution in the environment, and food additives. Genes determine susceptibility to complex common disorders such as cancer, heart disease, diabetes mellitus, Alzheimer disease, emphysema, mental illness, and others. Genetic risk factors are also important in preventing disease in the workplace.

Nurses in virtually all practice divisions and sites can therefore expect to encounter either individuals or families who are affected by genetic disease or are contemplating genetic testing. Nurses must be able to understand the implications of human genetic variation and gene–environment interaction, as well as overt disease, as they assist clients in maintaining and promoting health, and preventing and treating disease. Each person has his/her own relative state of health, and not all persons are at similar risk for developing disease because of variation in genetic makeup, for example, in regard to cancer. Thus, optimal planning, intervention, and health teaching in the appropriate educational and cultural context for a given client or family must make use of this knowledge in order to be effective. It is with these points in mind that the third edition of *Clinical Genetics in Nursing Practice* was written. This third edition is even more of a labor of love than the prior editions, and provides current information while maintaining a reasonable size and scope.

Nurses and other health professionals generally are still not educated in genetics. This educational deficit presents a barrier for receiving optimal services when it occurs in the consumer but is even more serious when it is present in those individuals *providing* health services. As far back as 1983, there was a call for the inclusion of genetics content in the curricula of Schools of Nursing, Medicine, and other health professions. With the efforts spearheaded by the National Human Genome Research Institute, National Institutes of Health, through the National Coalition for Health Professional Education in Genetics (NCHPEG), attention has been focused anew on the need for health professional competency in genetics. Today genetics is a topic discussed widely in the lay media—therefore health professionals must be able to understand this material and use it appropriately in their practices.

Clinical Genetics in Nursing Practice is written so that it can either be read in sequence, or, once the terminology is understood, as individual chapters out of sequence, because each chapter can stand on its own. The comprehensive bibliography includes the most up-to-date literature at the time of this writing as well as classic references and special older articles and books that are either still the standard or contain special examples or material that is unique. Genetic information and clinical implications are integrated for the nurse to use in practice as the topic is discussed. Illustrative examples from my own experience and practice in genetics, genetic counseling, and nursing are given throughout. In this book, the term "normal" is used as it is by most geneticists—to mean free from the disorder or condition in question. The term "practitioner" is used to mean the appropriately educated nurse or other health care provider. Genetic terminology does not generally use apostrophes (i.e., Down syndrome rather than Down's syndrome), and this pattern has been followed. In some cases, detailed information is provided that may be more useful as the reader becomes familiar with a topic. For example, a reader may not be interested in transcription factors until he/she encounters a client with Denys Drash syndrome. Ethical, social, and legal implications are integrated throughout the book and are highlighted where they are particularly vital.

The first part of the book discusses the broad scope of human genetic disease including the Human Genome Project and future directions; gives an introduction to basic information in genetics for those who need either an introduction or a review; discusses human variation and diversity as it pertains to health, disease, and molecular applications in forensics and society; and covers the various types of genetic disorders, gene action, and patterns of inheritance. Part II discusses major genetic disorders in three categories—cytogenetic or chromosomal disorders, inherited biochemical disorders, which are usually single-gene disorders, and congenital anomalies. The third part discusses assessing and intervening with clients and families at genetic risk. This section covers the impact of genetic disease on the family, assessment of genetic disorders, genetic counseling, genetic testing and screening including essential elements in such programs as prenatal detection and diagnosis, agents and conditions affecting the fetus, the reproductive and genetic effects of environmental agents, and treatment of genetic disorders. The taking of family histories, an important early-assessment tool, especially for nurses, is emphasized. Part IV discusses the burgeoning role of genetics in common situations, conditions, and diseases. It discusses the common complex disorders, twins, drug therapy, the immune system and infectious diseases, mental retardation, aging and Alzheimer disease, alpha-1-antitrypsin deficiency and its role in emphysema and liver disease, cancer, diabetes mellitus, mental illness, and behavior and heart disease. Part V discusses the ethical impact of genetics on society and future generations. Included in this section is information on assisted reproduction. The last section provides listings of Web sites for groups providing genetic information and services for professionals and clients. A glossary and detailed index are also included. Illustrations, tables, and photographs are liberally used to enrich the text.

In thanking all the people who helped bring this book to fruition, there are so many that to name them runs the risk of omitting someone. Therefore, I am acknowledging my long-time friend and colleague, Dr. Wendy Nehring, who was always there with an encouraging word when work bogged me down. I also want to acknowledge Dr. Ursula Springer and Ruth Chasek at Springer Publishing Company, who not only believed in this project but also are so wonderful to work with.

Nurses, depending on their education, preparation, and jobs, play a variety of roles in aiding the client and family affected by genetically determined conditions. All nurses, as both providers and as citizens, must understand the advances in genetics and their implications for health care and societal decisions. Future health care has become more and more influenced by genetic knowledge and the understanding of how genetic variation influences human responses. No health professional can practice without such knowledge.

—FELISSA ROSE LASHLEY, RN, PHD, FAAN, FACMG

List of Tables

List of Figures

I

Basics of Genetics and Human Genetics

1

Human Genetic Disease

enetic disease knows no age, social, economic, racial, ethnic, or religious barriers. Although many still think of genetic disorders as primarily affecting those in infancy or childhood, genetic disorders can be manifested at any period of the life cycle. The contribution of genetics to the common and complex diseases that usually appear in the adult such as cancer, Alzheimer disease, and coronary disease has become more evident in the past few years. The advances in genetic testing that are increasingly rapidly transferred to clinical practice, and innovative genetically based treatments for some of these diseases have changed the practice of health care. Improved therapeutic modalities and earlier detection and diagnosis have resulted in patient survival into adulthood with what were formerly considered childhood disorders. For example, about one third of patients with familial dysautonomia (an autosomal recessive disorder with autonomic and sensory nervous system dysfunction) are adults, the median survival age for persons with cystic fibrosis is over 30 years, and more than half of persons with sickle cell disease are adults.

In addition to the affected individual, genetic disorders exact a toll from all members of the family, as well as on the community and society (see chapter 8). Although mortality from infectious disease and malnutrition has declined in the United States, the proportion due to disorders with a genetic component has increased, assuming a greater relative importance. Genetic disorders can occur as the result of a chromosome abnormality, mutation(s) in a single gene, mutations in more than one gene, through disturbance in the interaction of multiple genes with the environment, and the alteration of genetic material by environmental

agents. Depending on the type of alteration, the type of tissue affected (somatic or germline), the internal environment, the genetic background of the individual, the external environment, and other factors, the outcome can result in no discernible change, structural or functional damage, aberration, deficit, or death. Effects may be apparent immediately or may be delayed. Outcomes can be manifested in many ways, including abnormalities in biochemistry, reproduction, growth, development, immune function, behavior, or combinations of these.

A mutant gene, an abnormal chromosome, or a teratologic agent that causes harmful changes in genetic material is as much an etiologic agent of disease as is a microorganism. Certain genetic states are definitely known to increase an individual's susceptibility and resistance to certain specific disorders, whereas others are suspected of doing so. Genes set the limits for the responses and adaptations that individuals can make as they interact with their environments. Genes never act in isolation; they interact with other genes against the individual's genetic background and internal milieu, and with agents and factors in the external environment. Conneally (2003, p. 230) expresses this by saying, "No gene is an island." For example, persons who have glucose-6-phosphate dehydrogenase (G6PD) deficiency (present in 10%–15% of Black males in the United States) usually show no effects, but they can develop hemolytic anemia when exposed to certain drugs such as sulfonamides. In another example, the child with phenylketonuria develops signs and symptoms after exposure to dietary phenylalanine. In the same manner, diseases thought of as "environmental" do not affect everyone exposed. Not all individuals who are exposed to a certain amount of trauma develop fractures. One of the determining factors is bone density, about 85% of which is normally governed by genetic factors. An extreme example of genes' effect on bone density is that of osteogenesis imperfecta type III in which the affected person is prone to fracture development with little or no environmental contributions.

Genes are important in an individual's susceptibility, predisposition, and resistance to disease. Some examples include the following.

- persons who are Duffy negative (one of the blood groups) are resistant to malaria caused by *Plasmodium vivax;*
- persons in Papua, New Guinea, who develop tinea imbricata, a fungus infection, must inherit a susceptibility gene and must also be exposed to the fungus *Trichophyton concentricum* in order for that susceptibility to manifest itself;
- possession of HLA-B27 leads to susceptibility for development of ankylosing spondylitis;
- the association of increased levels of pepsinogen I and the development of duodenal ulcer but protection against some extrapulmonary tuberculosis;
- the association of a certain homozygous defect ($\Delta 32$) in *CCR5* (the gene that encodes a coreceptor for HIV formerly called *CKR5*) in Whites results in high resistance to HIV infection, and in its heterozygous form delays the onset of AIDS in persons already infected, as does the more-recently recognized *CCR2* V64I variation;
- heterozygosity of the human prion protein gene appears protective, as most persons developing iatrogenic Creutzfeldt-Jakob disease are homozygotes at position 129;
- West Africans persons with certain variants of *NRAMP1* (the natural-resistance-associated macrophage protein 1 gene) appear more susceptible to tuberculosis;
- persons with alpha-1-antitrypsin deficiency are susceptible to the development of emphysema and/or certain hepatic disorders; and
- boxers who possess an apolipoprotein E ε4 allele appear more susceptible to chronic traumatic encephalopathy than those who do not possess it.

The concept of genetic risk factors, as well as the environmental risk factors usually considered, has thus become important.

EXTENT AND IMPACT

Results of surveys on the extent of genetic disorders vary based on the definitions used, the time of life at which the survey is done, and the composition of the population surveyed. More data are discussed in chapter 9. Researchers have estimated the incidence of chromosome aberrations to be 0.5% to 0.6% in newborns, the frequency of single gene disorders to be 2% to 3% by 1 year of age, and the frequency of major and minor malformations to range from 4% to 7% and 10% to 12%, respectively, at the same time. It is estimated that overall about 50% of spontaneous abortions are caused by chromosome abnormalities as are 5% to 7% of stillbirths and perinatal deaths. These are discussed in chapter 5. Rimoin, Connor, Pyeritz, and Korf (2002) cite the lifetime frequency of chromosomal disorders at 3.8/1,000 livebirths; single gene disorders at 20/1,000; multifactorial disorders at 646.4/1,000; and somatic cell (cumulative) genetic disorders (including cancer) at 240/1,000, meaning that deleterious genetic changes ultimately affect disease in nearly everyone!

Historic studies are still relevant because they provide information that predates the advent of prenatal diagnosis (which allows for the option of selective termination of pregnancy, preimplantation genetic diagnosis, and embryo selection) thus distorting information about genetic disorders at birth and after because of selection. A 1981 longitudinal study by Christianson, van den Berg, Milkovich and Oeshsli (1981) of pregnant women enrolled in the Kaiser Foundation Health Plan followed offspring to 5 years of age. Their definition of "congenital anomalies" was very broad and encompassed conditions of prenatal origin including "structural defects, functional abnormalities, inborn errors of metabolism, and chromosome aberrations" that were definitely diagnosed. They classified these anomalies as severe, moderate, and trivial. "Trivial" included conditions such as supernumerary nipples, skin tags, and umbilical hernias, and are excluded from consideration. Obviously, late-appearing disorders were not included.

Twenty-seven percent of those offspring who died before 1 year of age had an anomaly, as did 59% of those who died between 1 year of age and 5 years of age. There was a fivefold increase in the cumulative incidence of congenital anomalies between 6 days of age and 5 years of age. At 5 years of age, the incidence rate of severe and moderate congenital anomalies as defined was 15%. The incidence was higher among children weighing 2,500 g or less at birth. As high as this may seem, it still does not include conditions usually developing later (e.g., hypercholesterolemia, diabetes mellitus, Huntington disease). Another study by Myrianthopoulos and Chung (1974) found an overall incidence of congenital anomalies of 15.56% in infants at 1 year of age. These researchers included minor anomalies. In a New Zealand study of 4,286 infants, Tuohy, Counsell and Geddis (1993) recorded the prevalence of birth defects defined as "a significant structural deviation from normal that was present at birth" in infants alive at 6 weeks of age. The prevalence was 4.3% of live births.

According to the charts of patients evaluated between July 1981 and February 1995 at a medical center covering central and eastern Kentucky, 4,212 patients were seen. As classified by Cadle, Dawson, and Hall (1996), the most common chromosomal syndromes were Down syndrome, trisomy 18, Prader-Willi syndrome, fragile X syndrome, Turner syndrome and trisomy 13. The most common single-gene defects were Marfan syndrome, Noonan syndrome, neurofibromatosis, ectodermal dysplasia and osteogenesis imperfecta. The most common teratogenic diagnoses were fetal alcohol syndrome, infant of a diabetic mother, fetal hydantoin syndrome, and maternal PKU effects. In the category of other congenital anomalies, unknown multiple congenital anomaly syndromes were followed by spina bifida, cleft lip and palate, and microcephaly. Sever, Lynberg, and Edmonds (1993) estimated that in the United States 100,000 to 150,000 babies are born each year with a major birth defect and, of these, 6,000 die during the first 28 days of life and another 2,000 die before 1 year of age. In active surveillance of malformations in newborns in Mainz, Germany from 1990 to 1998, major malformations and minor errors of morphogenesis were found to be 6.9% and 35.8% respectively. Risk factors significantly associated with malformations were: parents or siblings with malformations,

parental consanguinity, more than three minor errors of morphogenesis in the proband, maternal diabetes mellitus, and using antiallergic drugs during the first trimester (Queisser-Luft, Stolz, Wiesel, Schlaefer, & Spränger, 2002). Koster, McIntire, & Leveno, (2003) examined minor malformations as part of their study, finding an incidence of 2.7%. They also detected a recurrence risk for minor malformations of about 7% in women whose index pregnancy had a mild malformation.

Genetic factors therefore play a role in both morbidity and mortality. Various studies have attempted to define more closely the extent of such involvement. Again, estimates are influenced by definition, population, type of hospital (community or medical center), and methodology. A 1978 study by Hall, Powers, McIlvaine, and Ean divided diseases into 5 categories: (1) single gene or chromosome disorders, (2) multifactorial/polygenic conditions, (3) developmental anomalies of unknown origin, (4) familial disorders, and (5) nongenetic disorders. The first four categories accounted for 53.4% of all admissions, whereas the first two categories alone accounted for 26.6% of all admissions. A 1981 Canadian study by Soltan and Craven classified diagnosis at discharge into four categories—chromosomal, single gene, multifactorial, and others, classifying such conditions as atopic sensitivity and hernias under others. In regional hospitals, patients with genetic conditions were 17.7% and 16.3% of the total in the pediatric and acute medical services, respectively. The average length of stay for pediatric patients with disorders with a genetic component was about twice that of the nongenetic, but on the medical service the length of stay was about the same for both genetic and nongenetic disorders. Older studies have had the following results: In a Canadian pediatric hospital, Scriver, Neal, Saginur, and Clow found that genetic disorders and congenital malformations accounted for 29.6% of admissions, whereas about another 2% were "probably genetic." In 1973 Day and Holmes found that 17% of pediatric inpatients and 9% of pediatric outpatients had primary diagnoses of genetic origin, and in 1970 Roberts, Chavez, and Court found that genetic conditions were involved in over 40% of hospital deaths among children. Yoon and colleagues (1997) in as well as Harris and James (1997), Hobbs, Cleves, and Simmons (2002) and

McCandless, Brunger, and Cassidy (2004) found that patients with birth defects and/or genetic disorders had longer hospital stays, greater morbidity, greater inpatient mortality, and higher expenses. In the United States overall, congenital malformations, deformations, and chromosomal abnormalities accounted for: 1–4 years of age, 10.9%; 5–9 years of age, 5.9%; and 10–14 years of age, 4.8%. These did not include most Mendelian disorders (Arias, MacDorman, Strobino, & Guyer, 2003). In Israel, Zlotogora, Leventhal, and Amitai, (2003), reported that in the period from 1996 to 1999, malformations and/or Mendelian disorders accounted for 28.3% of the total infant deaths among Jews and 43.6% of non-Jews. This did not account for pregnancy terminations. Hudome, Kirby, Senner, and Cunniff (1994) in examining neonatal deaths in a regional neonatal intensive care unit found 23.3% of the deaths were due to a genetic disorder. Review of the deaths during the five year period indicated that the contribution of genetic disorders was underrecognized. Further classification of mortality was: single primary developmental defect (42%), unrecognized malformations pattern, (29%), chromosome abnormality (18.8%), and Mendelian condition (10.1%). Cunniff, Carmack, Kirby, and Fiser (1995) examined the causes of deaths in a pediatric intensive care unit in Arkansas. They found that about 19% of deaths were in patients with heritable disorder. Stevenson and Carey (2004) found that 34.4% of mortality in a childrens hospital in Utah were due to malformations and genetic disorders while another 2.3% had such conditions but died of an acquired cause such as a patient with trisomy 21 who died of pneumonia. Classification of mortality in their study included malformations of unknown causes (65.6%), chromosome disorders (16.7%), malformations/dysplasia syndromes, (11.7%), and single gene and metabolic defects (6.1%). McCandless and colleagues (2004) examined admissions in a childrens hospital. They found that 71% of admissions had an underlying disorder known to be at least partly genetically determined. Genetically determined diseases were divided into those with a well-recognized genetically determined predisposition (51.8%) and those with clear cut genetic determinants (48.2%) and 96% of those with a chronic illness had a disorder that was in part, genetically determined. They also found that the 34% of admissions that had a clear genetic underlying disorder accounted for 50% of the total hospital charges and had a mean length of stay that was 40% longer.

An important outcome of some of these studies has been the realization that, from chart audit, relatively few patients or families received genetic counseling and this is still true to some extent today. To ensure that this shortcoming is recognized, the discharge protocol should include the following questions that address the issue: Does the disorder have a genetic component? Was the patient or family so advised? Was genetic information provided? Was genetic counseling provided? The latter two questions could be deferred if the time was not appropriate, but part of the discharge plan for that patient should include referral for genetic counseling, and the family should be followed up to ensure that this was accomplished. A summary of the genetic information and counseling provided should be recorded on the chart or record, so that others involved with the patient or family will be able to reinforce, reinterpret, or build on this information. Recognition of genetic condition can also provide the opportunity for appropriate treatment and guidance.

GENETIC DISEASE THROUGH THE LIFESPAN

Genetic alterations leading to disease are present at birth but may not be manifested clinically until a later age, or not at all. The time of manifestation depends on the following factors: (a) type and extent of the alteration, (b) exposure to external environmental agents, (c) influence of other specific genes possessed by the individual and by his/her total genetic make-up, and (d) internal environment of the individual. Characteristic times for the clinical manifestation and recognition of selected genetic disorders are shown in Table 1.1. These times do not mean that manifestations cannot appear at other times, but rather that the timespan shown is typical. For example, Huntington disease may be manifested in the older child, but this is very rare. Other disorders may be diagnosed in the newborn period or in infancy instead of at their usual later time because of participation in screening programs (e.g., Klinefelter

TABLE 1.1   Usual Stages of Manifestation of Selected Genetic Disorders

Disorder	Newborn	Infancy	Childhood	Adolescence	Adult
Achondroplasia	X				
Down syndrome	X				
Spina bifida	X				
Urea cycle disorders	X				
Menkes disease		X			
Tay-Sachs disease		X			
Lesch–Nyhan syndrome		X	X		
Cystic fibrosis		X	X		
Ataxia-telangiectasia			X		
Hurler disease			X		
Duchenne muscular dystrophy			X		
Homocystinuria			X		
Torsion dystonia			X	X	
Gorlin syndrome			X	X	
Acute intermittent porphyria				X	
Klinefelter syndrome				X	
Refsum disease				X	X
Wilson disease			X	X	X
Acoustic neuroma (bilateral)				X	X
Polycystic renal disease (adult)					X
Adenomatous polyposis					X
McArdle disease					X
Huntington disease					X

(Column header spanning Newborn, Infancy, Childhood, Adolescence, Adult: "Life cycle stage")

syndrome), or because of the systematic search for affected relatives due to the occurrence of the disorder in another family member, rather than because of the occurrence of signs or symptoms (e.g., Duchenne muscular dystrophy). Milder forms of inherited biochemical disorders are being increasingly recognized in adults.

HISTORICAL NOTES

Human genetics is an excellent example of how the interaction of clinical observation and application with basic scientific research in genetics, cytology, biochemistry, and immunology and today's bioinformatics and technological advances can result in direct major health benefits and influence the formation of health and social policies. Examples of the use of genetics in plant and animal breeding can be found in the bible and on clay tablets from as early as circa 3000 B.C. The Talmud (Jewish law clarifying the Old Testament) contains many references indicating familiarity with the familial nature of certain traits and disorders, but it reveals little or no awareness of basic principles. In the 1800s, patterns of disorders such as hemophilia and polydactyly were observed. In 1866 Mendel published his classic paper, which remained largely unappreciated until its "rediscovery" in 1900 by Correns, DeVries, and Tschermak. In the late 19th century, Galton made contributions to quantitative genetics and described use of the twin method. In the early 1900s, Garrod's concepts of the inborn errors of metabolism led eventually to Beadle and Tatum's development of the one-gene/one-enzyme theory in 1941. The 1950s, however, marked the beginning of "the golden age" of the study of human genetics. During this period, the correct chromosome number in humans was established, the first association between a chromosome aberration and a clinical disorder was made, the first enzyme defect in an inborn error of metabolism delineated, the structure of deoxyribonucleic acid (DNA) determined, the fine structure of the gene determined, and the first treatment of enzyme deficiency by a low phenylalanine diet attempted. What has been called a new golden age is now evolving in genetics due to the knowledge and applications arising from the various initiatives of the Human Genome Project discussed below.

Genetics has moved rapidly in applying basic knowledge from gene hybridization, sequencing, cloning, and synthesis; recombinant DNA and gene probes; determination of the molecular basis of disease; gene expression information; information about proteomics; human variation; somatic cell hybridization; and the development of newer, more sensitive cytogenetic techniques to clinical applications including testing, screening, counseling, prenatal diagnosis, assisted reproduction, intrauterine and postnatal treatment, transplantation of tissues and organs, gene therapy, pharmacogenomics; genetic surveillance and monitoring, and increased understanding of the basis for genetic susceptibility to disease. The term "genomics," the interface of the study of complete human genome sequences with the informatic tools with which to analyze them (Strauss & Falkow, 1997), has entered common vocabulary. Health professional education must keep pace with the explosion of this knowledge. To this end, various groups have determined core knowledge, and within the auspices of the National Human Genome Research Institute (NHGRI) the National Coalition for the Health Professional Education in Genetics (NCHPEG) was formed to address the integration of genetic content in health professional curricula and continuing education for those in practice, and various health professional disciplines as well as primary and secondary schools have acted to incorporate genetic knowledge into their disciplines and teaching. The International Society of Nurses in Genetics (ISONG) has set standards for genetic nursing. ISONG has served as a focal point for nurses involved with genetics and for leadership in nursing around genetic issues and information. Through a subsidiary, the Genetic Nursing Credentialing Commission, nurses with a baccalaureate or master's degree, respectively may apply to be recognized as a Baccalaureate Genetics clinical Nurse or an Advanced Practice Nurse in Genetics. Many other organizations of individual types of health practitioners and geneticists have been active in translating genetic findings into the specific clinical practice and education of various disciplines. In another project, British scientists have embarked on the "frozen arc" project, which aims to preserve and bank the DNA of various endangered species.

FEDERAL LEGISLATION:
A BRIEF HISTORICAL LOOK

The National Genetic Diseases Program was initiated in fiscal year (FY) 1976 under Public Law (PL) 94-278—The National Sickle Cell Anemia, Cooley's Anemia, Tay-Sachs and Genetic Diseases Act. This act, commonly known as the Genetic Diseases Act, grew out of individual legislation for sickle cell disease and Cooley's anemia and attempted to eliminate the passage of specific laws for individual diseases. Its purpose was to "establish a national program to provide for basic and applied research, research training, testing, counseling, and information and education programs with respect to genetic diseases including sickle cell anemia, Cooley's anemia (now called thalassemia), Tay-Sachs disease, cystic fibrosis, dysautonomia, hemophilia, retinitis pigmentosa, Huntington's chorea, and muscular dystrophy." To do this, support was available for research, training of genetic counselors and other health professionals, continuing education for health professionals and the public, and for programs for diagnosis, control, and treatment of genetic disease. In 1978, PL 95-626 extended the legislation which also added to the diseases specified "and genetic conditions leading to mental retardation or genetically caused mental disorders." Various research programs and services relating to genetic disorders are now located under various government agencies. Today, major federal legislation efforts are concerned with genetic privacy and genetic discrimination prevention. The Genetic privacy and Nondiscrimination Act of 2003 was introduced to the U.S. House of Representatives in November 2003, while the Genetic Information Nondiscrimination Act of 2003 was introduced to the U.S. Senate in May, 2003. A review of information in regard to genetics privacy, antidiscrimination laws and other legislation may be found at http://www.doegenomes.org (the U.S. Department of Energy).

THE HUMAN GENOME PROJECT

In the mid-1980s formal discussions began to emerge to form an international effort to map and sequence every gene in the human genome. The resultant Human Genome Project was begun in 1990, and in the United States was centered in the National Center for Human Genome Research at the National Institutes of Health (NIH) and the Department of Energy. David Smith directed the program at the Department of Energy while James Watson and Francis Collins were the first and second directors at NIH respectively. Various centers (22) were designated as Human Genome Project Research Centers across the United States. Major goals of this project were: genetic mapping; physical mapping; sequencing the 3 billion DNA base pairs of the human genome; the development of improved technology for genomic analysis; the identification of all genes and functional elements in genomic DNA, especially those associated with human diseases; the characterization of the genomes of certain non-human model organisms such as *Escherichia coli* (bacterium), *Drosophila melanogaster* (fruit fly), *Saccharomyces cerevisiae* (yeast); informatics development including sophisticated databases and automating the management and analysis of data; the establishment of the Ethical, Legal, and Social Implications (ELSI) programs as an integral part of the project; and the training of students and scientists.

ELSI issues included research on "identifying and addressing ethical issues arising from genetic research, responsible clinical integration of new genetic technologies, privacy and the fair use of genetic information, and professional and public education about ELSI issues". (Genome project finishes," 1995 . . ., p. 8). International collaborations such as the Human Genome Organization (HUGO), supported in part by The Wellcome trust and other private monies and those through United Nations Education, Social and Cultural Organization (UNESCO) were also developed. The Human Genome Project has made significant contributions to the understandings of the genetic contribution to genetic and common diseases such as polycystic kidney disease, Alzheimer disease, breast cancer and colorectal cancer. James Watson has been quoted as saying about the Human Genome Project, "I see an extraordinary potential for human betterment ahead of us. We can have at our disposal the ultimate tool for understanding ourselves at the molecular level" (quoted in Caskey, Collins, Juengst, & McKusich, 1994, p. 29). Of concern has been the specter of the potential eugenic purposes to which knowledge obtained by sequencing the genome could be put. In regard to this, Saunders (1993) has asked, "whether the project will be a scientific justification for neo-eugenics and a societal tool for discrimination or a grail to heal many inherited diseases." (p. 47) These issues are discussed further in chapter 27. Gerard, Hayes and Rothstein (2002) state that "genomics will be to the 21st century what infectious disease was to the 20th century for public health."

The Project finished sequencing 99% of the gene-containing part of the human genome sequence to 99.99% accuracy in April, 2003. One future aim is to look at human variation in DNA sequence in the form of the single nucleotide polymorphism (SNP). Millions of SNPs occur in each human genome. Sets of these are inherited as a haplotype or block, and the individual SNPs and their constellations are being examined to create pattern "maps" across populations in the United States, Asia and Africa. One concern is that the documentation of genetic differences could lead to discrimination on the basis of genetic makeup (see chapter 27).

Building on the foundation of the human genome project, three major themes are envisioned for the future, each with what are called grand challenges within them, as well as six crosscutting elements. See Collins, Green, Guttmacher and Guyer, (2003) for a detailed description. The three major themes and challenges are described in brief below:

1. *Genomics to biology*—includes the elucidation of the structure and function of genomes, including how genetic networks and protein pathways are organized and contribute to cellular and organismal phenotypes; understanding and

cataloguing common heritable variants in human populations; understanding the dynamic nature of the genome in relation to evolution across species; and developing policy options for data access, patenting, licensing, and use of information.

2. *Genomics to health*—includes identifying genetic contributions to disease and drug response; developing strategies to identify gene variants that contribute to good health and resistance to disease; developing genome-based approaches to prediction of disease susceptibility and drug response, early detection of illness, and molecular taxonomy of disease states including the possibility of reclassifying illness on the basis of molecular characterization; using these understandings to develop new therapeutic approaches to disease; investigating how genetic risk information is conveyed in clinical practice, how it influences health behaviors and affects outcomes and costs; and developing genome-based tools to improve health for all.

3. *Genomics to society*—includes developing policy options for the uses of genomics that include genetic testing and genetic research with human subject protection; appropriate use of genomic information; understanding the relationships between genomics, race and ethnicity as well as uncovering the genomic contributions to human traits and behaviors and the consequences of uncovering these types of information; and assessing how to define the appropriate and inappropriate uses of genomics. The six crosscutting elements are the generation of resources such as databases; technology development including nanotechnology and microfluidics; new and improved computational methods and approaches; training scientists, scholars and clinicians; investigation of ethical, legal, and social implications of genomics; and effective education of the public and health professionals.

The completion of the Human Genome Project also spawned what has become known as the -omics revolution. Proteomics refers to all of the proteins in the genome and is of interest because genes may code for more than one protein due to posttranslational modification. Proteomics involves the characterization of proteins and their complex interactions and bridges the gap between genetics and physiology. Metabolomics is the study of metabolites, particularly within a given cell, and involves cell signaling and cell-to-cell communication. Tran-

scriptomics refers to the study of mRNA and gene expression largely through the use of microarray technology to create profiles. Nutrigenomics looks at interactions between dietary components and genetic variations with an eye towards individualized nutrition to prevent or treat disease. Toxicogenomics is concerned with the effect of various chemical compounds on gene expression. Pharmacogenomics involves the interface between genetics and drug therapy both in regard to genetic variation as it influences the response to drugs and also using information regarding the underlying genetic defect in targeting treatment (see chapter 18). Scriver (2004) refers to study of the phenome referring to individuality in phenotypes. Further, a prospective research study examining the interaction between genetics and the environment has been called for by Collins (2004).

RELEVANCE TO NURSING

It is difficult to imagine that any nurse who is practicing today would not have contact with clients or families affected by a genetic disorder. As discussed in brief previously, and in more detail throughout this book, genetic disorders and variations are important in all phases of the life cycle, and span all clinical practice divisions and sites, including the workplace, school, hospital, clinic, office, mental health facility, and community health agency. It is time to integrate genetics into nursing education and practice and to encourage nursing personnel to "think genomically." The Task Force on Genetic Testing (Holtzman, Murphy, Watson, & Barr, 1997) recommended that schools of nursing, medicine, and other professional schools strengthen "training" in genetics. The National Human Genome Research Institute has a National Coalition for Health Professional Education in Genetics (NCH-PEG) whose major mission is the implementation of health professional education in genetics. As one looks at the future of nursing, health care, and genetics/genomics, there are basic assumptions involving the use of genomics in all of health care, and nurses must be prepared to meet these. Thus core understandings are needed and ways to integrate information into educational programs are essential (see Lashley, 2000, 2001, and NCHPEG Core competencies at http://www.nchpeg.org).

All nurses need to be able to understand the language of genetics, be able to communicate with others using it appropriately, interview clients and take an accurate history over three generations, recognize the possibility of a genetic disorder in an individual or family, and appropriately refer that person or family for genetic evaluation or counseling. They should also be prepared to explain and interpret correctly the purpose, implications and results of genetic tests in such disorders as cancer and Alzheimer disease. Nurses will be seeing adults with childhood genetic diseases, and will have to deal with how those disorders will influence and be influenced by the common health problems that occur in adults as they age, as well as seeing the usual health problems of adults superimposed on the genetic background of a childhood genetic disorder such as cystic fibrosis. Nurses will also see more persons with identified adult-onset genetic disorders, such as hemochromatosis and some types of Gaucher disease. The precise role played by the nurse varies depending on the disorder, the needs of the client and family, and the nurse's expertise, role, education, and job description. Advanced practice nurses will have additional skills to offer. Depending on these, he/she may be providing any of the following in relation to genetic disorders and variations, many of which are extensions of usual nursing practice:

- direct genetic counseling;
- planning, implementing, administering, or evaluating screening or testing programs;
- monitoring and evaluating clients with genetic disorders;
- working with families under stress engendered by problems related to a genetic disorder;
- coordinating care and services;
- managing home care and therapy;
- following up on positive newborn screening tests;
- interviewing clients;
- assessing needs and interactions in clients and families;
- taking comprehensive, relevant, family histories;
- drawing and interpreting pedigrees;
- assessment of genetic risk especially in conjunction with genetic testing options;

- assessing of the client and family's cultural/ethnic health beliefs and practices as they relate to the genetic problem;
- assessing of the client and family's strengths and weakensses and family functioning;
- providing health teaching and education related to genetics and genetic testing;
- serving as an advocate for a client and family affected by a genetic disorder;
- participating in public education about genetics;
- developing an individualized plan of care;
- reinforcing and interpreting genetic counseling and testing information;
- supporting families when they are receiving counseling and making decisions;
- recognizing the possibility of a genetic component in a disorder and taking appropriate referral action; and
- appreciating and ameliorating the social impact of a genetic problem on the client and family.

Recognizing the importance of genetics in health care and policy allows new ways to think about health and disease. Early in my genetic counseling career (1973), a man in his mid-40s made an appointment. He told me that he had decided to get married, and wanted his genes, "screened and cleaned." At that time the request seemed fantastic. Today, the possibility is just over the horizon. We are not far from the time when, at birth or even before, we will be able with one set of genetic testing to determine the genetic blueprint for the life of that infant and design an individualized health profile. This profile could then be used to develop a comprehensive personalized plan of health focusing on prevention based on his/her genes. Among our challenges will be developing these options with the consideration of the ethical and social issues and of ensuring access to these various options for various populations. Perhaps nowhere else is it as important to focus on the family as the primary unit of care, because identification of a genetic disorder in one member can allow others to receive appropriate preventive measures, detection, and diagnosis or treatment, and to choose reproductive and life options concordant with their personal beliefs. The demand for genetic services continues to grow. Only a small percentage of those who should receive them are actually receiving them. Health disparities especially among the poor and disadvantaged of various ethnic backgrounds may also occur in regard to genetic services and needs to be addressed. Nurses as a professional group are in an ideal position to apply principles of health promotion, maintenance, and disease prevention coupled with an understanding of cultural differences, technical skills, family dynamics, growth and development, and other professional skills to the person and family unit who is threatened by a genetic disorder in ways that can ensure an effective outcome.

BIBLIOGRAPHY

Acheson, L. (2003). Fostering applications of genetics in primary care: What will it take? *Genetics in Medicine, 5,* 63–65.

Almarsdottir, A. B., Bjornsdottir, I., & Traulsen, J. M. (2005). A lay prescription for tailor-made drugs—Focus group reflections on pharmacogenomics. *Health Policy, 71,* 233–241.

Arias, E., MacDorman, M. F., Strobino, D. M., & Guyer, B. (2003). Annual summary of vital statistics—2002. *Pediatrics, 112,* 1215–1230.

Austin, C. P. (2004). The impact of the completed human genome sequence on the development of novel therapeutics for human disease. *Annual Review of Medicine, 55,* 1–13.

Behnke, A. R., & Hassell, T. M. (2004). Need for genetics education in U.S. dental and dental hygiene programs. *Journal of Dental Education, 68,* 819–822.

Bell, J. I. (2003). The double helix in clinical practice. *Nature, 421,* 414–416.

Bellamy, R., Ruwende, C., Corrah, T., McAdam, K. P. W. J., Whittle, H. C., & Hill, A. V. S. (1998). Variations in the *NRAMP1* gene and susceptibility to tuberculosis in West Africans. *New England Journal of Medicine, 338,* 640–644.

Cadle, R. G., Dawson, T., & Hall, B. D. (1996). The prevalence of genetic disorders, birth defects and syndromes in central and eastern Kentucky. *Kentucky Medical Association Journal, 94,* 237–241.

Carrington, M., & O'Brien, S. J. (2003). The influence of *HLA* genotype on AIDS. *Annual Review of Medicine, 54,* 535–551.

Caskey, C. T., Collins, F. S., Juengst, E. T., & McKusick, V. T. (1994). Human genes: The map takes shape. *patient Care, 28*(1), 28–43.

Centers for Disease Control and Prevention. (2004). *Genomics and population health: United States 2003.* Atlanta, GA: Office of Genomics and Disease Prevention, Centers for Disease Control and Prevention.

Chakravarti, A., & Little, P. (2003). Nature, nurture and human disease. *Nature, 421,* 412–414.

Christianson, R. E., van den Berg, B. J., Milkovich, L., & Oechsli, F. W. (1981). Incidence of congenital anomalies among white and black live births with long-term follow-up. *American Journal of Public Health, 71,* 1333–1341.

Cobb, J. P., & O'Keefe, G. E. (2004). Injury research in the genomic era. *Lancet, 363,* 2076–2083.

Collins, F. S. (2004). The case for a U.S. prospective cohort study of genes and environment. *Nature, 429,* 475–477.

Collins, F. S., Morgan, M., & Patrinos, A. (2003). The human genome project: Lessons from large-scale biology. *Science, 300,* 286–290.

Collins, F. S., Green, E. D., Guttmacher, A. E., & Guyer, M. S. (2003). A vision for the future of genomics research. *Nature, 422,* 835–847.

Conneally, P. M. (2003). The complexity of complex diseases. *American Journal of Human Genetics, 72,* 229–232.

Cook, S. S., Kse, R., Middleton, L., & Monsen, R. B. (2003). Portfolio evaluation for professional competence: Credentialing in genetics for nurses. *Journal of Professional Nursing, 19,* 85–90.

Cunniff, C., Carmack, J. L., Kirby, R. S., & Fiser, D. H. (1995). Contribution of heritable disorders to mortality in the pediatric intensive care unit. *Pediatrics, 95,* 678–681.

Darnton-Hill, I., Margetts, B., & Deckelbaum, R. (2004). Public health nutrition and genetics: Implications for nutrition policy and promotion. *Proceedings of the Nutrition Society, 63,* 173–185.

Darvasi, A. (2003). Gene expression meets genetics. *Nature, 422,* 269–270.

Davis, C. D., & Milner, J. (2004). Frontiers in nutrigenomics, proteomics, metabolomics and cancer prevention. *Mutation Research, 551,* 51–64.

Day, N., & Holmes, L. B. (1973). The incidence of genetic disease in a university hospital population. *American Journal of Human Genetics, 25,* 237–246.

De Maio, A., Torres, M. B., & Reeves, R. H. (2005). Genetic determinants influencing the response to injury, inflammation, and sepsis. *Shock, 23,* 11–17.

Elkin, P. L. (2003). Primer on medical genomics. Part V: Bioinformatics. *Mayo Clinic Proceedings, 78,* 57–64.

Forsman, I. (1994). Evolution of the nursing role in genetics. *Journal of Obstetric, Gynecologic, and Neonatal Nursing, 23,* 481–487.

Frazier, M. E., Johnson, G. M., Thomassen, D. G., Oliver, C. E., & Patrinos, A. (2003). Realizing the potential of the genome revolution: The genomes to life program. *Science, 300,* 290–293.

Gerard, S., Hayes, M., & Rothstein, R. A. (2002). On the edge of tomorrow: Fitting genomics into public health policy. *Journal of Law, Medicine and Ethics, 30*(Suppl. 3), 173–176.

Hall, J. G., Powers, E. K., McIlvaine, R. T., & Ean, V. H. (1978). The frequency and financial burden of genetic disease in a pediatric hospital. *American Journal of Medical Genetics, 1,* 417–436.

Hamosh, A., Scott, A. F., Amberger, J. S., Bocchini, C. A., & McKusick, V. A. (2005). Online Mendelian Inheritance in Man (OMIM), a knowledgebase of human genes and genetic disorders. *Nucleic Acids Research, 33,* D514–D517.

Harris, J. A., & James, L. (1997). State-by-state cost of birth defects—1992. *Teratology, 56,* 17–23.

Hobbs, C. A., Cleves, M. A., & Simmons, C. J. (2002). Genetic epidemiology and congenital malformations. *Archives of Pediatrics and Adolescent Medicine, 156,* 315–320.

Holtzman, N. A., Murphy, P. D., Watson, M. S., & Barr, P. A. (19997). Predictive genetic testing: From basic research to clinical practice. *Science, 278,* 602–605.

Hudome, S. M., Kirby, R. S., Senner, J. W., & Cunniff, C. (1994). Contribution of genetic disorders to neonatal mortality in a regional intensive care setting. *American Journal of Perinatology, 11,* 100-103.

International Society of Nurses in Genetics. (1998). *Statement on the scope and standards of clinical genetics in nursing practice.* Washington, DC: American Nurses Publishing.

Jordan, B. D., Relkin, N. R., Ravdin, L. D., Jacobs, A. R., Bennett, A., & Gandy, S. (1997). Apolipopro-

tein E ε4 associated with chronic traumatic brain injury in boxing. *Journal of the American Medical Association, 278,* 136–140.

Kaput, J., & Rodriguez, R. L. (2004). Nutritional genomics: The next frontier in the postgenomic era. *Physiological Genomics, 16,* 166–177.

Kaslow, R. A., Dorak, T., & Tang, J. J. (2005). Influence of host genetic variation on susceptibility to HIV type 1 infection. *Journal of Infectious Diseases, 191*(Suppl. 1), S68–S77.

Koonin, S. E. (1998). An independent perspective on the Human Genome project. *Science, 279,* 36–37.

Korf, B. R. (2002). Integration of genetics into clinical teaching in medical school education. *Genetics in Medicine, 4*(Suppl. 6), 33S–38S.

Koster, E. L., McIntire, D. D., & Leveno, K. J. (2003). Recurrence of mild malformations and dysplasias. *Obstetrics & Gynecology, 102,* 363–366.

Lashley, F. R. (1997). Thinking about genetics in new ways. *Image, 29,* 202.

Lashley, F. R. (1998). Integrating genetic knowledge into community college nursing education. In M. R. Mays (Ed.), *The genetics revolution* (pp. 69–72). Washington, DC: Community College Press.

Lashley, F. R. (1999). Integrating genetics content in undergraduate nursing programs. *Biological Research in Nursing, 1,* 113–118.

Lashley, F. R. (2000). Genetics in nursing education. *Nursing Clinics of North America, 35,* 795–805.

Lashley, F. R. (2001). Genetics and nursing: The interface in education, research, and practice. *Biological Research in Nursing, 3,* 13–23.

Lashley, F. R. (2001). Ethical, social, and cultural implications for nursing education in the postgenomic era. *Chart, 98*(5), 4, 10.

Liu, R., Paxton, W. A., Choe, S., Ceradini, D., Martin, S. R., Horuk, R., et al. (1996). Homozygous defect in HIV-1 coreceptor accounts for resistance of some multiply-exposed individuals to HIV-1 infection. *Cell, 86,* 367–377.

McCandless, S. E., Brunger, J. W., & Cassidy, S. B. (2004). The burden of genetic disease on inpatient care in a children's hospital. *American Journal of Human Genetics, 74,* 121–127.

Myrianthopoulos, N. G., & Chung, C. S. (1974). Congenital malformations in singletons: Epidemiologic survey. *Birth Defects, X*(11), 1–58.

Nair, K. S., Jaleel, A., Asmann, Y. W., Short, K. R., & Raghavakaimal, S. (2004). Proteomic research:

Potential opportunities for clinical and physiological investigators. *American Journal of Physiology, Endocrinology and Metabolism, 286,* E863–874.

Noonan, A. S. (2002). Key roles of government in genomics and proteomics: A public health perspective. *Genetics in Medicine, 4*(Suppl. 6), 72S–76S.

Omenn, G. S. (2002). The crucial role of the public health sciences in the postgenomic era. *Genetics in Medicine, 4*(Suppl. 6), 21S–26S.

Patterson, S. D., & Aebersold, R. H. (2003). Proteomics: The first decade and beyond. *Nature Genetics Supplement, 33,* 311–323.

Prows, C. A., Hetteberg, C., Johnson, N., Latta, K., Lovell, A., Saal, H. M., et al. (2003). Outcomes of a genetics education program for nursing faculty. *Nursing Education Perspectives, 24,* 81–85.

Queisser-Luft, A., Stolz, G., Wiesel, A., Schlaefer, K., & Spränger, J. (2002). Malformations in newborn: Results based on 30,940 infants and fetuses from the Mainz congenital birth defect monitoring system (1990-1998). *Archives of Gynecology and Obstetrics, 266,* 163–167.

Ravine, D., Turner, K. J., & Alpers, M. P. (1980). Genetic inheritance of susceptibility to tinea imbricata. *Journal of Medical Genetics, 17,* 342–348.

Rimoin, D. L., Connor, J. M., Pyeritz, R. E. & Korf, B. R. (2002). Nature and frequency of genetic disease. In D. L. Rimoin, J. M. Connor, R. E. Pyeritz, & B. R. Korf (Eds.), *Emery and Rimoin's principles and practice of medical genetics* (4th ed., pp. 55–59). New York: Churchill Livingstone.

Roberts, D. F., Chavez, J., & Court, S. D. M. (1970). The genetic component in child mortality. *Archives of Diseases in Childhood, 45,* 33–38.

Robins, R., & Metcalfe, S. (2004). Integrating genetics as practices of primary care. *Social Science & Medicine, 59,* 223-233.

Saunders, R. S., Jr. (1993). Review of the book *Code of Codes.* In D. J. Kevles & L. Hood (Eds.). *National Forum, LXXIII*(2), 47–48.

Schmidt, C. W. (2004). Metabolomics: What's happening downstream of DNA. *Environmental Health Perspectives, 112,* A410–A4115.

Scriver, C. R. (2004). After the genome—the phenome? *Journal of Inherited Metabolic Disease, 27,* 305–317.

Scriver, C. R., Neal, J. L., Saginur, R., & Clow, C. (1973). The frequency of genetic disease and congenital malformation among patients in a pediatric hospital. *Canadian Medical Association Journal, 108,* 1111–1115.

Sever, L., Lynberg, M. C., & Edmonds, L. D. (1993). The impact of congenital malformations on public health. *Teratology, 48,* 547–549.

Soltan, H. C., & Craven, J. L. (1981). The extent of genetic disease in hospital populations. *Canadian Medical Association Journal, 124,* 427–429.

Stephenson, J. (1998). Group drafts core curriculum for 'what docs need to know about genetics.' *Journal of the American Medical Association, 279,* 735–736.

Stevenson, D. A., & Carey, J. C. (2004). Contribution of malformations and genetic disorders to mortality in a children's hospital. *American Journal of Medical Genetics, 126A,* 393–397.

Strauss, E. J., & Falkow, S. (1997). Microbial pathogenesis: Genomics and beyond. *Science, 276,* 707–712.

Sturtevant, A. H. (1965). *A history of genetics.* New York: Harper & Row.

Tuohy, P., Counsell, A. M., & Geddis, D. C. (1993). The Plunket National Child Health Study: Birth defects and sociodemographic factors. *New Zealand Medical Journal, 106,* 489–492.

Watson, J. D. (1990). The Human Genome Project: Past, present, and future. *Science, 248,* 44–99.

Watson, J. D., & Cook-Deegan, R. M. (1990). The Human Genome Project and international health. *Journal of the American Medical Association, 263,* 3322–3324.

Yankaskas, J. R., Marshall, B. C., Sufian, B., Simon, R. H., & Rodman, D. (2004). Cystic fibrosis adult care. Consensus conference report. *Chest, 125*(Suppl.), 1S–39S.

Yoon, P. W., Olney, R. S., Khoury, M. J., Sappenfield, W. M., Chavez, G. F., & Taylor, D. (1997). Contribution of birth defects and genetic diseases to pediatric hospitalizations. A population-based study. *Archives of Pediatrics & Adolescent Medicine, 151,* 1096–1103.

Zlotogora, J., Leventhal, A., & Amitai, Y. (2003). The impact of congenital malformations and Mendelian diseases on infant mortality in Israel. *Israeli Medical Association Journal, 5,* 416–418.

2

Basic and Molecular Biology:
An Introduction

Basic terms and genetic processes are introduced in this chapter as are the molecular methodologies used in genetic testing. Concepts are also integrated into chapters 3, 4, 5, 13, 14 and 17, which include discussion of human variation patterns of transmission for single gene disorders, factors that influence gene action and expression, the interaction of genes and environment, normal and abnormal chromosome numbers and structures, chromosome analysis, mutation, environmental insults, and the effects of environmental agents on the fetus.

GENES, CHROMOSOMES,
AND TERMINOLOGY

Genes are the basic units of heredity. In the early 1900s, the term "gene" was used to mean the hereditary factor(s) that determined a characteristic or trait. Today, a gene can be more precisely defined as a segment of deoxyribonucleic acid (DNA) that encodes or determines the structure of an amino acid chain or polypeptide. A polypeptide is a chain of amino acids connected to one another by peptide bonds. It may be a complete protein or enzyme molecule, or one of several subunits that undergo further modification before completion. After the first estimates made by the human genome project, it was believed that there were between 30,000 and 35,000 genes in a person's genome (total genetic complement or makeup), a number that seemed very small when compared to the genomes of other organisms, but which was held up. The haploid genome in humans (found in the egg and sperm) consists of about 3 billion base pairs. There are also stretches of DNA that are not known to contain genes. These are said to be noncoding DNA. Humans have in common a DNA sequence that is about 99.9% the same. Genes range in size. For example, the Duchenne muscular dystrophy gene is about 2,000 kilobases (kb) while the globin gene is 1.5 kb. The vast majority of genes are located in the cell nucleus but genes are also present in the mitochondria of the cells. Genes direct the process of protein synthesis; thus they are responsible for the determination of such products as structural proteins, transport proteins, cell membrane receptors, gap junction proteins, ion channels, hormones, and enzymes. Genes not only determine the structure of proteins and enzymes, but are also concerned with their rate of synthesis and regulatory control. Ultimately genes guide development of the embryo. One consequence of altered enzyme or protein structure can be altered function. The capacity of genes to function in these ways means that they are significant determinants of structural integrity, cell function, and the regulation of biochemical, developmental, and immunological processes.

Chromosomes are structures present in the cell nucleus that are composed of DNA, histones (a basic protein), nonhistone (acidic) proteins, and a small amount of ribonucleic acid (RNA). This chromosomal material is known as "chromatin." The precise role of chromatin and variations in it and its associated proteins in transcription is a subject of current interest. The coiling of DNA and histone complexes forms beadlike complexes called "nucleosomes" along the chromatin. Genes are located on chromosomes. Chromosomes can be seen under the light microscope and appear threadlike during certain stages of cell division, but they shorten and condense into rodlike structures during other stages, such as metaphase. Each chromosome can be individually identified by means of its size, staining qualities, and morphological characteristics (see chapter 5). Chromosomes have a centromere, which is a region in the chromosome that can be seen as a constriction. During cell division, the spindle fibers use the centromere as the point of attachment on the chromosome to perform their guiding function. Telomeres, which are specialized structures at the ends of chromosomes and which have been likened to the caps on shoelaces, consist of multiple tandem repeats (many adjacent repetitions) of the same base sequences. Telomeres are currently believed to have important functions in cell aging and cancer. The normal human chromosome number in most somatic (body) cells and in the zygote is 46. This is known as the diploid (2N) number. Chromosomes occur in pairs; normally one of each pair is derived from the individual's mother and one of each pair is derived from the father.

There are 22 pairs of autosomes (chromosomes common to both sexes) and one pair of sex chromosomes. The sex chromosomes present in the normal female are two X chromosomes (XX). The sex chromosomes present in the normal male are one X chromosome and one Y chromosome (XY). Gametes (ova and sperm) each contain one member of a chromosome pair for a total of 23 chromosomes (22 autosomes and one sex chromosome). This is known as the haploid (N) number or one chromosome set. The fusion of male and female gametes during fertilization restores the diploid number of chromosomes (46) to the zygote, normally contributing one maternally derived chromosome and one paternally derived chromosome to each pair, along with its genes.

Genes are arranged in a linear fashion on a chromosome; each with its specific locus (place). However, less than 5% of the DNA in the genome consists of gene-coding sequences. The areas between genes contain DNA that were once called "junk" DNA and are now known as "spacer," "intergenic," or "noncoding" DNA. These areas that in some way may be necessary for complete function of the genome consist of noncoding regions,

including repeated sequences of various types and sizes, non-repetitive sequences, and pseudogenes (additional copies of genes that are nonfunctional because they are not translated into protein). These repeat sequences may, over time, act to rearrange the genome, creating new genes or modifying or reshuffling existing genes. Autosomal genes are those whose loci are on one of the autosomes. Each chromosome of a pair (homologous chromosomes) normally has the identical number of arrangement of genes, except, of course, for the X and Y chromosomes in the male. Nonhomologous chromosomes are members of different chromosome pairs. Only one copy of a gene normally occupies its given locus on the chromosome at one time. The reason is that in somatic cells the chromosomes are paired, two copies of a gene are normally present—one copy of each one of a chromosome pair (the exception are the X and Y chromosomes of the male, or certain structural abnormalities of the chromosome). Genes at corresponding loci on homologous chromosomes that govern the same trait may exist in slightly different forms or alleles. Alleles are, therefore, alternative forms of a gene at the same locus.

For any given gene under consideration, if the two gene copies or alleles are identical, they are said to be homozygous. For a given gene, if one gene copy or allele differs from the other, they are said to be heterozygous. The term "genotype" is most often used to refer to the genetic makeup of a person when discussing a specific gene pair, but sometimes it is used to refer to a person's total genetic makeup or constitution. "Phenotype" refers to the observable expression of a specific trait or characteristic that can either be visible or biochemically detectable. Thus, both blond hair and blood group A are considered phenotypic features. A trait or characteristic is considered dominant if it is expressed or phenotypically apparent when one copy or dose of the gene is present. A trait is considered recessive when it is expressed only when two copies or doses of the gene are present, or if one copy is missing, as occurs in X-linked recessive traits in males. Dominance and recessivity are concepts that are becoming more complex as more is learned about the genome. Codominance occurs when each one of the two alleles present are expressed when both are present, as in the case of the AB blood group. Those genes located on the

X chromosome (X-linked) are present in two copies in the female but only in one copy in males, since males only have one X chromosome. Therefore, in the male, the genes of his X chromosome are expressed for whatever trait they determine. Genes on the X chromosome of the male are often referred to as "hemizygous," because no partner is present. In the female, a process known as X-inactivation occurs so that there is only one functioning X chromosome in somatic cells (see chapter 4). Very few genes are known to be located on the Y chromosome, but they are only present in males. Information related to disorders caused by single gene errors and pertaining to gene function is discussed in chapters 4 and 6. The interaction of genes and the environment is discussed in chapters 4 and 14.

Standards for both gene and chromosome nomenclature are set by international committees (see chapter 5 for chromosomes). To describe known genes at a specific locus, genes are designated by uppercase Latin letters, sometimes in combination with Arabic numbers, and are italicized or underlined. Alleles of genes are preceded by an asterisk. Some genes have many or multiple alleles that are possible at its locus. This can lead to slightly different variants of the same basic gene product. For any given gene, any individual would still normally have only two alleles present in somatic cells, one on each chromosome. Thus in referring to the genes for the ABO blood groups, *ABO*A1*, *ABO*O*, and *ABO*B* are examples of the formal ways for identifying alleles at the ABO locus. As an example, genotypes may be written as *ADA*1/ADA*2* or *ADA*1/*2* to illustrate a sample genotype for the enzyme, adenosine deaminase. Further shorthand is used to more precisely describe mutations and allelic variants. These describe the position of the mutation, sometimes by codon or by the site. For example, one of the cystic fibrosis mutations, deletion of amino acid 508, phenylalanine, is written as PHE508DEL or ΔF508. See Wain et al. (2002) for more details. However, to explain patterns of inheritance more simply, geneticists often use capital letters to represent genes for dominant traits and small letters to represent recessive ones. Thus a person who is heterozygous for a given gene pair can be represented as Aa, one who is homozygous for two dominant alleles, AA, and one who is homozygous for two recessive alleles, aa. For autosomal recessive traits, the homozygote (AA) and the heterozygote (Aa) may not be distinguishable on the basis of phenotypic appearance, but they may be distinguishable biochemically because they may make different amounts or types of gene products. This information can often be used in carrier screening for recessive disorders to determine genetic risk and for genetic counseling (see chapters 10 and 11). Using this system, when discussing two different gene pairs at different loci, a heterozygote may be represented as AaBb. When geneticists discuss a particular gene pair or disorder, normality is usually assumed for the rest of the person's genome, and the term "normal" is often used, unless stated otherwise.

DNA, RNA, THE GENETIC CODE, AND PROTEIN SYNTHESIS

When early work on the definitive identification of the genetic material was being done, geneticists identified essential properties that such material would have to possess. These included the capacity for accurate self-replication through cell generations; general stability, but with the capacity for change; and the ability to store, retrieve, transport, and relay hereditary information. Through elaborate work, geneticists identified the genetic material in humans as DNA, determined its structure, and determined how information coded within the DNA was eventually translated into a polypeptide chain. The usual pattern of information flow in humans in abbreviated form is as follows:

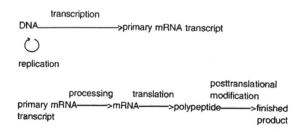

It is known that information can flow in reverse in certain circumstances, from RNA to DNA, by means of the enzyme, reverse transcriptase, a finding of special importance in cancer and human immunodeficiency virus (HIV) research. These terms and the process are defined and discussed next.

DNA AND RNA

DNA and RNA are both nucleic acids with similar components—a nitrogenous purine or pyrimidine base, a five-carbon sugar, and a phosphate group that together comprise a nucleotide. In DNA and RNA, the purine bases are adenine (A) and guanine (G). In DNA, the pyrimidine bases are cytosine (C) and thymine (T), while in RNA they are C and uracil (U) instead of T. RNA may also have some rare other bases. The human genome is believed to contain about 3 billion nucleotide bases. The sugar in DNA is deoxyribose and in RNA it is ribose. These nucleotides are formed into chains or strands. DNA is double stranded and RNA is single stranded. Each DNA strand has polarity or direction (5' to 3' and 3' to 5'), and two chains of opposite polarity are antiparallel and complementary. When a gene structure is represented diagrammatically, usually it is shown with the 5' end upstream on the left and the 3' end downstream on the right. The well-known three dimensional conformation of DNA is the double helix. This may be visualized as a flexible ladder in which the sides are the phosphate and sugar groups, and the rungs of the ladder are the bases from each strand that form hydrogen bonds with the complementary bases on the opposite strand. This flexible ladder is then twisted into the double helix of the DNA molecule. In DNA, A always pairs with T, forming two bonds (A:T), and G always pairs with C forming three bonds (G:C), although it does not matter which DNA strand a given base is on. However, a given base on one strand determines the base at the same position in the other DNA strand because they are complementary. If G occurs in one chain, then its partner is always C in the other strand. If one thinks of these bases as being similar to teeth in a zipper, then the two sides with the teeth can only fit together to zip in one way, A matched with T and G matched with C. Thus the sequence of bases in one strand determines the position of the bases in the complementary strand. In RNA, U pairs with A because T is not present. There are three major classes of RNA involved in protein synthesis—messenger RNA (mRNA), ribosomal RNA (rRNA), and transfer RNA (tRNA). The RNA that receives information from DNA, and serves as a template for protein synthesis, is mRNA. Ribosomal RNA is one of the structural components of ribosomes, the RNA-protein molecule that is the site of protein synthesis. Transfer RNA is the clover-leaf shaped RNA that brings amino acids to the mRNA and guides them into position during protein synthesis. The middle of the clover leaf contains the anticodon, and one end attaches the amino acid discussed later in this chapter. A transposable element (jumping gene or transposon) is a segment of DNA that moves from place to place within the genome of a single cell. These elements can alter the activity of other genes, and can cause mutations in a variety of ways. An example is the movement of a transposon or long interspersed element (LINE) during gametogenesis that, when moved from normal position into a specific exon in the factor VIII gene, disrupts the coding sequence and prevents the encoding of a functional factor VIII protein, thus resulting in hemophilia A. There are other noncoding RNAs such as small nucleolar RNAs, vault RNA, and small nuclear RNAs.

THE GENETIC CODE

The position or sequence of the bases in DNA ultimately determines the position of the amino acids in the polypeptide chain whose synthesis is directed by the DNA. Therefore, the structure and properties of body proteins are determined by the DNA base sequence of a person's genes. It does this by means of a code. Each amino acid is specified by a sequence of three bases called a "codon." There are 20 major amino acids and 64 codons or code words. Sixty-one of the codons specify amino acids, and three are "stop" signals that terminate the genetic message. One codon that specifies an amino acid usually begins the message. Because the genetic code was first worked out in mRNA, it is usually given in terms of these bases, although, of course, the code is originally read from the DNA. The first code word discovered was UUU, which specifies phenylalanine. More than one code word may specify a given amino acid, but only one amino acid is specified by any one codon; thus the code is said to be degenerate. For example, the codons that code for the amino acid, leucine, are UAG, UUG, CUU, CUC, CUA, and CUG, but none of these code for any other amino acid. The relationship between the base sequence in DNA, mRNA, the anticodon in tRNA, and the translation into an amino acid is shown in Figure 2.1. The code is nonoverlapping. Therefore, CACUUUAGA is read as CAC UUU AGA and specifies histidine, phenylalanine, and arginine, respectively. A shorthand way of referring to a specific amino acid is to use either a specified group of three letters or a single letter to denote a specific amino acid. In this system, for example, arginine may be referred to as arg or simply as "R," while the symbols for phenylalanine are either phe or "F." General genetics references in the bibliography provide more information about the code.

DNA REPLICATION

When a cell divides, the daughter cell must receive an exact copy of the genetic information that the original cell contains. Thus DNA must replicate itself. In order to do this, double-stranded DNA must unwind or relax first, and the strands must separate. Then, each parental strand serves as a template or model for the new strand that is formed. After replication of an original DNA helix, two daughter helices will result. Each daughter will have one original parental strand and one newly synthesized one. DNA replication is highly accurate, and needs to be, because, otherwise, mutations would frequently occur. After replication is complete, a type of "proofreading" for mutations occurs, and repair takes place if needed. Many enzymes, including DNA polymerases, ligases, and helicases, mediate the process. Replication of DNA is an important precursor of cell division. Despite several repair mechanisms, sometimes errors remain and are replicated, being passed to daughter cells.

DNA template	3'... AAA	TGA	CTG... 5'
mRNA	5'... UUU	ACU	GAC... 3'
tRNA anticodon	3'... AAA	UGA	CUG... 5'
Polypeptide chain	NH₂... phe	thr	asp... COOH

FIGURE 2.1   Relationship between the nucleotide base sequence of DNA, mRNA, tRNA, and amino acids in the polypeptide chain produced.
A = adenine, *C* = cytosine, *G* = guanine, *T* = thymine, *U* = uracil, *phe* = phenylalanine, *thr* = threonine, *asp* = aspartic acid.

PROTEIN SYNTHESIS

Basically, protein synthesis is the process by which the sequence of bases in DNA ends up as corresponding sequences of amino acids in the polypeptide chain produced. It is not possible to give a full discussion of protein synthesis here. The process is a complex one that involves many factors (e.g., initiation, elongation, and termination), RNA molecules, and enzymes that will not all be mentioned in the brief discussion below. The process is illustrated in Figure 2.2.

First, the DNA strands that are in the double helix formation must separate. One, the master or antisense strand, acts as template for the formation of mRNA. The nontemplate strand is referred to as the "sense strand." An initiation site indicates where transcription begins. Transcription is the process by which complementary mRNA is synthesized from a DNA template. This mRNA carries the same genetic information as the DNA template, but it is coded in complementary base sequence. Translation is the process whereby the amino acids in a given polypeptide are synthesized from the mRNA template, with the amino acids placed in an ordered sequence as determined by the base sequence in the mRNA. Posttranslational modifications occur, making it possible for a given gene to code for more than one final protein product.

Not long ago, it was believed that all regions of DNA within a gene were both transcribed and translated. It is now known that in many genes there are regions of DNA both within and between genes that are not transcribed into mRNA, and are therefore not translated into amino acids. In other words, many genes are not continuous but are split. Therefore, transcription first results in an mRNA that must then undergo processing in order to remove intervening regions or sequences that are known as "introns." This can influence mRNA metabolism, gene expression, and translation (see Le Hir, Nott, & Moore, 2003, for more information). Structural gene sequences that are retained in the mRNA and are eventually translated into amino acids are called "exons." Therefore, transcription first results in a primary mRNA transcript or precursor that must then undergo processing in order to remove the introns. Introns are recognized because they almost always begin with GT and end with AG. During processing a "cap" structure is

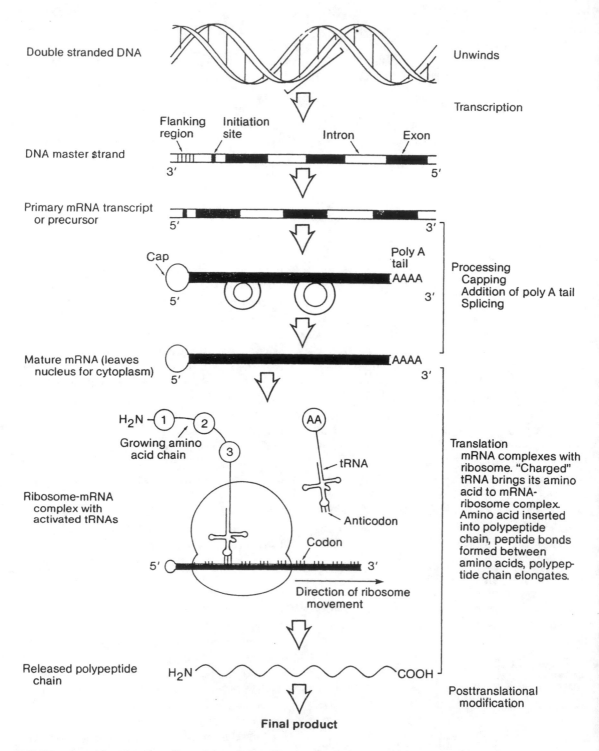

FIGURE 2.2   Abbreviated outline of steps in protein synthesis shown without enzymes and factors.

added at one end that appears to protect the mRNA transcript, facilitate RNA splicing, and enhance translation efficiency. A sequence of adenylate residues called the "poly-A tail" is added to the other end that may increase stability and facilitate translation. Splicing then occurs. The splice junction areas near intron/exon boundaries appear important in correct splicing. Introns almost always start with GT and end with AG. All this occurs in the nucleus.

The mature mRNA then enters the cell cytoplasm where it binds to a ribosome. There is a point of initiation of translation, and the coding region of the mRNA is indicated by the codon AUG (methionine). Methionine is usually cleared from the finished polypeptide chain. Sections at the ends of the mRNA transcript are not translated. Amino acids that are inserted into the polypeptide chain are brought to the mRNA-ribosome complex by activated tRNA molecules, each of which is specific for a particular amino acid. The tRNA contains a triplet of bases that is complementary to the codon in the mRNA that designates the specific amino acid. This triplet of bases in the tRNA is called an "anticodon." The anticodon of tRNA and the mRNA codon pair at the ribosome complex. The amino acid is placed in the growing chain, and as each is placed, an enzyme causes peptide bonds to form between the contiguous amino acids in the chain. Passage of mRNA through the ribosome during translation has been likened to that of a punched tape running through a computer to direct the operation of machinery. When the termination codon is reached, the polypeptide chain is released from the ribosome. After release, polypeptides may undergo posttranslational modification (i.e., carbohydrate groups may be added to form a glycoprotein, assembly occurs, as well as folding and new conformations). Proteins that are composed of subunits are assembled, and the quaternary structure (final folding arrangement) is finalized. In addition, epigenetic modifications may occur. The study of proteomics, defined as the large-scale characterization of the entire protein complement of a cell line, tissue, or organism (Graves & Haystead, 2002, p. 40), has evolved to give a broader picture of protein modifications and mechanisms involved in protein function and interactions and allows for the study of entire complex systems. This is important because it is increasingly realized that neither genes nor proteins function in isolation but are interconnected in many ways, and so it is important to understand the complex functioning of cells, tissues, and organs.

GENE ACTION AND EXPRESSION

Although the same genes are normally present in every somatic cell of a given individual, they are not all active in all cells at the same time. They are selectively expressed or "switched" on and off. For example, the genes that determine the various chains that make up the hemoglobin molecule are present in brain cells, but in brain cells hemoglobin is not produced because the genes are not activated. Some genes, known as "housekeeping genes," are expressed in virtually all cells. This selective activation and repression is important in normal development and is influenced by age as well as by cell type and function. As development of the organism proceeds, and specialization and differentiation of cells occur, genes that are not essential for the specialized functions are switched off and others may be switched on. Epigenetics refers to alterations of genes that do not involve the DNA sequence. Epigenetic mechanisms may be involved in gene expression control that includes modifications of chromatin and methylation. "Methylation" occurs in most genes that are deactivated or silenced, and demethylation occurs as genes are activated during differentiation of specific tissues. Methylation refers to a modification whereby a methyl group is added to a DNA residue. Methylation is not yet well understood, but it plays a role in imprinting (see chapter 4). Transcription factors play a role in demethylation. Certain genes (and their products) regulate and coordinate all of these functions. Gene expression and how it is controlled and regulated is of great interest in understanding various processes such as tissue differentiation and development as well as disease.

One control of gene expression occurs in the initiation of transcription. An external signal molecule such as a hormone binds to the cell membrane receptor, resulting in the activation of transcription factors. Transcription factors are proteins in the nucleus that play a role in the regulation of gene expression. Some are general and some are regulatory. These factors bind to promoters located close to the beginning of the transcription site and to enhancers. Enhancers, often located at a distant point downstream from the promoter, augment transcription. Silencers are regulatory elements that can inhibit transcription. Genes also control the number of cell membrane receptors, and can increase or decrease them according to needs. An area rich in AT bases known as the TATA box appears necessary in some genes for correctly positioning RNA polymearase II, a transcribing enzyme. Transcription factors may be classified into families on the basis of their structural motifs. For example, the thyroid hormone, steroid and retinoic acid receptors all belong to the zinc finger class. Motifs that characterize transcription factor families include the helix-turn-helix (HTH), zinc finger domains, helix-loop-helix, and leucine zippers. Mutations of a zinc finger in the Wilms tumor suppressor gene have been identified in people with Denys-Drash syndrome (an autosomal dominant disorder including Wilms tumor pseudohermaphroditism, nephropathy, and renal failure). The homeobox is a region that encodes a transcription factor ensuring correct embryonic development and patterning including HTH. In addition, histones (described above) can be modified by chemical interactions such as phosphorylation, acetylation, and methylation, also playing a role in gene expression and interaction with other epigenetic systems influencing development. The term "transcriptome" has been applied to the collection of mRNA in a cell (Bunney et al., 2003).

DNA VARIATION

Some DNA is highly repetitive, consisting of short sequences that are repeated many times. These sequences may vary from individual to individual. These differences in DNA sequence are sometimes polymorphic, and thus useful as markers. A site is traditionally considered polymorphic when a variation occurs in at least 1% of the population. The more alternate forms or variations present at a given site, the more useful a polymorphism is for genetic and medical applications. The following variations are among those identified:

1. single nucleotide polymorphisms (SNPs);
2. restriction fragment length polymorphisms (RFLPs);
3. minisatellites or variable number tandem repeats (VNTRs);
4. microsatellites or short tandem repeats (STRs, also called short sequence repeats or SSRs);
5. variants in mitochondrial DNA; and
6. others, such as the presence or absence of retroposons, LINES (long interspersed repetitive elements), or *Alu* repeats (repetitions of certain DNA sequences that have been conserved through evolution).

MUTATION

A mutation may be simply defined as a change (usually permanent) in the genetic material. A mutation that occurs in a somatic cell affects only the descendants of that mutant cell. If it occurs early in division of the zygote, it would be present in a larger number of cells than if it appeared late. If it occurred before zygotic division into twins, then the twins could differ for that mutant gene or chromosome. If mutation occurs in the germline, then the mutation will be transmitted to all the cells of the offspring, both germ and somatic cells. Mutations can arise *de novo* (spontaneously), or they may be inherited. Mutations can involve large amounts of genetic material, as in the case of chromosomal abnormalities, or they may involve very tiny amounts, such as only the alteration of one or a few bases in DNA. About 40% of small deletions are of one base pair (bp) and an additional 30% are of two to three bp. Different alleles of a gene can result in the formation of different gene products. These products can differ in qualitative or quantitative parameters, depending on the nature of the change. For example, some mutations of one base in the DNA still result in the same amino acid being present in its proper place, whereas others could cause substitution, deletion, duplication, or termination involving one or more bases. The gene product can be altered in a variety of ways that can include: (1) impairment of its activity, net charge, binding capability, or other functional parameter; (2) availability of a decreased or increased amount to varying degrees; (3) complete absence; or (4) no apparent change. Enzymes that differ in electrophoretic mobility (separation of protein by its charge across an electrical field, usually on a gel) because of different alleles at a gene locus are called "allozymes." Other types of mutations can result in other aberrations. Sometimes the effects of mutations are mild, and these can have more of an effect on the population at large because they tend to be transmitted, whereas a mutation with a very large effect may be eliminated because the affected person dies or does not reproduce.

Alteration of the gene product may have different consequences, including the following:

1. It may be clinically apparent in either the heterozygous or homozygous state (as in the inborn metabolic errors).
2. It might not be apparent unless the individual is exposed to a particular extrinsic agent or different environment (as in exposure to certain halogenated general anesthetics in malignant hyperthermia and in other pharmacogenetic disorders and environmental exposure, which are discussed in chapters 14 and 18).
3. It may be noticed only when individuals are being screened for variation in a population survey (as in allozymes in enzyme studies).
4. It may be noticed only when a specific variation is being looked for (as in specific screening detection programs among Ashkenazi Jews for Tay-Sachs disease carriers, or when specific genetic testing among individual family members is done).

Because the codons are read as triplets, an addition or deletion of only one nucleotide shifts the entire reading frame and can cause: (a) changes in the amino acids inserted in the polypeptide chain after the shift, (b) premature chain termination, or (c) chain elongation, resulting in a defective or deficient product. A base substitution in one codon may or may not change the amino acid specified, because it may change it to another codon that still codes for the specified amino acid. A point mutation is one in which there is a change in only one nucleotide base. This is also called a single-nucleotide substitution or polymorphism (SNP). There can be different SNP variations in the two alleles of a different gene. The consequences of these types of mutation are illustrated in Figure 2.3. Other types of mutations can occur. These include expansion of trinucleotide repeats, creating instability (see chapter 4); RNA processing, splicing, or transcriptional mutations (splicing mutations can arise within the splice site or within an exon or intron, creating new splice sites); regulatory mutations such as of the TATA box; and others as well as larger mutations such as deletions, insertions, duplications, and inversions that may be visible at the chromosomal level. Complex mutational events may occur as well, such as a combination of a deletion and an inversion. Sometimes mutations are described in terms of function. Thus a null mutation is one in which no phenotypic effect is seen. A "loss of function" mutation is said to occur when it results in defective, absent, or deficient function of its products. Mutations that result in new protein products with altered function are often called "gain of function" mutations. This term is also used to describe increased gene dosage from gene duplication mutations. Gene duplication has become of greater interest since new genes may be created by this mechanism. New mosaic genes may also be created by duplication from parts of other genes. Mutant alleles may also code for a protein that interferes with the product from the normal one, sometimes by binding to it, resulting in what is known as a "dominant negative" mutation.

CELL DIVISION

It is essential that genetic information be relayed accurately to all cell descendants. This occurs in two ways—through somatic cell division, or mitosis, and through germ cell division, or meiosis, leading to gamete formation. Recently the substances that hold the sister chromatids together and which allow them to separate during division and which regulate them have been of interest.

Mitosis and the Cell Cycle

Mitosis is the process of somatic cell division, whereby growth of the organism occurs, the embryo develops from the fertilized egg, and cells normally repair and replace themselves. Such division maintains the diploid chromosome number of 46. It normally results in the formation of two daughter cells that are exact replicas of the parent cell. Therefore, daughter cells have the identical genetic makeup and chromosome constitution of the parent cell unless a mutation has occurred. Somatic cells have a cell cycle composed of phases whose length varies according to cell type, age, and

1. Original or normal pattern

DNA	TTT	AGC	CTG	ATT
mRNA	AAA	UCG	GAC	UAA
Amino acid chain	lys	ser	asp	stop

    (Chain terminates here)

2. Deletion of T in first triplet of DNA

DNA	TTA	GCC	TGA	TT
mRNA	AAU	CGG	ACU	AA
Amino acid chain	ileu	leu	thr	no stop command

    (Chain elongates until stop reached)

3. Addition of T in first triplet of DNA

DNA	TTT	TAG	CCT	GAT	T
mRNA	AAA	AUC	GGA	CUA	A
Amino acid chain	lys	ileu	gly	his	no stop command

    (Chain elongates until stop reached)

4. Substitution of T for G in second triplet of DNA. This substitution of a pyrimidine for a purine base is called a transversion.

DNA	TTT	ATC	CTG	ATT
mRNA	AAA	UAG	GAC	UAA
Amino acid chain	lys	stop		

    (Chain is prematurely terminated)

5. Substitution of G for C in second triplet of DNA. This substitution of one purine base for another is called a transition.

DNA	TTT	AGG	CTG	ATT
mRNA	AAA	UCC	GAC	UAA
Amino acid chain	lys	ser	asp	stop

    (Note that there is no change in the amino acid inserted because both UCC and UCG code for serine.)

FIGURE 2.3   Examples of the consequences of different point mutations (SNPs).
lys = lysine, ser = serine, asp = aspartic acid, ileu = isoleucine, leu = leucine, thr = threonine, gly = glycine, his = histidine.
Note: Numbers 2 and 3 are examples of frame-shift mutations.

other factors. These phases are known as G_0, G_1, S, G_2, and M. During the G_1 phase, materials needed by the cell for replication and division, such as nucleotide bases, amino acids, and RNA, are accumulated. During the S phase, DNA synthesis occurs and the cell content of DNA doubles in preparation for the M phase. Mitosis occurs during the M phase. The term "interphase" is used to describe the phases of the cell cycle except for the M phase. Selected cells in the liver and brain have more than the usual number of chromosome sets and more DNA than other somatic cells. This has been attributed to the high metabolic needs of these cells. The cell cycle and mitosis are illustrated and further discussed in Figure 2.4.

Meiosis, Gamete Formation, and Fertilization

Meiosis is the process of germ cell division in which the end result is the production of haploid gametes from one diploid germ cell. Meiosis consists of two sequential divisions: the first is a reduction division, and the second is an equational one. In males, four sperm result from each original germ cell, and in females, the end result after the second meiotic division is three polar bodies and one ovum. As a result of meiosis, the daughter cells that are formed have 23 chromosomes, one of each pair of autosomes, and one sex chromosome, which in normal female ova will always be an X

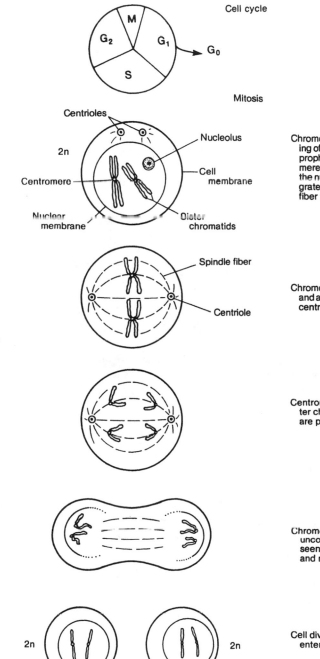

Cell cycle

Mitosis

Prophase

Chromosomes are doubled, each consisting of two sister chromatids as they enter prophase. They are joined at the centromere. In late prophase/prometaphase, the nuclear membrane begins to disintegrate; centrioles separate and spindle fiber formation is seen.

Metaphase

Chromosomes line up on metaphase plate and are attached to spindle fibers at their centromere.

Anaphase

Centromeres divide, single-stranded sister chromatids (now chromosomes) are pulled to opposite poles

Telophase

Chromosomes reach poles and begin to uncoil and elongate; division furrow is seen at cell membrane; nucleolus and nuclear membrane reform at end

Cell divides and new daughter cells enter interphase

FIGURE 2.4   Mitosis and the cell cycle. *(Top)* Cell cycle. G = gap; S = synthesis; M = mitotic division; G_1 = synthesis of mRNA, rRNA, and ribosomes; S = DNA and histone synthesis, chromosome replication sister chromatids form; G_2 = spindle formation. G_0, G_1, S, G_2 are all interphase periods. M is the period of mitotic division shown in the bottom figure. the time a cell spends in each phase depends on its age, type, and function. When a cell enters G_0 it is usually in differentiation, not growth, and needs a stimulus such as hormones to enter G_1. *(Bottom)* Mitosis (shown with one autosomal chromosome pair).

chromosome. Meiosis is shown in Figure 2.5. Fusion of the male and female gametes at fertilization restores the diploid number of chromosomes of 46. The zygote then begins a series of mitotic divisions as embryonic development proceeds.

In the males, meiosis takes place in the seminiferous tubules of the testes and begins at puberty. In females, oogenesis takes place in the ovaries. It is initiated in fetal development, and develops through late prophase. It is then dormant until maturation, usually at about 12 years of age, when the first meiotic division is completed at the time of the release of the secondary oocyte from the Graffian follicle at ovulation. The second meiotic division normally is not completed until the oocyte is penetrated by a sperm. During the process of fertilization, the female contributes most of the cytoplasm containing messenger RNA, the mitochondria, and so forth to the zygote.

In the process of meiosis, each homologous chromosome, with its genes, normally separates from the other (Mendel's Law of Segregation) so that only one of a pair normally ends up in a given gamete. Then, each member of the chromosome pair assorts independently. It is normally a matter of chance as to whether, for example, a chromosome number 1, which was originally from the person's mother, and a chromosome number 2, which was originally from the person's father, end up in the same gamete or not, or whether, by chance, all maternally derived chromosomes end up in the same gamete (Mendel's Law of Independent Assortment). During meiosis, the phenomenon of crossing over occurs. This process involves the breaking and rejoining of DNA and allows the exchange of genetic material and recombination to occur. This allows for new combinations of alleles and maintains variation. Assuming heterozygosity at only one locus per chromosome, 2^{23}, or more than 8 million possible different gametes, could be produced by one individual.

MITOCHONDRIAL GENES

The cell nucleus is not the only site where DNA and genes are present. These are also present in mitochondria and in chloroplasts (in plants only). The mitochondria are cell organelles located in the cytoplasm that are concerned with energy production and metabolism, and are thus known as the "power plants" of the cell. One of the functions of the mitochondrial oxidative phosphorylation system (OXPHOS) is to generate adenosine triphosphate (ATP) for cell energy. Cells contain hundreds of mitochondria and each mitochondrium can contain up to 10 copies of mtDNA, meaning that thousands of copies of mtDNA are present in some cells. The amount of DNA present in mitochondria is far less than in the nucleus—up to 1% of the cell total—and it is arranged circularly. Genes coding for proteins, tRNAs and mRNAs have been identified in human mitochondria. The mitochondrial genes are virtually only maternally transmitted (see chapter 4). Genes in the nucleus also influence certain mitochondrial functions. Diseases resulting from mtDNA mutations are discussed in chapter 6.

GENE MAPPING AND LINKAGE

The assignment of genes to specific chromosomes, specific sites on those chromosomes, and the determination of the distance between them is known as "gene mapping." One geneticist has likened the importance of mapping genes to their chromosomal location to the discovery that the heart pumps blood or that the kidney secretes urine. Both genetic and physical approaches have been used to map genes to specific locations on chromosomes. Gene mapping took on particular impetus with the initiation and funding of the Human Genome Project, described in chapter 1. A major goal of the Human Genome Project was to place all of the genes on a physical map. Thus the complete draft DNA sequence for each chromosome has essentially been determined. Within segments of DNA, the exact identity and order of nucleotides can be determined to sequence a gene. Human mapping databases can be accessed through the Internet.

In the genetic approach to mapping, the distance between genes on the same chromosome is commonly expressed in terms of map units or centimorgans (after the geneticist Thomas Morgan), while physical mapping uses measures such as bases and kilobases (kb). Many techniques are used to map genes. Genes located on the same chromosome are called "syntenic." Those located 50 or less map units apart are said to be "linked." Genes that

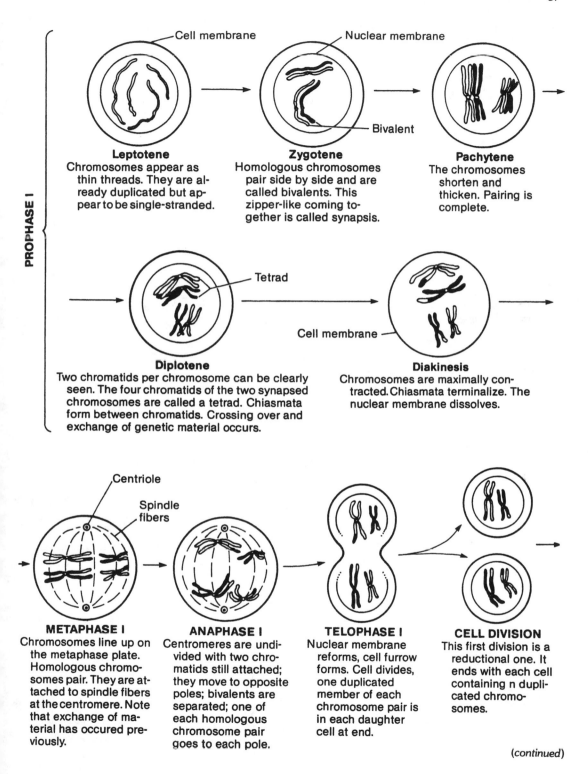

PROPHASE I

Leptotene
Chromosomes appear as thin threads. They are already duplicated but appear to be single-stranded.

Zygotene
Homologous chromosomes pair side by side and are called bivalents. This zipper-like coming together is called synapsis.

Pachytene
The chromosomes shorten and thicken. Pairing is complete.

Diplotene
Two chromatids per chromosome can be clearly seen. The four chromatids of the two synapsed chromosomes are called a tetrad. Chiasmata form between chromatids. Crossing over and exchange of genetic material occurs.

Diakinesis
Chromosomes are maximally contracted. Chiasmata terminalize. The nuclear membrane dissolves.

METAPHASE I
Chromosomes line up on the metaphase plate. Homologous chromosomes pair. They are attached to spindle fibers at the centromere. Note that exchange of material has occured previously.

ANAPHASE I
Centromeres are undivided with two chromatids still attached; they move to opposite poles; bivalents are separated; one of each homologous chromosome pair goes to each pole.

TELOPHASE I
Nuclear membrane reforms, cell furrow forms. Cell divides, one duplicated member of each chromosome pair is in each daughter cell at end.

CELL DIVISION
This first division is a reductional one. It ends with each cell containing n duplicated chromosomes.

(continued)

FIGURE 2.5   Meiosis with two autosomal chromosome pairs. *(Top)* Prophase I. *(Bottom)* Prometaphase—nuclear membrane disintegrates, nucleololus disappears, and spindle apparatus forms. This is followed by the rest of meiosis I—metaphase I, anaphase I, telophase I, and cell division.

As cells enter the second part of meiosis, chromosomes elongate, the nuclear membrane disintegrates after prophase II; no DNA replication occurs. Each cell contains 1 set (n) of duplicated chromosomes.

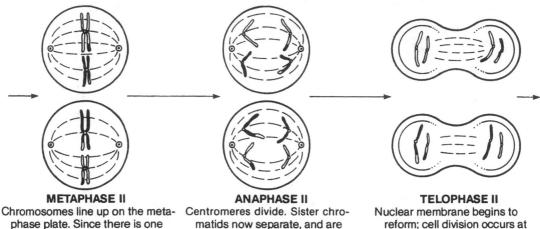

METAPHASE II
Chromosomes line up on the metaphase plate. Since there is one of each homologous chromosome pair in each cell, lining up is random.

ANAPHASE II
Centromeres divide. Sister chromatids now separate, and are called chromosomes. One of each goes to each pole.

TELOPHASE II
Nuclear membrane begins to reform; cell division occurs at end of stage.

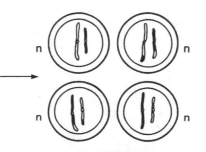

GAMETES
The end result of this division is four haploid gametes with one unduplicated member of each chromosome pair in each gamete, or n single chromosomes.

Dark = maternal origin
Light = paternal origin

FIGURE 2.5   Meiosis with two autosomal chromosome pairs—meiosis II *(continued)* .

are linked (located on the same chromosome, 50 map units or closer), are not likely to assort independently. The closer together or the more tightly linked they are, the greater the chance that they will "travel" together during meiosis and end up in the same gametic cell. Although direct detection of mutations, such as through DNA analysis, is the preferred method of diagnosis of genetic disease,

this is not always possible. Direct methods can be used to detect many known mutations, such as the one for sickle cell anemia, where one mutation, the substitution of the amino acid valine for glutamic acid, is known. When direct methods cannot be used, linkage analysis that depends on polymorphic markers can be used to figure out the inheritance of a given mutant allele within a family. This indirect method depends on the availability of an appropriate number of family members, informative polymorphisms or markers, and the absence of nonparenthood. Thus, if the marker is tightly linked to the gene mutation of interest, it will almost always predict the location of the gene mutation. This information can sometimes be used in specific situations to provide information for genetic risk determination and genetic counseling when direct prenatal diagnosis is not possible, if the gene in question is known to be linked to one for detectable trait, and the parental genotypes are such that essential information for calculating risks is available. The linkage phase of the two linked genes in question must be known before such linkage analysis can be done. A heterozygote for two linked genes (AaBb) may have them arranged so that both dominant alleles are on the same homologous chromosome and both recessive alleles are on the other (e.g., AB/ab, which is known as coupling or cis phase), or they may be arranged so that each homologous chromosome has one dominant and one recessive allele of each pair (e.g., Ab/aB, which is known as repulsion or trans phase). By meeting the criteria discussed previously, and others as detailed in the references, and by making appropriate mathematical calculations, the risk for a given fetus to be affected can be indirectly determined with varying degrees of accuracy. Segregation analysis plays a role in genetic linkage studies (see Spence & Hodge, 2002). One of the early linkage determinations was the ABO blood group locus, which was used as a marker gene for families at risk for nail-patella syndrome. Linkage calculations use the likelihood of a given pedigree under certain assumptions and a lod score is calculated. The lod score is the logarithm of the likelihood ratio. For an autosomal disorder, if the lod score exceeds 3, it is considered significant, while for an X-linked situation, a lod score of 2 or more denotes significant linkage. Today most linkage calculations are done by computer programs, as detailed by Anderson (2002).

In physical mapping, the major approaches used are positional cloning and functional cloning. To accomplish mapping, sequence-tagged sites are often used as markers. Overlapping cloned sets of DNA fragments, called contigs, may be used in mapping as they represent a continuous DNA region.

Functional cloning refers to the identification and location of a disease gene on the basis of knowledge of the basic biochemical defect in that disorder. In this instance, a cDNA probe is produced from the aberrant gene product and used to search the genome for this sequence, in hopes of locating the gene. Another technique, positional cloning, begins with the chromosome location of the gene and examines that DNA stretch for functional genes. High gene transcription activity in undermethylated areas may provide a clue to an active gene location. DNA samples from multiple affected families and normals are needed. The located area is treated with restriction enzymes, and patients affected by the disease are compared with those who are not. DNA probes are then used to locate the potential gene that can then be sequenced. A strategy that somewhat combines these methods is positional-candidate cloning, in which a disease is mapped to a small region of a chromosome and that area is searched for a candidate gene for that disease. Newer methods for positional cloning using linkage and linkage disequilibrium are being used for both Mendelian and complex diseases.

MOLECULAR TECHNIQUES AND TOOLS FOR DETECTION AND DIAGNOSIS OF GENETIC DISEASES

Molecular techniques in genetics have allowed for more precise diagnosis and counseling. Appropriate molecular methods can be applied to: (1) include the determination of whether or not a specific mutant gene(s) are present in persons who are at risk but are asymptomatic; (2) diagnose those who are symptomatic; (3) detect carriers; (4) differentiate between disorders producing a similar phenotype; (5) detect similarities and differences in specific pieces of DNA; and (6) have applications in other areas, such as in determining the microbial etiology of a person's infectious disease and in tracing variations in microbes to determine origins and patterns of spread. For the DNA sample, usually white blood cells or epithelial cells from the buccal mucosa can be used, thus eliminating the need for tissue biopsy. For prenatal diagnosis, chorionic villus or amniotic fluid cells can be used. A brief look at some of these techniques is given next. For more information, the reader is referred to Ross (2002).

One of the basic tools in molecular genetics is the use of restriction enzymes or restriction endonucleases for recombinant DNA or other technology. These enzymes recognize a specific nucleotide sequence (recognition site) and cut the DNA where that sequence occurs. Different restriction enzymes have different known recognition sites, and thus the number of fragments produced by the process depends on which enzyme is used. In brief, the procedure is as follows: The DNA is extracted from the sample and is incubated with a specific restriction enzyme that digests or cuts the DNA into thousands of fragments of varying lengths (RFLPs, as described earlier). The fragment length varies not only in regard to the specific restriction enzyme used but also in regard to individual variation, resulting in differences in the size of segments of DNA when a particular restriction enzyme cut site is present or absent. These are then subjected to another technique such as the Southern Blot or polymerase chain reaction (PCR), depending on the purpose of the analysis.

DNA profiling or fingerprints has uses, including criminal and paternity applications. After using a particular restriction enzyme to obtain DNA fragments from a sample, fragments are placed on a gel and into an electrical field to separate the fragments by size. This process, called "electrophoresis," depends on the more rapid migration of smaller fragments and the slower migrations of larger fragments. Fragments are rendered single stranded. They are then transferred to a membrane or filter, and a specific labeled probe is added, and washing occurs. Hybridization of the labeled probe will occur to the DNA with a complementary sequence. If radioactively labeled, then autoradiography is used to create an X-ray film showing a band pattern. Fluorescent dyes may also be used as labels with appropriate detectors for fluorescence instead of autoradiography. The process can be repeated for multiple probes. Specific fragments of samples from two or more different sources can be compared to see if they are from the same individual (with certain probabilities). Northern and Western blots are similar but are for messenger RNA and proteins, respectively. A variation is the use of in situ hybridization. With in situ hybridization, a prepared, labeled DNA probe is incubated with a cell or tissue sample and later examined.

Another major advance has been the ability to clone DNA. When a segment of DNA or a gene is isolated and cloned (copies made), a particular gene or DNA segment can be used as a DNA probe or in genetic engineering or gene or pharmacological therapy. During the cloning procedure, DNA fragments can be inserted into plasmids or other vectors to produce many copies of the specific fragment or gene as well as to produce large quantities of products for treatment, such as human growth hormone, insulin or alpha interferon (see chapter 15). Cloning systems may use bacterial artificial chromosomes (BAC), yeast artificial chromosomes (YAC), or others as vectors for insertion of a gene. Often, mRNA is used to synthesize a DNA copy by use of reverse transcriptase, which is know as "complementary" or "cDNA." cDNA made in this way does not contain the introns of the gene, only the exons. Once obtained, DNA probes can then be labeled in some way (either radioactively or with a dye) and made single stranded. A DNA probe can then be used to locate its complementary sequence in a target DNA sample, and visualized by autoradiography, fluorescence or other techniques. These are sometimes done on dot blots or DNA microarrays. Eventually thousands of mutations can be sought using one microarray. In this technology, single strands of DNA with certain genes are fixed in an array pattern. DNA from the specimen of interest is labelled with fluorescent tags and applied to the chip. During incubation, DNA in the sample binds to the fixed DNA strands that are a match and the presence of fluorescence is detected, usually by laser. The array is read as to sequences present, patterns of gene expression, and quantities. Collections of DNA probes are often called "libraries."

Another technique is PCR, which amplifies a chosen DNA segment rapidly and exponentially with each cell cycle, making up to millions of copies. Its inventor (Dr. Kary Mullis) was awarded the 1993 Nobel prize in chemistry. It can do this rapidly from as small a source of DNA as one nucleated cell. Thus DNA can be obtained from such sources as one hair, dried blood spots, saliva traces, or decayed DNA sources. PCR is so sensitive that it is important that no contamination occur, which can happen if proper precautions are not taken. It uses two oligonucleotide primers complementary to the flanking sequence of the DNA stretch that is of interest in amplification, and is usually used for smaller DNA regions. After enough DNA copies are generated, analysis can take place, which can include digesting the amplified DNA with a restriction enzyme, hybridizing the product by using allele-specific oligonucleotides (ASO) (these are short, usually 7 to 30 nucleotide long, probes) or other probes, direct nucleotide sequencing of the PCR product, and others. PCR is also being used in archaeological DNA studies because only very tiny amounts of DNA obtained from sources such as mummies can be used for analysis. Multiplex PCR refers to the analysis of more than one sample at the same time. Another application of PCR use is in chronic myeloid leukemia (CML). PCR can be used to detect the presence of *BCR-ABL* transcripts after bone marrow transplant to detect whether minimal residual disease remains (see chapter 23). Various advances and variations occur in the types of molecular diagnoses used as new techniques become available. Flow cytometry and fluorescence in situ hybridization (FISH) are discussed in chapter 5.

Microarray (or chip) technology has allowed the detection and analysis of thousands genes simultaneously as to patterns of expression and interaction of pathways. A microarray consists of a solid surface such as a glass slide or silicon wafer on which each spot on the array corresponds to an immobilized DNA target sample that can represent a gene. A fluorescent labelled sample (usually mRNA or DNA) is then applied, and incubated with the microarray allowing binding or hybridization to the immobilized target DNA. The fluorescent signal is measured so that information about gene expression can be obtained. Gene expression profiles can be developed. This technique is useful in many studies in cancers and in infectious diseases. For example, in leukemia, different expression profiles are seen with different genetic mutations and may be used in diagnosis, prognosis, and we hope, someday, prevention.

BIBLIOGRAPHY

Abbott, C. M., & Proud, C. G. (2004). Translation factors: In sickness and in health. *Trends in Biochemical Sciences, 29,* 25–31.

Alekseyenko, A. A., & Kuroda, M. I. (2004). Filling gaps in genome organization. *Science, 303,* 1148–1149.

Allshire, R. (2004). Guardian spirit blesses meiosis. *Nature, 427,* 495–497.

Anderson, N. H. (2002). Analysis of genetic linkage. In D. L. Rimoin, J. M. Connor, R. E. Pyeritz, & B. R. Korf (Eds.), *Emery and Rimoin's principles and practice of medical genetics* (4th ed., pp. 133–148). New York: Churchill Livingstone

Antonarakis, S. E., Krawczak, M., & Cooper, D. N. (2002). Mutations in human disease: Nature and consequences. In D. L. Rimoin, J. M. Connor, R. E. Pyeritz, & B. R. Korf (Eds.), *Emery and Rimoin's principles and practice of medical genetics* (4th ed., pp. 83–103). New York: Churchill Livingstone.

Ashkenas, J. (1997). Gene regulation by mRNA editing. *American Journal of Human Genetics, 60,* 278–283.

Barsh, G., Epstein, C. J., & Peltonen, L. (2002). Genome structure and gene expression. In D. L. Rimoin, J. M. Connor, R. E. Pyeritz, & B. R. Korf (Eds.), *Emery and Rimoin's principles and practice of medical genetics* (4th ed., pp. 60–82). New York: Churchill Livingstone

Beaudet, A. L., Scriver, C. R., Sly, W. S., & Valle, D. (2001). Genetics, biochemistry, and molecular basis of variant human phenotypes. In C. R. Scriver, A. L. Beaudet, W. S. Sly, & D. Valle (Eds.), *The metabolic and molecular bases of inherited disease* (8th ed., pp. 3–125). New York: McGraw-Hill.

Bryant, P. A., Venter, D., Robins-Browne, R., & Curtis, N. (2004). Chips with everything: DNA microarrays in infectious diseases. *Lancet Infectious Diseases, 4,* 100–111.

Bunney, W. E., Bunney, B. G., Vawter, M. P., Tomita, H., Li, J., & Evans, S. S. (2003). Microarray technology: A review of new strategies to discover candidate vulnerability genes in psychiatric disorders. *American Journal of Psychiatry, 160,* 657–666.

Chan, S. W-L., Zilberman, D., Xie, Z., Johansen, L. K., Carrington, J. C., & Jacobsen, S. E. (2004). RNA silencing genes control de novo DNA methylation. *Science, 303,* 1336–1337.

Conneally, P. M. (2003). The complexity of complex diseases. *American Journal of Human Genetics, 72,* 229–232.

Feinberg, A., Cui, H., & Ohlsson, R. (2002). DNA methylation and genomic imprinting: Insights from cancer into epigenetic mechanisms. *Seminars in Cancer Biology, 12,* 389–398.

Glick, B. R., & Pasternak, J. J. (2003). *Molecular biotechnology: Principles and applications of recombinant DNA* (3rd ed.). Washington, DC: American Society for Microbiology.

Graves, P. R., & Haystead, T. A. J. (2002). Molecular biologist's guide to proteomics. *Microbiology and Molecular Biology Reviews, 66,* 39–63.

Hampton, T. (2004). With RNA interference, silence is golden. *Journal of the American Medical Association, 291,* 2803–2804.

Hughes, S., Arneson, N., Done, S., & Squire, J. (2005). The use of whole genome amplification in the study of human disease. *Progress in Biophysics and Molecular Biology, 88,* 173–189.

Jaenisch, R., & Bird, A. (2003). Epigenetic regulation of gene expression: How the genome integrates intrinsic and environmental signals. *Nature Genetics Supplement, 33,* 245–254.

Kornberg, R. D., & Lorch, Y. (2002). Chromatin and transcription: Where do we go from here? *Current Opinion in Genetics & Development, 12,* 249–251.

Kreahling, J., & Graveley, B. R. (2004). The origins and implications of *Alu*ternative splicing. *Trends in Genetics, 20,* 1–4.

Kruglyak, L., & McAllister, L. (1998). Who needs genetic markers? *Nature Genetics, 18,* 200–202.

Le Hir, H., Nott, A., Moore, M. J. (2003). How introns influence and enhance eukaryotic gene expression. *Trends in Biochemical Sciences, 28,* 215–220.

Lewis, R. (2003). *Human genetics: Concepts and applications* (5th ed.). New York: McGraw Hill.

Liu, E. T., & Karuturi, K. R. (2004). Microarrays and clinical investigations. *New England Journal of Medicine, 350,* 1595–1597.

Mantripragada, K. K., Buckley, P. G., de Ståhl, T. D., & Dumanski, J. P. (2004). Genomic microarrays in the spotlight. *Trends in Genetics, 20,* 87–94.

Maquat, L. E. (1996). Defects in RNA splicing and the consequence of shortened translational reading frames. *American Journal of Human Genetics, 59,* 279–286.

Morton, N. E., & Collins, A. (2002). Toward positional cloning with SNPs. *Current Opinion in Molecular Therapy, 4,* 259–264.

Naraveneni, R., & Jamil, K. (2005). Rapid detection of food-borne pathogens by using molecular techniques. *Journal of Medical Microbiology, 54*(Pt. 1), 51–54.

Naslund, K., Saetre, P., von Salome, J., Bergstrom, T. F., Jareborg, N., & Jazin, E. (2005). Genome-wide prediction of human VNTRs. *Genomics, 85,* 24–35.

Ostrer, H. (1998). *Non-mendelian genetics in humans.* New York: Oxford University Press.

Reik, W., Santos, F., & Dean, W. (2003). Mammalian epigenomics: Reprogramming the genome for development and therapy. *Theriogenology, 59,* 21–32.

Rieger, R., Michaelis, A., & Green, M. M. (1991). *Glossary of genetics* (5th ed.). Berlin: Springer-Verlag.

Ross, D. W. (2002). *Introduction to molecular medicine* (3rd ed.). New York: Springer-Verlag.

Sancar, A., Lindsey-Boltz, L. A., Ünsal-Kaçmaz, K., & Lynn, S. (2004). Molecular mechanisms of mammalian DNA repair and the DNA damage checkpoints. *Annual Review of Biochemistry, 73,* 39–85.

Shows, T. B., McAlpine, P. J., Boucheix, C., Collins, F. S., Conneally, P. M., Frezal, J., et al. (1987). Guidelines for human gene nomenclature. An international system for human gene nomenclature (ISGN, 1987). *Cytogenetics and Cell Genetics, 46,* 12–28.

Sinclair, A. (2002). Genetics 101: Polymerase chain reaction. *Canadian Medical Association Journal, 167,* 1032–1033.

Sinclair, A. (2002). Genetics 101: Detecting mutations in human genes. *Canadian Medical Association Journal, 167,* 275–279.

Snyder, M., & Gerstein, M. (2003). Defining genes in the genomics era. *Science, 300,* 258–260.

Spence, M. A., & Hodge, S. E. (2002). Segregation analysis. In D. L. Rimoin, J. M. Connor, R. E. Pyeritz, & B. R. Korf (Eds.), *Emery and Rimoin's principles and practice of medical genetics* (4th ed., pp. 125–132). New York: Churchill Livingstone

Strachan, T., & Read, A. P. (2004). *Human molecular genetics* (3rd. ed.). London: Garland Science.

Steinmetz, L. M., & Davis, R. (2004). Maximizing the potential of functional genomics. *Nature Reviews Genetics, 5,* 190–201.

Tufarelli, C., Stanley, J. A. S., Garrick, D., Sharpe, J. A., Ayyub, H., Wood, W. G., et al. (2003).

Transcription of antisense RNA leading to gene silencing and methylation as a novel cause of human genetic disease. *Nature Genetics, 34,* 157–165.

Vastag, B. (2003). Gene chips inch toward the clinic. *Journal of the American Medical Association, 289,* 155–157.

Wain, H. W., Bruford, E. A., Lovering, R. C., Lush, M. J., Wright, M. W., & Povey, S. (2002). Guidelines for human gene nomenclature (2002). *Genomics, 79,* 464–470.

Watson, R. E., & Goodman, J. I. (2002). Epigenetics and DNA methylation come of age in toxicology. *Toxicological Sciences, 67,* 11–16.

Westover, K. D., Bushnell, D. A., & Kornberg, R. D. (2004). Structural basis of transcription: Separation of RNA from DNA by RNA polymeraser II. *Science, 303,* 1014–1016.

Wolfe, K. H., & Li, W-H. (2003). Molecular evolution meets the genomics revolution. *Nature Genetics Supplement, 33,* 255–265.

3

Human Variation and Its Applications

Each individual has a unique genetic constitution that makes him/her genetically and biochemically distinct from all other individuals (except for monozygous twins, triplets, and other multiples). No individuals, with the exceptions mentioned, have the exact same genotype or phenotype. Garrod noticed this back in 1902 when he stated ". . . just as no two individuals . . . are absolutely identical in bodily structure, neither are their chemical processes carried out on exactly the same lines." (Garrod, 1902). Because a person's genetic constitution determines the limits of the range of responses and potentials within which he/she can interact with the environment, each person has his/her own relative state of health, and all persons are not at equivalent risk for developing disease. A person's genetic makeup plays a pivotal role in the maintenance of homeostasis and in susceptibility and resistance to disease as well as response to treatment. In this context, no disease process can be said to be wholly genetic or wholly environmental. This chapter builds on information provided in chapter 2.

GENETIC DIVERSITY IN INDIVIDUALS AND POPULATIONS

Randomly occurring mutations in genes appear responsible for the occurrence of genetic variation. Mutation is an ongoing process that influences evolution. Genes may be thought of at the population level as well as at the individual level. Most genes in humans are shared by all members of the human species. Differences have more to do with variation in frequency of certain alleles than in whether or not the gene is present or absent. A genetic variation is called a "polymorphism" when two or more alleles are maintained in a population so that the frequency of the most common one is not more than 99%, or stated another way, in which the frequency of one of the uncommon alleles is maintained at a frequency of at least 1%. The ABO, MN, and Rh blood groups and the human leukocyte antigen (HLA) system are some of the best known examples of classic genetic polymorphisms. The clinical use of the knowledge of these polymorphisms has been amply demonstrated by the ability to perform compatible transfusions and tissue transplants. Glucose-6-phosphate dehydrogenase (G6PD) deficiency, of which there are more than 400 known variants, is the most common enzyme polymorphism in humans and is discussed in detail in chapter 18. The newer polymorphisms being identified may involve only one nucleotide change in a gene, and are known as single gene polymorphisms or SNPs. Information from the Human Genome Project has revealed that there are about 3 million places in the genome where SNPs occur. The reasons for such a high degree of variation or of its effects (if not known to be related to dysfunction) are speculative only. Most polymorphisms appear neutral or cause benign variations. However, the meaning of much of this variation is not yet known. It may be that the preservation of individual and population genetic diversity allows a species to adapt to environmental changes and challenges and thus to survive.

One of the major thrusts of future directions of the Human Genome Project is to establish a catalogue of common variants in the human population and characterize SNPs, patterns of linkage disequilibrium and haplotypes across the human genome, as well as to examine genomic function in relation to evolutionary variation and in understanding genetic variation in relation to race and ethnicity in various populations. SNPs and their constellations are being examined to create pattern "maps" across populations in the United States, Asia and Africa. These can give information about population history; patterns of migration; the evolution of the human genome; the geographic distribution of human variation; the age of populations; disease susceptibility in and among populations; and relationships among genetic, cultural, linguistic, and ecological variables. Ethical concerns such as informed consent, confidentiality, the possible exploitation of indigenous peoples, and the potential for abuse have resulted in the delay of the project. Ethical questions have also been raised about the uses of a genetics research database of the Icelandic population.

VARIATIONS AND POLYMORPHISMS IN DNA AND CHROMOSOMES

DNA varies among individuals and populations. Variation may be seen at the gene level and at the chromosome level (heteromorphisms). At the chromosomal level, variations are especially evident in certain chromosomes such as 1, 9, and the Y. In most cases, the significance is not known, and some of these may serve as "private" (within a family) markers. Others may be "public." DNA sequence polymorphisms may occur within the coding (exon) regions or noncoding (such as introns). Polymorphisms may occur in every 1:200 to 1:300 base pairs overall. Polymorphisms occur more often outside of coding genes. These polymorphisms may be single or multiple. The more alternate forms present, the more useful a polymorphism is for genetic and medical applications. The following variations are among those identified: 1. restriction fragment length polymorphisms (RFLPs), 2. minisatellites or variable number tandem repeats (VNTRs), 3. microsatellites or short tandem repeats (STRs), 4. single nurcleotide polymorphisms (SNPs), and 5. others such as *Alu* repetitions (see chapter 2) and variants in mitochondrial DNA. RFLPs are single-base pair changes in noncoding DNA areas that result in removal or addition of a recognition site for a restriction enzyme. This causes an increase or decrease in the length of

the restriction fragment due to differences in the number of cleavage sites cut by certain restriction endonucleases. The VNTRs are short DNA sequences that are repeated in tandem order a varying number of times, usually ranging in size from 6 to 60 or more base pairs. The size can change during cell division and, in some cases, expansion can lead to disease expression such as in fragile X syndrome (see chapter 20). The STRs usually comprise pairs such as CG of two bases (although three to five pairs have been noted) that are repeated a few to many times. SNPs are single nucleotide changes in DNA. Patterns of SNPs are also being used to look at particular phenotypic variations as haplotypes and across populations and ethnic groups. The variants mentioned previously are the basis of various DNA tests used for genetic parentage, individual identification in legal and forensic cases, and for genetic testing. Each person has his or her own distinct "fingerprint" of DNA.

MAINTENANCE OF VARIATION AND POLYMORPHISM

The rare, inherited, biochemical disorders are extreme examples of the spectrum of genetic diversity. Variations that are too rare to meet the criteria for a polymorphism in the human population at large may assume such allelic frequencies within particular groups. Population groups that have shared a common ancestry may be isolated from the population at large for cultural, social, religious, economic, political, linguistic, or geographic reasons. Members thus pick a mate or intermarry within the group. They therefore have more specific rare alleles in their gene pool (the collection of genes in a particular population) than that of the general population. Examples of such groups are the Finns, Icelanders, Pacific Islanders, and Ashkenazi Jews. This has clinical significance (1) in targeting groups for establishing screening or prenatal detection programs, and (2) for identifying individuals who are at the highest risk for adverse outcomes from exposure to certain drugs, foods, or external agents so that preventative measures can be taken. Some of the genetic diseases known to be present in higher frequencies or even in polymorphic proportions in certain groups are shown in Table 3.1. The presence of these rare alleles and

TABLE 3.1   Distribution of Selected Genetic Traits and Disorders by Population or Ethnic Group

Ethnic or Population Group	Genetic or Multifactorial Disorder Present in Relatively High Frequency
Åland Islanders	Ocular albinism (Forsius-Erikson type)
Amish	Limb-girdle muscular dystrophy (IN—Adams, Allen counties) Ellis-van Creveld (PA—Lancaster County) Pyruvate kinase deficiency (OH—Mifflin County) Hemophilia B (PA—Holmes County)
Armenians	Familial Mediterranean fever Familial paroxysmal polyserositis
Asians	Dubin-Johnson syndrome (Iran) Ichthyosis vulgaris (Iraq, India) Werdnig-Hoffmann disease (Karaite Jews) G6PD deficiency, Mediterranean type Phenylketonuria (Yemen) Metachromatic leukodystrophy (Habbanite Jews, Saudi Arabia)
Blacks (African)	Sickle cell disease Hemoglobin C disease Hereditary persistence of hemoglobin F G6PD deficiency, African type Lactase deficiency, adult β-thalassemia
Burmese	Hemoglobin E disease
Chinese	G6PD deficiency, Chinese type Lactase deficiency, adult
Costa Ricans	Malignant osteopetrosis
Druze	Alkaptonuria
English	Cystic fibrosis Hereditary amyloidosis, Type III
French Canadians (Quebec)	Morquio syndrome
Finns	Congenital nephrosis Generalized amyloidosis syndrome, V Polycystic liver disease Retinoschisis Aspartylglycosaminuria Diastrophic dwarfism
Gypsies (Czech)	Congenital glaucoma
Hopi Indians	Tyrosinase positive albinism
Icelanders	Phenylketonuria (PKU)
Inuit	Congenital adrenal hyperplasis Pseudocholinesterase deficiency Methemoglobinemia
Irish	Phenylketonuria Neural tube defects
Japanese	Acatalasemia Cleft lip/palate Oguchi disease
Jews Ashkenazi	Tay-Sachs disease (infantile Niemann-Pick disease (infantile) Gaucher disease (adult type) Familial dysautonomia Bloom syndrome Torsion dystonia Factor XI (PTA) deficiency

TABLE 3.1 *(Continued)*

Ethnic or Population Group	Genetic or Multifactorial Disorder Present in Relatively High Frequency
Sephardi	Familial Mediterranean fever
	Ataxia-telangiectasia (Morocco)
	Cystinuria (Libya)
	Glycogen storage disease III (Morocco)
Lapps	Congenital dislocation of hip
Lebanese	Dyggve-Melchior-Clausen syndrome
Mediterranean people (Italians, Greeks)	G6PD deficiency, Mediterranean type
	β-thalassemia
	Familial Mediterranean fever
Navaho Indians	Ear anomalies
Polynesians	Clubfoot
Polish	Phenylketonuria
Portuguese	Joseph disease
Nova Scotia Acadians	Niemann-Pick disease, Type D
Scandinavians (Norwegians, Swedes, Danes)	Cholestasis-lymphedema (Norwegians)
	Sjögren-Larsson syndrome (Swedes)
	Krabbe disease
	Phenylketonuria
Scots	Phenylketonuria
	Cystic fibrosis
	Hereditary amyloidosis, Type III
Thailanders	Lactase deficiency, adult
	Hemoglobin E disease
Zuni people	Tyrosinase positive albinism

disorders in higher frequency in some population groups is not "good" or "bad." They probably evolved, in some cases, because in the homozygous or carrier state they offered some type of protection, such as from malaria in sickle cell anemia heterozygotes in Africa. These rare alleles also evolved because of founder effects or population "bottlenecks," as described later in this chapter. As members of specific racial and ethnic groups intermarry, intermate, and become less isolated, there will be fewer definable genetic disorders occurring with greater frequency within given groups.

The population geneticist is interested in reasons for the maintenance of certain variations and polymorphisms in populations. Many complicated mathematical formulas are used to determine such things as mutation rates, to measure the effects of migration, and so forth. One of the fundamental principles in population genetics is that of the Hardy-Weinberg law. This law was developed in 1908 by the English mathematician G. H. Hardy and the German physician W. Weinberg. This law is useful for different types of population problems and has had practical application in genetic counseling for the determination of the risk of a counselee being a carrier for a certain gene when only the frequency of the homozygous disorder is known. An explanation and an example of the Hardy-Weinberg law is given in Figure 3.1.

Frequencies of alleles in populations change because of effects such as mutation, selection, migration, random genetic drift, nonrandom mating, and other factors such as meiotic drive (forces that change Mendelian segregation ratios in meiosis), differential gamete survival, and linkage to a favorable or unfavorable gene (hitchhiker effect). Differential gamete survival occurs when gametes with a certain composition are favored over the others with a different composition in survival. *Selection* is the process by which certain alleles become more or less frequent in a population because of the occurrence of events making their possession more or less advantageous. It is a powerful force in evolution. *Fitness* is the ability of a

The basic principle of the Hardy-Weinberg Law states that in a large, randomly mating population with no selection, mutation, migration, or linkage, with two alleles, A and a (at frequencies p and q), and three possible genotypes AA, Aa, and aa (at frequencies p^2, 2pq, and q^2), gene and genotype frequencies will attain equilibrium in one generation and remain constant from generation to generation. For a population meeting the conditions in the text and two autosomal alleles,* one dominant and one recessive (A and a), and 3 possible genotypes (AA, Aa, and aa),

p = proportion of allele A in the population (gene frequency of A)
q = proportion of allele a in the population (gene frequency of a); then the sum of alleles at one locus is p + q = 1; and if

genotype		genotype frequency
AA	=	p^2
Aa	=	2pq
aa	=	q^2

then by using algebraic process of binomial expansion, $p^2 + 2pq + q^2 = 1$.

Example: A rare autosomal recessive disorder occurs in 1 in 10,000 individuals (q^2)
            What is the heterozygous carrier frequency in this population?

Solution: Frequency of the recessive allele (q) = $\sqrt{q^2} = \sqrt{1/10{,}000} = 1/100$
            Frequency of the dominant allele (p) = 1 – q = 1– 1/100 = 99/100
            The frequency of heterozygote carrier (2pq) = 2 x 99/100 x 1/100 = approximately 1/50

This example also illustrates that in the general population, the heterozygote is much more frequent than is the affected individual.

FIGURE 3.1   Hardy-Weinberg Law.
*Other formulas are used for multiple alleles and X linked inheritance, etc.

person to reach reproductive age and pass on his or her genes to the next generation. Individuals who do not do this are genetically dead. An example is individuals who are homozygous for the gene for infantile Niemann Pick disease (an autosomal recessive disorder characterized by mental and physical retardation, neurological effects, and hepatosplenomegaly) and who die in childhood, or males with cystic fibrosis who are usually infertile, although assisted reproductive techniques can influence this situation. They are said to have genotypes with a low degree of fitness.

The fact that some alleles are rapidly eliminated from the gene pool in the homozygous recessive state, but may enjoy a higher frequency in the heterozygous state than could be maintained by mutation alone, suggests that their presence confers some type of selective advantage to the heterozygote over the normal homozygote. In the case of sickle cell disease, various lines of evidence indicate that the sickle cell heterozygotes (SA) in endemic malarial areas in Africa are less severely affected by *Plasmodium falciparum* (one type of malarial parasite) than are either the normal homozygote (AA) or the homozygote with sickle cell disease (SS), particularly for severe complications such as cerebral involvement. A positive correlation between the endemic malarial areas in Africa and the distribution of the hemoglobin (Hb) S gene was demonstrated years ago by Allison (1964), Livingstone (1971), and others. The same appears to be true for the Hb C allele in West Africa, the Hb E allele in Southeast Asia, β-thalassemia in the formerly endemic malarial areas in parts of Italy and Greece, and for one type of G6PD deficiency in Mediterranean populations. Those heterozygotes are not at an advantage once they have changed their environment and have settled in a malaria-free area such as the United States. It can be demonstrated that the frequency of the sickle cell gene in Blacks of African descent is decreasing in this country, as would be expected once the heterozygous advantage is removed.

Another polymorphism appears to have developed in response to malaria in Papua New Guinea. There, a defect known as "ovalocytosis," an erythrocyte membrane defect involving a mutation in erythrocyte band 3, results in rigidity of the membrane. The malarial parasite thus cannot pull the membrane around itself when it enters the blood. Because of this, in heterozygotes, there is resistance to invasion by malarial parasites. This situation has the potential for drug development to protect against malaria by mimicking this defect to some degree. The homozygous state is lethal in utero.

A selective advantage conferring resistance to various infectious and other diseases has been proposed for other genetic disorders such as cystic fibrosis (protection against asthma, diarrheal epidemics and others have been proposed) and Tay-Sachs disease (protection against tuberculosis, typhus and others have been proposed) in which there is a higher than expected frequency of heterozygotes in certain populations. Heterozygosity in the prion protein gene at codon 129 appears to confer relative resistance to prion diseases such as kuru in the Fore people of Papua New Guinea. Molecular genetic advances have provided new information. For example, it can now be determined that a particular allelic mutation such as the 1277ins4 allele of *HEXA* which results in Tay-Sachs disease is in particularly high frequency in Ashkenazic Jews who may have been resistant to tuberculosis. Most selective advantage theories for heterozygotes remain speculative.

Other interesting interactions between certain genes and environment exist for various blood components and for lactase. The Duffy antigen is a receptor site on the red cell to which *Plasmodium vivax* (a malarial parasite) attaches itself. About 85% of American Blacks lack the Duffy allele and are Fy (a-b-), whereas Caucasians possess alleles for it. Those who are Duffy negative because they lack the receptor site are resistant to the type of malaria caused by *P. vivax*. In another study, women with nonsecretor Lewis phenotypes and the recessive phenotype were more prone to recurrent urinary tract infections, perhaps because they provide a specific receptor for uropathogenic organisms so they can attach to these cells. Haptoglobin polymorphisms of the Hp 2-2 type seem more frequently associated with autoimmune disorders than the others. Variations in bone mineral density are associated with polymorphisms at the Vitamin D receptor locus on chromosome 12. In mammals, lactase activity is highest in the newborn and then declines; by adulthood, the recessive allele for lactase is "switched off" in most adults, but in some there is a hereditary persistence of lactase, and this does not occur. This may have conferred a selective advantage on societies who had cow's milk available for food. Individuals who lack lactase activity

may experience gastrointestinal symptoms such as flatulence, abdominal pain, and diarrhea after ingesting small to moderate amounts of lactose in dairy products. Analysis indicates that groups in Northern Europe and certain nomadic groups in Africa and Southwest Asia who were milking societies dating back 7,000 years have a high frequency of hereditary persistence of lactase activity while the Chinese, Arabs, Melanesians, Thais, American Blacks, and Native Americans do not. Others are intermediate. In the U.S., persons with low lactase activity can adjust to their changed environment by consuming less lactose or taking supplements, and thus minimizing annoying symptoms. Another interesting area has to do with inherited taste, which is genetically determined and reflected in taste buds. In regard to bitterness there are nontasters, regular tasters and supertasters that can be detected by 6-*n*-propylthiouracil. Supertasters have approximately 1,100 taste buds per square cm, whereas nontasters have as few as 11. Supertasters are sensitive to fats and strong tastes of fruit and vegetables. It has been suggested that those who are supertasters dislike bitter foods and avoid cruciferous vegetables, such as broccoli, which confer some chemoprotection against cancer. Thus the type of taster one is may confer an advantage or disadvantage. Some variation may be associated with sex differences. It appears as if males and females may process pain signals differently in part because of sex differences in μ-opioid receptors, eventually leading to tailoring analgesic medications differently according to sex. Likewise, persons with variants of the melanocortin-1 receptor gene, as seen in women with red hair and fair skin, appeared to have greater analgesia from pentazocine than other women or even men with red hair.

Besides selection, other influences that alter the frequency of alleles in certain population groups include the following:

1. *Random genetic drift* is said to occur when variation in gene frequency from one generation to another occurs because of chance fluctuations. It has its greatest effect in small groups. Genetic drift may also be produced by mortality, population size, and failure to find mates. Weiss (1995) describes the result as a steady stream of new variation moving in and existing variation moving out of a population like a river, "ever flowing, ever changing, always the same, never the same."

2. *Migration* refers to movement of a population into the territory of another with different allelic frequencies from the migrant one. Migration causes an exchange of alleles through interbreeding, and results in altered ratios from the original population in future generations. This gene flow can be measured by the application of certain formulas to the original population and the one to which the original one has migrated. Blood group frequency changes can be mapped geographically to examine such effects.

3. *Founder effect* is a special type of drift that occurs when a small group from a large population migrates to another locale, and one or more members of the founding group possess a variant allele that is rare in the original population. That variant now assumes a greater proportion. If allele A has a frequency of 1/10,000 in the original population, and a person who possesses A is one of 10 founders of a new community, the frequency of allele A is now $^1\!/_{20}$ (remember alleles come in pairs). The rare allele becomes more frequent and leads to the high frequency of genetic diseases in future generations, especially if the group is isolated in its new location for a time. Porphyria variegata is particularly common among Afrikaaners in South Africa and is an example of the founder effect. It is believed to have originated in South Africa from one Dutch settler who went there in the late 1600s. Another example is cerebral cavernous malformation, in which familial cases in Mexican Americans have been linked to inheritance from a common Mexican ancestor.

For more information, interested readers may refer to a reference on population genetics such as Ewens (2004), Gillespie (2004), Cavalli-Sforza and Feldman (2003), Epperson, (2003), Vogel and Motulsky (1997), or Weiss (1995).

ECOGENETICS AND PUBLIC HEALTH GENETICS

Ecogenetics may be defined as individual variation in response to agents in the environment causing genotoxic and other effects. Its importance lies in implications for policies that affect the public health. Because most individuals have some genetic differences from others, they may react in varying ways to their environment which, in a broad sense, includes all chemical exposures, food and drug intake, exposure to infectious agents and the like. Aspects of individual susceptibility and response are discussed in chapters 14 and 18. In many instances, the person who has an unexpected response to a particular food (e.g., persons with G6PD deficiency to fava bean ingestion) can easily avoid the food. A person who is susceptible to a certain drug such as barbituates in acute intermittent porphyria can avoid the drug.

In the case of food additives, the picture is more complex. For example, supplementing commercial bread and baked goods with iron may be beneficial to those with a mild iron deficiency anemia. However, it can cause adverse effects in patients with hemochromatosis because iron overload damages their liver, heart, and pancreas. Individuals who carry the gene for thalassemia also absorb more iron and can suffer damage to those organs. Another substance that is widely supplemented is folic acid. Folic acid supplementation has been shown to be protective against neural tube defects in the fetus when taken periconceptionally and during pregnancy. Folic acid supplementation also appears to reduce levels of homocyteine, an amino acid that, when elevated, predisposes to arteriosclerotic vascular disease. About 1:200–1:300 persons are heterozygotes for homocystinuria and have elevated homocyteine levels that predispose them to arteriosclerotic vascular disease. Thus, the widespread supplementation of foods with folate was originally recommended by some and opposed by others mainly on the grounds that in persons with pernicious anemia, the consumption of large amounts of folate masks the hematologic signs while neurological damage progresses. Thus, whether the best way to deliver folate supplementation for disease prevention is through widespread food addition is not entirely resolved but it has been implemented in grains and cereals in the United States in 1998.

Food additives such as dyes and preservatives may act to modify the metabolism of chemicals. Well-known examples of individual responses include that to monosodium glutamate (Chinese restaurant syndrome) and to foods containing nitrates and tyramine. The addition of tartrazine (FD&C yellow no. 5), a color additive to food, drink, and pharmaceuticals, may cause the response of asthma, urticaria, rhinitis, or angioedema in susceptible persons. The Food and Drug Administration (FDA) estimates that 50,000 to 100,000 persons in the United States are intolerant to tartrazine. About 15% of those who are intolerant to aspirin are also affected by tartrazine. Recent labeling requirements have made products containing tartrazine easier to identify. However, the public health issue is whether or not additives that may benefit one group should be added to a wide range of food when they may not be tolerated by some individuals. Truly, "one man's meat can be another's poison."

Such concerns are not limited to foods. As an example, a child who used an insect repellant containing N,N-diethyltoluamide (DEET) developed a Reye-like syndrome and died. She was heterozygous for ornithine carbamoyltransferase deficiency (a urea cycle enzyme disorder), which caused her to have a lower level of this enzyme. These decreased levels apparently did not allow her to metabolically process the chemicals in the repellant properly. Yet most people use the product without apparent effect, and it is particularly effective in repelling mosquitoes, some of which may carry diseases such as the West Nile virus. Should such products be removed from the market? Should warning labels be used? How many other products cause severe effects in a few susceptible individuals? Do most chemicals carry some risk to a few individuals? Many public health applications to genomic discoveries are emerging such as the application of genetic variation to disease prevention and health promotion as well as to susceptibility to environmental exposures, such as chemical sensitivity, as discussed in chapter 14. There are also applications to genetic screening programs discussed in chapter 11.

Hemochromatosis

Hemochromatosis is a very common autosomal recessive genetic disorder with a frequency of 1:200 to 1:400 and a carrier frequency of as high as 1:8–10 in White populations. The gene that is most commonly mutated in classic hereditary hemochromatosis, also known as hemochromatosis type 1, is located on chromosome 6 (6p21.3), and is designated HFE (formerly HLA-H). Most affected North Americans have a mutational change known

as C282Y which substitutes tyrosine for cysteine at position 282 of the HFE protein. Another mutational change, H63D (in which aspartic acid replaces histidine at position 63), may either produce disease in a homozygous form or as a compound heterozygote form with C282Y. The mutational variant S65C (in which cysteine replaces serine at position 65 may also be found in a compound heterozygous form with C282Y. Other hereditary forms include juvenile hereditary hemochromatosis in which type 2, subtype A involves a mutation in the gene encoding hemojuvelin, known as HJV (formerly $HFE2$) on chromosome 1q21, and type 2, subtype B in which the mutation is in the gene coding for hepciden $(HAMP)$ on chromosome 19q13.1. In both of these, inheritance is autosomal recessive and organ damage can occur to the liver, heart and endocrine glands, often presenting in the second or third decade of life with heart disease and/or hypogonadism. Another non-HFE-related form of hereditary hemochromatosis (type 3) is mutation of the transferrin receptor-2 gene $TFR2)$, on chromosome 7q22, which is also autosomal recessive. Ferroportin-related iron overload (type 4) results from mutation in ferroportin $(SLC11A3$ gene), is on chromosome 2q32, and is an autosomal dominant form. The latter two usually appear in the fourth or fifth decade of life as does the classic type.

Normally, all dietary iron is not absorbed; of the 15–20 mg of iron present in the average U.S. diet, males and reproductive age females absorb 1 mg and 2 mg, respectively. In classic hemochromatosis, iron overload develops, and the iron saturation of serum transferrin of 45–50% or higher in females and 60% or higher in males indicates the need for genetic testing, as is elevated serum ferritin. Men may show more serious disease than women, probably because of the physiological loss of iron due to menstruation and pregnancy in women. In heterozygote carriers, up to 1/4 may show biochemical evidence of iron metabolism abnormalities but do not usually develop disease, unless they inherit another gene that also increases iron absorption or increases alcohol or iron intake significantly. In hemochromatosis, iron is deposited into the liver, joints, heart, pancreas, and endocrine glands. The usual initial symptoms are somewhat vague— lethargy, weakness, abdominal and/or joint pain. Later, loss of libido, cardiac complaints, liver disease, diabetes mellitus, arthritis, skin pigmentation, and hypogonadism and infertility may be seen. Homozygotes for hemochromatosis are relatively common among those with diabetes mellitus or arthritis, and should be looked for.

Treatment is relatively straight-forward—lifelong phlebotomy of 500 ml of blood, usually weekly initially, and then every 3 to 4 months, depending on iron levels and tolerance. If early treatment is not initiated, cirrhosis, liver failure, portal hypertension, carbohydrate intolerance, and diabetes may occur as may cardiomegaly, dysfunction and arthopathy. It has been suggested that hemochromatosis is so common because it once conferred some type of selective advantage. For example, heterozygous women might have a reproductive advantage because of less likelihood of iron deficiency anemia, and for both men and women, survival in times of starvation might have been enhanced. The ecogenetic implications of this disorder relate to iron supplementation of food and to intake of certain foods. Vitamin C supplementation can increase iron overload as can supplemental iron. Thus, supplementing food with iron can accelerate iron deposition and be damaging to those with hemochromatosis. In addition, persons with hemochromatosis are susceptible to infection with *Vibrio vulnificus*, a bacterium present in raw oysters that thrives in iron rich blood and organs, and deaths have occurred from ingestion. In Africa, iron overload is correlated with heavy consumption of beer brewed in nongalvanized iron containers. Hemochromatosis has been suggested for population screening because of the potential for prevention of damage, however, the degree of clinical penetrance and variation in expressivity has raised questions by some about the cost versus benefits for general population screening as opposed to in specific populations (Pietrangelo, 2004).

DETERMINING GENETIC PARENT-HOOD AND FORENSIC AND OTHER APPLICATIONS OF VARIATION

Paternity suits are the most frequent reason for the determination of genetic parenthood, but it may also be done to determine maternity, especially in cases where infants may have been exchanged in the hospital, or to establish parenthood in inheritance cases. The following discussion focuses on paternity because it is expected that paternity suits will become more common in the future in order to enforce paternal support for ones own children instead of using public welfare funds. Unless a rare inherited variant is present in both the child and the putative father, but not the mother (except for rare recessive disorders), it is more difficult to attribute paternity than to exclude it. Tests, therefore, are usually based on exclusion.

There are two basic approaches to determine genetic parenthood: (1) DNA analysis or (2) a combination of genetic marker systems found in the blood. DNA testing may use blood or buccal cell samples from the inside of the mouth. Usually, at least four specific regions of DNA from the child and each parent are analyzed through comparing fragments by restriction fragment length polymorphism (RFLP) testing, which takes several weeks, or by using polymerase chain reaction (PCR), which generally takes only a week or less. The test is capable of excluding between 99% and 99.9% of the random population from the possibility of being the biological father. An example is shown in Figure 3.2. If using an approach of blood groups and HLA, the more genetic markers used, the higher the probability for the exclusion of someone who is not the father. Red cell antigen tests (ABO, MNSs, Rh, Kell, Duffy, and Kidd) plus HLA typing, serum proteins such as haptoglobin, Gm, and

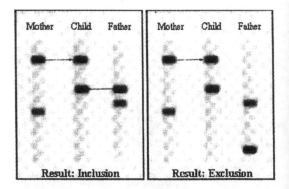

FIGURE 3.2   Paternity test showing two putative fathers, the mother, and the child in question. The father on the left has a given marker that matches that of the child in question, whereas the father on the right does not.

From ReliaGene Technologies, Inc., New Orleans, LA. Design by Shantanu Sinha. Printed by permission.

transferrin and red cell enzymes such as acid phosphatase, phosphoglucomutase, adenylate kinase, and adenosine deaminase may be used. All of these tests together result in a theoretical exclusion rate of 99.95%, but in practice the rate can be less because their genotypes may not be revealing for each marker. This approach is being used less and less frequently because of the availability of DNA testing. Other factors such as circumstances, access, and timing are usually also taken into account. Some pitfalls in the determination of genetic parenthood have included the receiving of blood transfusions, cases in which the mother and putative (suspected) father or two putative fathers were relatives, inaccurate laboratory determinations or errors, and the use of markers that are not fully developed in the infant. For example, at birth not all of an infant's antigens are fully developed and some are maternally derived. For full reliability, it is recommended that testing be postponed until the infant is 6 months of age. These issues are readily addressed by DNA testing, which is widely available. Information on such testing is widely available through billboard advertising and the internet.

Aside from parenthood determination, molecular techniques are also used in forensics. Saliva, blood, semen, and sweat all yield DNA that can be used for analysis. DNA databases are now being assembled in various states, although there is some controversy regarding who must submit to testing and who has access to the results. For example, in South Dakota, DNA samples are taken on arrest, and Virginia takes samples from all convicted felons. DNA samples from various suspects may be compared with a sample that was found on a victim. DNA profiling or fingerprinting techniques, which capitalize on variations, may be used. Opportunity is another consideration. For example, a case that came to my attention several years ago involved the rape and murder of an 80-year-old woman. The defense attorney tried to claim that it was chance that a DNA match of his client was found in fluids in her vagina. However, in addition to this suspect matching the DNA profile found (in addition to her own), the suspect was also in possession of the woman's TV set! The combination of evidence was enough to convince the jury to convict the suspect.

The use of DNA evidence received wide publicity in the murder trial of O. J. Simpson. Improvements

in techniques and more data on DNA polymorphism patterns in various ethnic groups have removed many of the earlier concerns about accuracy of a given match. Mitochondrial DNA (mtDNA) is increasingly used in forensic applications particularly for material where nuclear DNA is low such as old bones and teeth. A number of issues have been raised with this technique including the very rare situation of paternal leakage (paternal inheritance of the mitochondrial genome) and recombination. See Budowle et al. (2003) for detailed discussion of mtDNA in forensics.

There are also anthropological applications of DNA analysis. The Y chromosome is passed from father to son, essentially retaining its integrity. Some researchers examined a cultural characteristic—the passing down of Jewish priesthood from father to son, originating with Aaron and reflected in certain last names such as Kohn or Cohen—and examined variation in the Y chromosome. In a sample of such men, two marker sites with variable DNA sequences on the Y chromosome were examined. Those who identified themselves as priests had different marker patterns from those who were not. Such a finding has potential implications. Men who come from this priestly lineage are not permitted to marry divorced women, and such testing might have a social effect if used for that purpose. The Y chromosome markers such as the *Alu* element have been used to study whether the Jomon or the Yayoi people were the origins of the modern Japanese.

Mitochondrial DNA (mtDNA) is passed from a woman to her children (see chapter 4). The degree of similarity between humans cam be quantitated by comparing the number of mutations in the mitochondrial genome. Theoretically, a human evolutionary tree could be developed. Cann, Stoneking, and Wilson (1987) examined mtDNA from many diverse groups and used extensive RFLP mapping for comparative analysis. Their controversial finding, debated by many, was that all of the mtDNAs originated from one woman, nicknamed "mitochondrial Eve," who they postulated lived in Africa about 200,000 years ago. MtDNA has also been used to examine the evolution from Neanderthals.

Another application of DNA variation is in individual identification in times of war or disaster. In the United States, storage of the DNA of armed service personnel for such use has been the subject of controversy (see chapter 11). This method has been used to identify remains and reunite families. In the unfortunate aftermath of the terrorist attack on the World Trade Center in New York City on September 11, 2001, DNA analysis was used in victim identification. In another application example, in some Central and South American countries, children of dissidents were considered war booty and were often placed with families who were connected to the military regime. Children who were kidnapped by the Salvadoran military in 1982 were reunited with their families 13 years later by use of DNA fingerprinting. DNA techniques have also been used to identify remains in airline disasters and during combat by comparison with DNA samples of the individual or comparison with relatives. On a darker note, Germany was using saliva to screen Turkish and Iraqi visa applicants who said they had relatives in Germany so as to verify the claim by DNA comparisons.

END NOTES

Humans are remarkably alike—they are similar in 99.95 of their genes. The study of human variation is important in susceptibility and resistance to both genetic and complex diseases. What is known about human genetic variation is being applied for forensic uses such as genetic parenthood, certain criminal acts, identification in times of war and disaster and anthropological studies. Population genetics has provided information about the maintenance of certain variations and polymporphisms in specific groups.

BIBLIOGRAPHY

Allison, A. C. (1964). Polymorphism and natural selection in human populations. *Cold Spring Harbor Symposia on Quantitative Biology, 29,* 137–149.

Bowman, J. E., & Murray, R. F. Jr. (1998). *Genetic variation and disorders in peoples of African origin.* Baltimore: Johns Hopkins University Press.

Bradbury, J. (2003). Why do men and women feel and react to pain differently? *Lancet, 361,* 2052–2053.

Bradbury, J. (2004). Ancient footsteps in our genes: Evolution and human disease. *Lancet, 363,* 952–953.

Budowle, B., Allard, M. W., Wilson, M. R., & Chakraborty, R. (2003). Forensics and mitochondrial DNA: Applications, debates, and foundations. *Annual Review of Genomics and Human Genetics, 4,* 119–141.

Cann, R. L., Stoneking, M., & Wilson, A. C. (1987). Mitochondrial DNA and human evolution. *Nature, 325,* 31–36.

Cardon, L. R. & Palmer, L. J. (2003). Population stratification and spurious allelic association. *Lancet, 361,* 598–604.

Cavalli-Sforza, L. L. & Feldman, M. W. (2003). The application of molecular genetic approaches to the study of human evolution. *Nature Genetics Supplement, 33,* 266–275.

Cipollaro, M., Galderisi, U., & Di Bernardo, G. (2005). Ancient DNA as a multidisciplinary experience. *Journal of Cell Physiology, 202,* 315–322.

Collins, F. S., Green, E. D., Guttmacher, A. E., & Guyer, M. S. (2003). A vision for the future of genomics research. *Nature, 422,* 835–847.

Drewneowski, A., & Rock, C. L. (1995). The influence of genetic taste markers on food acceptance. *American Journal of Clinical Nutrition, 62,* 506–511.

Epperson, B. K. (2003). *Geographical genetics.* Princeton: Princeton University Press

Ewens, W. J. (2004). *Mathematical population genetics.* New York: Springer-Verlag.

Garrod, A. E. (1902). The incidence of alcaptonuria: A study in chemical individuality. *Lancet, 2,* 1616–1620.

Gillespie, J. H. (2004). *Population genetics: A concise guide.* Baltimore: Johns Hopkins University Press.

Gochfeld, M. (1997). Factors influencing susceptibility to metals. *Environmental Health Perspectives, 105*(Suppl. 4), 817–822.

Goldberg, C. (1998, February 19). DNA databanks giving police powerful weapon: The instant hit. *New York Times.* Retrieved from http://www.nytimes.com/yr/mo/day/news/national/dna-crime-database.html

Günel, M., Awad, I. A., Finberg, K., Anson, J. A., Steinberg, G. K., Batjer, H. H., et al. (1996). A founder mutation as a cause of cerebral cavernous malformation in Hispanic Americans. *New England Journal of Medicine, 334,* 946–951.

Gwinn, M., & Khoury, M. J. (2002). Research priorities for public health sciences in the postgenomic era. *Genetics in Medicine, 4,* 410–411.

Hardy, J., Singleton, A., & Gwinn-Hardy, K. (2003). Ethnic differences and disease phenotypes. *Science, 300,* 739–740.

Hirvonen, A. (1995). Genetic factors in individual responses to environmental exposures. *Journal of Occupational and Environmental Medicine, 37,* 37–43.

Immigrants are genetically tested to prove claims of kin in Germany. (1998, January 24). *Chicago Tribune,* Section 1, p. 3.

Individual susceptibility. (1981). *Lancet, 1,* 368.

Kan, Y. W., & Dozy, A. M. (1980). Evolution of the hemoglobin S and C genes in world populations. *Science, 209,* 388–391.

Kelada, S. N., Eaton, D. L., Wang, S. S., Rothman, N. R., & Khoury, M. J. (2003). The role of genetic polymorphisms in environmental health. *Environmental Health Perspectives, 111,* 1055–1064.

Lashley, F. R., & Durham, J. D. (Eds.). (2002). *Emerging infectious diseases: Trends and issues.* New York: Springer Publishing Co.

Limdi, J. K., & Crampton, J. R. (2004). Hereditary haemochromatosis. *Quarterly Journal of Medicine, 97,* 315–324.

Livingstone, F. B. (1971). Malaria and human polymorphisms. *Annual Review of Genetics, 5,* 33–64.

M'Charek, A., Rabinow, P., & Rodr, N. (Eds.). (2005). *The Human Genome Diversity Project: An ethnography of scientific practice.* Cambridge: Cambridge University Press.

McKeigue, P. M. (2005). Prospects for admixture mapping of complex traits. *American Journal of Human Genetics, 76,* 1–7.

Mead, S., Stumpf, M. P. H., Whitfield, J., Beck, J. A., Poulter, M., Campbell, T., et al. (2003). Balancing selection at the prion protein gene consistent with prehistoric kurulike epidemics. *Science, 300,* 640–643.

Merz, J. F., McGee, G. E., & Sankar, P. (2004). "Iceland Inc."?: On the ethics of commercial population genomics. *Social Science & Medicine, 58,* 1201–1209.

Meyerson, M. (2003). Human genetic variation and disease. *Lancet, 362,* 259–260.

Miller, L. H. (1994). Impact of malaria on genetic polymorphism and genetic diseases in Africans and African-Americans. *Proceedings of the National Academy of Sciences, USA, 91,* 2415–2419.

Mogil, J. S., Wilson, S. G., Chester, E. J., Rankin, A. L., Nemmani, K. V., Lariviere, W. R., et al. (2003). The melanocortin-1 receptor gene mediates female-specific mechanisms of analgesia in mice and humans. *Proceedings of the National Academy of Sciences, USA, 100,* 4867–4872.

Olaisen, B., Stenersen, M., & Mevåg, B. (1997). Identification by DNA analysis of the victims of the August 1996 Spitsbergen civil aircraft disaster. *Nature Genetics, 15,* 402–405.

Penchaszadeh, V. B. (1997). Genetic identification of the children of the disappeared in Argentina. *Journal of the American Medical Women's Association, 52,* 16–21, 27.

Pietrangelo, A. (2004). Hereditary hemochromatosis—a new look at an old disease. *New England Journal of Medicine, 350,* 2183–2197.

Salisbury, B. A., Pungliya, M., Choi, J. Y., Jiang, R., Sun, X. J., & Stephens, J. C. (2003). SNP and haplotype variation in the human genome. *Mutation Research, 526,* 53–61.

Schroeder, S. A., Gaughan, D. M., & Swift, M. (1995). Protection against bronchial asthma by *CFTR* ΔF508 mutation: A heterozygote advantage in cystic fibrosis. *Nature Medicine, 1,* 703–705.

Sheinfeld, J., Schaffer, A. J., Cordon-Cardo, C., Rogatko, A., & Fair, W. R. (1989). Association of the Lewis blood-group phenotype with recurrent urinary tract infections in women. *New England Journal of Medicine, 320,* 773–777.

Tse, C. S. T. (1982). Food products containing tartrazine. *New England Journal of Medicine, 306,* 681–682.

van Leeuwen, J. P. T. M., Uitterlinden, A. G., Birkenhäger, J. C., & Pols, H. A. P. (1996). Vitamin D receptor gene polymorphisms and osteoporosis. *Steroids, 61,* 154–156.

Vogel, F., & Motulsky, A. G. (1997). *Human genetics: Problems and approaches* (3rd ed.). Berlin, Germany: Springer-Verlag.

Weiss, K. M. (1995). *Genetic variation and human disease* (paper ed.). Cambridge, MA: Cambridge University Press.

4

Gene Action and Patterns of Inheritance

Genetic disorders generally fall into the following categories: (a) chromosomal abnormalities, (b) inherited biochemical disorders (most of which are single gene disorders), (c) multifactorial/polygenic disorders, and (d) environmental causes known as "teratogenic effects" when they affect the fetus. This is somewhat of an oversimplification. For example, small chromosomal deletions on one chromosome can result in the expression of a single or multiple gene disorder. The chromosome abnormalities and their transmission are considered in chapter 5. In addition to the chromosomal aberrations, patterns of transmission of inherited disorders include single gene disorders transmitted in Mendelian and non-Mendelian manners, multiple gene disorders, and multifactorial inheritance. Influences on gene expression and inheritance are discussed next. Further details about the inheritance of the common or complex disorders such as cancer are discussed in later chapters. Teratogenesis and mutations from environmental agents are discussed in chapters 13 and 14.

INFLUENCES ON GENE ACTION AND EXPRESSION

Because genes operate within an integrated body system, their expression can be affected by internal and external variables. The most important of these variables are discussed next.

Age of Onset

In the inherited biochemical disorders, the mutant gene itself is present from fertilization onward, but the appearance of its effects may not be seen immediately but can occur at different times in the lifespan (see chapter 1). Such appearance may be caused or influenced by any of the factors discussed in this section or by factors in the external environment. A correct diagnosis, which is important not only for treatment of the individual but also for genetic counseling, prenatal diagnosis, and life and reproductive planning for both the family and the affected person, is complicated by the fact that the same disorder may show different clinical pictures at different ages. Age of onset is also influenced by a phenomenon known as "anticipation," which is discussed below.

One of the most notorious diseases for late age of onset is Huntington disease. Less than 10% of affected individuals show any symptoms before age 30. By age 40, about 50% of those who will become affected have developed disease; by age 50, 75%; by age 60, 95%; and by age 70, almost 100%. It was not too long ago that there was no available method to distinguish individuals with the gene mutation from those without it. Individuals with a family history of Huntington disease in a parent used to have no way of knowing whether or not they had inherited the mutant gene until symptoms occurred. By the time it was known if a parent in fact had Huntington disease, their children may already have had their own children. This situation is often true as a prototype for other late-onset inherited disorders such as autosomal dominant polycystic kidney disease, which is discussed in more detail later in this chapter and in chapter 6.

Heterogeneity, Allelism, and Phenocopies

The same or similar phenotype may result from different mutant alleles at the same locus (i.e., glucose-6-phosphate dehydrogenase (G6PD) deficiency variants), mutant genes at different loci that affect the same product (i.e., Hb variants with mutations in different chains), or mutant alleles at different loci that affect different products (i.e., coagulation factor defects). For example, both a deficiency in factor VIII and one in factor IX produce coagulation defects and hemophilia, but biochemically and genetically they are different. Different types of mutation within a gene may lead to dysfunction and disease. For example, cystic fibrosis can result from deletions, point mutation, and splicing errors within the *CFTR* gene. Different mutant alleles can also result in gene mutation leading to the same genetic disorder but which may result in differences in severity and/or prognosis. Biochemical, genetic, molecular, and clinical analyses can all be used to demonstrate heterogeneity. Other examples of disorders that can arise from genes at different loci but with similar clinical appearances include albinism, hyperphenylalaninemia, methylmalonic acidemia (an inborn error of metabolism), and congenital blindness. Sometimes, such differences are not detected until appropriate matings, molecular analysis or cell complementation techniques demonstrate that two individuals do not have the same genetic disorder. If two persons with albinism with the same mutation at the same gene locus have children, all of them will also be albino, but if the mutations are in genes at different loci, then none of their children will be affected (except possibly by a rare mutation). In cell culture, fibroblasts (cells found in connective tissue) from two patients with the same apparent enzyme mutation can be fused. If the same abnormal phenotype (e.g., lack of enzyme activity) remains, the defect is presumed identical. If correction occurs, the defects are assumed to be different. This technique has been used to distinguish complementation groups in such disorders as xeroderma pigmentosum or Cockayne disease, which are (discussed in chapters 23 and 21 respectively).

Some genetic disorders may show the same apparent phenotype but different modes of inheritance. On close examination or detailed molecular analysis, they may actually be a similar group of disorders. Examples of this are Ehlers-Danlos syndrome (a group of connective tissue disorders), and Charcot-Marie-Tooth disease (a group of peripheral nervous system disorders) that can show autosomal dominant, autosomal recessive, or X-linked inheritance. It is important to determine the correct inheritance pattern within a given family in order to provide accurate genetic counseling.

Different mutant alleles at the same locus can cause different changes to occur in the resultant defective enzyme, causing differences in functioning (e.g., different degrees of stability and activity). This can result in different clinical pictures, although the same enzyme is affected, as in the mucopolysaccharide disorders, Hurler and Scheie syndromes. In each of these examples, the enzyme α-L-iduronidase is defective, but the clinical course of Scheie syndrome has a later onset and is different from and milder than Hurler. Thus some disorders caused in this way show different forms and degrees of severity at different points in the life cycle. Such disorders may show an acute, severe, progressive infantile form; a subacute juvenile form; and a milder chronic adult form. This may be because a less severe enzyme alteration may allow the person to function adequately for years unless he or she encounters a stressor such as infection, or even aging, or when a substance that has been accumulating finally reaches a toxic level. Notable examples of such disorders include Tay-Sachs disease, metachromatic leukodystrophy, fucosidosis, Niemann-Pick disease, citrullinemia, GM1 gangliosidosis, and Gaucher disease. Sometimes disorders resulting from environmental factors mimic those caused by single gene mutations. These are called "phenocopies." An example is prenatal use of the drug, thalidomide, in which the resulting limb defects closely resemble those of Robert syndrome or pseudothalidomide (SC) syndrome, which are inherited in an autosomal recessive manner.

Penetrance

In the case of a mutant gene, individuals either have it or they don't. "Penetrance" refers to the percentage of persons known to possess a certain mutant gene who actually show the trait. Incomplete or nonpenetrance occurs when a person is known to have a specific gene and shows no phenotypic manifestations of that gene. As an example, if in a specific family a person's parent and offspring both had tuberous sclerosis, the person would be assumed to have the gene even if he or she was clinically unaffected. Incomplete penetrance is a frequent finding in the autosomal dominant disorders. Estimates of penetrance have been calculated for certain autosomal dominant genes so that they can be used in calculating risks for genetic counseling. For example, the penetrance for otosclerosis is 40%, 80% for retinoblastoma, and nearly 100% for achondroplasia. One of the effects of incomplete penetrance is that the gene appears to skip a generation. This characteristic can be responsible for errors in genetic counseling if care is not exercised, although the use of molecular diagnostic techniques allows greater precision. The risk for a person to manifest a specific disorder is equal to the risk for inheriting the gene multiplied by the penetrance (see chapter 10).

Variable Expressivity

Variable expressivity occurs when an individual has the gene in question and is clinically affected, but the degree of severity of the manifestations of the mutant gene varies. As a simple example, in the case of polydactyly, the extra digit present may be full size or just a finger tag. Such variation may occur within a single family and may be caused by the influence of other factors on the major defective gene. It is most obvious in autosomal dominant disorders. Careful examination or testing is necessary before deciding that someone is free of the manifestations of a genetic disorder. The extent of severity of a disorder in one family member is not related to its severity in another. This means that if a parent is mildly affected with only minor manifestations of a disorder, his/her offspring could be severely, moderately, or mildly affected. The severity cannot be predicted reliably by the gene's expression in another family member.

Several years ago, the author counseled a 30-year-old man whose younger sister, who lived in another state, had been diagnosed at 8 years of age as having facioscapulohumeral muscular dystrophy and who was severely incapacitated. The man was not contemplating a family. This uncommon type of dystrophy is an autosomal dominant disorder with wide variation in expression within families, ranging from slight muscle weakness of one muscle group that develops later in life, to complete inability to walk by late adolescence. Although he showed no obvious clinical symptoms of muscle dysfunction on gross examination, the referral to a neurologist revealed a minimal weakness of the scapular muscles that was believed to represent a "forme fruste" or minimal manifestation of the disorder. Thus, at that time, he was considered to have the gene and his risk of transmitting it to his offspring, regardless of sex, was 50%. It could not be predicted to what degree his offspring would be affected. Counseling was continued on that basis.

New Mutation

If no other cases exist in a family and neither parent can be found to have any subclinical signs of the disorder, it may be caused by a new mutation. Such a case is often called "de novo" or "sporadic". The affected person with the new mutation can transmit the disorder to his or her offspring in the same manner as an affected individual with an affected parent. When truly unaffected parents have had a child with a genetic disease caused by a new mutation, the risk of having another child with the same disorder is no greater than that for the general population (except in rare cases of gonadal mosaicism explained below). New mutations are most frequently seen immediately in the dominantly inherited syndromes, because only one mutant gene is necessary to produce a phenotypic effect. When a recessive single gene disorder appears in a person and both parents are not heterozygous (meaning they are not carriers, see later discussion), this should prompt cytogenetic analysis of the affected individual, because a microdeletion that includes the normal gene may be present that allows expression of a single recessive mutant gene without the countering effect of the normal gene that is missing. The more incapacitating the disorder, the more likely for a large percentage to be due to new mutations because the person is less likely to reproduce. Disorders in which a high proportion of cases are caused by new mutations include Apert syndrome (an autosomal dominant disorder with craniostenosis, shallow ocular orbits, and syndactyly), and achondroplasia (a type of disproportionate dwarfism) (see chapter 8).

Genetic and Environmental Background

Genes never act in isolation. As Conneally (2003, p. 230), has said, "No gene is an island." They function against the background of other genes and the internal and external environment. A mutant gene may interact differently with different genetic constitutions or within different tissue types. This helps to explain the varying degree of clinical severity seen in individuals with the same genetic disorder. The sex constitution of the individual is one part of the genetic background that regulates the internal environment through hormonal and other changes, and can influence the expression of genes in varying degrees. An example of modifying genes is the milder disease seen in persons homozygous for the sickle cell gene who also have hereditary persistence of fetal hemoglobin. Thus, although mutation in one gene may be the major determinant, mutations at one or more other loci may be necessary for either pathogenesis or influencing severity. In rare instances, diseases thought to be typical Mendelian recessive disorders may be complex in some families. In some families with Bardet-Biedl syndrome (obesity, polydactyly, renal malformations, developmental delay, pigmentary retinal dystrophy) six loci are involved, and it appears that it is necessary to have three mutations at two loci to see the phenotypic effects but in other families it appears inherited as a simple Mendelian recessive disorder.

A simple example of environmental influence is seen in classical phenylketonuria (PKU). The individual can have the mutant genes, but if dietary phenylalanine is restricted, the individual may not show obvious clinical manifestations such as severe mental retardation. He or she still has the gene mutations, but the environment has been manipulated so that substrate is limited and toxic products do not build up. Other environmental influences may include maternal nutrition, infection, noise, drugs, pressure, radiation, temperature, and amniotic fluid characteristics. Further, the way in which all proteins function together in cells, tissues, and organs and differential gene expression also influences ultimate functioning.

Epistasis

One way in which the genetic background can affect gene action is illustrated by epistasis, which is the masking of the effect of one set of genes by a different set at another locus. As an example, if an individual is homozygous for genes for albinism, then any alleles at another locus for brown hair would not be expressed and the person would have white hair. Thus, one can say that the albinism genes are epistatic to the genes for hair pigment.

X Chromosome Inactivation (The Lyon Hypothesis or Principle)

Because there are many genes known to be on the X chromosome, and because females have two Xs whereas males have only one X, visible differences due to inequality in gene dosage would be expected. Normal females and males were shown to have equivalent amounts of enzymes coded by X-linked genes, such as G6PD, hypoxanthine-guanine-phosphoribosyl transferase (HPRT) (deficiency resulting in Lesch-Nyhan syndrome), clotting factor VIII (deficiency resulting in hemophilia A) (see chapter 6), and others. Mary Lyon, in 1961, hypothesized that in female somatic cells, only one X is active, thus "compensating" for any male and female gene dosage difference. Although there are some deviations from it, the basic tenets of the now well-accepted Lyon hypothesis were as follows: (1) in any female somatic cell, only one of the two Xs is active. In karyotypes with several Xs, all but one X is inactivated. (2) X chromosome inactivation occurs early in embryonic development, probably at the early blastocyst stage. (3) The inactive X (or Xs) can be seen in interphase nuclei as sex chromatin, heterochromatin, or the Barr body (see chapter 5). (4) In any given cell it is generally random whether it is the maternal or paternal X chromosome that is inactivated. (5) Once it occurs, all descendants of the original cell will have the same X chromosome inactivated. (6) Inactivation is irreversible (except perhaps in the oocyte).

A common, easily visible example of this principle is seen in calico cats. These females have a gene for black color on one X and one for yellow color on the other. X inactivation results in random patches of black and yellow fur, for a mottled appearance. Male calico cats are of an XXY constitution. The inactivation of one of the X chromosomes in the female essentially leads to a mosaic condition or two cell populations in females who are heterozygous for X-linked recessive disorders.

Because X-inactivation is generally a random occurrence, in the population at large there is a 50:50 chance as to whether the maternal or paternal

X is inactivated. But any given individual may have ratios that deviate. Occasionally the percentage of cells that have the X with the normal gene turned off is very high. This leads to a skewed population in which the preponderance of cells having the X bearing the mutant gene is the active one. This explains why hemophilia can clinically manifest itself in a female known to be a heterozygous carrier, although this can also result from chromosomal microdeletions of the normal gene. It also explains why traditional methods of carrier detection are difficult for X-linked recessive disorders, as the possible range for enzyme activity values can vary greatly, depending on the genetic constitution of the X chromosome inactivated. Some genes appear to escape inactivation, being expressed in both active and inactive X chromosomes. There are genes that control X inactivation. There is an X inactivation center believed to be responsible for initiation of inactivation. The gene, *XIST* (X-inactivation-specific transcript), apparently controls it. *XIST* RNA apparently silences the X chromosome, which is expressed from the inactive X. There have been suggestions that other factors may be involved in interaction with *XIST* RNA to initiate transcriptional silencing, perhaps involving histone or chromatin modifications. In cases where there is an unbalanced nonreciprocal X-autosome translocation, the abnormal X is usually inactivated, and this inactivation may "spread" to part of the autosome. When a gene on the X chromosome is needed for cell survival, the normal allele will be on the active X chromosome, and the defective allele on the inactive X. Nonrandom or skewed X inactivation can also result from (1) chance, (2) imprinting (discussed later), (3) monozygotic twinning with unequal distribution of the X with the mutant gene, (4) cytogenetic abnormalities, (5) gene expression, (6) clonal selection in which there is nonrandom inactivation of the X chromosome with the mutant allele, (7) preferential selection that is either positive or negative for the X chromosome with the abnormal gene, and (8) a specific gene mutation affecting X inactivation. Methylation (discussed in chapter 2) maintains the X inactivation. Because a female may express an X-linked recessive disorder because of a chromosomal abnormality, such as a deletion, an X-autosome translocation, or an isochromosome, such females should have chromosome analysis done.

Sex-Limited Traits

Autosomal genes that are normally expressed phenotypically in either males or females but not in both are sex limited. The sex that does not express the gene may still possess and transmit it. Examples of such traits are milk production and menstruation in females.

Sex-Influenced Traits

Sex-influenced genes act differently in males and females and are often frequent in one sex and rare in the other. Pattern baldness is an autosomal dominant trait in males, requiring only one copy of the gene. In females it appears to be recessive and expressed only when two copies are present, probably due to hormonal influences such as androgen levels. Rare homozygous females can thus manifest the trait. Sometimes it is not expressed until menopause.

Parental-Age Effect

The frequency of some gene mutations in offspring rises with parental age, especially that of the father, whereas some chromosome abnormalities are associated with advanced maternal age (discussed in chapter 5). The data are clearest for autosomal dominant mutations because they only need one mutant allele for effects to be manifested, whereas recessive mutations need two and may, therefore, be unseen for several generations, whereas dominants can be shown in the next generation. Mutation is an ongoing event in the human gene pool, but many cause little noticeable effect individually, especially in recessive conditions. In the normal course of events, older individuals would have more exposure to mutagenic agents such as environmental radiation and chemical exposure than would younger individuals. In older males, the continuous production of sperm may result in errors in DNA replication or an inability to repair DNA damage. In some X-linked recessive disorders, the advanced age of the maternal grandfather was found to be significant when compared with controls. Those disorders that have an advanced paternal age association are shown in Table 4.1. The current population mean paternal age is about 27 years. The risk for sporadic autosomal domi-

TABLE 4.1   Genetic Disorders Associated with Increased Paternal Age

Disorder	Description of major features	Inheritance mechanism
Achondroplasia	Short-limbed type of dwarfism with large head (see chapter 8)	AD
Acrodysostosis	Mental retardation, short limbs with deformities, especially in arms and hands; growth deficiency; small head, nose, and maxilla	AD
Apert syndrome	Craniofacial deformities such as craniostenosis; skeletal deformities, especially "sock" feet and syndactyly	AD
Basal cell nevus syndrome	Nevi that become malignant, rib and spine anomalies, variable degrees of mental retardation, eye abnormalities	AD
Crouzon craniofacial dysostosis	Hypoplasia and abnormalities of skull and face; craniosynostosis; premature suture closure, shallow eye orbits	AD
Marfan syndrome	Elongated thin extremities; cardiovascular complications, especially of aorta; ocular anomalies, especially of lens	AD
Oculodentodigital dysplasia	Digital anomalies such as incurved 5th finger (camptodactyly) or syndactyly; tooth enamel hypoplasia, other dental abnormalities; microphthalmos, glaucoma possible	AD
Treacher Collins syndrome (mandibulofacial dysostosis)	Malar and mandibular hypoplasia; conductive deafness; ear malformations; lower eyelid defects; limb abnormalities. Caused by mutations in *TCO1* gene	AD
Waardenburg syndrome 1	Bilateral perception deafness; pigment disturbances of hair and eyes (e.g., white lock of hair and uniform light-colored irises or heterochromic irises), lateral displacement of inner canthus of eye; may have other anomalies	AD
Progeria	Thin skin, alopecia, growth deficiency, atherosclerosis, appearance of premature aging (see chapter 21)	AD AR(?)
Duchenne muscular dystrophy	Progressive degenerative muscle disease with weakness (see chapter 6)	XR
Hemophilia A	Coagulation disorder with deficiency of factor VIII (see chapter 6)	XR

Note: AD = autosomal dominant; AR = autosomal recessive; XR = X-linked recessive.

nant single gene mutations is 4 to 5 times greater for fathers aged 45 years and older than for fathers 20 to 25 years old. Most sperm banks will not accept the sperm of older men for artificial insemination and other assisted reproductive techniques for this reason. The American Society for Reproductive Medicine (2004b) gives detailed guidelines for sperm donation including that "the donor should be of legal age but younger than 40 years of age (p. S10). The recommended age for oocyte donors by this group is between 21 and 34 years of age (American Society for Reproductive Medicine, 2004a). Under various statistical conditions, with adjusted maternal age, there was an effect of increased paternal age in relation to risk of Down syndrome (Kazaura & Lie, 2002). A study by McIntosh, Olshan, and Baird (1995) noted that men

below 20 years of age were at increased risk for fathering children with some birth defects such as hypospadias and Down syndrome, and Abel, Kruger, & Burd (2002) found that they also had an increased risk of fathering low birth weight and preterm infants. Nurses can encourage male clients to complete their families after age 20 and before 40–45 years of age, and to avoid unnecessary radiation and drug exposure. Males should avoid conception for a few months after exposure to radiation, cytotoxic drugs, or chemical mutagens. Women are at increased risk for adverse pregnancy outcomes below age 15 years as well as over 35 years of age. In the younger age groups, this may be because of nutritional competition between a fetus and their own growth or for some other reason.

Linkage and Synteny

Genes that are located on different chromosomes are said to assort independently and are unlinked. Genes that are located close together (50 map units or less) on the same chromosome are linked; and those that are on the same chromosome but are more than 50 map units apart are syntenic. The closer together that two pairs of genes are, the more likely it is that the two alleles that are together on the same chromosome will remain together when gametes are formed without any exchange or recombination between them. This information can be used to study families who have a genetic disorder for which there is no means of detection, and who also have a detectable trait linked to the mutant gene in question. For example, the ABO blood group locus is linked to that for the nail-patella syndrome; the myotonic dystrophy locus is linked to the blood group secretor locus; and hemophilia is linked to the deutan locus for color blindness. For information to be applicable clinically, families must be large enough for accurate study and possess different allele combinations at the linked loci that allow for accurate genetic study and analysis. Linkage analysis today is often accomplished using various computer programs (see chapter 2). Haplotype refers to several linked genes on a segment of chromosome, and is frequently used in relation to HLA (see chapter 19). The phenomenon of linkage disequilibrium occurs when two or more of alleles occur together in a haplotype significantly more frequently than would be expected by chance alone.

Consanguinity

Concern about consanguinity relates mostly to marriage between blood relatives. Although most individuals would be distantly related to their mate, if one went back far enough in time, only relationships closer than first cousins are usually genetically important. Each individual carries from five to seven harmful recessive genes that are not usually apparent. Individually, each of these is extremely rare (except for a few, like cystic fibrosis), so that the likelihood of selecting a mate with the same harmful recessive genes is remote. This chance becomes less remote if the two individuals are related to each other by blood or are from the

same ethnic group or population isolate. The consequence of consanguineous mating results from the possible bringing together of two identical recessive alleles that are inherited by descent from a common ancestor, thus bringing out deleterious genes in the homozygous (aa) state. The resulting homozygous phenotypes that are deleterious are more obvious than those that are neutral or favorable. This effect may also operate for single nucleotide polymorphisms (SNPs) or variations in genes. Effects that determine one trait are more evident than those contributing to a complex trait, such as body size or intelligence. Many cultures and groups have actively encouraged consanguineous marriages. These have included the ancient Egyptians, Incas, royalty, and many modern societies, such as Japan, various Hindu groups in India, Muslim groups especially in the Eastern Mediterranean, and groups in which arranged marriages are an accepted custom. The frequency of consanguineous marriages depends on social custom, religious customs and laws, socioeconomic concerns, family ties and traditions, the degree of geographic isolation of a village, and the degree of isolation of a specific group within a community. It is estimated that in parts of Asia and Africa, consanguineous marriages account for about 20 to 50% of all marriages. Other groups oppose it. In South Korea, it is frowned upon to marry someone with the same family name and same-clan marriages are barred. Every 10 years or so there is an amnesty period during which such marriages can occur. Among certain followers of the Koran, there are taboos against marriage between a boy and a girl who were breast-fed by the same woman more than a certain number of times during the first 2 years of life. Thus consanguinity may be perceived differently among different cultures.

In one study by Bennett, Hudgins, Smith, and Motulsky (1999), about genetic counseling in consanguineous couples, great variation in quoted risk figures for mental retardation and birth defects was found among counseling providers. The author has had several genetic counseling clients who were contemplating cousin marriages. Myths abound about such matings, particularly those between first cousins. One client reported that he had been told by a health professional that all of their children would be crazy or retarded. In actuality, the risks are associated with the chance of bringing together the same recessive gene possessed by each one of them in their offspring, as previously discussed. If no known genetic disease exists in the family, and the persons do not belong to an ethnic group with a genetic disease that is above the usual population frequency, then the risk for homozygosity at a gene locus is 1/16 for first cousins. In the absence of a positive family history and under good economic conditions, empiric risk estimates for a genetic disease, malformation, or early mortality among the offspring of first cousin marriages are about 3–4% over the general population risk. For first cousins once removed and second cousins, the observed risk is about 1 1.5% over that of the general population. An uncle-niece mating would carry about a 10% risk. Individuals may be related to one another in more than one way. A formula is available that calculates the probability of homozygosity at a given locus, or the coefficient of inbreeding.

Confusion about exact familial relationships is common to many people. Accurate risk estimates cannot be made unless the correct relationship is known, and so it may be up to the nurse to clarify it. For example, first cousins once removed refers to the relationship between the grandchild of one sibling and the child of another sibling, whereas second cousins refers to the relationship between the grandchildren of two siblings. These relationships are illustrated in Figure 4.1.

Incest in the legal sense refers to matings between related individuals who cannot be legally married, whereas in the genetic sense it refers to matings between persons more closely related by blood than double first cousins (those who have both sets of grandparents in common). All states prohibit parent–child, grandparent–grandchild and brother–sister marriages, and the vast majority prohibit uncle–niece and aunt–nephew marriages. The most frequent form of genetic incest is father–daughter followed by brother–sister. Nurses encountering female adolescents who are victims of incest may notice a loss of self-esteem and an attitude of aggression or hostility toward the mother, who is perceived as allowing the relationship. Family counseling is imperative.

The degree of genetic risk for an infant born of an incestuous mating between first-degree relatives is an important concern to adoption agencies and prospective adoptive parents. Data indicate that the risk is approximately one-third for serious abnormality or early death, with an added risk of mental retardation. Most abnormalities become evident within the first year of life, and a reasonable suggestion is that the finalization of adoption wait until this time.

A marriage between blood relatives that takes place in a state in which it is legal is still legal if the couple then moves to a state in which it would be illegal to marry. Legal restrictions on marriages are based not only on genetic-related concerns, but also on legal, social, and moral concerns. Thus in some states a man may not, for example, marry his stepmother, although they are not blood relatives.

Anticipation

Anticipation is said to occur when the severity of a genetic disease increases with each generation, and/or the age at which the disorder manifests itself becomes earlier and earlier with each vertical generation. Anticipation is generally seen in autosomal dominant disorders. This phenomenon was observed in Huntington disease, and eventually the reason was found to be unstable triplet repeat expansion of the nucleotides cytosine, adenosine, and guanine (CAG). The expanding repeats accounted for the anticipation phenomenon, which is described in detail later in this chapter.

Parent-of-Origin Effect

In some cases, a parent-of-origin effect has been described. For example, a disorder might appear more severe, or show different expression, if inherited through either the maternal or paternal line. Many parent-of-origin effects are now known to be due to uniparental disomy, imprinting, and/or unstable nucleotide expansion, discussed later.

Gonadal or Germline Mosaicism

Gonadal or germline mosaicism occurs when one parent has a mutant allele that results from mutation in the gonads, which occurs after fertilization, resulting in mosaicism. Clinical manifestations in that parent may not be seen because it may occur in the cells of the developing gonad in either the male and female, and be present in few, if any, somatic cells. Gonadal mosaicism is most clinically

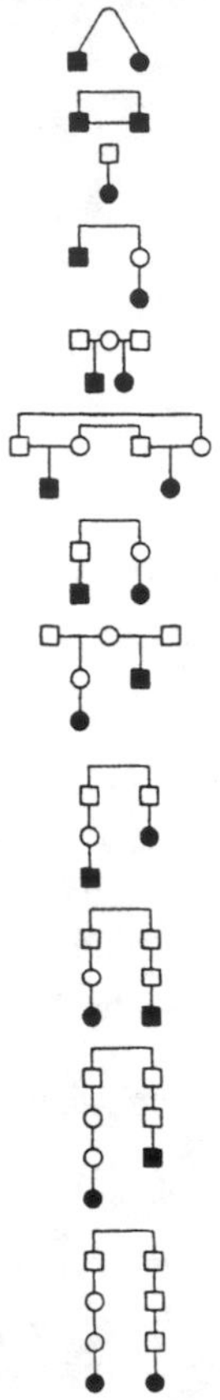

Relationship (between shaded individuals		Degree of Relationship	Proportion of Genes Shared	Chance of Homozygosity by Descent
	Dizygotic twins	First	1/2	1/4
	Sibs	First	1/2	1/4
	Parent-child	First	1/2	1/4
	Uncle-niece (aunt-nephew)	Second	1/4	1/8
	Half sibs	Second	1/4	1/8
	Double first cousins		1/4	1/8
	First cousins	Third	1/8	1/16
	Half-uncle-niece (or similar)	Third	1/8	1/16
	First cousins once removed	Fourth	1/16	1/32
	Second cousins	Fifth	1/32	1/64
	Second cousins once removed		1/64	1/128
	Third cousins		1/128	1/256

■ = male; ● = female.

FIGURE 4.1   Patterns of relationships.
Source: Harper, P. S. *Practical genetical counseling* (4th ed.). Oxford, England: Butterworth Heinemann, 1993. Reproduced with permission of Edward Arnold.

evident in both autosomal dominant and X-linked inheritance. One example is the case in which a clinically normal father had two children with osteogenesis imperfecta by two different women. The children both had the same point mutation in type I collagen, and it could be detected in their hair root bulbs, lymphocytes, and sperm. It has also occurred in the apparent sporadic occurrence of a male with Duchenne muscular dystrophy where the apparent noncarrier mother may have had gonadal mosaicism. Ostrer (1998) estimates that the aggregate risk that a mother who is thought to be a noncarrier of Duchenne muscular dystrophy may run of having a second affected child is 14%. Gonadal mosaicism is important because if it is present, there is a risk of a second affected child following the birth of a first with an apparent new mutation. Thus genetic counseling and evaluation for apparent new or sporadic mutation should take the possibility of gonadal mosaicism into account. In one instance FISH analysis (see chapter 5) of sperm in a couple with a history of three spontaneous abortions revealed paternal gonadal mosaicism although peripheral blood cytogenetic studies were normal (Somprasit et al., 2004).

TRADITIONAL OR MENDELIAN PATTERNS OF INHERITANCE IN SINGLE GENE DISORDERS

Most of the inherited biochemical disorders are determined by a single nuclear gene mutation that follows the inheritance patterns of autosomal recessive, autosomal dominant, X-linked recessive, and X-linked dominant. Few conditions are known to be Y-linked. These are typically referred to as Mendelian disorders. It has been relatively recently that it has been discovered that mutations in genes located in the mitochondria of the cell cause certain genetic diseases, as discussed later. A trait is considered dominant if it is expressed (phenotypically apparent) when one dose or copy of the gene is present. A trait is considered recessive when it is normally expressed only when two copies or doses of the gene are present. Dominance and recessiveness refer to phenotypes expressed by alleles, not to the gene locus. For example, in osteogenesis imperfecta, different mutations in the same gene can have dominant or recessive effects. Codominance occurs when each one of the two alleles at a locus is expressed when both are present, as in the case of the AB blood group antigens. Those genes located on the X chromosome (X-linked) are present in only one copy in the male because males have only one X chromosome, and therefore are expressed whether dominant or recessive. Very few genes are known to be on the Y chromosome, but they are present only in males. A person who has two mutant alleles at the same locus is sometimes referred to as a compound heterozygote.

An international committee has established formal ways of referring to genes and gene loci, as shown in chapter 6. However, to more simply explain and illustrate patterns of transmission, capital letters will represent dominant genes and small letters will represent recessive genes. The same letter is used to describe genes at the same locus on the chromosome. Thus, a person who is heterozygous for one gene pair is represented Aa, whereas homozygotes for two dominant alleles and for two recessive alleles are AA and aa, respectively. The homozygous normal person (AA) and the heterozygous person (Aa) are usually distinguishable only biochemically, not clinically. Different letters are used for genes at different loci. If two gene pairs are being discussed and the person is heterozygous

at both, he or she could be represented as AaBb. Many gene loci are known to have more than two alternate forms of genes (alleles) that can be present at each site (although each chromosome can normally only have one allele present at a time). These multiple alleles can cause different forms of a gene product to be produced. When a particular gene pair or disorder is being discussed, or its pattern of inheritance are diagrammed, only one pair is represented and normality is assumed for the rest of the genome, unless otherwise stated.

Each major type of inheritance pattern, its characteristics, and examples are discussed below. The reader is also referred to the section on pedigrees in chapter 9 for a discussion on how pedigree analysis and interpretation help to determine patterns of transmission within a family for use in genetic counseling. The traditional knowledge regarding transmission of genetic disorders is still basically correct; however new knowledge and exceptions that are relatively rare have been identified. These include uniparental disomy, imprinting, unstable or expanding triplet repeat mutations, mitochondrial inheritance, gonadal mosaicism, and others. Discussion of the traditional mechanisms will not mention each exception but they will be considered separately in this chapter.

Autosomal Recessive

In autosomal recessive (AR) inheritance, the mutant gene is located on an autosome rather than on a sex chromosome. Therefore, males and females are affected in equal proportions. The affected person usually inherits one copy of the same mutant gene from each heterozygous (Aa), or carrier, parent, and is thus homozygous (aa) at that locus, having two copies of the mutant gene. Parents who have had a child with an AR disease are sometimes referred to as "obligate heterozygotes" meaning that each must have one copy of the mutant gene, even if no test for detection exists. Occasionally, a rare recessive disorder is manifested in a person when only one parent is a carrier. This can result in one of two ways, either because of a small deletion of the chromosome segment involving the normal gene, thus allowing expression of the mutant gene, or because the person inherits two copies of the same chromosome from the parent with the mutant gene (uniparental disomy). These disorders are discussed further later in this chapter. Because normal gene function is dominant to the altered function of the mutant recessive gene, the heterozygote usually shows no obvious phenotypic manifestations but, depending on the disorder, may show biochemical differences that form the basis for heterozygote detection using blood, hair bulbs, or skin fibroblasts (see chapter 11), although DNA testing is now commonly used where possible. Enzyme defects and deficiencies are frequent.

In practice, most situations involving AR inheritance come to attention in a variety of ways, (1) recent birth of an affected child, (2) couples who have been identified as carriers of a specific disorder (e.g., Tay-Sachs disease) and are contemplating marriage or children, (3) one member of a couple has a sibling or cousin known to have a genetic disorder and are concerned that they may be carriers, (4) their child has recently been diagnosed as having an inherited biochemical disorder, (5) both members of a couple belong to a population group in which a specific genetic disorder is frequent (e.g., thalassemia in Mediterranean people), (6) a couple is contemplating pregnancy after an earlier birth of an affected child who may be either living or deceased. Therefore, such individuals may have different immediate and long-range needs, ranging from genetic testing and carrier detection to genetic counseling to prenatal diagnosis, and the nurse should refer such individuals to a geneticist. If a couple has had a child with an AR disorder, the family history for the genetic disease may be completely negative, due in part to the trend to smaller family size and in part because two copies of a rare gene are needed in order to be affected. If there are other affected individuals, they are usually members of the same generation. If the parents of the affected child are related to each other by blood, this suggests AR inheritance but it does not prove it. The more common the disorder is in the general population, the less relevant is the presence of consanguinity.

The mechanics of transmission of autosomal recessively inherited genes are shown in Figure 4.2. The most common situation is when both parents are heterozygotes (carriers). The theoretical risks for their offspring, regardless of sex, are to be (1) affected with the disorder (aa), 25%; (2) carriers like their parents (Aa), 50%; and (3) normal, without inheriting the mutant gene (AA), 25%. Of the phenotypically normal offspring (AA and Aa), two thirds will be carriers. These risks hold true for each pregnancy. Because "chance has no memory," each pregnancy is, in essence, a throw of the genetic dice, so that the outcome of the past pregnancy has no effect on a future one. This is a point that clients often need clarified and reinforced. Nurses should therefore be able to understand it and explain it. If two carriers have had three unaffected children in three sequential pregnancies, it does not mean that their next child will be affected; it has no bearing on the outcome of the next pregnancy.

These theoretical risks hold true with large numbers of families. Within an individual family at risk with two carrier parents, the actual number of affected children can, by chance, range from none that are affected to all that are affected. This does not change their risks for another pregnancy from those described previously. In general, most AR disorders tend to have an earlier, more severe, onset than do diseases with other inheritance modes. Many are so severe that they are incompatible with a normal lifespan, and many affected individuals do not reach reproductive age. Due to recent advances in diagnosis and treatment in certain AR diseases, such as sickle cell anemia and cystic fibrosis, individuals who formerly died in childhood now are reaching young adulthood and having their own children, creating obligatory transmission of the mutant gene to all of their offspring. If the affected person mates with someone who does not carry the same mutant gene, then all of their children, regardless of sex, will be carriers but none will be affected (see Figure 4.2). If the affected person mates with someone who is a carrier for the same recessive gene, then there is a 50% risk for having an affected child and a 50% risk for having a child who is a heterozygous carrier, regardless of sex for each pregnancy. This risk is most likely to materialize for a disorder such as cystic fibrosis where the frequency of carriers in the White population is about 5%, or for sickle cell disease where the frequency of carriers in the American Black population is 7% to 9%. If the mother is the one who has the genetic disease in question, there may be effects on the fetus that result from an altered maternal environment, as in PKU (see chapter 13). The salient characteristics of autosomal recessive inheritance are summarized in Table 4.2. Examples

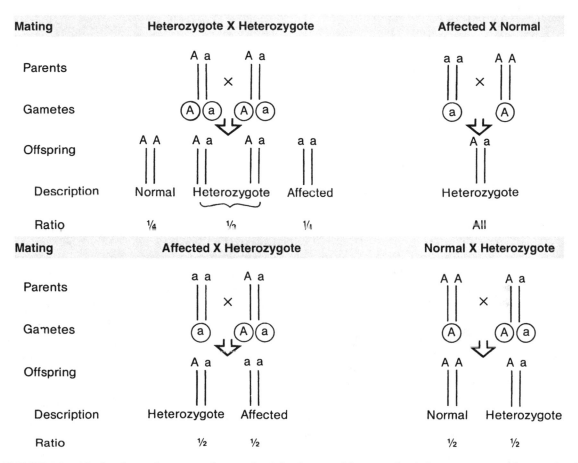

FIGURE 4.2   Mechanisms of autosomal recessive inheritance with one pair of chromosomes and one pair of genes. *AA* = normal, *Aa* = heterozygous carrier, *aa* = affected individual.

of different genetic disorders inherited in this manner are given in Table 4.3, and many of these disorders are explained in greater detail in chapter 6.

Autosomal Dominant

As in AR inheritance, the mutant gene is on an autosome, so males and females are equally affected. Only one copy of the dominant gene is necessary for the detrimental effects to be evident; the affected individual is heterozygous, and there is no carrier status. It is believed that most homozygous individuals who have inherited two genes for an autosomal dominant disorder are so severely affected that they die in utero or in infancy. An example of an exception is familial hypercholesterolemia where the homozygote survives but shows the very early onset of severe effects. In con-

trast to AR inheritance, structural protein defects are common rather than those involving enzymes. Autosomal dominant (AD) disorders are usually less life-threatening than AR ones, although they may involve more evident physical malformations. A later age of onset of symptoms and signs is frequent and may not become evident until adulthood. In practice, persons usually seek counseling because 1) they or their mate are affected with a particular AD disorder; 2) someone in their family (often a parent, aunt or uncle, or sibling) has an AD disorder; or 3) they have had a previous child with an AD disorder.

The recognition of an autosomal dominant disorder in a child may indicate the presence of that disorder in one of the parents as well. However, there are exceptions to this. When the parents appear normal, several possibilities exist including: (1) the

TABLE 4.2   Major Characteristics of Autosomal Recessive Inheritance and Disorders

- Gene is located on autosome.
- Two copies of the mutant gene are needed for phenotypic manifestations.
- Males and females are affected in equal numbers on average.
- No sex difference in clinical manifestations is usual.
- Family history is usually negative, especially for vertical transmission (in more than one generation).
- Other affected individuals in family in same generation (horizontal transmission) may be seen.
- Consanguinity or relatedness is more often present than in other types of inherited conditions.
- Fresh gene mutation is rare.
- Age of disease onset is usually early—newborn, infancy, early childhood.
- Greatest negative effect on reproductive fitness.

gene can be present but nonpenetrant, (2) the gene expression may be minimal and not have been detected by the practitioner, (3) the disorder can be caused by a new mutation, or (4) the child is not the natural offspring of both parents. Careful examination of both parents is extremely important. In one case of a child brought for counseling with full-blown Waardenburg syndrome type 1 (deafness, heterochromic irises, partial albinism, and broad facial appearance [before subgrouping of this syndrome was known]), no evidence was at first seen in either parent. If the disorder was actually caused by a new mutation, then the risk for those parents to have this syndrome appear in another child would be negligible. If, however, one of the parents actually had the syndrome, then the risk for recurrence in another child would be 50%. It turned out that the only manifestation that the mildly affected mother had was a white forelock of hair, which she usually dyed. This is an example of variable expression in which the parent was only mildly affected but the child had severe manifestations. Such cases represent a challenge to the practitioner. In this case, the counselor, knowing the full constellation of the syndrome, specifically asked her if anyone in the family had premature white hair. If not directly asked, such information may not have been volunteered, because (1) the relevance of it was not recognized by the client, (2) there may be guilt feelings when only one parent transmits a disorder, (3) there may be fear of stigmatization or being blamed for transmission of the disorder, or (4) of other reasons.

The mechanisms of transmission of autosomal dominant traits are shown in Figure 4.3. In matings in which one partner is affected and one is normal, the risk for their child to inherit the gene, and therefore the disorder too (except in disorders with less than 100% penetrance), is 50%, regardless of sex. The chance for a normal child is also 50%. This holds true for each pregnancy, regardless of the outcomes of prior pregnancies. Unless nonpenetrance has occurred, those truly unaffected individuals run no greater risk than the general population of having an affected child or grandchild of their own. Risk calculations that include the possibility of nonpenetrance can be made by the geneticist. If a woman were an affected heterozygote for a rare AD disorder with 60% penetrance, and she was planning a family with a normal man, the risk for each child to both inherit the mutant gene and to manifest the disorder is as follows: the risk to inherit the mutant gene from each parent (50% from the mother and the population mutation rate from the father, which in this case is disregarded because of rarity), multiplied by the penetrance (60%) or (.5 x .6 = .3). Therefore, the risk for the child to inherit the gene is 50% and to both inherit the gene and manifest the disorder is 30%.

If two individuals affected with the same AD disorder have children, as is frequently seen in achondroplasia, then for each pregnancy the chance is 25% for having a child who is an affected homozygote; 50% for having an affected heterozygote like the parents; and 25% for having a normal child without a mutant gene (see Figure 4.3). The homozygote is usually so severely affected that the condition is lethal in utero.

In many autosomal dominant disorders the primary defect is still unknown, so that diagnosis of

TABLE 4.3   Selected Genetic Disorders Showing Autosomal Recessive Inheritance

Disorder	Occurrence	Brief description
Albinism (tyrosinase negative)	1:15,000–1:40,000 1:85–1:650 (Native Americans)	Melanin lacking in skin, hair, and eyes; nystagmus; photophobia; susceptible to neoplasia; strabismus, impaired vision
Argininosuccinic aciduria (ASA)	1:60,000–1:70,000	Urea cycle disorder; hyperammonemia, mild mental retardation, vomiting, seizures, coma, abnormal hair shaft
Cystic fibrosis	1:2,000–1:2,500 (Caucasians) 1:16,000 (American Blacks)	Pancreatic insufficiency and malabsorption; abnormal exocrine glands; chronic pulmonary disease (see chapter 8)
Ellis-van Creveld syndrome	Rare, except among eastern Pennsylvania Amish	Short limbed dwarfism, polydactyly, congenital heart disease, nail anomalies.
Glycogen storage disease Ia (von Gierke disease)	1:200,000	Glucose-6-phosphatase deficiency, bruising, hypoglycemia, enlarged liver, hyperlipidemia, hypertension, short stature
Glycogen storage disease II (Pompe disease)	3:100,000–4.5:100,000	Infant, juvenile, and adult forms; acid maltase deficiency. In infant form, cardiac enlargement, cardiomyopathy, hypotonia, respiratory insufficiency, developmental delay, macroglossia, death from cardiorespiratory failure by about 2 years of age.
Hemochromatosis	1:3,000 (Whites)	Iron storage and tissue damage can result in cirrhosis, diabetes, pancreatitis, and other diseases. Skin pigmentation seen (see chapter 3)
Homocystinuria	1:40,000–1:140,000	Mental retardation, skeletal defects, lens displacement, tall, risk for myocardial infarction. Caused by cystathionine β-synthase deficiency
Metachromatic leukodystrophy	1:40,000	Arylsulfatase A deficiency leading to disintegration of myelin and accumulation of lipids in white matter of brain; psychomotor degeneration, hypotonia. There are adult, juvenile, and infantile forms.
Sickle cell anemia	1:400–1:600 (American Blacks)	Hemoglobinopathy with chronic hemolytic anemia, growth retardation, susceptibility to infection, painful crises, leg ulcers, dactylitis (see chapter 5)
Tay-Sachs disease	1:3,600 (Ashkenazi Jews) 1:360,000 others	Progressive mental and motor retardation with onset at about 6 months, poor muscle tone, deafness, blindness, convulsions, decerebrate rigidity, and death usual by 3 to 5 years of age (see chapters 6 and 11)
Usher syndromes	Rare	A group of syndromes characterized by congenital sensorineural deafness, visual loss due to retinitis pigmentosa, vestibular ataxia, occasionally mental retardation, speech problems. There are several subtypes.
Xeroderma pigmentosa (Complementation groups A-G)	1:60,000–1:100,000	Defective DNA repair; sun sensitivity, freckling, atrophic skin lesions, skin cancer develops; photophobia and keratitis; death usually by adulthood. Some types have CNS involvement (see chapter 23).

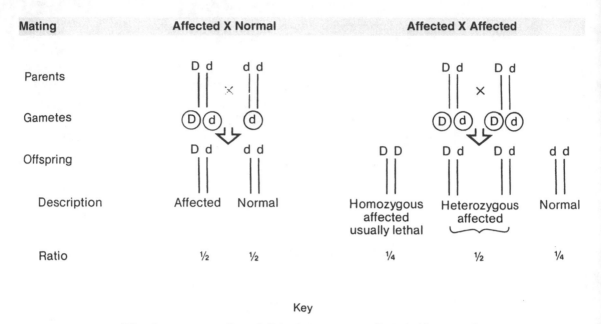

Mating	Affected X Normal		Affected X Affected		
Parents	D d × d d		D d × D d		
Gametes	Ⓓ ⓓ ⓓ		Ⓓ ⓓ Ⓓ ⓓ		
Offspring	D d	d d	D D	D d D d	d d
Description	Affected	Normal	Homozygous affected usually lethal	Heterozygous affected	Normal
Ratio	½	½	¼	½	¼

Key

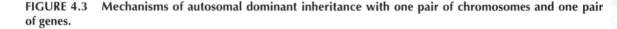

DD = homozygous affected, *Dd* = heterozygous affected, *dd* = normal.

FIGURE 4.3   Mechanisms of autosomal dominant inheritance with one pair of chromosomes and one pair of genes.

the individual who is known to be at risk for having the disorder before symptoms become clinically evident or prenatal diagnosis for their offspring may not be possible, although gene mapping and DNA technology are making this situation less common. In those disorders where the onset is characteristically late and diagnosis is not available, individuals with a family history of such a disorder have difficulty in making reproductive and life plans because they may not know whether or not they have inherited the mutant gene. Where possible, many choose alternate reproductive options such as artificial insemination, in vitro fertilization, embryo implantation, or adoption rather than run a possible 50:50 risk; but others only become aware of the hereditary nature of the disease after they have had children or choose to "take a chance." Nurses should encourage each individual to talk with their partners about available options and, if possible, both should also talk with a counselor to clarify feelings and options. Such supportive counseling may need to be ongoing.

A summary of the major characteristics of autosomal dominant inheritance is given in Table 4.4.

Examples of disorders inherited in an autosomal dominant manner are shown in Table 4.5.

X-Linked Inheritance

In both dominant and recessive X-linked disorders, the mutant gene is located on the X chromosome. Because males have only one X chromosome, there is no counterpart for its genes, and so the gene is expressed when present in one copy regardless of whether it is dominant or recessive in females. Therefore, males cannot be carriers; they will show the effects of the gene in question and are said to be "hemizygous." A female receives one X chromosome from each of her parents for a normal sex constitution of XX. A male receives his single X chromosome from his mother and his Y chromosome from his father for a normal sex constitution of XY. Whether it is the X chromosome that a woman gets from her father or the X she gets from her mother that is passed to her sons and daughters is random. Figure 4.4 illustrates X and Y chromosome transmission. Dobyns et al. (2004) have suggested that the inheritance of X-linked disorders

TABLE 4.4   Major Characteristics of Autosomal Dominant Inheritance and Disorders

- Gene is on autosome.
- One copy of the mutant gene is needed for effects.
- Males and females are affected in equal numbers on average.
- No sex difference in clinical manifestations.
- Vertical family history through several generations may be seen.
- There is wide variability in expression.
- Penetrance may be incomplete (gene can appear to "skip" a generation).
- Increased paternal age effect may be seen.
- Fresh gene mutation is frequent.
- Later age of onset is frequent.
- Male-to-male transmission is possible.
- Normal offspring of an affected person will have normal children, grandchildren, etc
- Least negative effect on reproductive fitness.
- Structural protein defect is often involved.
- In general, disorder tends to be less severe than the recessive disorders.

be redefined because of various exceptions to the rules involved in the concept of X-linked recessive and X-linked dominant inheritance.

X-Linked Recessive

The most common pattern of X-linked transmission is that in which the female partner is a heterozygous carrier for the mutant gene (see Figure 4.5). If her partner is normal, then for each pregnancy the couple runs a 25% chance for the offspring to be one of the following: (1) a female carrier like the mother, (2) a normal female without the mutant gene, (3) a normal male without the mutant gene, or (4) a male who is affected with the disease in question. Thus the risk for a male offspring to be affected is 50%. As in the other types of single gene inheritance, the outcome of one pregnancy does not influence the others; these odds remain the same. The carrier female usually shows no obvious clinical manifestations of the mutant gene, unless X inactivation is skewed (see earlier discussion). In such an instance she may be a "manifesting heterozygote." For example, if the mutant gene was for Duchenne muscular dystrophy, she might demonstrate muscle weakness, enlarged calves, and moderately elevated serum creatine kinase levels. If the mutant gene were for hemophilia A, she might demonstrate prolonged bleeding times. Females with X chromosome abnormalities, such as even microscopic deletions, may also manifest X-linked recessive (XR) disorders if

the normal gene on the counterpart chromosome was deleted. Such individuals should have cytogenetic analysis.

In practice, individuals usually seek genetic counseling (1) before marriage or before planning children when they have a male family member such as an uncle or brother who has a known XR disorder, or (2) after the birth of an affected child. In some cases, the woman will know she is a carrier or a man will know he is affected with an XR disorder such as hemophilia. A woman who needs to determine whether or not she is a carrier because of the presence of one affected brother or maternal uncle can be in a difficult situation. Because about one third of the cases of X-linked disorders are caused by new mutations, the trend toward smaller family size does little to clarify carrier status by family history. Detection of the carrier state in females is often difficult because of the overlapping of test results between normal, carrier, and affected women that is possible due to inequality of X inactivation. A geneticist can account for factors such as ambiguous testing and history in part by the use of Bayes theorem, which is beyond the scope of this text, and molecular techniques may be useful in establishing heterozygosity. The birth of an affected child to such a woman (who has another affected male relative) would establish her as a carrier. The use of DNA probes and linkage analysis is proving useful in certain families with X-linked disorders in which the mother is a known carrier

TABLE 4.5   Selected Genetic Disorders Showing Autosomal Dominant Inheritance

Disorder	Occurrence	Brief description
Achondroplasia	1:10,000–1:12,000	Short-limbed dwarfism, large head, narrowing of spinal canal.
Adult polycystic kidney disease	1:250–1:1,250	Enlarged kidneys, hematuria, proteinuria, renal cysts, abdominal mass; eventual renal failure may be associated (adult) with hypertension, hepatic cysts, diverticula; cerebral hemorrage may occur. See cystic kidneys on X-ray films (see also chapter 6).
Aniridia	1:100,000–1:200,000	Absence of the iris of the eye to varying degrees; glaucoma may develop. May be associated with other abnormalities in different syndromes.
Facioscapulohumeral muscular dystrophy 1A	1:100,000–5:100,000	Facial weakness, atrophy in facial, upper limb, shoulder girdle, and pelvic girdle muscles; speech may become indistinct; much variability in progression and age of onset.
Familial hypercholesterolemia	1:200–1:500	LDL receptor mutation resulting in elevated LDL, xanthomas, arcus lipoides corneae, and coronary disease (see chapter 26).
Hereditary spherocytosis	1:4,500–1:5,000	Red cell membrane defect leading to abnormal shape, impaired survival, and hemolytic anemia.
Huntington disease	1:18,000–1:25,000 (United States) 1:333,000 (Japan)	Progressive neurologic disease due to trinucleotide repeat expansion of CAG. Involuntary muscle movements with jerkiness, gait changes, lack of coordination; mental deterioration with memory loss, speech problems, personality changes, confusion, and decreased mental capacity. Usually begins in mid-adulthood (see chapter 6).
Nail-patella syndrome	1:50,000	Nail abnormalities, hypoplasia or absent patella, and iliac horns; elbow dysplasia, renal lesions and disease, iris and other eye abnormalities, glaucoma, gastrointestinal problems.
Neurofibromatosis 1	1:3,000–1:3,300	Café-au-lait spots, neurofibromas, and malignant progression are common; complications include hypertension. Variable expression (see chapter 6).
Osteogenesis imperfecta Type IA	1:30,000	Blue sclera, fragile bones with multiple fractures, mitral valve prolapse, short stature in some cases, progressive hearing loss, wormian bones (see chapter 8).
Polydactyly	1:100–1:300 (Blacks) 1:630–1:3,300 (Caucasians)	Extra (supernumerary) digit on hands or feet.
Tuberous sclerosis-1	about 1:10,000	White leaf-shaped macules, seizures, mental retardation, facial angiofibromas, erythemic nodular rash in butterfly pattern on face; learning and behavior disorders; shagreen patches. May develop retinal pathology and rhabdomyoma of the heart.
van der Woude syndrome	1:80,000–1:100,000	Cleft lip and/or palate with lower lip pits, missing premolars, variable expression.
von Willebrand disease	1:1,000–30:1,000	Deficiency or defect in plasma protein called von Willebrand factor, leading to prolonged bleeding time; bleeding from mucous membranes.

and the status of her daughters is in doubt. In certain circumstances, it can be determined whether or not the X chromosome with the mutant gene was passed to a given daughter.

Because better treatment has increased the lifespan for many XR disorders such as hemophilia, affected males are now reproducing. If the female is normal in such a mating, all of their female children will be carriers and all the males will be normal; stated otherwise, the theoretical risk for each pregnancy is that there is a 50% chance that the offspring will be carrier females and a 50% chance that they will be normal males. If the male is affected and the female is a carrier for the same disorder, as may occur in the very common X-linked recessive disorders such as G6PD deficiency and color blindness, then with each pregnancy there will be a theoretical risk of 25% for the birth of each of the following offspring: an affected female, a carrier female, a normal male, an affected male (see Figure 4.5).

A much rarer mating is that of an affected female and normal male in which with each pregnancy there is a 50% chance that the child will be a female carrier and a 50% chance that the child will be an affected male.

In the past, little could be accomplished in the way of prenatal detection for X-linked recessive disorders except to determine the sex of the fetus. For the more common types of matings, this often resulted in the loss of normal, as well as affected, male offspring due to termination of those pregnancies in which the fetus was a male. It is now possible to provide more accurate prenatal diagnosis for many of the XR disorders by using molecular technology, so the nurse should be sure to refer such couples to a genetic counselor for the latest information and not rely on older printed material. A summary of the characteristics of XR disorders is given in Table 4.6 and examples of these disorders are in Table 4.7.

X-Linked Dominant

The X-linked dominant (XD) type is less frequently seen than the other modes of inheritance discussed. Because the mutant gene is dominant, only one copy is necessary for its effects to be manifested phenotypically. Both males and females can be affected, and both can transmit the gene. Because of the gene's location on the X chromosome, there

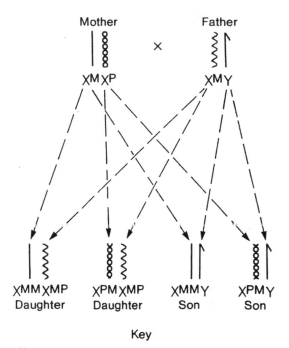

FIGURE 4.4 Transmission of the X and the Y chromosomes.

are several differences between this type of inheritance and autosomal dominant inheritance:

1. An affected male (except in cases of new mutation) has an affected mother because males inherit their X chromosome from their mother and not their father.
2. Some affected females may be less severely affected than males because of X-inactivation, as previously discussed.
3. There may be an excess of female offspring in the family tree or pedigree, as some X-linked dominant genes are lethal in the male.
4. Male-to-male transmission is not seen because males transmit their X chromosome only to their daughters, not to their sons. Thus an affected male would transmit the disorder to all of his daughters and none of his sons.

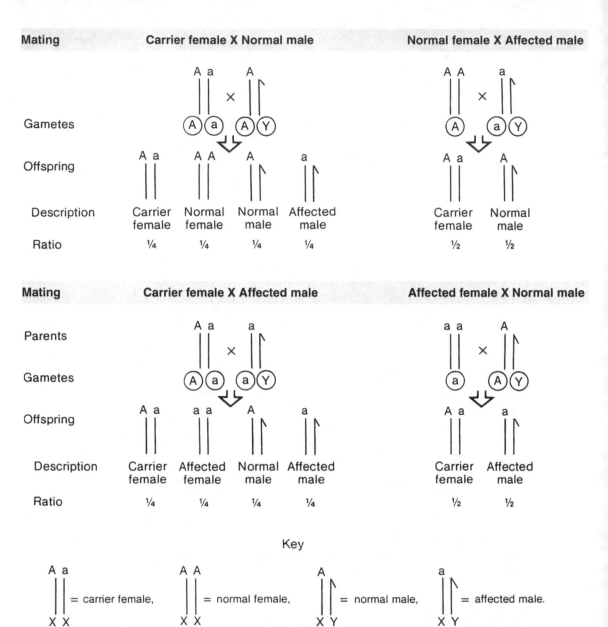

FIGURE 4.5   Mechanisms of X-linked recessive inheritance with one pair of chromosomes and one pair of genes.

Affected females are more likely to transmit the gene to their offspring because the gene is less severe in females due to X inactivation. If her mate is not affected, the theoretical risk for each pregnancy to her offspring is a 25% chance for each of the following: (1) an affected female, (2) an affected male, (3) a normal female, or (4) a normal male. Put a different way, there is a 50% chance that the offspring of each pregnancy will be affected without considering sex.

Because the gene is often lethal in males since they have no normal gene counterpart, the mating of an affected male and normal female is uncommon. For each pregnancy there is a 50% risk for an affected female and a 50% risk for a normal male. Thus all female children would be affected,

TABLE 4.6   Major Characteristics of X-Linked Recessive Inheritance and Disorders

- Mutant gene is on the X chromosome.
- One copy of the mutant gene is needed for phenotypic effect in males (hemizygous).
- Two copies of the mutant gene are usually needed for phenotypic effect in females.
- Males are more frequently affected than females.
- Unequal X inactivation can lead to "manifesting heterozygote" in female carriers.
- Transmission is often through heterozygous (carrier) females.
- All daughters of affected males will be carriers if the mother is normal.
- All sons of affected males will be normal if mother is normal.
- There is no male-to-male transmission.
- There are some fresh gene mutations.

although severity might differ, and all male children would be normal (see Figure 4.6). In such cases, prenatal determination of fetal sex would be all that would be necessary in order to allow the parents to make reproductive choices.

The very unlikely event of two affected individuals mating would result in a 25% risk of each of the following: (1) a homozygous affected female (probably lethal in utero), (2) a heterozygous female, (3) an affected male, and (4) a normal male. The fragile X syndrome is considered to be inherited in an XD fashion with incomplete penetrance. The features of X-linked dominant inheritance are summarized in Table 4.8 and a list of disorders inherited in this way is given in Table 4.9.

Y-Linked (Holandric)

Relatively few genes are known to be located on the Y chromosome, and so this type of inheritance has little clinical significance. Most Y-linked genes have to do with male sex determination. Y-linked genes manifest their effect with one copy and show male-to-male transmission exclusively. All sons of an affected male would eventually develop the trait, although the age at which they do so varies. None of the affected male's daughters would inherit the trait. It can be hard to distinguish Y-linked inheritance from autosomal dominant disorders that are male sex limited. Some genes on the Y chromosome are for determining height, male sex determination such as the *SRY* gene for the testis-determining factor, tooth enamel and size, RNA binding motif protein 1 gene, hairy ears, and a zinc finger protein.

MITOCHONDRIAL INHERITANCE

As described in chapter 2, genes are also present in the mitochondria of cells. Mitochondria are cell organelles that use oxygen in the process of energy production. The mutation rate is much higher in mitochondria than in the nucleus. This may be because they lack histones, do not have some DNA repair systems found in the nucleus, and may be more vulnerable to free oxygen radicals entering the cell because more than 90% of the entering oxygen is consumed by mitochondria (mt). MtDNA can replicate in postmitotic cells and is compact, having no known introns or large noncoding sequences. Mitochondria are transmitted along maternal lines (matrilinearity). Paternal mitochondria may be transferred to the egg during fertilization, but are lost very early in embryogenesis. Therefore, virtually all mitochondria that are passed along to the fetus are maternally-derived. An mtDNA mutation can be present in all mtDNA copies (homoplasmy) or in some (heteroplasmy). The percent of mtDNA mutations necessary to cause dysfunction is believed to vary depending upon the type of tissue affected, and even among cells in the same tissue. Cells with high energy demands such as nerve and muscle have many more mitochondria present than others. Mutation may be present in mtDNA somewhere in the cell but disease will not be evident until the mutation is present in a sufficient number of the mitochondria. Mitochondrial genes encode subunits of enzyme complexes of the respiratory chain and oxidative phosphorylation system, while some subunits are encoded by nuclear genes. Thus

TABLE 4.7   Selected Genetic Disorders Showing X-Linked Recessive Inheritance

Disorder	Occurrence	Brief description
Color blindness (deutan)	8:100 Caucasian males 4:100–5:100 Caucasian females 2:100–4:100 Black males	Normal visual acuity, defective color vision with green series defect
Duchenne muscular dystrophy	1:3,000–1:5,000 male births	Muscle weakness with progression, eventual respiratory insufficiency, and death (see chapter 6).
Fabry disease (diffuse angiokeratoma)	1:40,000 males	Lipid storage disorder. Ceramide trihexosidase deficiency, α-galactosidase deficiency. Onset in adolescence to adulthood. Angina, pain attacks, autonomic dysfunction, angiokeratoma.
G6PD deficiency	1:10 Black American males 1:50 Black American females	Enzyme deficiency with subtypes shows effects in RBC; usually asymptomatic unless under stress or exposed to certain drugs or infection (see chapter 18)
Hemophilia A	1:2,500–1:4,000 male births	Coagulation disorder due to deficiency of factor VIII. Severity varies with factor VIII levels. In severe cases, spontaneous bleeding in deep tissue (see chapter 6).
Hemophilia B (Christmas disease)	1:4,000–1:7,000 male births	Coagulation disorder caused by deficiency of factor IX similar to hemophilia A
Hunter syndrome (Mucopolysaccharidosis II)	1:100,000 male births	Mucopolysaccharide storage disorder with iduronate 2-sulfatase deficiency; mental retardation usual, hepatomegaly, splenomegaly, course facies, dwarfing, stiff joints, hearing loss, mild and severe forms (see chapter 6)
Lesch-Nyhan syndrome	Rare	Deficiency of purine metabolism enzyme HPRT; hyperuricemia, spasticity, athetosis, self-mutilation, developmental delay (see chapter 6)
Menkes disease	1:200,000 male births	Copper deficiency caused by defective transport; short stature, seizures, spasticity, hypothermia; kinky, sparse hair (pili torti); mental retardation
X-linked ichthyosis	1:5,000–1:6,000	Symptoms usual by 3 months. May be born with sheets of scales (collodion babies); dry scaling skin, often appears as if unwashed; developmental delay; bone changes; vascular complications; corneal opacities; steroid sulfatase deficiency.

mutations in either or both can affect ultimate enzyme function. Most nuclear gene defects resulting in mitochondrial disorders are associated with abnormalities of oxidative phosphorylation (OXPHOS). Mitochondrial disease (see chapter 6) can result from mtDNA mutation, nuclear gene mutation, or both. Diseases due to mtDNA mutations often involve tissues dependent on large amounts of adenosine triphosphate (ATP) for energy, such as the skeletal and heart muscles, central nervous system, kidney, liver, pancreas, and retina, and sensorineural hearing loss is frequent.

During division of cells containing both mutant and normal mtDNAs, individual cells can accumulate varying proportions of each. A mother with a homoplasmic mtDNA mutation can transmit only that mutant mtDNA to her offspring, while a mother with varying levels of mutated mtDNA may not always transmit mutated mtDNA, depending on the percentage of mutated mtDNA present. However, above a certain level, it is likely that all children will receive some mutated mtDNA. Susceptibility of specific tissue types to impaired mitochondrial function as a result of an mtDNA

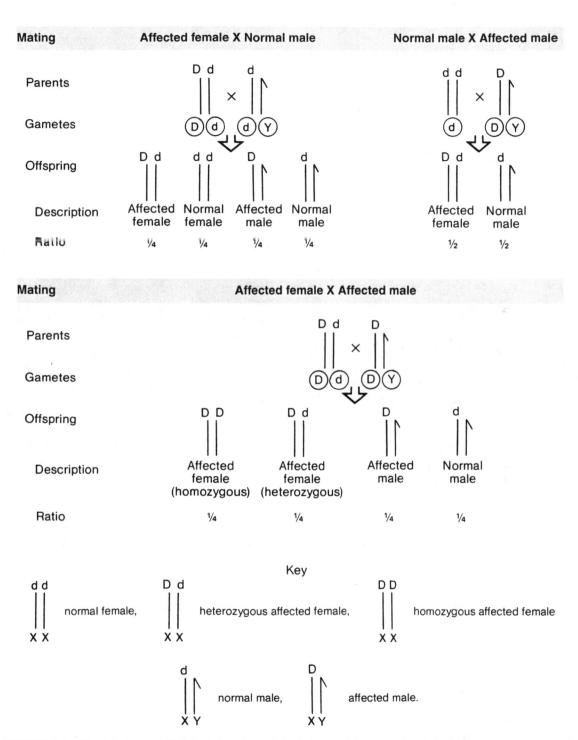

FIGURE 4.6   Mechanisms of X-linked dominant inheritance with one pair of chromosomes and one pair of genes.

TABLE 4.8   Major Characteristics of X-Linked Dominant Inheritance and Disorders

- Mutant gene is located on X chromosome.
- One copy of the mutant gene is needed for phenotype manifestation.
- X inactivation modifies the gene effect in females.
- Often lethal in males, and so may see transmission only in the female line.
- Affected families usually show excess of female offspring (2:1).
- Affected male transmits gene to all of his daughters and to none of his sons.
- Affected males have affected mothers (unless new mutation).
- There is no male-to-male transmission.
- There is no carrier state.
- Disorders are relatively uncommon.

mutation, the proportion of mutated mtDNA in a given cell or tissue type, and the severity of the specific mutation determine the phenotype. This may explain why some disorders show a childhood form with early onset, rapid progression, and multiple organ effects while others lead to an adult form with late onset, slower progression, and effects mainly confined to the nervous and muscular systems. Various types of mutations in mtDNA may be found including single base changes, deletions, and duplications.

Accumulating damage to mtDNA in somatic tissues over time appears important in aging and in Parkinson's disease development. External influences are known to have effects, some of which are reversible. For example, zidovudine, which is used in the treatment of HIV infection, can inhibit mtDNA replication and cause mtDNA depletion, resulting in mitochondrial myopathy that is usually reversible when it is discontinued.

Like mutations in nuclear DNA, those in mtDNA may be sporadic or inherited. Because mtDNA mutations are inherited through the female, a mother would potentially transmit the mutation to all of her offspring while an affected father would not transmit it to any of his offspring. Some disorders due to mitochondrial mutation include Leber optic neuropathy, Leigh syndrome, mitochondrial myopathy with encephalopathy, lactic acidosis and stroke-like episodes (MELAS syndrome), and myoclonic epilepsy with ragged red fibres (MERRF). Mutations in certain nuclear genes may predispose to mtDNA aberrations and thus result in mitochondrial disorders. Mitochondrial diseases are discussed further in chapter 6. Characteristics of mitochondrial inheritance are summarized in Table 4.10. Empiric recurrence risk figures for true mitochondrial diseases are about 3% for siblings and 6% for offspring, but in some families, where a mother is known to have a point mutation for a mitochondrial disorder, or where more than one child has been affected, the risk is estimated at 1 in 2. These figures should be interpreted cautiously. With more information about these disorders, more precise information will become available.

MULTIFACTORIAL INHERITANCE

"Multifactorial" refers to the interaction of several genes (often with additive effects) with environmental factors. Some have used the terms "multifactorial" and "polygenic" synonymously, but the latter does not imply any environmental component and is not recommended for such use. Many morphologic features and developmental processes are believed to be under multifactorial control, with minor differences determining variability in the characteristic they determine. The spectrum ranges from different degrees of normal to abnormal outcomes. The concept of this gene-environment interaction is well illustrated by congenital dislocation of the hip and the interruption of the development of the palate, leading to a cleft. Each of these is discussed in chapter 7.

Some of the more common congenital anomalies that are inherited in a multifactorial manner are listed in Table 7.1. One must, however, be careful to exclude specific identifiable causes before counseling on this basis. One way to accomplish this is to always seek diagnosis in an infant with

TABLE 4.9   Selected Genetic Disorders Showing X-Linked Dominant Inheritance

Disorder	Occurrence	Brief description
Albright hereditary osteodystrophy	Rare	Short stature, delayed dentition, brachydactyly hypocalcemia, pseudohypoparathyroidism, many endocrine problems, muscular atrophy, mineralization of skeleton, round facies, possible mental retardation; hypertension
Focal dermal hypoplasia	Very rare, exact rate unknown	Atrophy; linear pigmentation; papillomas of skin on lips, and umbilicus; digital anomalies; hypoplastic teeth; ocular anomalies (coloboma, microphthalmia), may have mental retardation
Incontinentia pigmenti	Very rare	Irregular swirling pigmentation of skin (whorled look), progressing to other skin lesions, dental anomalies, alopecia, mental retardation common, seizures, uveitis, retinal abnormalities
Ornithine transcarbamylase (OTC) deficiency	1:80,000 in Japan Very rare elsewhere	Inborn error in urea cycle metabolism; failure to thrive, hyperammonemia, vomiting, headache, confusion, rigidity, seizures, coma lethargy; many males die in neonatal period
Orofaciodigital syndrome Type I	1:50,000	Cleft palate, tongue, jaw and/or lip; facial hypoplasia; mental retardation, syndactyly, short digits, polycystic kidneys with renal failure
X-linked hypophosphatemia or vitamin D resistant rickets	1:25,000	Disorder of renal tubular phosphate transport. Rickets, bowed legs, growth deficiency rickets with ultimate short stature, possible hearing loss.

congenital anomalies, especially if they are multiple. This includes chromosome analysis, detailed histories, and complete physical examination. As an example, a child at the local cleft palate center was noticed to have lip pits in addition to the cleft (Figure 4.7). He was found to have van der Woude syndrome, an autosomal dominant disorder with a 50% recurrence risk, instead of isolated cleft palate with an approximate 5% recurrence risk (see chapter 7). Careful assessment is important.

An example of a normal trait inherited in a multifactorial manner is stature, in which ultimate height may be constrained within a range by genetic factors; but environmental factors (especially nutrition) play an important role in the final achievement of the genetic potential. This has been demonstrated in studies of immigrant families coming to the United States where the height of the first generation of offspring is above the mean height of the first generation of the offspring of siblings who remained behind.

Many normal multifactorial traits show a tendency to regress towards the mean of the population, as allele combinations and environmental factors favoring extremes tend to be relatively rare. Mathematical calculations of additive multiple gene effects show a normal bell-curve distribution within the population. To arrive at the concept of the presence or absence of a birth defect, one only needs to postulate a threshold beyond which the abnormal trait is manifested (Figure 4.8). In the case of some types of hypertension, the bell curve may represent the distribution of blood pressure in the general population, with the upper end of the continuous distribution representing hypertension, the exact threshold depending on the definition of "hypertension" used.

When parents each have several unfavorable alleles with minor effects that never encounter an unfavorable environment, they themselves may fall below the threshold. But when one of their children by chance inherits a genetic constitution with

TABLE 4.10   Major Characteristics of Mitochondrial Inheritance and Disorders

- Mutant gene is located in the mitochondrial DNA.
- Each mitochondrion contains multiple DNA molecules.
- Cells contain multiple mitochondria.
- Normal and mutant mitochondrial DNA for the same trait can be in the same cell (heteroplasmy).
- Inheritance is through the maternal line.
- Males and females are affected in equal numbers on average.
- Variability in clinical expression is common.
- There is no transmission from a father to his children.
- Disorders are relatively uncommon.

a large number of these unfavorable alleles from each parent, and also encounters some environmental insult that someone without that particular genetic susceptibility could handle, a malformation results. Because relatives share a certain number of their genes in common, depending on their degree of relationship as described in chapter 9, they are at greater risk for the same defect than are others in the general population.

A theoretical example to help conceptualize the process is given in Figure 4.9. Consider 5 gene pairs with 10 possible alleles per person that are

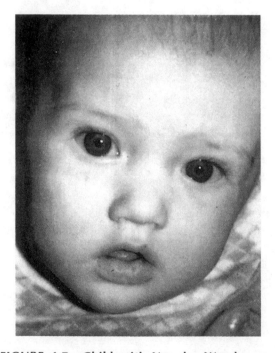

FIGURE 4.7   Child with Van der Woude syndrome. Note the lip pits. (Courtesy of Dr. Antonio Carbonell, Peoria, Illinois.)

responsible for the determination of a certain developmental process. In our example, each parent has 4 abnormal alleles out of the 10. Theoretically, the way the example is composed, their offspring could inherit from 0 to 8 of the abnormal alleles. Two offspring are shown in Figure 4.9, top. People in the general population might have from 0 to 10 abnormal alleles and be distributed in the bell curve as shown in Figure 4.9, bottom. Perhaps this hypothetical developmental process can function without apparent problems to result in a normal organ or part, as long as a certain minimal normal number is retained or, conversely, until 8 unfavorable alleles are present. Then liability is too great, the threshold is passed, and a defect is manifested.

An analogy (although not an exact one) often used to explain this type of inheritance to the lay person is to ask them to imagine two glasses of water, each of which is three-fourths full. These represent the unfavorable genes of the parents, whereas the airspace represents the favorable genes for the trait. They are below the threshold, which is the rim of the glass. When the water is poured into a glass (representing the child), which has an ice cube in it (representing unfavorable environmental factors), the water overflows, thus exceeding the threshold (Figure 4.10). It must be emphasized that this is what occurred with this pregnancy, that the genetic factors may be combined differently next time, and that the unfavorable environmental factors may not be present. The actual recurrence risk figures for their specific trait should be presented along with this.

The characteristics of multifactorial inheritance are summarized in Table 4.11. For the most part, only empiric (observed) recurrence risk figures are

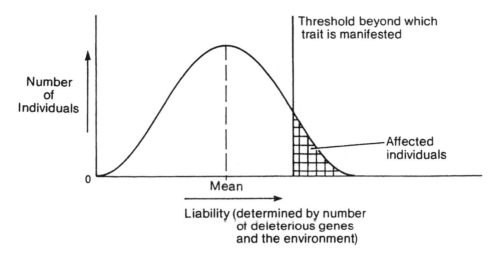

FIGURE 4.8   Distribution of individuals in a population according to liability for a specific multifactorial trait.

available for use in counseling. In contrast to the single gene disorders, in which the recurrence risk for subsequent pregnancies remains the same regardless of the number of affected offspring, in multifactorial inheritance the risks increase with the number of affected individuals. For congenital heart disease, if one child is affected, the risk to the next is 2% to 4%, and if 2 siblings are affected (or one parent and one sibling), this rises to 8%. The risk for recurrence after one affected child is higher if the population incidence is higher. For example, neural tube defects are especially prevalent in Northern Ireland. Thus the recurrence risk for a child with a neural tube defect is higher after one affected child born in Northern Ireland than it is for one born in the United States.

For defects in which one sex is affected more frequently than others, the risk to the relatives is greater when the defect occurs in the less-frequently affected sex. This is because it is assumed that the threshold is higher for that sex and that it takes a greater number of unfavorable factors to exceed it. For example, in pyloric stenosis, males are usually more frequently affected than females.

TABLE 4.11   Major Characteristics of Multifactorial Inheritance Assuming a Threshold

- The genetic component is assumed to be polygenic, quantitative, and additive in nature.
- The more severe the defect in the proband (index patient), the greater the recurrence risk in first-degree relatives.
- When the person with a congenital anomaly is of the least commonly affected sex, the greater the recurrence risk in first-degree relatives.
- The more affected individuals in a family, the greater the recurrence risk for additional members.
- The frequency of the defect in first-degree relatives is approximately equal to the square root of the frequency in the general population.
- There is a sharp drop in the frequency of affected persons between first- and second-degree relatives, and a less sharp one between second- and third- degree relatives.
- The consanguinity rate is often higher in affected families than in the general population.
- The risk for recurrence is higher if consanguinity is present.
- The risk for an affected parent to have an affected child is similar to the risk for unaffected parents with one affected child to have another affected child.
- If concordance for the defect in monozygotic twins is more than four times higher than that in dizygotic twins, the defect is likely to be multifactorial.

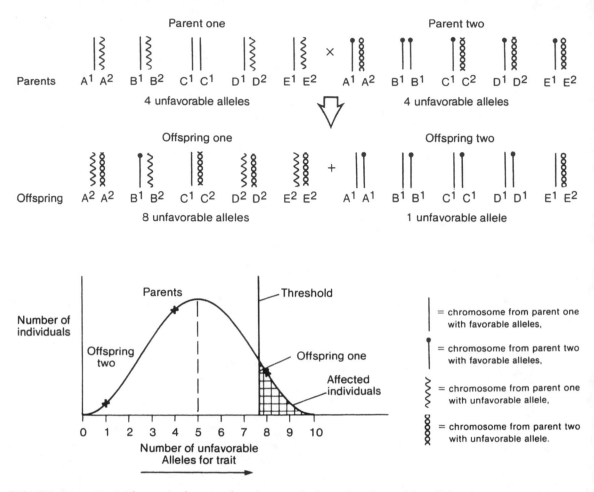

FIGURE 4.9   *(Top)* **Theoretical example of transmission of unfavorable alleles from normal parents demonstrating chance assortment of normal and unfavorable alleles in two possible combinations in offspring. *(Bottom)* Position of parents and offspring from the example above is shown for a specific theoretical multifactorial trait.**

The recurrence risk for first-degree relatives of female patients with pyloric stenosis has been estimated as about 18% for first-degree male relatives and about 8% for first-degree female relatives. It is presumed that not as many unfavorable factors are necessary in males for them to show this defect (Figure 4.11). The risk for first-degree relatives of male patients is about 4.6% and about 2.6% for first-degree male and first-degree female relatives, respectively. The biological basis for the sex difference seen has not yet been identified.

The extent of the severity of the disease also influences the recurrence risk estimates. The more severely the child is affected, the more unfavorable factors are presumed to be operating and

the higher will be the risk for recurrence. In Hirschsprung disease, it has been observed that the risk for subsequent siblings of an affected child is about 4% for siblingss of male index patients who have a short aganglionic segment affected and about 16% if a long aganglionic segment was affected.

Another characteristic is that the frequency of the defect in first-degree relatives (parents, siblings, offspring) is approximately equal to the square root of the frequency in the general population. Thus, if the population frequency for a specific defect was 1:10,000, it would be 1:100 among first-degree relatives. In addition, there is a sharp drop in the frequency of affected persons between first- and second-degree relatives and less between second- and third-degree relatives (Figure 4.11). For example, for cleft lip, the expected risks for first-, second- (aunts, uncles, nephews, nieces) and third-degree (first cousins) relatives are 40, 7, and 3 times that of the 1:1000 incidence in the general population. Risks for relatives less closely related are essentially the same as for the rest of the population.

The usual risk for recurrence of a multifactorial defect after one affected child is often cited as between 2% and 6%. However, those figures do not take into consideration all of the factors above, and thus they are not as accurate as they should be. Each family should be individually evaluated and counseled.

NONTRADITIONAL MECHANISMS AND INHERITANCE

A number of assumptions underly the basic tenets of patterns of inheritance. Although these are correct in the majority of instances, there are exceptions to those assumptions that have been elucidated relatively recently. These include differential gene expression, uniparental disomy, imprinting, and unstable mutations involving expanding repeats that often include the phenomenon of anticipation. Mitochondrial inheritance has already been discussed. Epigenetic mechanisms include "all meiotically and mitotically heritable changes in gene expression not coded in the DNA sequence itself" (Egger, Liang, Aparicio, & Jones, 2004, p. 457). DNA methylation, RNA-associated silencing and histone modification interact and if disrupted can lead to inappropriate silencing or expression of genes that can result in what are known as epigenetic diseases. These include disorders resulting from imprinting, such as Beckwith-Wiedemann syndrome (an overgrowth disorder involving organ overgrowth, hemihypertrophy, macroglossia, and increased cancer incidence). Assisted reproductive technologies may be associated with an increased risk for epigenetic disorders in the fetus. "Contiguous gene syndromes" is the term given when a usually very small chromosomal abnormality such as microdeletion results in alteration of gene dosage. It involves more than one adjacent gene so that a specific complex phenotype is seen. Individual components may be previously recognized

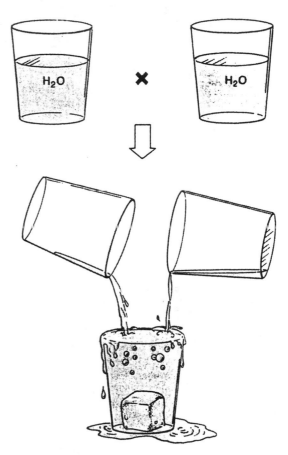

FIGURE 4.10   Water glass analogy for explaining multifactorial inheritance. In the first illustration, the water represents the parents' unfavorable alleles. The rim of the glass is the threshold. In the second illustration, the child inherits a large number of unfavorable alleles, plus unfavorable environmental factors (represented by the ice cube), and therefore "overflows" the threshold and manifests the anomaly.

Mendelian conditions when they occur singly. An example is the Smith-Magenis syndrome resulting from an interstitial deletion of 17p11.2 consisting of mental retardation, sleep disturbances, low adaptive functioning and behavioral difficulties. Rubinstein-Taybi syndrome [del(16p13.10)] consisting of mental retardation, dysmorphic features and broad toes and thumbs.

In the normal course of events, a child inherits one of each pair of genes and chromosomes from the mother and one from the father. In uniparental disomy, however, both chromosomal homologues are inherited from the same parent

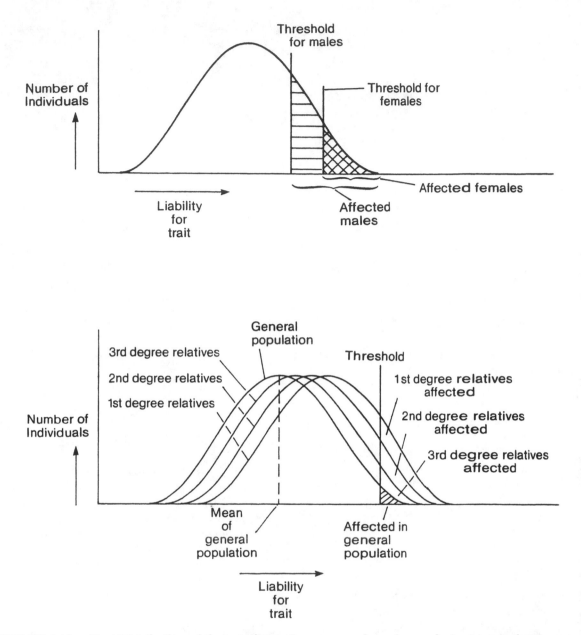

FIGURE 4.11 *(Top)* Distribution of the population for an anomaly such as pyloric stenosis that is more frequent in males than females. Note the difference in the position of the thresholds. The threshold for males is lower than that for females. *(Bottom)* Differences in the distribution of liability for a multifactorial trait due to the degree of relatedness after birth of an affected infant.

(e.g., two paternal chromosome 9 homologues and no maternal chromosome 9 homologues). The child has a normal total number of chromosomes. Uniparental disomy (UPD) may apply to all or part of a chromosome. If all the genes involved are normal then this may occur without being recognized, although growth retardation and other effects may result. However, if a mutant allele for an AR disorder was present on one parental chromosome, and this is the one inherited, then it now will be present in two copies and will be manifested. UPD was first recognized in a person who had inherited two maternal copies of chromosome 7 and came to attention with cystic fibrosis, short stature, and growth hormone deficiency. Uniparental maternal disomy for chromosome 7 may be responsible for up to 10% of cases of Silver-Russell syndrome, as well as some cases of intrauterine growth retardation. UPD may in some instances result because an embryo may be trisomic for a given chromosome, and one of the three may be eliminated, leaving two from the same parent of origin (trisomy rescue), or may result from other events including postfertilization nondisjunction. Chromosomes may contain paternally or maternally imprinted genes. In some cases, no apparent phenotypic effect is noted, for example from either maternal or paternal UPD of chromosome 1.

Another nontraditional inheritance mechanism is genomic imprinting, also called "parental imprinting" and "genetic imprinting." Normally, one of an identical pair of alleles from one parent is expressed in the same way as the other of the pair from the other parent. In imprinting, the alleles of a given pair of genes are not expressed in an equivalent manner depending upon the parent of origin. A gene is said to be maternally imprinted if the allele derived from the mother is the one that is silenced, repressed, or inactivated, and paternally imprinted if it is the allele contributed by the father that is inactivated. Thus certain genes may be expressed from either the maternal or paternal chromosome, depending on imprinting. Methylation is involved in imprinting, which is thought to occur before fertilization and confers transcriptional silencing for that gene. Imprinting is transmitted stably through mitosis in somatic cells and is reversible on passage through the opposite parental germline. Genomic imprinting may be suspected when:

- in looking at a pedigree, a given genetic disorder is always expressed when transmitted by only the male or only the female parent;
- the sex of persons affected by the disorder in a pedigree will be approximately equal, and not show a differentiation;
- a disorder is present in one monozygous twin but not the other.

Clinically, uniparental disomy and imprinting have been predominantly recognized in disorders of growth and behavior.

The best-known examples of differential gene expression, due to parent-of-origin effects, uniparental disomy, and imprinting are Prader-Willi and Angelman syndromes. Both Angelman and Prader-Willi syndromes can result from the absence of a maternal or paternal imprinted gene or because of deregulation of an imprinted gene. Prader-Willi syndrome (PWS) is a disorder that includes early obesity, hypotonia, hypopigmentation, small hands and feet, and mental retardation ranging in degree. Angelman syndrome (AS) is marked by severe mental retardation, inappropriate laughter, decreased pigmentation, ataxia and jerky arm movements, and seizures. In about 60–70% of cases, PWS results from an interstitial deletion (15q11-q13) in the paternally derived chromosome, in about 28% because of maternal uniparental disomy, and in the rest there is the presence of one chromosome 15 from each parent both of which are maternally imprinted. In contrast, in AS, most cases have an interstitial deletion (15q11-q13) in the maternally contributed chromosome; about 2 to 5% are caused by paternal uniparental disomy, and some are due to unknown single gene mutations and an imprinting abnormality. AS results from deficient maternal expression of the *UBE3A* gene, which encodes E6-AP ubiquitin-protein ligase resulting in a loss of function mutation. Recommended diagnostic testing includes methylation analysis, high-resolution chromosome analysis, FISH with appropriate probes, and PCR within a recommended protocol. Beckwith-Wiedemann syndrome (BWS) is an overgrowth disorder with macroglossia, embryonic tumor occurrence, hemihypertrophy, omphalocele or other abdominal wall defects, and hypoglycemia. The genetics of BWS are complex involving a domain on 11p15 with two imprinted subdomains. Most commmonly it results from uniparental paternal disomy for chromosome 11p15, but other mechanisms can result in BWS such as genomic imprinting dysregulation resulting from defective or absent maternally derived alleles in the 11p15 region due to microdeletions as well as other chromosomal rearrangements and loss of imprinting of the insulin-like growth factor 2 *(IGF2)* gene in which the maternal allele is activated, as well as other gene dysregulation such as for *LIT1*, an antisense RNA. See Niemitz et al. (2004) for more information.

Present throughout the human genome are short repeated segments usually in tandem that contribute to polymorphism, and thus are useful as markers. The most common repeats associated with disease to date are repeated units of three nucleotides that are arrayed contiguously and known as "triplet repeats" or "trinucleotide repeats." The nucleotides are cytosine (C), guanine (G), thymine (T), and adenine (A). Usually, there are fewer than 20–40 of any given repeat. When these nucleotides become unstable and expand or lengthen, usually during meiosis, they may cause disease. Many of these show anticipation and a parent-of-origin effect, and some have a length associated with premutation. Some of the diseases so far known to be associated with this type of mutation at specific sites are fragile X syndrome (CCG, see chapter 20), Huntington disease (CAG, see chapter 6), myotonic dystrophy (CTG), Machado-Joseph disease (CAG), and spinocerebellar ataxia type 1 (CAG). As knowledge of this type of disorder increases, variations are noticed. For example, repeat expansions in RNA may result in an abnormal gene product and this mechanism may occur in myotonic dystrophy types 1 and 2 and certain types of spinocerebellar ataxia. Dinucleotide expansions can also occur, and in the cystic fibrosis transmembrane conductance regulator *(CFTR)* gene appear to be involved in determining the clinical phenotype expression (see chapter 8).

END NOTES

Knowledge of mechanisms of gene inheritance continues to expand. Complexities of epigenetic and other mechanisms that influence the regulation of gene expression and the influence of the modifying effects of other genes in the genome as well as environmental factors add to knowledge and understanding.

BIBLIOGRAPHY

Abel, E. L., Kruger, M., & Burd, L. (2002). Effects of maternal and paternal age on Caucasian and Native American preterm births and birth weights. *American Journal of Perinatology, 19,* 49–54.

American College of Medical Genetics. (1996). *Statement on guidance for genetic counseling in advanced paternal age.* Available on line at http://www.acmg.ent.

American Society of Human Genetics/American College of Medical Genetics Test and Technology Transfer Committee. (1996). Diagnostic testing for Prader-Willi and Angelman syndromes: Report of the ASHG/ACMG Test and Technology Transfer Committee. *American Journal of Human Genetics, 58,* 1085–1088.

American Society for Reproductive Medicine. (2004a). Guidelines for oocyte donation. *Fertility and Sterility, 82*(Suppl. 1), S13–S15.

American Society for Reproductive Medicine. (2004b). Guidelines for sperm donation. *Fertility and Sterility, 82*(Suppl. 1), S9–S12.

Bennett, R. L., Hudgins, L., Smith, C. O., & Motulsky, A. G. (1999). Inconsistencies in genetic counseling and screening for consanguineous couples and their offspring: The need for practice guidelines. *Genetics in Medicine, 1,* 286–292.

Berry, R. J., Leitner, R. P., Clarke, A. R., & Einfeld, S. L. (2005). Behavioral aspects of Angelman syndrome: A case control study. *American Journal of Medical Genetics A, 132A,* 8–12.

Bjornsson, H. T., Fallin, M. D., & Feinberg, A. P. (2004). An integrated epigenetic and genetic approach to common human disease. *Trends in Genetics, 20,* 350–358.

Clayton-Smith, J., & Laan, L. (2003). Angelman syndrome: A review of the clinical and genetic aspects. *Journal of Medical Genetics, 40,* 87–95.

Conneally, P. M. (2003). The complexity of complex diseases. *American Journal of Human Genetics, 72,* 229–232.

Cook, J., Lam, W., & Mueller, R. F. (2002). Mendelian inheritance. In D. L. Rimoin, J. M. Connor, R. E. Pyeritz, & B. R. Korf (Eds.), *Emery and Rimoin's principles and practice of medical genetics* (4th ed., pp. 104–124). New York: Churchill Livingstone.

DiMauro, S., & Schon, E. A. (2003). Mitochondrial respiratory-chain diseases. *New England Journal of Medicine, 348,* 2656–2668.

Dobyns, W. B., Filauro, A., Tomson, B. N., Chan, A. S., Ho, A. W., Ting, N. T., et al. (2004). Inheritance of most X-linked traits is not dominant or recessive, just X-linked. *American Journal of Medical Genetics, 129A,* 136–143.

Egger, G., Linag, G., Aparicio, A., & Jones, P. A. (2004). Epigenetics in human disease and prospects for epigentic therapy. *Nature, 429,* 457–463.

Eggermann, T., Zerres, K., Eggermann, K., Moore, G., & Wollmann, H. A. (2002). Uniparental disomy: Clinical indications for testing in growth retardation. *European Journal of Pediatrics, 161,* 305–312.

Hefferon, T. W., Groman, J. D., Yurk, C. E., & Cutting, G. R. (2004). A variable dinucleotide repeat in the CFTR gene contributes to phenotype diversity by forming RNA secondary structures that alter splicing. *Proceedings of the National Academy of Sciences USA, 101,* 3504–3509.

Jansen, R. C., & nap, J-P. (2004). Regulating gene expression: Surprises still in store. *Trends in Genetics, 20,* 223-225.

Jones, J. L. (1997). *Smith's recognizable patterns of human malformation* (5th ed.). Philadelphia: W.B. Saunders.

Kazaura, M. R., & Lie, R. T. (2002). Down's syndrome and paternal age in Norway. *Pediatric and Perinatal Epidemiology, 16,* 314–319.

Knight, J. C. (2004). Allele-specific gene expression uncovered. *Trends in Genetics, 20,* 113–116.

Kotzot, D. (2004). Advanced parental age in maternal uniparental disomy (UPD): Implications for the mechanism of formation. *European Journal of Human Genetics, 12,* 343–346.

Kuhnert, B., & Nieschlag, E. (2004). Reproductive functions of the ageing male. *Human Reproductive Update, 10,* 327–339.

Lau, J. C. Y., Hanel, M. L., & Wevrick, R. (2004). Tissue-specific and imprinted epigenetic modifications of the human *NDN* Gene. *Nucleic Acids Research, 32,* 3376–3382.

Leiter, R. A. (1993). *National survey of state laws.* Detroit, MI: Gale Research.

Lewis, R. (2003). *Human genetics: Concepts and applications* (5th ed.). New York: McGraw Hill.

McIntosh, G. C., Olshan, A. F., & Baird, P. A. (1995). Paternal age and the risk of birth defects in offspring. *Epidemiology, 6,* 282–288.

Murakami, T., Garcia, C. A., Reiter, L. T., & Lupski, J. R. (1996). Charcot-Marie-Tooth disease and related inherited neuropathies. *Medicine, 75,* 233–250.

Niemitz, E. L., & Feinberg, A. P. (2004). Epigenetics and assisted reproductive technology: A call for investigation. *American Journal of Human Genetics, 74,* 599-609.

Ostrer, H. (1998). *Non-Mendelian genetics in humans.* New York: Oxford University Press.

Paldi, A. (2003). Genomic imprinting: Could the chromatin structure be the driving force? *Current Topics in Developmental Biology, 53,* 115–138.

Peters, S. U., Goddard-Finegold, J., Beaudet, A. L., Madduri, N., Turcich, M., & Bacino, C. A. (2004). Cognitive and adaptive behavior profiles of children with Angelman syndrome. *American Journal of Medical Genetics, 128A,* 110–113.

Petronis, A. (2004). Epigenetics and bipolar disorder: New opportunities and challenges. *American Journal of Medical Genetics, Part C (Seminars in Medical Genetics), 123C,* 65–75.

Port, K. E., Mountain, H., Nelson, J., & Bittles, A. H. (2005). Changing profile of couples seeking genetic counseling for consanguinity in Australia. *American Journal of Medical Genetics A, 132A,* 159–163.

Puck, J. M., & Willard, H. F. (1998). X inactivation in females with X-linked disease. *New England Journal of Medicine, 338,* 325–328.

Pulver, A. E., McGrath, J. A., Liang, K.-Y., Lasseter, V., Nestadt, G., & Wolyniec, P. S. (2004). An indirect test of the new mutation hypothesis associating advanced paternal age with the etiology of schizophrenia. *Amerian Journal of Medical Genetics, Part B (Neuropsychiatric Genetics), 124B,* 6–9.

Ranum, L. P. W., & Day, J. W. (2002). Dominantly inherited, non-coding microsatellite expansion disorders. *Current Opinion in Genetics & Development, 12,* 266–271.

Reynolds, R. M., Browning, G. G. P., Nawroz, I., & Campbell, I. W. (2003). Von Recklinghausen's neurofibromatosis: Neurofibromatosis type 1. *Lancet, 361,* 1552–1554.

Somprasit, C., Agunaga, M., Cisneros, P. L., Torsky, S., Carson, S. A., Buster, J. E., et al. (2004). Paternal gonadal mosaicism detected in a couple with recurrent abortions undergoing PGD: FISH analysis of sperm nuclei proves valuable. *Reproductive Biomedicine Online, 9,* 225–230.

Stoltenberg, C., Magnus, P., Lie, R. T., Daltveit, A. K., & Irgens, L. M. (1997). Birth defects and parental consanguinity in Norway. *American Journal of Epidemiology, 145,* 439–448.

Sweeney, E., Fryer, A., Mountford, R., Green, A., & McIntosh, I. (2003). Nail patella syndrome: A review of the phenotype aided by developmental biology. *Journal of Medical Genetics, 40*, 153–162.

Thacker, P. D. (2004). Biological clock ticks for men, too. *Journal of the American Medical Association, 291*, 1683–1684.

Van Heyningen, V., & Yeyati, P. L. (2004). Mechanisms of non-Mendelian inheritance in genetic disease. *Human Molecular Genetics, 13*, R225–R233.

Varcia, M., Kok, F., Setian, N., Kim, C., & Koiffmann, C. (2005). Impact of molecular mechanisms, including deletion size, on Prader-Willi syndrome phenotype: Study of 75 patients. *Clinical Genetics, 67*, 47–52.

Vu, T. H., Hirano, M., & DiMauro, S. (2002). Mitochondrial diseases. *Neurologic Clinics, 20*(3), 809–839.

Wain, H. W., Bruford, E. A., Lovering, R. C., Lush, M. J., Wright, M. W., & Povey, S. (2002). Guidelines for human gene nomenclature. *Genomics, 79*, 464–470.

Willard, H. F. (2001). The sex chromosomes and X chromosome inactivation. In C. R. Scriver, A. L. Beaudet, W. S. Sly, & D. Valle (Eds.), *The metabolic and molecular bases of inherited disease* (8th ed., pp. 1191-1211). New York: McGraw-Hill.

WuDunn, S. (1996, September 11). In Korea, same-name marriage is still taboo. *New York Times*, online edition.

Zeviani, M., Spinazzola, A., & Carelli, V. (2003). Nuclear genes in mitochondrial disorders. *Current Opinion in Genetics & Development, 13*, 262–270.

Zlotogora, J. (2004). Parents of children with autosomal recessive diseases are not always carriers of the respective mutant alleles. *Human Genetics, 114*, 521–526.

II

Major Genetic Disorders

5

Cytogenetic Chromosome Disorders

The progress made in human cytogenetics is remarkable when one realizes that it was only in 1956 that Tjio and Levan established the number of human chromosomes as 46 instead of 48. Today, application has been made of new techniques to detect and diagnose suspected errors more rapidly, to identify new syndromes, to relate chromosome changes to certain abnormalities, to provide accurate genetic counseling, to allow prenatal diagnosis for chromosome disorders, to determine the parental origin of some chromosome errors, to elucidate the meaning of chromosomal abnormalities and cancer, to map genes, to do anthropological studies, and to investigate chromosome structure and function. Basic information about chromosomes and their structure is necessary before discussing chromosome analysis and abnormalities.

CHROMOSOME NUMBER AND STRUCTURE

The normal human chromosome number in most body (somatic) cells and in the zygote is 46. This is known as the diploid (2N) number. Gametes (eggs and sperm) each contain 23 chromosomes. This is known as the haploid (N) number or one chromosome set. There are 22 pairs of autosomes (chromosomes common to both sexes) numbered from 1 to 22, and 2 sex chromosomes. Females possess two X chromosomes, and males have one X and one Y chromosome.

Chromosomes are composed of chromatin, which includes DNA, RNA, histones (a basic protein), and nonhistone proteins. The genes are arranged in a linear fashion on the chromosome. The actual arrangement of the chromatin has become a subject of interest especially in regard to gene expression. Each chromosome of a pair (homologous chromosome) normally has the identical number and arrangement of genes, except for the X and Y chromosomes in males. When a somatic cell enters metaphase of mitosis, the chromosome is seen to be doubled, consisting of two arms (sister chromatids). The chromatids are joined at the centromere, a primary constriction, that also separates the long (designated q) and short (designated p) arms of the chromosome and is where the spindle fibers attach during cell division (Figure 5.1). Banding techniques, which are discussed later, allow more precise descriptions of sites on chromosomes. For example, each arm is divided into regions and given numbers, with region number 1 closest to the centromere, each region is further divided into bands, and some bands into sub-bands. Sub-bands are indicated by a decimal point before it and are numbered from the centromere outward. Thus the designation Xq22 refers to band 2 of region 2 of the long arm of the X chromosome while 4p32.1 means chromosome 4, short arm, region 3, band 2, sub-band 1. Sometimes bands need to be defined within sub-bands such as 4q21.23. Each chromosome pair is unique and can be identified. Chromosome errors are of two basic types—changes in number and changes in structure. Chromosome abnormalities may be constitutional or acquired. Constitutional chromosome abnormalities arise during gametogenesis or early embryo development and affect all or nearly all of the cells. Acquired chromosome abnormalities arise later, usually in adulthood, most often affecting one or more somatic cells and their descendants, thus having a limited distribution in the body.

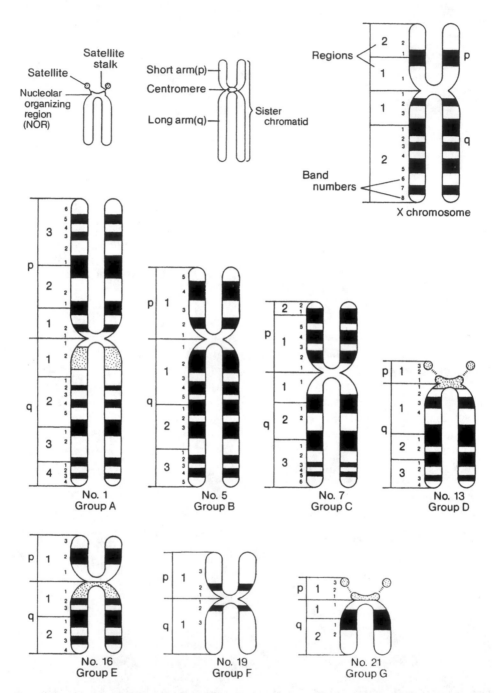

FIGURE 5.1 *(Top)* **Diagrammatic representation of chromosome structure at mitotic metaphase.** *(Bottom)* **Diagrammatic representation of chromosome bands as observed with Q, S, and R staining methods. Centromere is representative of Q staining methods only.** ☐ = negative or pale staining Q and G bands, positive R bands; ■ positive Q and G bands, negative R bands: ▒ variable bands.

(The bottom figure is redrawn from Paris Conference 1971, Supplement 1975: Standardization in Human Cytogenetics. In D. Bergsma (Ed.): White Plains: The National Foundation—March of Dimes, BD: OAS, XI(9), 1975. Used with permission.

CHANGES IN CHROMOSOME NUMBER

The term used to denote the correct complete chromosome set is *euploidy*. Deviations from that number can be of the following two types: (1) *polyploidy*, in which the deviation is an exact multiple of the haploid set [e.g., a triploid (3N) cell has 69 chromosomes with 3 copies of each chromosome (and, of course, its genes) instead of 2, and a tetraploid (4N) cell has 92 chromosomes with 4 copies of each chromosome]; and (2) *aneuploidy*, in which numerical deviation is not an exact multiple of the haploid set (e.g., 2N+1, 2N+2, . . ., or 2N-1, 2N-2, . . .). *Monosomy* (2N-1) refers to the presence of 45 chromosomes with one member of one pair being absent; whereas *trisomy* (2N+1) refers to the presence of 47 chromosomes with one extra member of a chromosome pair being present. *Mosaicism* refers to the presence of two or more cell lines that differ in chromosome or gene number or structure but are derived from a single zygote. The only monosomies (in nonmosaic form) known to be compatible with life are of the X chromosome 45,X, (Turner syndrome), and monosomy 21 (rare). Polyploidy is common in plants, but in humans it is generally incompatible with life. Triploids and tetraploids together account for about one fourth of all spontaneous abortions caused by chromosome abnormalities. Rare infants with triploidy have been live born, but most die within a few days, unless they are mosaic. Most triploidy occurs as a result of two sperm fertilizing the same egg, but the re-union of an egg and polar body or failure of a meiotic reduction in sperm or egg can also be responsible. Tetraploids occur most often from failure of the first cleavage division in the zygote (mitotic). These are usually, but not always, lost early in gestation. One case report details features of a 26-month-old girl with tetraploidy (92,XXXX). Extra structurally abnormal chromosome (ESAC) is a term synonomous with supernumerary marker chromosome. These are very small extra chromosomes of unknown origin that do not follow the usual pattern of cell division. Their incidence in newborns is 0.2 to 0.72 per 1,000, and are estimated in prenatal studies as 0.6 to 1.5 per 1,000. Some are associated with known chromosomal syndromes such as isochromosome 9p. It is estimated that about 40% of ESACs determined by prenatal cytogenetic analysis are inherited. In these cases, if the carrier parent has a normal phenotype then the risk of an abnormal phenotype in the fetus is low.

CHANGES IN CHROMOSOME STRUCTURE

Variations in chromosome structure (heteromorphisms) are widespread. These variations are observed particularly in chromosomes 1, 9 and the Y chromosome, and especially in satellite and short-arm areas of acrocentric chromosomes as well as the heterochromatic regions near the centromeres of all chromosomes. It is becoming more obvious that while most have little or no known effect, others do. Those with little or no effect mainly affect those portions of chromosomes where few active genes are found. There are four major classifications of alterations in chromosome structure: (1) deletions or deficiencies, (2) duplications, (3) inversions, and (4) translocations. Each leads to a change in the original linear order of genes on the chromosome that is involved (see Figure 5.2). Uniparental disomy is discussed in chapter 4.

Deletions

A deletion is the loss of part of a chromosome. Deletions can occur either at the ends of a chromosome (terminal deletion) as a result of a single break, or within the body of the chromosome (interstitial deletion), a process that requires two breaks and the reattachment of the broken chromosomal pieces (see Figure 5.2). The broken ends of chromosomes are generally considered "sticky," and thus allow for such reattachment. If the fragments that are displaced have no centromere, they are lost from the cell during division, and thus the genetic information carried on that fragment is lost. The best known human chromosome disorders resulting from a deletion are 5p- (cri-du-chat) and 4p- (Wolf-Hirschhorn syndrome), which are discussed below. Sometimes a deleted fragment can become inserted into another chromosome. When two terminal deletions occur in the same chromosome, the two "sticky" ends may form a ring, as shown in Figure 5.2. The two fragments

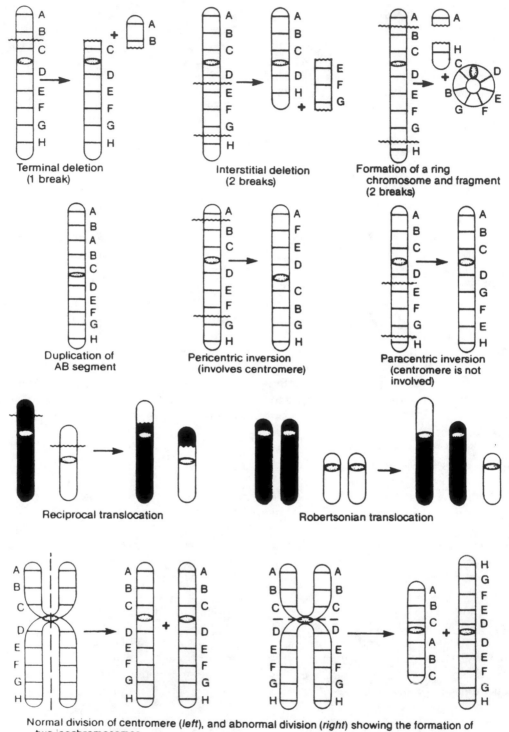

FIGURE 5.2   Diagrammatic representation of alterations in chromosome structure.

produced may stay separated, or they may fuse, but unless they include a centromere they are eventually lost. Ring chromosomes are seen in connection with many syndromes and have been reported for all chromosomes. Small interstitial deletions known as "microdeletions" have been found in certain genetic disorders that were originally believed to be single-gene disorders. For example, a microdeletion of chromosome 22 (del 22q11.2) has been found in the DiGeorge/velocardiofacial syndrome. This may also be called a contiguous gene syndrome. Microdeletions in the Y chromosome have been found in some men with infertility. The use of fluorescent in situ hybridization (FISH) with specific probes has enhanced detection of microdeletions, since most are not visible during routine cytogenetic studies.

Duplications

These refer to the presence of a segment that occurs more than the normal number of times in the same chromosome. Duplication can be a result of a primary structural change, or a defect in crossing over (the exchange of material by homologous chromosomes during cell division). The process can result in extra copies of genes (see Figure 5.2). Duplications may be in the same orientation or inverted. It is believed that this process protects organisms from the loss of vital genetic material due to mutation and is important in evolution. The results of the extra gene copies may or may not be phenotypically noticeable. Indirect effects may occur because of changes in chromosome folding caused by duplication. Duplications can involve large regions on the chromosome and may have flanking repeat sequences that permit unequal crossing over by homologous or asymmetric nonsister chromosome exchanges. Chromosome duplications result in the duplication of genes present there. An example of disorders of chromosome duplication is Charcot-Marie-Tooth disease 1A (an inherited peripheral neuropathy) in which the duplication is is tandem on chromosome 17 (17p11.2).

Inversions

Inversions are aberrations in which a portion of the chromosome has become rearranged in reverse order. This occurs as a result of two breaks, 180° rotation of the chromosomal piece between them, and its reinsertion. A pericentric inversion is one that includes the centromere, whereas a paracentric inversion does not (see Figure 5.2). In humans with inversions, problems can occur during meiotic crossing over, because chromosome pairing cannot proceed normally. It is suspected that increased infertility, increased incidence of spontaneous abortions, and perhaps an increased frequency of birth defects may result, but few abnormal births have been actually attributed to the presence of inversions. Fetuses with inversions have been prenatally detected. Inversions appear nonrandom—more than 40% of all inversions involve chromosome 9. Small inversions may be frequent in certain populations or families.

Translocations

A translocation is the transfer of a chromosome segment to another chromosome after breakage has occurred. An example is the translocation of material from chromosome 22 to chromosome 9 [t{9;22}] that results in the creation of a *BCR-ABL* fusion gene and chronic myelogenous leukemia (chapter 23). In reciprocal translocations, two chromosomes exchange pieces and no material is usually lost (see Figure 5.2). In the nonreciprocal type, one chromosome or a piece of one attaches itself to another so that little or no genetic material is lost. A Robertsonian or centric fusion translocation is a special type that occurs between the long arms of two acrocentric (D and G group) chromosomes (see Figure 5.2). Small fragments from the short arms may be lost, usually without any phenotypic effect. A balanced translocation is one in which no genetic material is added or lost, whereas in an unbalanced translocation, material is gained or lost. However, some phenotypic abnormalities have been found in persons with apparently balanced translocations and other rearrangements. Using newer techniques, small deletions have been found in some cases. The majority of persons with a balanced translocation appear normal and are only uncovered with chromosome analysis. The frequency of balanced translocations in the general population is about 1 in 500–625, while the frequency of Robertsonian translocations is about 1 in 900. Upon chromosome analysis, one of the parents of some children with multiple anomalies and unbalanced translocations is often found to have a balanced translocation. Such a finding is important for future genetic counseling of that couple and also of other family members. Translocations are further discussed under Down syndrome.

Isochromosome Formation

Isochromosomes result when the centromere splits in an abnormal way during cell division; instead of dividing so that each new cell contains one complete daughter chromosome, one cell contains both short arms, and the other contains both long arms (see Figure 5.2). Thus an isochromosome is one that consists of 2 identical chromosome arms. The most frequently found isochromosome in humans is of the X chromosome. If a female has one normal X chromosome, and one isochromosome composed of the long arms of the X, i(Xq), then she is monosomic or deficient for those genes on the short arm and trisomic for those on the long arm leading to phenotypic manifestations.

Position Effects

All of the previously mentioned structural alterations can produce position effects. This occurs when genes on a chromosomal segment are moved to a new chromosomal "neighborhood." Position effects may result in the activation or inactivation of genes on the involved chromosomes, and are important in the development of cancer and other disorders, for example in the activation of oncogenes after chromosome translocation. Certain genes are known to be inactivated in X-autosome translocations.

Chromosome Breakage, Sister Chromatid Exchange, and Fragile Sites

Before chromosomes can form structural rearrangements, breakage must occur in either one chromatid or the entire chromosome. This can lead to any of the abnormalities just discussed or to other more complex arrangements. A chromatid gap is a discontinuity in a single chromatid with minimal disalignment, while misalignment is present in a chromatid break. A number of known genetic disorders have accompanying spontaneous chromosome breakage and are discussed in chapter 23. Ionizing radiation and certain chemicals can also cause breakage. Exchange between sister chromatids (chromatids arising from the same chromosome during division) can be demonstrated by special techniques and can be used to ascertain the mutagenic potential of chemical compounds (see chapter 13).

Fragile sites are known on the X chromosome and on autosomes. Such sites manifest themselves cytogenetically only in special culture media, and can be influenced by external conditions. Molecular methods are now favored for detection and diagnosis. The fragile X syndrome is discussed in chapter 20.

INCIDENCE OF CHROMOSOME ERRORS

Large surveys of consecutive newborns have allowed the incidence of chromosome aberrations present at birth to be well-established at 0.5% to 0.6%, although prenatal diagnosis and selective termination of pregnancy has had an impact on decreasing this. The incidence of the specific chromosome abnormalities found is summarized in Table 5.1. Autosomal trisomies account for about 25%, sex chromosome abnormalities for about 35%, and structural rearrangements for about 40%. This figure represents only a small fraction of chromosomally abnormal conceptions. Nature exercises considerable selection, as only a small percentage of cytogenetically abnormal conceptions survive to term especially if severe, such as trisomy 2 and trisomy 16, as well as the majority of other autosomal trisomies, as discussed below. Between 10% to 20% of all recognized conceptions end in spontaneous abortion. Studies of the products of spontaneous abortion have indicated that, overall, between 50% and 60% have detectable chromosomal abnormalities. The distribution of specific errors in abortuses is somewhat different, as illustrated in Table 5.2. In various studies, a high percentage of tetraploid and triploid abortuses were detected, and the sex chromosome trisomies were rarely seen since most survive to term. Turner syndrome represents about 20% of the total cases. Approximately 95% to 99% of all Turner syndrome embryos are spontaneously aborted, as are about 95% of those with trisomy 18, and 65% to 75% of those with trisomy 21. These data support

TABLE 5.1   Incidence of Selected Chromosome Abnormalities in Live-Born Infants*

Abnormality	Incidence
Autosomal trisomies	
Trisomy 21 (Down syndrome)	1:650–1:1,000 live births
Trisomy 13 (Patau syndrome)	1:4,000–1:10,000 live births
Trisomy 18 (Edwards syndrome)	1:3,500–1:7,500 live births
Sex chromosome disorders	
45,X (Turner syndrome)	1:2,500–1:8,000 live female births
47,XXX (Triple X)	1:850–1:1,250 live female births
47,XXY (Klinefelter syndrome)	1:500–1:1,000 live male births
47,XYY	1:840–1:1,000 live male births
Other sex chromosome abnormalities	
(males)	~1:1,300 live male births
(females)	~1:1,300 live female births
Structural	
rearrangements (e.g., translocations, deletions)	~1:440 live births

*Based on statistics from surveys in different populations and not age adjusted. Data prior to use of prenatal diagnosis and selective termination of pregnancies became widespread.

the concept of not intervening therapeutically in cases of threatened spontaneous abortion. Chromosomal abnormalities account for 6% to 12% of stillbirths and perinatal deaths respectively, about 7% of deaths between 28 days and 1 year of age, and slightly over 7% of later infant deaths. In stillbirths, the karyotypic abnormalities seen most often are trisomy 21 (23%), Turner syndrome (23%), trisomy 18 (21%), trisomy 13 (8%), and unbalanced translocations and deletions each occurring in less than 1% (Wapner & Lewis, 2002). The different incidence figures reported from study to study reflect variety in gestational ages included, population differences, differences in chromosome preparation techniques, and different rates of culture failure, particularly in tissue obtained from autopsy material. Extrapolating from available data, it appears that chromosome abnormalities are present in 10% to 20% of all recognized conceptions. This may eventually be higher as techniques for determining cytogenetic causes in macerated tissue improve. More than 1,000 different chromosome abnormalities have been described in livebirths.

FACTORS IN CHROMOSOME ERRORS

Mechanisms that may result in chromosome errors include meiotic and mitotic nondisjunction, meiotic and mitotic anaphase lag, double fertilization, retention of second polar body, unequal crossing over, chromosome breakage and reunion, meiotic crossing over in inversion heterozygotes, and aberrant segregation in translocation heterozygotes.

Parental Age

The increased risk for trisomy 21 (Down syndrome) and other trisomies, although to a lesser extent, with advancing maternal age has long been known. This effect begins to assume more importance at about age 35 years, and that is the reason for the inclusion of maternal age of 35 years and older as one of the indications for amniocentesis. Mothers under 15 years of age may be at the same magnitude of risk as those over 35 years of age, but this is debated. Other studies have suggested that increased parity, especially at older maternal age,

TABLE 5.2   Distribution of Chromosome Aberrations Found in Spontaneous Abortions*

Chromosome aberration	Percentage found
Autosomal trisomies	49–52
Turner syndrome (45,X)	18–23
Triploid	15–20
Tetraploid	4–6
Structural rearrangements	3–7
Other	3–5

*Based on statistics from surveys in different populations and not age adjusted.

was independently associated with a higher risk for a child with trisomy 21 (Kallen, 1997; Schimmel, Eidelman, Zadka, Kornbluth, & Hammerman, 1997). Prenatal screening and diagnosis with selective pregnancy termination has had a considerable impact in reducing the number of liveborn children with Down syndrome. Without accounting for prenatal diagnosis and selective pregnancy termination, the overall incidence of Down syndrome is about 1 in 800 live births, regardless of maternal age. Age-specific risk figures for bearing a live-born infant with Down syndrome have been estimated in various ways. Using a newer statistical approach, Hecht and Hook (1996) calculated rates with confidence intervals (CI), however the traditional risk figures for giving birth to a child with Down syndrome are widely used as follows:

Age in years	Traditional risk
20	1/1667
25	1/1250
30	1/952
35	1/385
40	1/106
45	1/30
49	1/11

It is important for the nurse to note that these figures do not include conceptions that are not liveborn, or the risk of other trisomies (i.e., trisomy 13; trisomy 18; 47,XXX; 47,XXY). Thus, the risk for bearing a child with any of these trisomies may be as much as twice the age-specific risk for trisomy 21. Nurses also should recognize the implications of these data for health teaching. Chromosomally speaking, men and women should be encouraged to plan to complete their families before the age of 40–45 and 35 years, respectively; and women who plan to become, or are already pregnant by age 35 should be referred for genetic counseling and amniocentesis. Increased paternal age is associated with certain autosomal dominant mutations, which are discussed in chapters 4 and 6.

In 1970 it was estimated that women over 35 years of age had only 13% of all pregnancies but gave birth to about 50% of all infants with Down syndrome. Because of prenatal diagnosis for women aged 35 years and older with the option of selective termination of pregnancy, that trend has changed and (depending on the time and population surveyed) most infants with Down syndrome are now born to women under 35 years of age. However, maternal serum screening for Down syndrome is impacting upon these statistics (see chapter 12). The recent use of more precise techniques has revealed that in about 5% of trisomy 21 cases, the extra chromosome is of paternal origin. In one study by McIntosh, Olshan and Baird (1995), paternal age below 20 years was associated with an increased risk of birth defects such as Down syndrome in their offspring. The role of increased paternal age has been under investigation but is somewhat hampered by the high correlation of increased maternal age with increased paternal age, by the small proportion of trisomy caused by paternal nondisjunction, and by contradictory research findings. Under various statistical conditions, with adjusted maternal age, there was an effect of increased paternal age in relation to risk of Down syndrome (Kazaura & Lie, 2002). At the present time, the risk appears possibly significant only in males 55 years and above. The strength of a paternal effect is difficult to determine, and there is no definitive answer at this time. A paternal age effect may occur for XYY. It is desirable for sperm donors to be younger than 40 years of age. Egg donors are usually recruited to be between 21 and 32 years of age.

The association of increased maternal age with the increased risk of bearing a child with trisomy 21 has been thought to be caused by nondisjunction of chromosome 21 during oogenesis. When the extra chromosome is of paternal origin, nondisjunction in spermatogenesis is a possibility in older men. The precise reason for the nondisjunction remains to be found.

Nondisjunction and Mosaicism

There are two types of cell division—mitosis and meiosis. In mitosis (somatic cell division for growth and repair), normally each daughter cell ends up with the same chromosome complement as the parent. During oogenesis and spermatogenesis, meiosis (reduction division of 2N germ cells) normally results in gametes with the haploid (N) chromosome number. Nondisjunction can occur in anaphase 1 or 2 of meiosis, or in anaphase of mitosis.

If nondisjunction occurs in meiosis, the chromosomes fail to separate and migrate properly into the daughter cells, so that both chromosomes of a pair end up in the same daughter cell, leading to some gametes with 24 (N+1) chromosomes and some with 22 (N-1) chromosomes. When such gametes are fertilized by a normal gamete, trisomic or monosomic zygotes result, such as in trisomy 21 or in Turner syndrome (45,X), respectively. Offspring resulting from such fertilization generally have a single abnormal cell line. If nondisjunction occurs in the first meiotic division, only abnormal gametes result; but if it occurs in the second division, half of the gametes will be normal. Nondisjunction during meiosis is shown in Figure 5.3. Anaphase lag, in which the chromosomes of a pair separate but one member "gets left behind" and is lost, leads to monosomy. If this occurs in meiosis, it affects the gamete. Variation in crossing over or recombination may be associated with nondisjunction in oocytes. Another mechanism that is thought to lead to single chromatid nondisjunction is disturbance in sister-chromatid adhesion.

The occurrence of these errors during mitosis results in mosaicism in somatic cells, except in the first zygotic division which results in tetrasomy. An individual who is mosaic possesses two or more cell populations, each with a different chromosome constitution that (in contrast to a chimera) arises from a single zygote during somatic cell development. The number of cells that will have an abnormal chromosome makeup will depend on how early in the division of the zygote the error occurs, and the viability of the cell line. The earlier it occurs, the higher the percentage of abnormal cells there will be. The results of abnormal division in mitosis leading to mosaicism are shown in Figure 5.4. Chromosome abnormalities resulting from errors in mitosis are only seen in descendants of the initial cell with the error. Mosaicism is a common finding in chromosomal syndromes, and the degree to which a person is clinically affected depends on the percentage of cells with the abnormal chromosome makeup. Some persons with

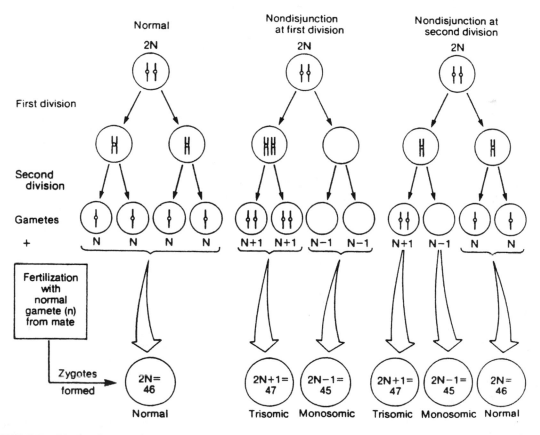

FIGURE 5.3   Mechanisms and consequences of meiotic nondisjunction at oogenesis or spermatogenesis.

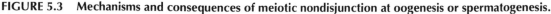

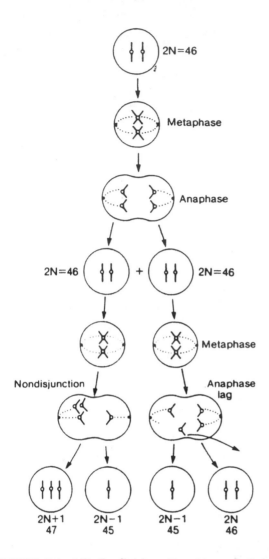

FIGURE 5.4   Mitotic division. *Top:* **Normal.** *Bottom:* **Nondisjunction and anaphase lag producing mosaicism with three types of cell lines—(45/46/47).**

mild mosaicism show few or no phenotypic changes. Chromosome analysis of too few cells can miss mosaic persons with a small percentage of abnormal cells.

Confined placental mosaicism (CPM) refers to a condition whereby mosaic abnormality is found in the placenta upon chorionic villus sampling. It is presumed to result from a trisomic conceptus and the loss of one of the extra chromosomes during mitosis, resulting in rescue to a disomic embryo. CPM is associated with increased fetal loss and intrauterine growth retardation.

Effects of Radiation, Chemicals, Viruses, and Specific Genes

The effect of these classes of agents capable of damaging chromosomes are discussed in detail in chapter 14. For many years ionizing radiation such as X-rays has been known to cause mutation, chromosome breaks, and rearrangements. A single large dose of radiation, as from an X-ray, is more mutagenic than chronic administration of the same total dose as might be found in natural background radiation. However, chronic low dose radiation may be reflected in cytogenetic changes. With an increase in radiation dosage, there is a linear increase in chromosome and point mutations. An increased frequency of both unstable (e.g., acentric fragments, ring chromosomes) and stable (e.g., translocations, inversions, some deletions) chromosomal aberrations is found in human lymphocytes immediately after a large enough dose of ionizing radiation. Although cells with unstable aberrations usually disappear in 3 to 5 years, those with stable aberrations may persist for over 20 years. How these somatic cell changes are reflected in gonadal cells is not fully known. Although there is difficulty in obtaining unbiased data with large enough samples on which to base conclusions, there are studies that link increased preconception radiation in mothers with subsequent chromosomally abnormal fetuses and studies that have found a significantly higher frequency of occupational exposure to radiation in fathers of chromosomally abnormal fetuses than in controls. Mothers who are older at the time of conception would also be more likely to have been exposed to more radiation. Radiation can induce chromosomal nondisjunction and other abnormalities in animals and cultured human lymphocytes. Chemicals, such as certain antibiotics, agents used in cancer chemotherapy, and toxic substances such as benzene, have been shown to produce chromosomal aberrations.

The phenomenon of potentiation, in which two or more agents cause greater damage together than the simple total of each individual effect, has only begun to be explored. Exposure to both radiation and chemicals is increasing, and together the effects could be substantial.

Viruses are also known to be capable of damaging chromosomes, chiefly causing breaks or gaps.

An increased frequency of chromosome breaks is found in children with congenital rubella syndrome when compared with controls. The relationship between such damage and congenital malformations remains to be firmly established. Other viruses known to cause breaks include varicella zoster (chickenpox), measles virus, mumps virus, herpesvirus, adenoviruses, and the Rous sarcoma virus, as well as mycoplasmas.

Because some families show an unusual clustering of several different trisomic disorders, it has been suggested that they may have genes segregating within the family that predispose the individuals in some way to the occurrence of nondisjunction. At the present time, this theory awaits confirmation, as such clustering may also be due to chance or some common environmental exposure. Chromosomes may also be differentially susceptible to aneuploidy.

CHROMOSOME ANALYSIS AND CELL CULTURE

The cells most commonly used for chromosome analysis are peripheral white blood cells. This is because they can undergo mitosis, can grow in culture in a relatively short period of time, and are easily obtained with a minimum of trauma (venipuncture) from the person from whom they are needed. The erythrocyte cannot be used because it has neither a nucleus nor chromosomes. Bone marrow cells, skin fibroblasts, amniotic fluid cells, and other tissue are also used in specific situations. Flow cytometry as another type of method for chromosome analysis, is a sorting technique whereby aneuploidy can be quickly detected but fine analysis is not yet available. It maybe combined with FISH (described in the next section).

The following is an abbreviated description of the traditional chromosome analysis process. Heparinized blood is centrifuged and sampled. Cells are grown in culture media containing human or fetal calf serum, amino acids, buffered salts, and occasionally antibiotics, to which phytohemagglutinin (PHA), which is a mitogenic plant extract that stimulates cell growth and mitosis, is added. This is incubated at constant temperature (37°C) for 72 hours, and the proper pH is maintained.

After 72 hours, colchicine is added in order to arrest cell division at metaphase when chromosomes are maximally contracted, have duplicated in preparation for division (have two sister chromatids), and are most visible. It does this by destroying the spindle, thus allowing chromosomes to spread throughout the cell. Cells are "harvested" after being centrifuged and then treated with a hypotonic solution that swells the cells and slightly separates the chromatids. Finally, the cells are fixed, spread on a slide, dried, and then stained. At this point they are examined under the microscope. Suitable "spreads" are then analyzed and photographed (see Figure 5.5). Each laboratory has developed a minimum number of spreads that they examine before karyotyping, usually 20. The chromosomes in a photograph can then be cut out and arranged into a karyotype arrangement of chromosomes by size and morphology according to a standard classification. Because these chromosomes have been arrested in metaphase of mitosis, they have already duplicated in preparation for division, and thus, two sister chromatids held together at the centromere are seen. The amount of time needed for preparing and interpreting the karyotype, the necessity for well-educated, skilled personnel, and the cost of equipment and materials have made this a relatively expensive procedure. Amniotic fluid cell and fibroblast cultures take longer to grow, and these and bone marrow preparations are more difficult to work with and to

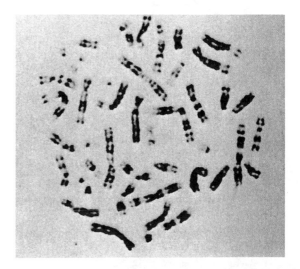

FIGURE 5.5   Giemsa banded chromosome spread.

interpret. The increasing use of automated and computerized systems decreases technician time and the time period necessary to obtain results. These include robotic harvesters and computerized imaging systems. In the latter, the computer can "cut" the chromosome images while the technician classifies them, or the computer can create the karyotype for review and correction if necessary. By knowing some of what the process entails, the nurse can be prepared to explain the reason for the long time it may take to get results and the high cost of the procedure. Sometimes rapid techniques are used so that cytogenetic information can be available in 24 to 48 hours. These are usually for fetal or neonatal problems. Much more detail for the interested reader can be found in Gersen and Keagle (1999), Rooney (2001), Czepulkowski (2001), and Keagle (2004).

A variety of staining methods can be used, depending on what type of information is needed from the chromosome analysis. Each chromosome has its own individual unique banding pattern and, therefore, can be identified with certainty. In the United States, the most frequent routine banding method used is Giemsa (G) banding, which produces light and dark bands on each chromosome in a unique manner. These bands are produced by using trypsin or another chemical to remove some chromosomal protein before staining. Quinacrine (Q) banding makes use of dyes that bind to the DNA in chromosomes and fluoresce in various degrees of brilliance under ultraviolet light. It has been especially useful for the identification of, and studies involving, the Y chromosome but has largely been replaced by other techniques. Other relatively common types of banding are C banding, which stains the centromere darkly and is useful for detecting some inversions; R banding, which produces a banding pattern that is the reverse of G and Q banding and was especially useful to visualize the terminal ends of chromosomes and detect terminal deletions; and silver staining that stains only the active nucleolar organizing regions (NOR), which are the areas that possess the DNA that codes for certain ribosomal RNA. Other more specialized techniques are available for specific purposes and in some cases newer techniques have replaced more traditional ones.

New methods of banding have made it possible to detect more subtle abnormalities such as microdeletions, small insertions, and those rearrangements that do not alter the size of the chromosome; to detect normal variants (polymorphisms) that occur within the population; and to identify fragments of chromosomes to determine their origin as well as other abnormalities. High resolution banding of prophase and prometaphase chromosomes allows a greater number of bands to be identified than the usual number (850 as opposed to 400 or 550). A karyotype with high resolution banding is shown in Figure 5.6.

Another technique is fluorescent in situ hybridization (FISH). This is a variation of in situ hybridization techniques using fluorescent dyes instead of labeled isotopes. A detailed description may be found in Rooney, 2001, and in Czepulkowski, 2001. Basically, a standard cytogenetic preparation is treated to remove excess RNA and protein, a fluorescent labeled single-stranded DNA probe is hybridized to these denatured chromosomes if there is a complementary sequence, and a signal results at the site of hybridization that can be visualized using fluorescence contrast microscopy. The fluorescent probes may be whole chromosome, satellite sequence probes, or unique sequence or gene-specific probes. Whole chromosome probes are mixtures of numerous smaller probes, and allow each chromosome to be "painted" a different color. Although FISH can be used in metaphase nuclei, it is also useful in interphase preparations, and interphase FISH can be used on uncultured cells or on direct buccal smear preparations. It requires a smaller sample than karyotyping. FISH is used to detect aneuploidy (this has made it useful for rapid screening of uncultured amniotic fluid cells in only 24 to 48 hours), the origin of marker chromosomes, detection of microdeletions, small translocations, and other small aberrations, and can be used prenatally to detect fetal cells in maternal serum. For example, FISH has been used to detect if microdeletion(s) of the *WT1* gene were present in children with aniridia to determine whether they were then at increased risk for Wilms tumor and needed ultrasound screening. Reverse painting, such as by using flow sorting or microdissection to isolate abnormal chromosomes and then label them and use them as probes in FISH on normal chromosomes, can be done. Comparative genomic hybridization (CGH) can detect chromosomal imbalances and has been used for

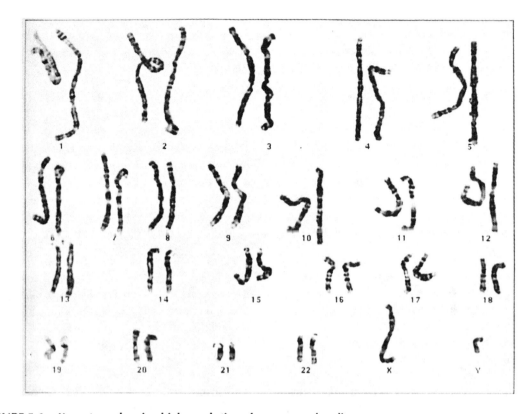

FIGURE 5.6   Karyotype showing high resolution chromosome banding.

Courtesy of Dr. Douglas Chapman, Cytogenetics Laboratory, University of Washington Medical Center, Seattle, WA.

preimplantation confirmations and in cancer cytogenetics as well as pre- and postnatally.

CGH arrays are a technique that will allow large numbers of samples to be analyzed and reduce time and cost.

DESCRIBING AND INTERPRETING THE KARYOTYPE

Karyotypes are arranged in a standardized way according to international agreement (ISCN, 1995): first, on the basis of chromosome size from the largest to smallest, and second, according to the location of the centromere (the constricted portion of the chromosome). The only exception to this is that chromosome 22 is longer than chromosome 21, but it was agreed to retain this order and nomenclature because chromosome 21 was already too well associated with Down syndrome to make such a change realistic. Chromosomes are classified according to the position of the centromere as follows: metacentric (the centromere is in the center of the chromosome); submetacentric (the centromere is slightly off center, resulting in one longer and one shorter arm); acrocentric (the centromere is very near one end of the chromosome with one very short and one very long arm); and telocentric (the centromere is at one end, but these are not seen in humans). In 1960, cytogeneticists at the first international conference on nomenclature designated the groups and the chromosome pairs belonging to each group (see Figure 5.1) as follows:

Group A	chromosomes 1 to 3	Large metacentrics
Group B	chromosomes 4 to 5	Large submetacentrics
Group C	chromosomes 6 to 12, the X	Medium-sized metacentrics and submetacentrics
Group D	chromosomes 13 to 15	Medium and large acrocentrics with satellites

Group E	chromosomes 16 to 18	Relatively short metacentrics or submetacentrics
Group F	chromosomes 19 to 20	Short metacentrics
Group G	chromosomes 21 to 22, the Y	Small acrocentrics with satellites except for the Y

It is conventional to place the sex chromosomes together at the bottom of the karyotype as shown in Figure 5.7.

To facilitate communication and to prevent confusion, a kind of shorthand system for describing the chromosome constitution of a karyotype was devised. Because these symbols are in international usage to describe the chromosome constitution of an individual, nurses should be able to interpret the meaning of at least the most commonly used symbols. These are illustrated in Table 5.3 and their usage is explained below. For some conditions, both simple and complex symbolism may be used according to the audience to which the communication is geared, or to the necessity of clarifying a precise point. For more detail, the reader is referred to ISCN (1995) which is still the accepted standard. New language that incorporates the FISH methodology (if used) has been added (see Rooney, 2001; Czepulkowski, 2001).

RULES AND EXAMPLES FOR INTERPRETING AND DESCRIBING KARYOTYPES

Both general rules and examples of their usage are given below.

1. The total number of chromosomes present is always given first, followed by the designation of the sex chromosome complement. Thus, the normal female is designated as 46,XX and the normal male as 46,XY.

Example 1: A triploid cell—69,XXY

Example 2: A tetraploid cell—92,XXYY

2. After the sex chromosome designation, it is customary to indicate chromosomes that are missing (–), extra (+), or structurally altered. The short arm of the chromosome is designated as p and the

long arm as q. If (+) or (–) is placed before the chromosome number, then this indicates extra or missing whole chromosomes (e.g., +21 or –4). If (+) or (–) is placed after the arm designation, they indicate a change in that arm length (e.g., p– is a decrease in the length of the short arm; q+ is an increase in length of the long arm). These latter designations are usually used in text rather than in a formal karyotype, and the examples of designations below may be shortened when used in text rather than in formal cytogenetic analysis. In formal cytogenetic analysis even greater detail than the examples given below may be used especially when precise breakpoints are being communicated and/or chromosome arrangements are complex.

Example 3: Trisomy 13 (Patau syndrome) in a female—47,XX+13

Example 4: Cri-du-chat or deletion of part of the short arm of chromosome 5 in a male—46, del(5)(p15.2)

Example 5: A male with monosomy 21—45, XY,–21

Example 6: A female with trisomy 18 and monosomy 22—46,XX,+18,–22

Example 7: A male with 46 chromosomes that includes a ring chromosome 3 that affects a single chromosome—46,XY,r(3)(p10q22)

Example 8: A female with a direct or interstitial duplication of the segment between bands q22 and 224 on the long arm of chromosome 1—46,XX,dup(1)(q22q24)

Example 9: In a male, a reciprocal translocation has occurred between the long arm of one chromosome 5, which has been exchanged with a segment from the short arm of one chromosome 8. The t(5;8) indicates the translocation between chromosomes 5 and 8 and the (q31.1;p23.1) indicates the breakpoints in chromosomes 5 (q31.1) and 8 (p23.1)—46,XY,t(5:8)(q31.1;p23.1)

Example 9B: A Robertsonian translocation is a particular type of tranlocation in which the long arms of the acrocentric chromosomes 13 through 15 and 21–22 are involved and centric fusion may occur. In a female, a Robertsonian translocation between the long arms of chromosomes 13 and 21 may be written as 45,XX,der(13;21)(q10:q10). This female has 45 chromosomes including one normal chromosome 13, and one normal

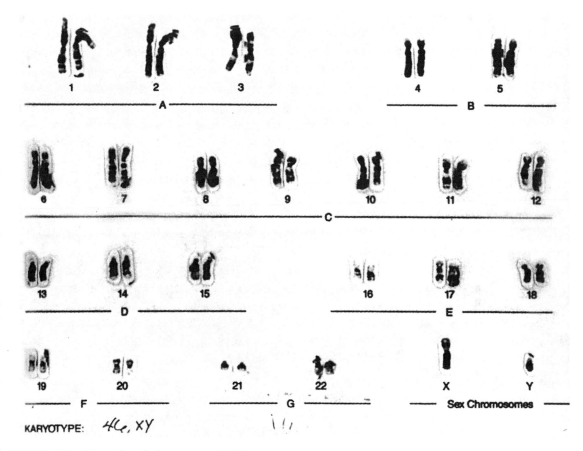

KARYOTYPE: 46, XY

FIGURE 5.7   Normal male karyotype, 46,XY.
Courtesy of Dr. V. Kimonis, Southern Illinois University School of Medicine, Springfield, IL.

chromosome 21 as well as one derivative or translocation chromosome replacing one chromosome 13 and one chromosome 21 instead of the usual two of each. The short arms of chromosomes 13 and 21 involved in the translocation may be lost.

3. Different cell lines in the same individual are separated by a slash.

Example 10: A male who is mosaic for trisomy 21—47,XY,+21/46,XY or mos 47,XY,+21/46,XY

Example 11: A female mosaic who has three cell lines—45,X/47,XXX/46,XX or mos 45,X/47,XXX/46,XX

4. If one wishes to indicate a specific point on a chromosome, this is done by giving, in the following order, the number of the chromosome, the chromosome arm (q or p), the region number, the band number, and in some cases, if a band is subdivided, a sub-band. If sub-bands are subdivided

further, there may be an additional digit but no period (see Figure 5.1). An example of both a short and a detailed way to indicate the same terminal deletion of chromosome 3 in a male with 46 chromosomes is as follows:

Example 12: 46,XY,del(3)(q22) or 46,XY,del(3) (pter→q22:) The single colon in the latter case indicates a break in the long arm of chromosome 3 with deletion of the rest of the segment, and the retention in the cell of all of the short arm of chromosome 3 and the portion of the long arm between the centromere and region 2, band 2.

Example 13: For 3 sub-bands in the short arm of chromosome 1 one would write 1p31.1, 1p31.2, 1p31.3 (sub-band 1p31.1 is closest or proximal to the centromere and 1p31.3 is distal). An example of further subdivision of sub-band 1p31.2 would be 1p31.21, 1p31.22 and so on.

TABLE 5.3   Symbols and Nomenclature Used to Describe Karyotypes

Symbol	Karyotype
A-G	the chromosome group
1-22	the autosome numbers
X,Y	the sex chromosome
diagonal (/)	separates cell lines in describing mosaicism
plus sign (+) or minus sign (−)	placed immediately before the autosome number, indicates that the chromosome is extra or missing; placed immediately after the arm, structural, or other designation, indicates an increase or decrease in length
(?)	questionable identification of chromosome or structure
(*)	chromosome or structure explained in text or footnote
:	break—no reunion, as in terminal deletion
::	break and join
→	from-to
( )	parentheses, used to enclose altered chromosomes
ace	acentric
cen	centromere
chi	chimera
cs	chromosome
del	deletion
der	derivative chromosome
dic	dicentric
dis	distal
dup	duplication
end	endoreduplication
e	exchange
f	fragment
g	gap
h	secondary constriction or negatively staining region
i	isochromosome
inv	inversion
inv ins	inverted insertion
inv (p−q+) or inv (p+q−)	pericentric inversion
mar	marker chromosome, unknown origin
mat	maternal origin
mn	modal number
mos	mosaic
p	short arm or chromosome (pter: end of short arm)
pat	paternal origin
prx	proximal
q	long arm of chromosome (qter: end of long arm)
r	ring chromosome
s	satellite
sce	sister chromatid exchange
t	translocation
rcp	reciprocal translocation
rob	Robertsonian translocation
tan	tandem translocation
ter	terminal or end

5. Sometimes "shorthand" forms are used in nontechnical literature.

Example 14: Cri-du-chat can be referred to as 5p− or del(5p) without any other designation, a translocation between chromosomes 8 and 22 is written as t(8;22) with no further designation. A semicolon is used to separate the chromosomes involved in the translocation. Another "shorthand" is to use a + or − sign to indicate an increase or decrease in the length of a chromosome arm. An inversion of chromosome 3 might be shortened to inv(2), or a ring chromosome 18 to (18),

while double satellites on the short arm of chromosome 22 may be designated as 21 pss.

CHROMOSOME STUDIES: WHEN AND WHY

Chromosome studies may be needed at any age depending on the indication. Reasons to recommend prenatal chromosome diagnosis are discussed in chapter 12. Current indications for other age groups are summarized in Table 5.4. Some of these reasons are discussed in more detail next.

TABLE 5.4   Current Indications for Chromosome Analysis in Different Phases of the Life Span*

Indication	Antenatal	Newborn/ Infant	Child	Adolescent	Adult
Two or more dysmorphic features or anomalies		X	X	†	†
Mental retardation		X	X	†	†
Infertility or premature menopause					X
History of two or more spontaneous abortions or stillbirths					X
Neonatal death		X			
Stillbirth or spontaneous abortion	X				
Confirmation of a suspected syndrome	X	X	X	X	X
Ambiguous genitalia		X	X	X	†
Inguinal masses/hernia in female		X	X		
Failure to thrive		X			
Short stature (especially female)			X	X	†
Low birth weight (small-for-date)		X			
Developmental delay		X	X		
Amenorrhea (female)				X	†
Failure to develop secondary sex characteristics				X	†
Structural chromosome error in family member			X	X	X
Small genitalia (males)				X	†
Cancer (varies with type)		X	X	X	X
Hydatidiform mole	X	X			
Gynecomastia (male)				X	
Cryptorchidism (male)			X	†	
Lymphedema (female)		X			
Unexplained appearance of an autosomal or X-linked recessive disorder (female)		X	X	X	X

*Prenatal indications are discussed in chapter 12.
X = primary indication
†If not previously investigated and explained.

Although the nurse may or may not be responsible for directly ordering chromosome studies, he or she should be able to identify individuals who may benefit from such studies and refer them to the geneticist or recommend such a course of action to the physician.

Some indications are most likely to be noticed at certain ages (e.g., dysmorphic features should be noticed and accounted for before adulthood), but they should not be ignored if present later in life, as sometimes individuals "slip through the cracks." General reasons for undertaking chromosome study common to all indications listed below are for genetic counseling of the individual and/or family members, reproductive planning, prenatal diagnosis, initiation of early treatment if needed, realistic life planning including anticipatory guidance, and goal setting for the affected individual and family. In addition, specific reasons are added where salient.

Suspicion of a Known Syndrome or Presence of a Known Chromosome Variant in Family Member, Parent, or Sibling

No one anomaly is exclusive to any one chromosome syndrome and many abnormalities such as growth retardation and mental retardation are common to most of the chromosomal syndromes. Therefore, even a suspected classic chromosome disorder such as Down syndrome must always be confirmed by chromosome diagnosis. The same disorder can arise from different chromosomal mechanisms (an example is translocation Down syndrome as opposed to trisomy 21), or from nongenetic mechanisms. It is important to distinguish among these in order to provide accurate genetic counseling and opportunity for prenatal diagnosis. For these same reasons, parents who have had a previous child or family member with an error or persons who have a family member with a chromosome error should have chromosome analysis for the reasons just given.

Unexpected Appearance of an Autosomal Recessive Disorder or of an X-linked Recessive Disorder in a Female

The unexpected appearance of an autosomal recessive disorder in cases where both parents are not carriers suggests the possibility of a chromosomal explanation, uniparental disomy or nonpaternity, adoption, or an assisted reproductive technology in which one or both parents is not the natural parent. Sometimes these disorders appear because the affected individual has one mutant gene for the recessive disorder, and a microdeletion involving the normal copy of that gene on another chromosome. Thus, one copy of the mutant gene is expressed and seen in the phenotype. The same can happen in an X-linked recessive disorder in which there is a small deletion of the chromosome section with the normal gene, allowing the carrier female to express the disorder because the mutant gene has, in effect, no opposition. Another explanation may be uniparental disomy. In this case, both chromosomal homologues are inherited from the same parent instead of inheriting one copy of each chromosome pair from the mother and one from the father (for example, two maternal chromosome 7 homologues amd no paternal chromosome 7). This is further explained in chapter 4.

Ambiguous Genitalia

Most ambiguous genitalia are detected at birth or in early infancy. Traditionally it has been considered a medical emergency because the sex in which to raise the child is seen as needing to be determined as quickly and early as possible, and because of psychological reasons for the parents and family. The establishment of chromosomal sex constitution is one component of this process that also may involve reconstructive surgery, psychological counseling, and ongoing support by the nurse. In recent years, some adult persons who had ambiguous genitalia have advocated waiting until adolescence or adulthood for the person to choose their preferred sex. A recent study of women with intersex conditions and ambiguous genitalia (Minto, Liao, Woodhouse, Ransley, & Creighton, 2003) indicated ongoing sexual problems into adulthood, thus underscoring the need for counseling and support.

Two or More Dysmorphic Features or Anomalies

Because it is unusual for two defects to occur in the same person, if chromosome analysis is not undertaken small abnormalities may go undiagnosed. Such analysis is needed to differentiate a defect related to a chromosome abnormality from one caused by intrauterine infection, teratogen exposure, a single-gene disorder, or another cause for counseling and prognostic purposes. One cannot conclude that such anomalies are isolated defects unless a chromosome error is excluded as one possibility.

Spontaneous Abortion, Stillbirth, or Neonatal Death

In cases of spontaneous abortion, stillbirth, or neonatal death, material should be obtained for chromosome study as quickly as possible. This should be done whether or not external malformations are visible. The rate of failure for tissue culture is higher than usual in these situations, so several samples from different tissues should be obtained since there will not be an opportunity for a second specimen. Blood samples can be placed in a heparinized tube, whereas other tissues, especially from the skin, pericardium, spleen, or thymus, can be placed in individual bottles to tissue culture medium, never in formalin. Nurses should ensure the availability of such equipment and either collect or recommend the collection of such specimens, depending on the circumstances. A specific protocol should be developed for the medical unit, inpatient or outpatient, with all equipment available. Photographs of the head, face, body, and especially of any unusual features should also be obtained; physical measurements, a detailed written description of the physical findings, and a complete pathologist's report are essential. Often radiology also needs to be done, and if there is doubt, then it should be carried out. An inadequate study at this time leads to the inability of the genetic counselor to discuss the couple's chance for a future affected child, another stillbirth, or spontaneous abortion. Ample protocols are given in American College of Obstetricians and Gynecologists (1996).

Infertility or Premature Menopause

Although chromosome disorders do not account for the majority of infertile couples, it has been determined that 10% to 15% have a chromosome anomaly present in one member, ranging from an undiscovered sex chromosome disorder to

chromosome rearrangements such as balanced translocations. Premature menopause/ovarian failure is discussed under 47,XXX. Breakpoints in chromosome 1 have been implicated in male infertility by Bache et al. (2004).

History of Two or More Spontaneous Abortions, Stillbirths, or Neonatal Deaths

The incidence of chromosome abnormalities in these cases was discussed earlier. About 10% of couples with recurrent abortions have a chromosome anomaly in one member. Among couples who have recurrent abortions plus a previous stillborn infant, the incidence of chromosome abnormalities has been estimated at 15–25%. The risk of another spontaneous abortion is about 25% after one, and greater if the couple has no live-born offspring. The risk is also greater if the embryo had a normal chromosome complement. Hogge and colleagues (2003) estimate that about 2% to 4% of couples have two spontaneous abortions by chance alone. Patients who had three or more spontaneous abortions had 50% chance for the next loss to be due to aneuploidy. They found an association with maternal age in that 80% of pregnancy losses in women over 35 years of age were due to chromosomal abnormalities. After a chromosomally abnormal pregnancy loss, the outcome for a successful future pregnancy exceeds 75% but, for example, a history of a trisomic pregnancy puts a woman at increased risk for an aneuploid conception (Munné et al., 2004)

Hernia/Inguinal Mass in the Female

It is possible that this may represent a Y-bearing gonad or testis as in the testicular feminization syndrome. The phenotype is female, but the chromosome constitution is male. Some believe the mass should be removed to prevent the common sequelae of neoplastic development, whereas others prefer to leave it in place until after puberty.

Hydatidiform Mole

Pregancies resulting in hydatidiform moles may be of normal or abnormal chromosome constitutions such as triploidy. Those with diploid chromosome constitutions have a risk for malignant transformation into choriocarcinomas. There is a recurrence risk of about 1% following a molar pregnancy.

Failure to Develop Secondary Sexual Characteristics, Amenorrhea (Females), Proportional Short Stature (Females), Gynecomastia (Males), Lymphedema or Webbed Neck (Female Infant), Cryptorchidism (Males), Small Genitalia (Males).

These findings are very common in a variety of chromosome abnormalities, particularly of the sex chromosomes, and therefore should be explored as soon as possible because an early diagnosis allows optimal management (for example, maximum height attainment in Turner syndrome) and in order to provide genetic counseling, treatment where indicated and possible, and the other aims discussed.

Cancer

More than 90% of persons with chronic myeloid leukemia have a characteristic translocation [t{9;22}] in their bone marrow. Other cancers also show distinct cytogenetic abnormalities. Such studies are useful for diagnosis, treatment choice, and prognosis (see chapter 23).

Mental Retardation, Failure to Thrive, Developmental Delay, and Low Birth Weight

These are found with such great frequency in so many of the chromosome disorders that they are an indication for chromosome analysis. An individual feature such as developmental delay is not itself diagnostic but the reason needs to be determined.

TELLING THE PARENTS THAT THEIR CHILD HAS A CHROMOSOME DISORDER

In the chromosome disorders, physical abnormalities are often readily apparent, with diagnostic procedures begun immediately after birth, or,

especially in the sex chromosome disorders, these abnormalities may not be detected until late childhood, adolescence, or even adulthood. The shock of diagnosis and the coping with this information is discussed fully in chapter 8.

Consecutive screening of newborns for chromosome abnormalities was often done in the 1960s without the informed consent or even the knowledge of the parent. These programs were largely discontinued in this country because of the debate over the ethical problems engendered, some of which are discussed in chapters 20 and 27. One major issue was what (if anything) to tell parents whose infant is found to have a sex chromosome abnormality or other variation but who appeared phenotypically normal. Because severe autosomal abnormalities are usually visible, the problems are different (see chapters 8 and 9).

Special Issues in Discussing Sex Chromosome Variation

One of the major problems involved is whether behavior associated with sex chromosome aneuploidy is (1) inevitable and not dependent on external influences, or (2) modifiable by developmental experience. If the latter is true, is it better to (1) tell the parents what has been found?, and (2) if so, when?, or (3) is it better to conceal this information? The results of several long-term developmental studies have now been reported that shed some light on the development of the individual with a sex chromosome disorder, but the question of whether or not to tell the parent, and what to tell them, still engenders debate in some arenas, particularly if the findings are incidental while testing for something else. Current trends favor disclosure with honesty about what is and is not known.

Some favorable aspects of disclosing the information include the following:

1. Health professionals can work with the family to minimize any risk (e.g., by counseling, remedial classes, provisions for special skill development, optimum treatment, etc.).
2. Genetic counseling and prenatal diagnosis options can be provided.
3. "Old wives' tales" and media distortion of syndromes can be discussed and counteracted.

4. There is an opportunity to confront feelings early and work them out.
5. Researchers can study individuals and obtain more reliable information about actual growth and development.
6. If information is concealed and the child later has problems that cause the disorder to come to light, the parents will direct hostility, anger, and mistrust against the health professionals.

Although current standards favor full disclosure, some reasons for nondisclosure have included the following.

1. Telling the parents about their child's condition can lead to rejection, failure of parent-infant bonding, and a situation of self-fulfilling prophecy.
2. Actual outcomes are not known in many cases so it is difficult to provide accurate predictions.
3. Parents may view the child as handicapped.
4. Confidentiality may be difficult to protect, especially in smaller communities.
5. Normal behavioral variation may be seen as abnormal.
6. The child may be stigmatized and treated as different.

Valentine (1982) stated that after watching the normal development of a 47,XYY boy to age 10 years, when the family refused further study, he wished that they had not been told of his altered sex-chromosome constitution. In what is said to be the last report on a small number of adults with certain sex-chromosome variations (45,X; 47,XXX; 47,XXY) followed from childhood, despite various described setbacks when compared with sibling controls, overall adaptation was positive (Bender, Linden, & Harmon, 2001).

Some basic points are relevant for nurses.

1. Family strengths should be noted and built upon.
2. Basic family dynamics should be observed, and care should be taken not to introduce new stresses e.g., from whom the abnormality might have arisen if not determined).

3. When the parent is told, the term chromosome "variation" can be stressed, instead of abnormality.
4. Because the only association parents may have with chromosomes is Down syndrome, the parent should be reassured that the child does not have Down syndrome.
5. Some recommend that the parents be told that their child has a chromosome variation in stages, several months after birth, so that bonding has already occurred. However, one danger is that families may not continue in the same health care system and may not get the full information.
6. Parental anxiety and guilt feelings require further discussion, repetition, and counseling.
7. A trust relationship should be carefully developed; this means that some team member must be easily accessible to them, even on weekends and evenings.
8. With the parents, a decision should be made on how much information should be given to the child at developmental stages so that the family does not develop a situation where there is an open "secret" that everyone knows but no one discusses.
9. It should be emphasized that sex chromosome variations have no bearing on determining the sexual preferences of the person. More specific points are discussed later in this chapter. A recent study (Mezei et al., 2004) examined parental decision making when prenatal diagnosis revealed sex chromosome aneuploidy. The choice of pregnancy termination was made more frequently for pregnancies with 45,X and 47,XXY fetuses than for 47,XXX, 47,XYY, and various mosaic karyotypes. This is largely attributed to more recent information about those conditions as discussed later in this chapter.

AUTOSOMES AND THEIR ABNORMALITIES

The severity of the consequences of numerical abnormalities in the autosomes is illustrated by their high percentage of loss before birth. Of the trisomies lost in spontaneous abortion, about 15% are trisomy 16, which is interesting because no live-born case (except for mosaics) has been confirmed. Defects of those chromosomes known to have the most active gene loci are more likely to be incompatible with life. Thus only three trisomies (13, 18, and 21) are relatively common among live-born infants. Other trisomies and the monosomies are almost always seen only as mosaics that include a normal cell line, the assumption being that enough normal cells are present to be compatible with life. A variety of structural changes of every chromosome has been reported. Each individual one is extremely rare. Relatively common ones (1:20,000 to 1:50,000) include cri-du-chat (5p−), DiGeorge/velocardiofacial syndrome [(del)22q11.2], and Wolf-Hirchhorn syndrome (4p−). Information about the rarer (less than 100 reported cases) chromosome abnormalities can be found in Jones (1997) and in Gorlin, Cohen, and Hennekam (2001).

In any of the trisomies, but especially Down syndrome, the actual error can be caused either by the presence of a free extra chromosome or by one that is translocated to another chromosome. In translocations, the chromosomal material of 47 chromosomes, and therefore three copies of each gene are present instead of the normal two, but the chromosome count is 46. This illustrates one reason that a full chromosome analysis is necessary. The risks for recurrence are very different for translocations as opposed to free trisomies. For example, in Down syndrome, if one parent has 45 chromosomes and a translocation of chromosome 21 to chromosome 14, then the gametes they produce can theoretically result in six possible combinations in a zygote, which are shown in Figure 5.8. In theory, the chance of each of these occurring is equal, and because three of the six outcomes result in nonviable offspring, the chances of a normal child, a balanced translocation carrier like the parent, or one with Down syndrome would each be one-third. In practice, the distribution is observed to be different. If the female is the translocation carrier, then the actual observed risk is 10% to 15% for having a child with Down syndrome; whereas if the male is the carrier, it is 5% to 8%. The risk for having a normal-appearing child who, like the parent, is a translocation carrier is about 45% to 50%. In either case, the option of prenatal diagnosis should be explained to the parents. If both chromosomes 21s are involved in the translocation in the parent, 45,XX, t(21;21) or 45,XY, t(21;21) then

only Down syndrome offspring can result because the monosomic alternative is nonviable; thus, the risks in this type for parents to have a child with Down syndrome is 100%. Such parents should have genetic counseling that includes discussion of other reproductive options. Although more children with translocation Down syndrome are born to women under 30 years of age than over 30 years of age, assumptions as to cause can never be made. Chromosome analysis *must* be done.

The birth of a child with multiple visible defects requires parents to mourn the loss of their imagined "perfect" child before they can accept their infant. Parent-child bonding is often impaired. These issues are discussed fully in chapter 8. In all the syndromes discussed next, the most commonly found features are given. Affected persons do not always have all of these together, and they may also have other abnormalities. Diagnosis cannot be made on a clinical basis alone; chromosome studies are essential. The degree of mosaicism, if present, can also act to modify findings and prognosis. For a karyotype illustrating the major autosomal and sex chromosome abnormalities, see Figure 5.9.

In the severe autosomal anomalies other than Down syndrome, many affected individuals die relatively soon after delivery or in the first year of life because multiple, severe, life-threatening problems are present. Some, particularly those who are less severely affected or who are mosaic, do survive, and parents often have angry feelings toward professionals who may have told them that their child would not live beyond a certain age. Thus it is important to provide accurate information in a sensitive manner. One parent organization specifically for the rare chromosome disorders is the Support Organization for Trisomy 18, 13, and Related Disorders (http://www.trisomy.org). Progress has been made in the prenatal detection of trisomies 13, 18, and 21 through maternal serum screening and ultrasonography (see chapter 12).

Trisomy 21 (Down Syndrome)

First described as mongolian idiocy by Dr. John Langdon Down in 1866, Down syndrome is the most common chromosome abnormality in liveborns. It was the first chromosome abnormality associated (by Lejeune) with a specific chromosome, three copies of chromosome 21. Clinical

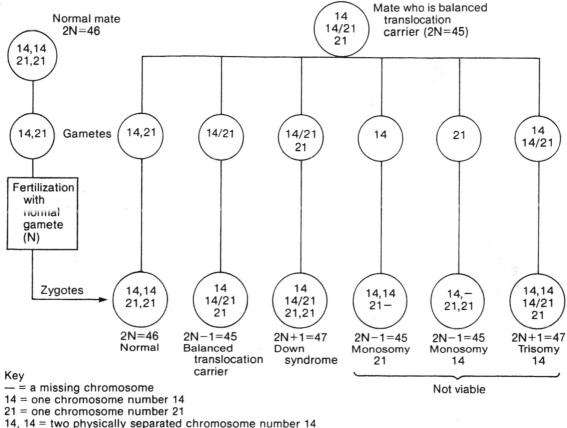

Key
— = a missing chromosome
14 = one chromosome number 14
21 = one chromosome number 21
14, 14 = two physically separated chromosome number 14
21, 21 = two physically separated chromosome number 21
14/21 = a translocation chromosome, consisting of the long arms of chromosome number 14 and the long
      arms of chromosome number 21

FIGURE 5.8   Possible reproductive outcomes of a 14/21 balanced translocation carrier.

features can vary greatly, as shown in Figure 5.10. There is no way, other than chromosome analysis, to tell if a free trisomy (about 95%), a translocation (about 5%), or mosaicism is present. About 90% of the time the extra chromosome is of maternal origin. The exact band responsible for the Down phenotype has been identified; the presence of the entire extra chromosome is not necessary in order to produce it. The karyotype of a patient with Down syndrome with a 14/21 translocation is shown in Figure 5.11. The author continues to stress the need for chromosome analysis because, even in recent years, a client was seen whose child with Down syndrome had never had chromosome study due to the assumption of the diagnosis because of the "characteristic appearance." Accurate genetic counseling before another pregnancy

could not be accomplished until chromosome studies were done.

Children with Down syndrome do tend to resemble each other, but no physical feature is in itself diagnostic. Hypotonia is a frequent early feature, and infants are often floppy. Mental retardation is consistent; the degree varies, and the typical IQ range is said to be mild to moderate impairment with some individuals achieving an IQ that is near low normal, and a few experiencing severe impairment. The limbs are typically short; the hands are often broad with an incurved 5th finger (clinodactyly) and a single transverse (simian) crease. This crease, commonly associated with Down syndrome, is found in about 50% of cases, and in 5% to 10% of the normal population (Figure 5.12). Features are usually flattened; the tongue

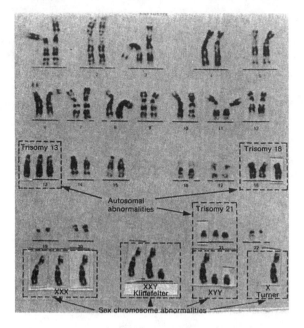

FIGURE 5.9 G-banded karyotype illustrating the major chromosome abnormalities in a composite.

may protrude because of the high arched narrow palate; and the nose is small with a flat nasal bridge, leading to feeding and breathing difficulties. Parents need assistance from the nurse in solving these problems. If the mother is breast-feeding, she needs additional patience and support from the nurse as sucking may be weak. Snuffling is common. Sleep apnea has also been noted. Epicanthic folds and Brushfield spots (light speckling of the edge of the iris) are found in about 50% but are also present in normal individuals. The eyes may slant upward (oblique palpebral fissure). The Moro reflex is usually absent. Joints are hyperflexible. The feet usually show wide spaces between the first and second toes. Otitis media and hearing impairment are relatively common and evaluation for hearing loss should begin in the newborn period and continue periodically throughout life. Ocular problems such as nystagmus, myopia, strabismus, glaucoma, and cataracts also may begin early so that screening should occur soon after birth. Examination by a pediatric ophthalmologist is desirable. Thyroid problems are also common and need to be observed for. Various dental problems such as missing or unusual teeth or orthodontic problems may occur later.

Congenital heart defects are present in 40% to 60%. The most common types are atrioventricular

septal defects, ventricular septal defects, and tetralogy of Fallot. Despite advances in surgical correction, they are a major cause of early death. The risk for leukemia is elevated, especially acute myeloid leukemia. A transient form of leukema (transient myeloproliferative disorder) develops in about 10% of newborns with Down syndrome. There is a high remission rate but some children experience a relapse. Duodenal atresia and other gastrointestinal problems such as megacolon may be seen. Orthopedic problems such as scoliosis, late hip dislocation, and foot deformities can occur. Seizures have also been noted to occur more often in children with Down syndrome.

Persons with Down syndrome require regular childhood care such as immunizations, and growth monitoring with standards appropriate to Down syndrome. In addition, special attention needs to be paid to the eyes (for problems such as strabismus, myopia, etc.), to the ears (for otitis media, and hearing loss), and for thyroid function in addition to monitoring for heart disease, hematologic problems, orthopedic problems, gastrointestinal disorders, and others as detailed. Thus persons

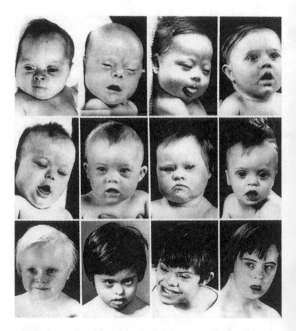

FIGURE 5.10 Photos of children with Down syndrome: A spectrum.

Source: From Tolksdorf, M., & Wiedemann, H-R. (1981). Clinical aspects of Down syndrome from infancy to adult life. *Human Genetics* (Suppl. 2, 3). Used with permission.

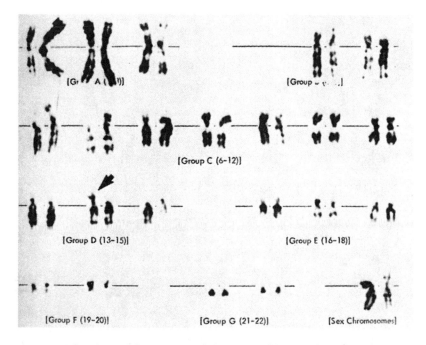

FIGURE 5.11   Karyotype of patient with Down syndrome caused by translocation of chromosome 21 to 14.
Courtesy of Dr. V. Kimonis, Southern Illinois University School of Medicine, Springfield, IL.

with Down syndrome require ongoing medical treatment and often surgical procedures, which may be difficult for both the affected person and the family. Referral should be made for such programs as Supplemental Security Income and other programs. Detailed guidelines for health management and for sports and activities have been developed by the American Academy of Pediatrics (2001), Cohen (1999), Roizen (2002), Saenz (1999) and Smith (2001). Early intervention programs and support can be very beneficial. A wide variety of lay publications are available for families. See Appendix B for support organizations.

Males are usually infertile, and have hypogonadism, whereas females can be fertile (although not frequently), and of those with free trisomy, about half of her offspring will have Down syndrome and half will be normal. At one time, involuntary sterilization of a person with Down syndrome was almost routinely carried out in many institutions and is still on the books as law in some states, although rarely invoked (see chapter 20). It is important to provide sex education appropriate to the developmental level of the person with

Down syndrome. Socially acceptable sexual behavior should also be taught. Many parents need help in recognizing the sexuality of their adolescent or young adult. Appropriate contraceptive information and care should also be provided. Guidelines for help in teaching sexuality to persons with Down syndrome for both parents and professionals should be obtained.

Premature aging and development of early Alzheimer disease is a notable feature of Down syndrome. Mortality due to respiratory infection has been reduced, but can still be significant in the first few years of life. The rest live to about age 50 to 55 years, and about 45% of live-born infants survive to 60 years of age. The majority who do so are employed in some setting. It is only relatively recently that health professionals have addressed attention to problems of adolescents and adults with Down syndrome. Examples of health promotional programs include those directed at weight control especially for those with Down syndrome. Many believe that persons with Down syndrome are uniformly happy, friendly, and "good." While most tend to be, others can be stubborn, mischievous,

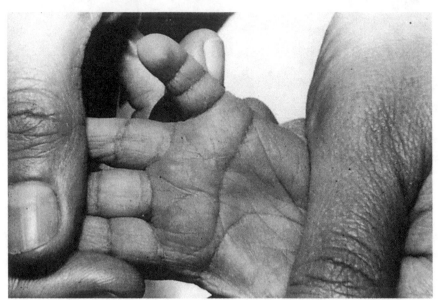

FIGURE 5.12   Mid-Palmar transverse crease.

and poorly coordinated. Smith (2001) estimates that 13% have serious emotional problems. Families may require ongoing psychological support and counseling.

The severity of the disorder and the degree of developmental delay is not as evident in the infant as it later becomes, making it hard for the parents to accept the diagnosis. Many parents I have seen have believed that their child would eventually be normal. It takes time for the impact of the diagnosis to sink in and for realistic decision making to occur. Support is essential, and it should be suggested to the parents that they enroll their baby in an early intervention program as part of the effort to maximize potential. Many persons with Down syndrome function at a higher social than intellectual level.

Various therapies have been proposed for use with children with Down syndrome. Human growth hormone to improve height has been used but is not standard practice. Detailed age-related health and prevention guidelines have been published specific for various ages that supplement standard pediatric care. New information for adults with Down syndrome is becoming available. Adults with Down syndrome require care from clinicians who understand the syndrome and its manifestations and can provide sensitive, coordinated care. As described in chapter 12, Down syndrome may be detected by maternal serum screening for multiple serum analytes and ultrasound. It can be diagnosed prenatally by chromosome analysis of material obtained by amniocentesis and chorionic villus sampling (CVS) as can other chromosomal variations.

Trisomy 18 (Edwards Syndrome)

Edwards syndrome is the second most common autosomal trisomy and more than 130 abnormalities have been recognized in patients who have this disease. There is a 3:1 ratio of females to males. The most common of the severe defects is congenital heart disease (90%). Birth weight is low, and infants are very feeble with a weak cry and poor sucking capacity, leading to failure to thrive. A small jaw (micrognathia), recessed chin, prominent occiput, extreme rigidity, overlapping fingers with hypoplastic nails, "rocker bottom" feet, low-set malformed ears, mental retardation, a short sternum, and a small pelvis are among the most common abnormalities found. Umbilical artery aneurysm with a single umbilical artery is an apparent prenatal feature identified by ultrasound as are others. The probability of survival to 1 month of age is about 39%, whereas 70% die by 3 months of age. Only about 10% usually survive the first year, and they are severely to profoundly retarded. Girls are significantly more likely than boys to live longer than 1 month. Most deaths result from cardiopulmonary arrest. The natural history is described by Baty, Blackburn, and Carey (1994), and in their series of 50 children with trisomy 18, some skills were acquired and survival to early adulthood did occur. Prenatal screening advances can now detect trisomy 18 at about 80% by second trimester ultrasound, and may also be detected by analysis of multiple maternal serum markers as described in chapter 12.

Trisomy 13 (Patau Syndrome)

Infants with Patau syndrome have more severe external malformations than do the other trisomies, and is the rarest autosomal trisomy that is liveborn. The most common constellation of symptoms is cleft lip and palate, polydactyly, and eye defects such as microphthalmia or absence of the eyes. Only 60% to 80% have all three present. The hands are often held in a clenched position, and various deformities of the hands and nails are common. The birth weight is low. Retardation is extremely severe, with many having incomplete forebrain development. The persistence of fetal hemoglobin is common. Most have congenital heart disease, renal and reproductive tract abnormalities, malformed ears and deafness, and hemangiomas. A "punched out" type of scalp defect that is sometime confused with damage from a fetal monitor may be seen. Patau syndrome is illustrated in Figure 5.13.

The defect is so profound that the probability to survival to 1 month of age is 30%, about 8.6% survive the first year, and by three years of age 95% die. A few survive to late childhood. In those who do survive, some skills may be acquired such as walking and toileting. Failure to thrive and periods of apnea are common in infancy. The appearance of such an infant is devastating to the parents, and much support is needed. Some believe that corrective surgery and prolongation of life by medical means should not be undertaken because of the severity of the defects and the poor prognosis. Others disagree. Baty, Blackburn and Carey (1994) studied development in 12 children with trisomy 13. They found a developmental deterioration from early to late childhood. However, some children were walking and had some toileting skills. One child in their study was 13 years of age.

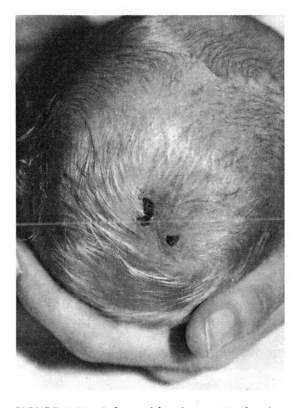

FIGURE 5.13   Infant with trisomy 13 showing characteristic scalp defect.

From "Genetic Diseases and Birth Defects," by R. M. Bannerman, 1981. In L. Iffy & H. A. Kaminetzky (Eds.), *Principles and Practice of Obstetrics and Perinatology* (Vol. 1). New York: John Wiley. Used with permission.

This syndrome results from having three copies of chromosome 13, either free or as a translocation. If of the translocation type, parents should have chromosome studies, even if they do not plan more children, because siblings may be translocation carriers as discussed previously. Nurses should explain the reason for the desirability of such analysis to the parents. Second trimester ultrasound screening can detect 90% or more.

Cri-du-chat Syndrome (5p- Syndrome, Deletion 5p Syndrome)

The most distinctive feature of this deletion of the short arm of chromosome 5 is the unusual catlike mewing cry of the infant. Valentine (1975) described the occasion when such an infant was in the hospital nursery and the "cleaning woman hearing the cry spent some time searching for the stray kitten." The cry, which arises from abnormal laryngeal development, normalizes after a few weeks. In typical cases, the birth weight is low, with severe mental and growth retardation. Microcephaly, hypotonia, round face with poorly formed, low-set ears, hypertelorism, epicanthic folds, and a transverse crease are the most common findings. These infants very closely resemble each other, more so than most other chromosomal syndromes. Nurses can anticipate the occurrence of respiratory and feeding problems that commonly occur and can take preventative precautions. Scoliosis and cardiovascular defects may be seen. Language delay, especially expressive, may occur. Self-injurious behavior such as headbanging and biting have been described but may be related to communication difficulties. Their lifespan is impaired only somewhat, and many reach adulthood. The IQ is usually below 30 but functioning may appear higher. Parents need assistance in long-term planning when they are ready. In about 10% to 15% of all cases, one parent is a translocation carrier, so again chromosome analysis is essential, as is the giving of information on prenatal diagnosis. The deleted chromosome is of paternal origin in 80% of cases. Some persons have deletions of the distal part of p15.3 and have profound speech delay but virtually none of the other features of cri-du-chat. Intellectual impairment is minimal in these cases. Other phenotypic variation has been found in persons with varying specific deletions of 5p15, although most features map to 5p15.2. The incidence is 1:37,000 to 1:50,000 live births.

DiGeorge/Velocardiofacial Syndrome

This syndrome has an incidence of about 1 in 3,500 live births and is due to a deletion in chromosome 22 (22q11.2). Other syndromes have also been associated with this deletion. Clinical findings vary and may include a characteristic facial appearance, palate abnormalities such as cleft palate (occult or overt), velopharyngeal incompetence, learning disabilities, conotruncal heart defects, speech and language problems, hypotonia, feeding problems, T-cell abnormalities, and thymus gland hypoplasia or aplasia. Persons with DiGeorge syndrome are at high risk for psychiatric disorders especially schizophrenia and depression as discussed

in chapter 25. The heart defects are very characteristic and many cardiologists will screen for this anomaly in children with conotruncal heart defects. Early educational, intervention, and therapeutic services are needed and Individualized Family Service Plans and Individualized Educational Plans can be helpful.

Wolf-Hirschhorn Syndrome (4p-)

This syndrome is due to deletion of a critical region on the short arm of chromosome 4, 4p16.3, and may be submicroscopic but typically involves 1/3 to 1/2 of the short arm. Clinical characteristics include microcephaly, mental retardation, congenital heart malformations, seizures, cleft palate with or without cleft lip, microcephaly, a characteristic face with hypertelorism and a wide nasal bridge, hypospadias in males, and growth retardation. The incidence is about 1 in 50,000 births and females are more commonly affected. About one-third of these children die in the first year, usually due to cardiac defects, but some survive to adulthood.

Other Autosomal Chromosome Abnormalities

Advances in cytogenetic techniques and their widespread availability have led to an increased rate of both pre- and postnatal identification of various chromosome abnormalities, including subtle changes such as microdeletions and mosaicism. Many of these abnormalities may be very rare; therefore the long-term outlook may be unknown or uncertain. This presents difficulties for both the health practitioner and for the families when attempting to make decisions about living arrangements, schooling, and so on. Literature searches may reveal some information or help to locate geneticists with experience in such care. Support groups (see Apprendix B) have arisen to help others, and such referrals can be useful for the family. Among the subtle autosomal chromosome variations that have been recently identified are microdeletions seen in (1) some cases of Sotos syndrome (syndrome with overgrowth, advanced bone age, pointed chin, macrocephaly, mental retardation due to mutation in NSD1 gene) that have microdeletions at 5q35; (2) some cases of Smith Magenis syndrome (mental retardation, sleep disturbances, low adaptive functioning, hearing impairment, short stature, cardiac anomalies) that have microdeletions at 17p11.2; and (3) some cases of idiopathic subtelomeric chromosome rearrangements such as del 22q13.3, which are associated with early hypotonia, autistic behavior, and speech and language delays; and microduplication of 22q11.2 which is a relatively new syndrome featuring velopharyngeal insufficiency as well as other features (Ensenauer et al., 2003). It is believed that as many as 6 to 10% of idiopathic mental retardation may be due to cryptic subtelomeric chromosome rearrangements (Manning et al., 2004). Deletions (some subtle or cryptic) have also been found to be a cause of phenotypic abnormalities that are seen in apparently balanced chromosomal rearrangements such as translocations or inversions probably due to gene disruption. FISH may be used for detection of subtle chromosome abnormalities and families should be referred for genetic counseling.

THE SEX CHROMOSOMES AND THEIR ABNORMALITIES

The sex chromosomes in humans are the X and the Y chromosome. Normal human females are 46,XX and normal human males are 46,XY. The X chromosome is believed to encode nearly 2,000 genes. As described in chapter 4, daughters normally receive one X chromosome from their father and one from their mother. Sons normally receive their X chromosome from their mother and their Y chromosome from their father. In females, as discussed in chapters 4 and 6, one of the two X chromosomes is inactivated within somatic cells, although a few genes apparently escape and X inactivation can be skewed. X inactivation may require a specific gene (XIST gene) to occur. The Y chromosome is one of the smallest, and has relatively few genes. The Y chromosome has been studied extensively for its use in anthropological studies through many generations (see chapter 3). The Y chromosome has a pseudoautosomal region and a Y specific region. The pseudoautosomal region on the Y has homologous sequences to the X chromosome for pairing during meiosis. Most of the Y chromosome is nonrecombining, and new genes are discovered within this region. As techniques

have advanced, it has been found that Y chromosome microdeletions are a relatively frequent genetic cause of infertility in men and is now considered to be essential to an infertility work-up.

There appears to be more tolerance to most aneuploidy in the sex chromosomes than in the autosomes (the exception being 45,X). Reasons for this include the following: (a) the very few genes known to be on the Y chromosome—examples are those for male sex determination such as the SRY gene for the testis-determining factor, one for tooth enamel, a zinc finger protein, and perhaps one for tooth size, hairy ears, and height influence; (b) only one active X chromosome is present in each somatic cell; all others are inactivated (see chapter 4).

Although nondisjunction gives rise to most of the sex chromosome abnormalities, neither 45,X nor 47,XYY is associated with increased parental age. The possible reproductive outcomes arising from meiotic nondisjunction at oogenesis and spermatogenesis are illustrated in Figure 5.14. First division nondisjunction results in no normal karyotype, whereas second division nondisjunction results in half normal and half abnormal gametes and offspring. This chart can be compared with Figure 5.3.

Considering all the sex chromosome aneuploidies together, their overall incidence is about 1 in 400 live births. The most common sex chromosome variations are those in which there is a single extra or missing X or Y chromosome, resulting in Turner syndrome (45,X), Triple X (47,XXX), Klinefelter syndrome (47,XXY), or XYY (47,XYY). Those in which more Xs or Ys are added, such as tetrasomy or pentasomy X (48,XXXX; 49,XXXXX), are rare and mental retardation is common. For sex chromosome variations, the most common mosaic conditions (some cells have a normal chromosome makeup whereas others do not) include 47,XXY/46,XX; 45,X/46,XX; 47,XXX/46,XX; and 47,XYY/46,XY. In general, those with mosaic sex chromosome abnormalities tend to show milder signs, and the degree tends to be related to the percent of abnormal cells. The identification of persons with sex chromosome abnormalities often occurs at the following points in the life cycle (examples are given in parenthesis):

- Prenatally—due to prenatal cytogenetic diagnosis (all types)

Nondisjunction in oogenesis

| | Ova | | | | | |
	First division nondisjunction		Second division nondisjunction			
Sperm	XX	O	XX	O	X	X
X	XXX	XO	XXX	XO	XX	XX
Y	XXY	YO*	XXY	YO*	XY	XY

Nondisjunction in spermatogenesis

| | Sperm | | | | | | | | | |
	First division nondisjunction		Second division nondisjunction (if of X chromosome)				Second division nondisjunction (if of Y chromosome)			
Ova	XY	O	XX	O	Y	Y	X	X	YY	O
X	XXY	XO	XXX	XO	XY	XY	XX	XX	XYY	XO
X	XXY	XO	XXX	XO	XY	XY	XX	XX	XYY	XO

FIGURE 5.14   Possible reproductive outcomes after meiotic nondisjunction of sex chromosomes.

*nonviable; X = X chromosome; Y = Y chromosome; O = no sex chromosome present.

- At birth—confirmation of prenatal diagnosis (all variations), clinical suspicion (45,X), or through newborn screening (all types)
- Childhood–due to establishing the cause of short stature (45,X), or speech or language disabilities (47,XXY)
- Adolescence—due to delayed development or absence of secondary sex characteristics (45,X; 47,XXY), delayed menarche (45,X), or short stature (45,X)
- Adulthood—due to fertility or reproductive problems (45,X; 47,XXY)

Mildly affected individuals, especially some with 47,XYY; 47,XXY; 47,XXX or mosaics may go unrecognized. Recently, a case report described the first-time diagnosis of Turner syndrome in an elderly woman, important because of predisposition to certain conditions. The relatively high frequency

of speech and language disorders in some sex chromosome disorders may indicate the desirability of screening for these disorders in these clinics.

The fact that two X chromosomes are needed sometime in development is evidenced by the abnormalities found when one is missing (Turner syndrome). The X chromosome contains determinants for ovarian function and for stature, apparently on both arms. The actual band regions that are essential for normal sex development have been identified (Xq13-q23). The four major sex chromosome variations (45,X; 47,XXX; 47,XXY; 47,XYY) are discussed below. Other disorders of sexual differentiation (e.g., testicular feminization syndrome) are not included. The major disorders are illustrated by karyotype in Figure 5.9. Sex chromosome variations appear more frequently after the use of intracytoplasmic sperm injection, a method of assisted reproductive technology.

Sex Chromatin

Barr Bodies

In 1949, observations by Barr and Bertram led to the discovery that in interphase cell nuclei of normal females, a dark staining body was present at the edge of the nucleus that was not present in normal males. It is now known that the Barr body of X chromatin is the condensed inactive X chromosome, and that it can be found in most female somatic cells. Epithelial cells from the buccal mucosa have been used for Barr body screening but other techniques are usually used currently. Nurses should be aware that certainly no genetic counseling, treatment, or decisions should be based on Barr body analysis; chromosome analysis must be done. Because, according to the Lyon hypothesis (chapter 4), only one active X chromosome can be present in a somatic cell, then in a given somatic cell:

The number of X chromosomes =
The number of Barr bodies + 1
and
The number of Barr bodies =
The number of X chromosomes − 1

Approximately 5% of polymorphonuclear leukocytes in normal females show a "drumstick," whereas males normally have none. The number of drumsticks is usually equal to the number of Barr bodies. This test is not very reliable.

Y Chromatin

The Y chromosome can also be detected in interphase cells by using the buccal smear technique and a quinacrine stain that allows the Y chromatin or bodies, if present, to brightly fluoresce as well as by FISH. The fluorescing Y bodies have a 1:1 relationship with the Y chromosome, so that normal females have none and normal males have one; whereas males with a 47,XYY constitution have two Y bodies. The reliability is not high because the Y body is seen in 25% to 50% of interphase cells in normal males, and because other chromosomes in either sex (e.g., chromosomes 3 and 13) may pick up the quinacrine dye and also fluoresce, leading to false interpretations. Y-bearing sperm can be differentiated from X-bearing sperm by this method.

Turner Syndrome (45,X)

This monosomy is usually written as 45,X. The complete absence of the X chromosome occurs in about 50%–60%, with the rest having various combinations of partial deletion, isochromosome formation, and mosaicism. In about 70% to 80% of the cases, the paternal X is missing. This may be due to paternal meiotic errors leading to abnormal sex chromosomes and their loss during mitosis. Chromosome analysis is necessary, not only for diagnostic confirmation but also because about 25% of mosaic individuals can menstruate and because those (5%–6%) with an XY cell line may be prone to malignancies such as dysgerminomas or gonadoblastomas. Patients are phenotypic females but have gonadal dysgenesis or streak ovaries. The ovaries begin to develop in the embryo but degenerate and connective tissue forms without ovarian follicles. Thus sex steroids, estrogen, and progesterone levels are low. The term "Turner syndrome" is reserved only for partial or complete X monosomy and not for other syndromes with gonadal dysgenesis. Short stature is the most consistent feature with an average untreated height attainment of about 144 cm (4'6"). Final height in those with Turner syndrome is influenced by other height-determining factors such as parental height and by the extent of ovarian failure and cardiovascular status, but may

ultimately be about 20 cm below the population mean for adult females. The genes involved are located on the short arm of the X chromosome at Xp11.2-p.22.1. The *SHOX* gene (short stature homeobox-containing gene), a member of the homeobox family discussed in chapter 2, contributes to some of the abnormalities found, such as short stature.

Many cases of Turner syndrome are detected at birth because (1) 60% to 80% show lymphedema of the hands and feet, which disappears shortly (see Figure 5.15); (2) presence of a webbed neck is noted; or (3) coarctation of the aorta or another cardiovascular anomaly is found (25%). In one case, seen by the author, an alert delivery room nurse initiated chromosome study because of lymphedema. Prenatal diagnosis is possible through chromosome analysis on amniocentesis or CVS or detection may occur through characteristics revealed on ultrasonography (see chapter 12). Other cases are detected in later childhood because of the short stature, or at puberty when secondary sex characteristics fail to develop and menstruation fails to occur. Some are not detected until

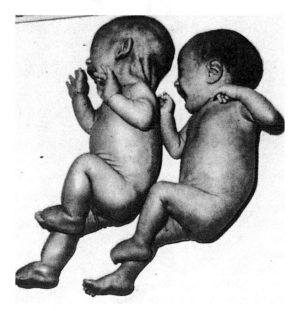

FIGURE 5.15 Dizygotic twins. Note the lymphedema and extra nuchal skin in the twin on the left with Turner syndrome.

Source: Nyhan, W. L. & Sakati, N. © 1976. *Genetic and malformation syndromes in clinical medicine.* Chicago: Year Book Medical Publishers, Inc. Reprinted with permission from Elsevier.

adulthood when they are noted to have amenorrhea or infertility. The external genitalia and vagina remain infantile without hormone therapy. Only 1% have had children; most are infertile. Intelligence is not impaired, but cognitive defects in spatial perception and orientation are common, resulting in difficulties in telling left from right and in reading maps, as detailed next. Many adults go on to college education and beyond.

Other common somatic characteristics are cubitus valgus (an increased carrying angle of the arms so that the arms turn out at the elbow), a broad "shield" chest with widely spaced nipples, short neck, low hairline, high narrow-arched palate, short fourth metacarpals, many pigmented nevi, and hypoplastic nails. It is important to thoroughly investigate for urinary tract anomalies because between 45% to 80% have some malformation such as horseshoe kidney, and a sonogram is recommended in infancy for detection. Cardiovascular anomalies occur in 20% to 44% with bicuspid aortic valve anomalies and coarctation of the aorta being most frequent. Mitral valve prolapse and other anomalies may be seen. Referral to a pediatric cardiologist with initial echocardiography, and perhaps, MRI is recommended. If this is normal, then probably repeat echocardiography and examination are not needed until adolescence at about 12 to 15 years of age. Consistent monitoring of blood pressure is necessary because hypertension, even without any accompanying cardiac or renal malformations, may be seen. Since females with Turner syndrome may develop primary hypothyroidism as well as antithyroid antibodies and Hashimoto thyroiditis, thyroid function measurements at diagnosis and every 1 to 2 years after is also needed. Other autoimmune phenomena, such as inflammatory bowel disease, may be seen. Growth velocity should be monitored, and specific growth charts for Turner syndrome should be used. Recurrent otitis media and progressive sensorineural hearing loss may occur and should be evaluated. Ophthalmic disorders such as strabismus and ptosis may be seen. Orthopedic evaluation should begin with detection of congenital hip dislocation. Scoliosis may be seen later in life and degenerative arthritis may occur in the older individual. Detailed medical management may be found in the references by Frías and Davenport (2003), Conway (2002), Saenger et al. (2001), and Sybert and McCauley (2004).

If untreated, the greatest problems reported by patients result from short stature and the nondevelopment of secondary sex characteristics. Early diagnosis, before cessation of bone growth, permits the use of recombinant growth hormone (GH) therapy often with oxandrolone, usually beginning at about age 9 or 10 years, to promote growth. Reports of degree of effectiveness vary across studies, some suggesting intermittent GH therapy and others uncertain. This may be followed by ethinyl estradiol with or without progesterone to induce breast development, menstruation, and vaginal maturation. It should be noted that Paterson, Hollman, and Donaldson (2002) found that oral estrogen therapy did not result in a mature uterine configuration and recommended that other ways of replacement be investigated. Ophthalmalogic evaluation is necessary because strabismus is relatively common.

Nursing Pointers

A diagnosis of Turner syndrome means lifelong ongoing health care that involves the parents as well as the patient. One of the most important aspects is to give them a chance to ask questions, to discuss problems they have encountered, and to assess how the family unit is coping and functioning. More in-depth counseling may be needed at times. Different points made here are appropriate at various developmental stages, depending on the individuals involved. Many of these points need to be emphasized and repeated many times, and the nursing plan should account for this. A specialized clinic can offer access to a variety of needed disciplines and continuity of care. It is important that coordinated interdisciplinary care be integral in the transition from adolescent to adult care. A detailed plan at each age group may be found in Frías and Davenport (2003). The following are some pointers for the nurse in addition to the information provided above.

1. The point that the occurrence is no one's fault and could not be predicted or prevented should be reemphasized, genetic counseling should be recommended if not already done, and the availability of prenatal diagnosis for future pregnancies should be reemphasized. A level of anxiety and guilt is present to some degree in every family.

2. Patients with Turner syndrome have a feminine gender identity. The lack of the X chromosome has no relationship to lesbianism, promiscuity, inadequateness as a female, or lack of maternal feelings. These types of concerns may be difficult to verbalize, but it has been the author's experience that these are often of great parental and client concern.

3. Selectivity should be used when deciding who should be told about the diagnosis. Some schools have a tendency to apply labels that stigmatize, so that it may or may not be desirable to use the term "Turner syndrome" in communications with them. The parents can decide how they wish to handle this, and perhaps one sympathetic counselor or nurse or the principal can be informed of the diagnosis. The parents also need to decide how much information should be given to relatives and friends. Parents can be advised that there is no reason to discuss the diagnosis with casual acquaintances, and no rush to make a decision to disclose the diagnosis. Sometimes parents later regret having revealed a diagnosis of Turner syndrome to others.

4. As the child grows, parents need to be able to give their daughter a few facts about Turner syndrome because she will begin to realize that there is excessive concern and that she is having more medical examinations than her peers. When appropriate, she should know that she does not need to tell anyone else about her condition except, perhaps, a very close friend or potential mate when she is older. If the client is an adult when she is first diagnosed with Turner syndrome, she may need to decide whether or not to tell her parents and other relatives.

5. The emphasis should always be on the normal aspects. When appropriate, it can be explained to the girl that she will be able to marry, enjoy sexual relations, and that other reproductive options such as adoption or receiving an egg donation are available.

6. Despite GH therapy, some degree of short stature usually remains, the degree of which also depends on the parents' stature. The nurse can help the family in realistic anticipation of GH results. Many aids are available for the short person if needed. In addition, ways to handle comments about her small size should be discussed with the parents so that they can help her if this becomes a problem with peers and with the child herself, if appropriate (see chapter 8).

7. Because of the problems with spatial orientation, parents can be advised that their daughter might get lost more easily or have difficulty in finding her way, so that, for example, when she starts school she may need to be shown the route more often or have more reliance on landmarks than unaffected siblings. She may also have difficulties in telling left from right, with handwriting, drawing shapes and figures, remembering numbers, and solving math problems. Intelligence is normal and the author is acquainted with several women with Turner syndrome who are nurses.

8. It is tempting to treat the patient as if she were younger than her true age because of the short stature. Eventually, she will have to realize that her behavior cannot be both that of a little girl and a mature individual at the same time; but guidance to achieve this will be ongoing and necessary. Parents have to resist the temptation to "baby" her. One way that they can give her responsibility is to suggest that she assume the responsibility for taking her own hormone medication.

9. Many girls with Turner syndrome become overweight. This not only causes them to have additional body image problems but also can contribute to the development of diabetes, to which there is a tendency. Careful attention to diet should begin in early childhood and always be maintained.

10. In late childhood and adolescence, the use of aids, such as a padded bra, may help the girl to feel more feminine. She should also be helped to make her physical appearance as attractive as possible. If plastic surgery is considered, it should be remembered that the female with Turner syndrome has a tendency to form keloids.

11. If cyclic estrogen therapy is used, the girl and the family should realize that results will not be seen immediately; rather, it takes months. The long-term adverse effects, if any, are not known and should be discussed with the family before therapy is undertaken.

12. Any respiratory infections should be treated promptly, as a tendency to otitis media and to resultant hearing loss is common. Hearing loss due to poorly treated otitiis media can result in speech problems.

13. Thyroid function should be evaluated periodically, as dysfunction is often found. Hypothyroidism occurs in about 10–30% of women with Turner syndrome early, and as many as 50% may

develop Hashimoto's thyroiditis. There is also an increased incidence of inflammatory bowel disease.

14. Written materials may be helpful. Booklets written for the patient are available.

15. Under the auspices of a clinic or counselor, parent or parent-child group meetings may be helpful, but names of affected persons should never be distributed or exchanged without their full consent.

16. In the older adolescent and young adult, it is important to reemphasize the potential for satisfying lives. Vaginal estrogen creams can be used for vaginal atrophy and dryness, but the client should be monitored for endometrial hyperplasia. In Hall's series (1997) more than 50% of adults were married.

17. The finding of an increased incidence of essential hypertension in girls with Turner syndrome means that careful monitoring of this parameter is necessary on a lifelong basis.

18. The high frequency of bicuspid aortic valve anomalies is important because it is the most common risk for significant cardiovascular disease from later aortic stenosis. Therefore, frequent examination by a cardiologist and echocardiography when indicated for this with appropriate actions are necessary.

19. Evaluation of fertility may be best achieved by referring the person to a center that specializes in such problems. Assisted reproduction techniques such as oocyte donation may be used to allow fertility options for the woman with Turner syndrome.

20. Referral to a Turner syndrome support group may be helpful (see Appendix B).

47,XXX (Triple X Syndrome)

In 47,XXX, in about 90% of cases, the extra X chromosome is of maternal origin arising from maternal nondisjunction at meiosis I. Females who have triple X syndrome do not demonstrate any consistent constellation, and most of them are not discovered unless they are picked up through chromosome screening programs or speech clinics. There is a tendency to tallness (above the 80th percentile), and increased height velocity has been noted particularly between 4 and 8 years of age. About one-fourth show mild congenital anomalies. Menstrual irregularities have been commonly reported by some investigators but not others. Fertility is not impaired, and in those cases studied, their offspring were usually chromosomally normal (instead of the expected half of the female offspring being XXX and half of the males being XXY as would be theoretically expected). Abnormal gametes are probably selected against, ending up in the polar bodies instead of the ovum. Females with 47,XXX often have IQs that average between 85 and 90 and that are 10 to 15 points below that of their siblings. Learning disabilities are common; however, there is wide variation, and some individuals have not graduated high school while others have completed college. They have some developmental delay, especially in walking. Clumsiness and poor coordination have been described. Receptive and expressive language deficits with decreased verbal ability are frequent. It may be that the presence of an extra X chromosome may be associated with defects in verbal ability. Some difficulties with interpersonal relationships have been noted. In a long-term study of persons with sex chromosome disorders, those with 47,XXX tended to have a lower educational achievement and hold less-skilled jobs than others, but the sample size was small and other studies indicate IQs in the normal range. Some differences may be due to the socioeconomic group of the affected person. Amniocentesis should be discussed with affected females planning pregnancy. Premature ovarian failure (before 40 years of age) and early menopause used to be considered associated with 47,XXX, but some current prospective studies do not support these earlier findings and this question remains unresolved. Tetrasomy X (48,XXXX) and pentasomy X (49,XXXXX) usually lead to multiple physical defects and mental retardation.

Klinefelter Syndrome (47,XXY)

In 47,XXY, about 50% of the time the extra X chromosome is of maternal origin and about 50% of the time it is paternally derived. Klinefelter syndrome is underdiagnosed. Most of these affected males are not ascertained until puberty, when incomplete development of secondary sex characteristics is noticed in the form of sparse body hair, gynecomastia occurs, or small testes are discovered during a physical examination. Often the condition is not diagnosed until help is sought in adulthood for infertility. In adults, 47,XXY men may account for 14% of the cases of azoospermia. Some reports indicate an increase in the presence of minor congenital anomalies, especially clinodactyly. If multiple anomalies are present, then these boys might be detected through chromosome analysis in infancy. Penile size is usually near normal in adolescence and adulthood, but may be small (below the 50th percentile) in children. Sexual functioning is normal. Although development of breast tissue may occur in normal male adolescents, it is more common and tends to persist in males with Klinefelter syndrome. In some patients, this gynecomastia is not seen until later in life. An increased risk of breast cancer and various germ cell tumors has been noted (see chapter 23). Mammoplasty or, in some cases, prophylactic mastectomy is recommended for patients with persistent gynecomastia. Males with Klinefelter syndrome tend to be tall, with increased leg length. They may be overweight with fat distribution resembling that of the female, and they may have an incomplete masculine body build. They usually have a normal sex drive and functioning. Head circumference may be decreased. Intelligence appears essentially in the low normal range but impaired coordination may give the impression of slowness. The most consistent problems are speech and language delays, reading deficiencies, and poor spelling. There may be more difficulties in verbal skills than in performance ability, with difficulties in processing, retrieving, and storing information. Walking may be delayed, and these boys exhibit clumsiness. There is some evidence that some personality impairment exists in the form of passivity, unassertiveness, and shyness. Although the timing of the use of testosterone therapy is in debate, some therapists advocate its use in childhood to increase penile size, and most advocate therapy in late childhood to ensure normal pubertal development and to prevent most of the behavioral problems. Therefore, it is important that adequate therapy be made available to such men so that problems of being "different" in appearance are minimized. Testosterone replacement therapy may be lifelong if testosterone levels are low. In a long-term study, as adults, men with XXY tended to prefer noncompetitive outside physical activities such as sailing, camping, or fishing more often than sibling controls.

Some other nursing points that should be stressed to the individual and family are the following: (1) Males with Klinefelter syndrome have a male gender identity. Normality should be emphasized. (2) They are not predisposed to feminine attributes or qualities, and there is no tendency to homosexuality (remember that the Y chromosome is male-determining). (3) Sexual adequacy is not impaired; most 47,XXY males marry and some (usually mosaics) can reproduce. If they are infertile, reproductive options such as adoption or artificial insemination can be discussed. (4) The use of testosterone can help to ameliorate any lack of puberty that can cause problems for the early adolescent. (5) In the preschool years, nursery school can provide good socialization experiences. (6) Parents are urged to be selective about who is given information about the disorder. Points relating to this under Turner syndrome also apply here. (7) Language delay or motor skill problems should be observed for and remedial intervention taken if they occur. (8) Specialists in fertility problems can be suggested in adulthood, if needed. (9) Gravitational leg ulcers often appear at an unusually early age and preventive teaching aimed at reducing hypostasis should be taught. These may be associated with plasminogen activator inhibitor-1 elevation. (10) Venous thromboembolic risk may occur due to androgen deficiency, and clinicians should be alert for preventive teaching. (11) It is not uncommon for parents to experience disappointment that their tall son is not athletically inclined, and they may need help to deal with these feelings. Well-meaning but misdirected instructors, parents, or coaches may try to persuade or direct these boys into sports. This is usually unsuccessful because of the boys' poor coordination and passivity, which may not be compatible with the aggressiveness of team sports. Late development may make the boy unwilling to expose himself to locker room situations. (12) Boys with 47,XXY whould be encouraged to participate in those activities in which they are likely to have strengths and a likelihood of success. (13) Additional problems may arise because of clumsiness, the gynecomastia, and the body-fat distribution that do not fit the image of a masculine body build. These problems can lead to teasing from classmates and difficult social interactions, and they may result in a lowered self-esteem. A vicious cycle may become established. Counseling may be necessary, but also a plan for handling any school problems should be arrived at in consultation with experts in health care, school officials, and teachers.

Nurses should consider the possibility of chromosome analysis for any male with small testes, significantly delayed sexual maturation, learning or language disabilities when combined with minor congenital anomalies, or males with severe or persistent gynecomastia. Klinefelter syndrome is underdiagnosed despite the fact that it is the most frequent form of male hypogonadism. Amniocentesis should be recommended to the mates of males with Klinefelter syndrome.

47,XYY

Contrary to popular opinion and early studies, the most frequent finding in males with XYY is not criminality but above-average height. Large teeth are also found, as is occasional acne. They usually are above the 75th to 90th percentile by 6 years of age. Most are not otherwise distinguishable from normal individuals. Sexual development and fertility appear normal, and there does not appear to be an increase in abnormalities in their offspring. The origin of the syndrome is obviously paternal, usually occurring at the second meiotic division, or nondisjunction of the Y may occur after fertilization. Past studies linking 47,XYY with deviant or criminal behavior have been flawed because of selection bias. The apparent prevalence of males with 47,XYY in prisons or in institutions for the criminally insane gave rise to the idea that criminality could be genetically predetermined. The idea of such a "criminal gene" has grave social and political implications. Publicity about the murders committed by Richard Speck falsely implied that he was XYY, and novels have characterized XYY males as criminals or, in one case, as the character of Spider Scott by Kenneth Royce, as a super male detective. Data from long-term prospective studies of newborns with XYY have shown some delayed speech development; some learning difficulties, especially in reading; poorer fine-motor coordination; and low normal to normal intelligence (average of about 105) when compared to controls, but no constant aggressive tendencies. There is a trend in some XYY persons for some behavioral difficulties that appear to be related to a low frustration threshold, immaturity, and impulsiveness that are nonspecific, and which may be manifested in childhood by temper tantrums. In discussing the syndrome with parents, caution and back-up counseling should be used because of the wide, incorrect, and adverse publicity associated with the XYY male. Amniocentesis should be recommended to the mates of males with 47,XYY. A few cases of Y trisomies, tetrasomies and pentasomies have been diagnosed.

SUMMARY

Chromosome disorders are responsible for a proportion of congenital anomalies, mental retardation, and behavioral difficulties. The majority of spontaneous abortions, particularly if early, are due to chromosome abnormalities. If looked for with the appropriate techniques, virtually all chromosomal disorders can be detected prenatally. Methods of chromosome analysis and karyotyping continue to advance. Nurses can play an important role in the detection and recognition of these disorders and in the education and anticipatory guidance of families in which one or more members have a chromosome variation.

BIBLIOGRAPHY

American Academy of Pediatrics. (2001). Health supervision for children with Down syndrome. *Pediatrics, 107*, 442–449.

American College of Obstetricians and Gynecologists (1996). Committee Opinion. Genetic evaluation of stillbirths and neonatal deaths. No. 178, November, 1996, 1–3.

Antonarakis, S. E., and the Down Syndrome Collaborative Group. (1991). Parental origin of the extra chromosome in trisomy 21 as indicated by analysis of DNA polymorphisms. *New England Journal of Medicine, 324*, 872–876.

Astbury, C., Christ, L. A., Aughton, D. J., Cassidy, S. B., Kumar, A., Eichler, E. E., et al. (2004). Detection of deletions in de novo "balanced" chromosome rearrangements: Further evidence for their role in phenotypic abnormalities. *Genetics in Medicine, 6*, 81–89.

Bache, I., Assche, E. V., Cingoz, S., Bugge, M.,

Turner, Z., Hjorth, M., et al. (2004). An excess of chromosome 1 breakpoints in male infertility. *European Journal of Human Genetics, 12,* 993–1000.

Baena, N., De Vigan, C., Cariati, E., Clementi, M., Stoll, C., Caballin, M. R., et al. (2003). Prenatal detection of rare chromosomal autosomal abnormalities in Europe. *American Journal of Medical Genetics, 118A,* 319–327.

Barr, M. L., & Bertram, E. B. (1949). A morphological distinction between neurones of the male and female, and the behavior of the nucleolar satellite during accelerated nucleoprotein synthesis. *Nature, 163,* 676–677.

Baty, B. J., Blackburn, B. L., & Carey, J. C. (1994). Natural history of trisomy 18 and trisomy 13. I and II. *American Journal of Medical Genetics, 49,* 175–194.

Bender, B., Fry, E., Penningon, B., Puck, M., Salbenblatt, J., & Robinson, A. (1983). Speech and language development in 41 children with sex chromosome anomalies. *Pediatrics, 7,* 262–267.

Bender, B. G., Linden, M. G., & Harmon, R. J. (2001). Life adaptation in 35 adults with sex chromosome abnormalities. *Genetics in Medicine, 3,* 187–191.

Bishop, J. B., Dellarco, V. L., Hassold, T., Ferguson, L. R., Wyrobek, A. J., & Friedman, J. M. (1996). Aneuploidy in germ cells: Etiologies and risk factors. *Environental and Molecular Mutagenesis, 28,* 159–166.

Bock, R. (1993). *Understanding Klinefelter syndrome. A guide for XXY males and their families.* Bethesda, MD: U.S. Department of Health and Human Services, NIH Pub. No. 93-3202.

Bojeson, A., Juul, S., & Gravholt, C. H. (2003). Prenatal and postnatal prevalence of Klinefelter syndrome: A national registry study. *Journal of Clinical Endocrinology and Metabolism, 88,* 622–626.

Brun, J.-L., Gangbo, F., Wen, Z. Q., Galant, K., Taine, L., Maugey-Laulom, B., et al. (2004). Prenatal diagnosis and management of sex chromosome aneuploidy: A report on 98 cases. *Prenatal Diagnosis, 24,* 213–218.

Bui, T-H. (2002). Prenatal diagnosis: Molecular genetics and cytogenetics. *Best Practice & Research Clinical Obstetrics and Gynecology, 16,* 629–643.

Cohen, W. I. for the Down syndrome Medical Interest Group. (1999). Health care guidelines for individuals with Down syndrome. 1999 revision. (Down syndrome preventive medical check list.) *Down Syndrome Quarterly, 4*(3), 1–10.

Conway, G. S. (2002). The impact and management of Turner's syndrome in adult life. *Best Practice & Research Clinical Endocrinology and Metabolism, 16,* 243–261.

Cornish, K., & Bramble, D. (2002). Cri du chat syndrome: Genotype-phenotype correlations and recommendations for clinical management. *Developmental Medicine & Child Neurology, 44,* 494–497.

Czepulkowski, B. (2001). *Analyzing chromosomes.* London: Bios.

de Kretser, D. M., & Burger, H. G. (1997). The Y chromosome and spermatogenesis. *New England Journal of Medicine, 336,* 576–578.

Dickens, B. M. (1982). Ethical and legal issues in medical management of sex-chromosome abnormal adolescents. *Birth Defects, 18*(4), 227 246.

Elsheikh, M., Dunger, D. B., Conway, G. S., & Wass, J. A. H. (2002). Turner's syndrome in adulthood. *Endocrine Reviews, 23,* 120–140.

Ensenauer, R. E., Adeyinka, A., Flynn, H. C., Michels, V. V., Lindor, N. M., Dawson, D. B., et al. (2003). Microduplication of 22q11.2, an emerging syndrome: Clinical, cytogenetic, and molecular analysis of thirteen patients. *American Journal of Human Genetics, 73,* 1027–1040.

Fisch, H., Hyun, G., Golden, R., Hensle, T. W., Olsson, C. A., & Liberson, G. L. (2003). The influence of paternal age on Down syndrome. *Journal of Urology, 169,* 2275–2278.

Forrester, M. B., & Merz, R. D. (2003). Epidemiology of triploidy in a population-based birth defects registry, Hawaii, 1986–1999. *American Journal of Medical Genetics, 119A,* 319–323.

Freed, M. D., Moodie, D. S., Driscoll, D. J., & Bricker, J. T. (1997). Health supervision for children with Turner syndrome. *Pediatrics, 99,* 146.

Frey-Mahn, G., Behrendt, G., Geiger, K., Sohn, C., Schäfer, D., & Miny, P. (2003). Y chromosomal polysomy: A unique case of 49,XYYYY in amniotic fluid cells. *American Journal of Medical Genetics, 118A,* 184–186.

Frías, J. L., Davenport, M. L., the Committee on Genetics, and the Section on Endocrinology. (2003). Health supervision for children with Turner syndrome. *Pediatrics, 111,* 692–702.

Fryns, J. P., Kleczkowska, A., Petit, P., & Van den Berge, H. (1983). X-chromosome polysomy in the female: Personal experience and review of the literature. *Clinical Genetics, 23,* 341.

Fryns, J. P., Kleczkowska, A., Kubien, E. & Van den Berge, H. (1995). XYY syndrome and other Y chromosome polysomies. Mental status and social functioning. *Genetic Counseling, 6,* 197–206.

Gerdes, M., Solot, C., Wang, P., McDonald-McGinn, D. M., & Zackai, E. H. (2001). Taking advantage of early diagnosis: Preschool children with the 22q11.2 deletion. *Genetics In Medicine, 3,* 40–44.

Gersen, S. L., & Keagle, M. B. (1999). (Eds.). *The principles of clinical cytogenetics.* Totowa, NJ: Humana Press.

Gorlin, R. J., Cohen, M. M., & Hennekam, R. C. M. (2001). *Syndromes of the head and neck* (4th ed.). Oxford, England: Oxford University Press.

Graham, E. M., Bradley, S. M., Shirali, G. S., Hills, C. B., & Atz, A. M. (2004). Effectiveness of cardiac surgery in trisomies 13 and 18 (from the Pediatric Cardiac Care Consortium). *American Journal of Cardiology, 93,* 801–803.

Griffin, D. K. (1996). The incidence, origin, and etiology of aneuploidy. *International Review of Cytology, 167,* 263–296.

Guc-Scekic, M., Milasin, J., Stevanovic, M., Stojanov, L. J., & Djordjevic, M. (2002). Tetraploidy in a 26-month-old girl (cytogenetic and molecular studies). *Clinical Genetics, 61,* 62–65.

Guidelines for optimal medical care of persons with Down syndrome. (1996). *Acta Paediatrica, 84,* 823–827.

Gurbuxani, S., Vyas, P., & Crispino, J. D. (2004). Recent insights into the mechanisms of myeloid leukemogenesis in Down syndrome. *Blood, 103,* 399–406.

Halac, I., & Zimmerman, D. (2004). Coordinating care for children with Turner syndrome. *Pediatric annals, 33,* 189–196.

Haverty, C. E., Lin, A. E., Simpson, E., Spence, M. A., & Martin, R. A. (2004). 47,XXX associated with malformations. *American Journal of Medical Genetics, 125A,* 108–111.

Hecht, C. A., & Hook, E. B. (1996). Rates of Down syndrome at livebirth by one-year maternal age intervals in studies with apparent close to complete ascertainment in populations of European origin: A proposed revised rate schedule for use in genetic and prenatal screening. *American Journal of Medical Genetics, 62,* 376–385.

Hill, D. A., Gridley, G., Cnattingius, S., Mellemkjaer, L., Linet, M., Adami, H. O., et al. (2003). Mortality and cancer incidence among individuals with Down syndrome. *Archives of Internal Medicine, 163,* 705–711.

Hitzler, J. K., & Zipursky, A. (2005). Origins of leukaemia in children with Down syndrome. *Nature Reviews Cancer, 5,* 11–20.

Hogge, W. A., Byrnes, A. L., Lanasa, M. C., & Surti, U. (2003). The clinical use of karyotyping spontaneous abortions. *American Journal of Obstetrics and Gynecology, 189,* 397–402.

Holland, C. M. (2001). 47,XXX in an adolescent with premature ovarian failure and autoimmune disease. *Journal of Pediatric and Adolescent Gynecology, 14*(2), 77–80.

Holmberg, K., Meijer, A. E., Harms-Ringdahl, M., & Lambert, B. (1998). Chromosomal instability in human lymphocytes after low dose rate gamma-irradiation and delayed mitogen stimulation. *International Journal of Radiation Biology, 73,* 21–34.

Hook, E. B. (1981). Rates of chromosome abnormalities at different maternal ages. *Obstetrics & Gynecology, 58,* 282–285.

Isaacs, H., Jr. (2003). Fetal and neonatal leukemia. *Journal of Pediatric Hematology and Oncology, 25,* 348–361.

ISCN. (1995). *An international system for human cytogenetic nomenclature.* Mitelman, F. (Ed.). Basel, S. Karger.

Jacobs, P. A., & Hassold, T. J. (1995). The origin of numerical chromosome abnormalities. *Advances in Genetics, 33,* 101–133.

Jones, K. L. (1997). *Smith's recognizable patterns of human malformation* (5th ed.). Philadelphia: W. B. Saunders.

Kallen, K. (1997). Parity and Down syndrome. *American Journal of Medical Genetics, 70,* 196–201.

Kamischke, A., Baumgardt, A., Horst, J., & Nieschlag, E. (2003). Clinical and diagnostic features of patients with suspected Klinefelter syndrome. *Journal of Andrology, 24,* 41–48.

Kazaura, M. R., & Lie, R. T. (2002). Down's syndrome and paternal age in Norway. *Pediatric and Perinatal Epidemiology, 16,* 314–319.

Kolettis, P. N. (2003). Evaluation of the subfertile man. *American Family Physician, 67,* 2165–2172.

Korenberg, J. R., & Mohandas, T. K. (2002). Chromosomal basis of inheritance. In D. L. Rimoin, J. M. Connor, R. E. Pyeritz, & B. R. Korf (Eds.), *Emery and Rimoin's principles and practice of medical genetics* (4th ed., pp. 149–173). New York: Churchill Livingstone.

Kucheria, K., Jobanputra, V., Talwar, R., Ahmad, M. E., Dada, R., & Sivakumaran, T. A. (2003). Human molecular cytogenetics: Diagnosis, prognosis, and disease management. *Teratogenesis, Carcinogenesis, and Mutagenesis Supplement 1*, 225–233.

Kuhnert, B., & Nieschlag, E. (2004). Reproductive functions of the ageing male. *Human reproduction Update, 10*, 327–339.

Lanfranco, F., Kamischke, A., Zitzman, M., & Nieschlag, E. (2004). Klinefelter's syndrome. *Lancet, 364*, 273–283.

Lapecorella, M., Marino, R., De Pergola, G., Scaraggi, F. A., Speciale, V., & De Mitrio V. (2003). Severe thromboembolism in a young man with Klinefelter's syndrome and heterozygosis for both G20210A prothrombin and factor V Leiden mutations. *Blood Coagulation and Fibrinolysis, 14*, 95–98.

Leonard, M. F., Schowalter, J. E., Landy, G., Ruddle, F. H., & Lubs, H. A. (1979). Chromosomal abnormalities in the New Haven newborn study: A prospective study of development of children with sex chromosome anomalies. *Birth Defects, 15*(1), 115–159.

Leonard, M. F., Sparrow, S., & Schowalter, J. E. (1982). A prospective study of development of children with sex chromosome anomalies— New Haven Study III. The middle years. *Birth Defects, 18*(4), 193–218.

Linden, M. G., Bender, B. G., & Robinson, A. (1996). Intrauterine diagnosis of sex chromosome aneuploidy. *Obstetrics & Gynecology, 87*, 468–475.

Management of Turner's syndrome. (2004). *Journal of Pediatric Endocrinology and Metabolism, 17*(Suppl. 2), 257–261.

Manning, M. A., Cassidy, S. B., Clericuzio, C., Cherry, A. M., Schwartz, S., Hudgins, L., et al. (2004). Terminal 22q deletion syndrome: A newly recognized cause of speech and language disability in the autism spectrum. *Pediatrics, 114*, 451–457.

Massey, G. V. (2005). Transient leukemia in newborns with Down syndrome. *Pediatric Blood Cancer, 44*, 29–32.

McDermid, H. E., & Morrow, B. E. (2002). Genomic disorders on 22q11. *American Journal of Human Genetics, 70*, 1077–1088.

McIntosh, G. C., Olshan, A. F., & Baird, P. A. (1995). Paternal age and the risk of birth defects in offspring. *Epidemiology, 6*, 282–288.

Melville, C. A., Cooper, S. A., McGrother, C. W., Thorp, C. F., & Collacott, R. (2005). Obesity in adults with Down syndrome: A case-control study. *Journal of Intellectual Disabilities Research, 49*(Pt. 2), 125–133.

Merrick, J., Kandel, I., & Vardi, G. (2004) Adolescents with Down syndrome. *International Journal of Adolescent Medicine and Health, 16*, 13–19.

Mezi, G., Papp, C., Tóth-Pál, E., Beke, A., & Papp, Z. (2004). Factors influencing parental decision making in prenatal diagnosis of sex chromosome aneuploidy. *Obstetrics & Gynecology, 104*,. 94–101.

Migeon, C. J., & Wisniewski, A. B. (2003). Human sex differentiation and its abnormalities. *Best Practice & Research Clinical Obstetrics & Gynaecology, 17*, 1–18.

Miller, O. J., & Therman, E. (2001). *Human chromosomes* (4th ed.). New York: Springer-Verlag.

Minto, C. L., Liao, K. L., Woodhouse, C. R., Ransley, P. G., & Creighton, S. M. (2003). The effect of clitoral surgery on sexual outcome in individuals who have intersex conditions with ambiguous genitalia: A cross-sectional study. *Lancet, 361*, 1252–1257.

Morton N. E., Hassold, T. J.,& Funkhouser, J., McKenna, P. W., & Lew, R. (1982). Cytogenetic surveillance of spontaneous abortions. *Cytogenetics Cell Genetics, 33*, 232–239.

Munné, S., Bahçe, M., Sandalinas, M., Escudero, T., Marquez, C., Velilla, E., et al. (2004). Differences in chromosome susceptibility to aneuploidy and survival to first trimester. *Reproductive BioMedicine Online, 8*, 81–90.

Nielsen, J., Sillesen, I., Sorensen, A. M., & Sorensen, K. (1979). Follow-up until age 4 to 8 of 25 unselected children with sex chromosome abnormalities, compared with sibs and controls. *Birth Defects, 15*(1), 15–73.

Nielsen, J., Sorensen, A. M., & Sorensen, K. (1982). Follow-up until age 7 to 11 of 25 unselected children with sex chromosome abnormalities. *Birth Defects, 18*(4), 61–97.

Nyhan, W. L., & Sakati, N. (1976). *Genetic and malformation syndromes in clinical medicine.* Chicago: Year Book Medical Publishers, Inc.

Page, D. C. (2004). On low expectations exceeded; or, the genomic salvation of the Y chromosome. *American Journal of Human Genetics, 74,* 399–402.

Pai, G. S., Borgaonkar, D. S., Lewandowski, R., & Lewandowski, R. C. (2002). *Handbook of chromosomal syndromes.* New York: John Wiley & Sons.

Palermo, G. D., Schlegel, P. N., Sills, E. S., Veeck, L. L., Zaninovic, N., Menendez, S., et al. (1998). Births after intracytoplasmic injection of sperm obtained by testicular extraction from men with nonmosaic Klinefelter's syndrome. *New England Journal of Medicine, 338,* 588–590.

Paris Conference. (1971), Supplement (1975). Standardization in human cytogenetics. *Birth Defects: Original Article Series XI, 9.* White Plains, NY: National Foundation.

Paterson, W. F., Hollman, A. S., & Donaldson, M. D. C. (2002). Poor uterine development in Turner syndrome with oral oestrogen therapy. *Clinical Endocrinology, 56,* 359–365.

Pellestor, F., Andréo, B., Arnal, F., Humeau, C., & Demaille, J. (2003). Maternal aging and chromosomal abnormalities: New data drawn from in vitro unfertilized human oocytes. *Human Genetics, 112,* 195–203.

Pryor, J. L., Kent-First, M., Muallem, A., Van Bergen, A. H., Nolten, W. E., Meisner, L., et al. (1997). Microdeletions in the Y chromosome of infertile men. *New England Journal of Medicine, 336,* 534–539.

Puck, J. M., & Williard, H. F. (1998). X inactivation in females with X-linked disease. *New England Journal of Medicine, 338,* 325–328.

Puck, M. H. (1981). Some considerations bearing on the doctrine of self-fulfilling prophecy in sex chromosome aneuploidy. *American Journal of Medical Genetics, 9,* 129–137.

Puck, M. H., Bender, B. G., Borelli, J. B., et al. (1983). Parents' adaptation to early diagnosis of sex chromosome anomalies. *American Journal of Medical Genetics, 16,* 71–79.

Ravisé, N., Dubourg, O., Tardieu, S., Aurias, F., Mercadiel, M., Coullin, P., et al. (2003). Rapid detection of 17p11.2 rearrangements by FISH *without cell culture* (direct FISH, DFISH): A prospective study of 130 patients with inherited peripheral neuropathies. *American Journal of Medical Genetics, 118A,* 43–48.

Reilly, P. R. (1987). Involuntary sterilization in the United States: A surgical solution. *The Quarterly Review of Biology, 62*(2), 153–170.

Rieser, P. A., & Underwood, L. E. (1992). *Turner syndrome: A guide for families.* The Turner Syndrome Society.

Robinson, A., Bender, B., Borelli, J., Puck, M. H., Salbenblatt, J., & Webber, M. L. (1982). Sex chromosome abnormalities (SCA): A prospective and longitudinal study of newborns identified in an unbiased manner. *Birth Defects, 18*(4), 7–39.

Robinson, A., Puck, M., Pennington, B., Borelli, J., & Hudson, M. (1979). Abnormalities of the sex chromosomes: A prospective study on randomly identified newborns. *Birth Defects, 15*(1), 203–241.

Roizen, N. J. (2002). Medical care and monitoring for the adolescent with Down syndrome. *Adolescent Medicine State of the Art Reviews, 13,* 345–358.

Roizen, N., & Patterson, D. (2003). Down's syndrome. *Lancet, 361,* 1281–1289.

Rooney, D. E. (Ed.). (2001). *Human cytogenetics: Constitutional analysis.* London: Oxford University Press

Ross, J. L., Roeltgen, D., Stefanatos, G. A., Feuillan, P., Kushner, H., Bondy, C., et al. (2003). Androgen-responsive aspects of cognition in girls with Turner syndrome. *Journal of Clinical Endocrinology and Metabolism, 88,* 292–296.

Saenger, P., Wikland, K. A., Conway, G. S., Davenport, M., Gravholt, C. H., Hintz, R., et al. (2001). Recommendations for the diagnosis and management of Turner syndrome. *Journal of Clinical Endocrinology and Metabolism, 86,* 3061–3069.

Saenz, R. B. (1999). Primary care of infants and young children with Down syndrome. *American Family Physician, 59,* 381–390.

Schimmel, M. S., Eidelman, A. I., Zadka, P., Kornbluth, E., & Hammerman, C. (1997). Increased parity and risk of trisomy 201. Review of 37 110 live births. *British Medical Journal, 314,* 720–721.

Schreck, R., & Silverman, N. (2002). Fetal loss. In D. L. Rimoin, J. M. Connor, R. E. Pyeritz, & B. R.

Korf (Eds.), *Emery and Rimoin's principles and practice of medical genetics* (4th ed., pp. 982–997). New York: Churchill Livingstone.

Sepulveda, W., Corral, E., Kottmann, C., Illanes, S., Vasquez, P., & Monckeberg, M. J. (2003). Umbilical artery aneurysm: Prenatal identification in three fetuses with trisomy 18. *Ultrasound in Obstetrics and Gynecology, 21,* 292–296.

Shipp, T. D., & Benacerraf, B. R. (2002). Second trimester ultrasound screening for chromosomal abnormalities. *Prenatal Diagnosis, 22,* 296–302.

Simoni, M., Bakker, E., & Krausz, C. (2004). EAA/EMQN best practice guidelines for molecular diagnosis of y-chromosomal microdeletions. State of the art 2004. *International Journal of Andrology, 27,* 240–249.

Simpson, J. L., de la Cruz, F., Swerdloff, R. S., Samango-Sprouse, C., Skakkebaek, N. E., Graham, J. M., Jr., et al. (2003). Klinefelter syndrome: Expanding the phenotype and identifying new research directions. *Genetics in Medicine, 5,* 460–468.

Simpson, J. L., & Elias, S. (2003). *Genetics in obstetrics and gynecology* (3rd ed.). Philadelphia: Saunders.

Skotko, B. (2005). Mothers of children with Down syndrome reflect on their postnatal support. *Pediatrics, 115,* 64–77.

Smith, D. S. (2001). Health care management of adults with Down syndrome. *American Family Physician, 64,* 1031–1038.

Spurbeck, J. L., Adams, S. A., Stupca, P. J., & Dewald, G. W. (2004). Primer on medical genomics. Part XI: Visualizing human chromosomes. *Mayo Clinic Proceedings, 79,* 58–75.

Stewart, D. A., Netley, C. T., & Park, E. (1982). Summary of clincal findings of children with 47,XXY, 47,XYY and 47,XXX karyotypes. *Birth Defects, 18*(4), 1–5.

Storeng, R. T., Plachot, M., Theophile, D., Mandelbaum, J., Belaisch-Allart, J., & Vekemans, M. (1998). Incidence of sex chromosome abnormalities in spermatozoa from patients entering an IVF or ICSI protocol. *Acta Obstetrica et Gynecologica Scandinavica, 77,* 191–197.

Sybert, V. P., & McCauley, E. (2004). Turner's syndrome. *New England Journal of Medicine, 351,* 1227–1238.

Taback, S. P., Collu, R., Deal, C. L., Guyda, J. H.,

Salisbury, S., Dean, H. J., et al. (1996). Does growth-hormone supplementation affect adult height in Turner's syndrome? *Lancet, 348,* 25–27.

Tease, C., Hartshorne, G. M., & Hultén, M. A. (2002). Patterns of meiotic recombination in human fetal oocytes. *American Journal of Human Genetics, 70,* 1469–1479.

Tjio, J. H., & Levan, A. (1956). The chromosome number in man. *Hereditas, 42,* 1–6.

Tolksdorf, M., & Wiedemann, H-R. (1981). Clinical aspects of Down's syndrome from infancy to adult life. *Human Genetics,* Suppl. 2, 3–31.

Toth, P. P., & Jogerst, G. J. (1996). Identification of Turner's syndrome in an elderly woman. Case report and review. *Archives of Family Medicine, 5,* 48–51.

Valentine, G. H. (1975). *The chromosome disorders* (3rd ed.). Philadelphia: J.B. Lippincott.

Valentine, G. H. (1979). The growth and development of six XYY children. *Birth Defects, 15*(1), 175–190.

Valentine, G. H. (1982). The growth and development of six XYY children: A continuative report. *Birth Defects, 18*(4), 219–226.

Verger, P. (1997). Down syndrome and ionizing radiation. *Health Physics, 73,* 882–893.

Verlinde, F., Massa, G., Lagrou, K., Froideceour, C., Bourguignon, J. P., Craen, M., et al. (2004). Health and psychosocial status of patients with Turner syndrome after transition to adulthood: The Belgian experience. *Hormone Research, 62,* 161–167.

Walzer, S., Graham, J. M., Jr., Bashir, A. S., & Silbert, A. R. (1982). Preliminary observations on language and learning in XXY boys. *Birth Defects, Original Article Series, 18*(4), 185–192.

Wapner, R. J., & Lewis, D. (2002). Genetic and metabolic causes of stillbirth. *Seminars in Perinatology, 26,* 70–74.

Warburton, D., Smith, Z., Kline, J., & Susser, M. (1980). Chromosome abnormalities in spontaneous abortion: Data from the New York City Study. In I. Porter, & E. B. Hook (Eds.), *Human embryonic and fetal death* (pp. 261–287). New York: Academic Press.

Warburton, D. (1991). De novo balanced chromosome rearrangements and extra marker chromosomes identified at prenatal diagnosis: Clinical significance and distribution of breakpoints. *American Journal of Human Genetics, 49,* 995–1013.

Wessels, M. W., Los, F. J., Frohn-Mulder, I. M. E., Niermeijer, M. F., Williams, P. J., & Wladimiroff, J. W. (2003). Poor outcome in Down syndrome fetuses with cardiac anomalies or growth retardation. *American Journal of Medical Genetics, 116A,* 147–151.

Wilkins, L. E., Brown, J. A, Nance, W. E., & Wolf, B. (1983). Clinical heterogeneity in 80 home-reared children with cri du chat syndrome. *Journal of Pediatrics, 102,* 528–533.

Willard, H. F. (2001). The sex chromosomes and X chromosome inactivation. In C. R. Scriver, A. L. Beaudet, W. S. Sly, & D. Valle (Eds.), *The metabolic and molecular bases of inherited disease* (8th ed., pp. 1191–1211). New York: McGraw-Hill.

Williams, J. K. (1983). Reproductive decisions: Adolescents with Down syndrome. *Pediatric Nursing, 9*(1), 43–44.

Xu, J., & Chen, Z. (2003). Advances in molecular cytogenetics for the evaluation of mental retarda-

tion. *American Journal of Medical Genetics, Part C, 117C,* 15–24.

Zhang, L., Lu, H. H., Chung, W. Y., Yang, J., & Li, W. H. (2005). Patterns of segmental duplication in the human genome. *Molecular Biology & Evolution, 22,* 135–141.

Zhang, X., Snijders, A., Segraves, R., Zhang, X., Niebuhr, A., Albertson, D., et al. (2005). High-resolution mapping of genotype-phenotype relationships in cri du chat syndrome using array comparative genomic hybridization. *American Journal of Human Genetics, 76,* 312–326.

Zipursky, A., Brown, E., Christensen, H., Sutherland, R., & Doyle, J. (1997). Leukemia and/or myeloproliferative syndrome in neonates with Down syndrome. *Seminars in Perinatology, 21,* 97–101.

Zlotogora, J. (2004). Parents of children with autosomal recessive diseases are not always carriers of the respective mutant alleles. *Human Genetics, 114,* 521–526.

6

Inherited Biochemical Disorders

Individually, the inherited biochemical disorders are each rare, but as a group they impose a considerable burden on the patient, family, community, and society (see chapters 8 and 27). The total reported incidence at birth varies from 1% to 2%, but accuracy is compromised by the delayed appearance of mutant gene effects (see age of onset) and failure to accurately diagnose certain inherited disorders, especially in newborns who die suddenly. Consequently, their frequency is underestimated. About 25% are apparent at birth; more than 90% are evident by puberty. Life span is decreased in about 60%. Biochemical disorders are important not only for their burden of disease but also for the knowledge about human metabolism that has been gained through their investigation. If the basic molecular defect has not been identified, then these disorders are characterized by their pathophysiologic consequences, clinical manifestations, secondary biochemical alterations, or mode of inheritance.

Most inherited biochemical disorders are single-gene defects, or Mendelian defects, and are caused by a heritable permanent change (mutation) occurring in the DNA, usually resulting in alteration of the gene product. Gene products are usually polypeptide chains composed of amino acid sequences that form an entire molecule or subunit of such entities as structural proteins, membrane receptors, transport proteins, hormones, immunoglobulins, regulatory proteins, coagulation factors, and enzymes. Thus, gene mutation results in defective, absent, or deficient function of these products (often known as "loss of function" mutations), or in some cases, in no discernable phenotypic effect. Mutations not showing a phenotypic effect are called "null" mutations.

Mutations that result in new protein products with altered function are often called "gain of function" mutations. Mutations may also code for a protein that interferes with a normal one, sometimes by binding to it resulting in what is known as a "dominant negative" mutation.

The consequences of altered function depend on the type of defect, the molecule affected, the usual metabolic reactions it participates in, its usual sites of action, how much (if any) residual activity remains, its interactions including those with other gene variants, the body milieu, external factors, and the degree of adaptation that is possible. Some proteins and enzymes are widely distributed in body cells, whereas others are confined to one type (e.g., hemoglobin is expressed only in red blood cells). Enzymes show different degrees of stability in different tissue. For example, glucose-6-phosphate dehydrogenase (G6PD, an enzyme), variants that are unstable can be compensated for in some tissues by an increased rate of synthesis, but this cannot occur in red cells because no protein synthesis occurs there.

GENE NOMENCLATURE

To describe known genes at a specific locus, genes are designated by uppercase Latin letters, sometimes in combinations with Arabic numerals and are italicized or underlined without superscripts or subscripts. Gene products of similar function coded for by different genes have the corresponding loci designated by Arabic numerals after the gene symbol. Thus 3 loci for phosphoglucomutase are designated as *PGM1*, *PGM2*, and *PGM3*. Alleles of genes are preceded by an asterisk. Thus in referring to the alleles for phosphoglucomutase 1 locus *(PGM1)*, one would write, for example, *PGM*1, PGM*2*. Genotypes are written with either a horozontal line or a slash and may be written as *ADA*1/ADA*2* or *ADA*1/*2* to illustrate a sample genotype for the enzyme, adenosine deaminase. In writing the phenotype, there is no underlining or italicization, and no subscripts or superscripts. The asterisk separating gene and allele characters is not used. A space separates gene and allele characters and a comma separates alleles. Thus the genotype *ADA*1/ADA*2* is written as a phenotype as ADA 1, 2. Greek letters are changed to Latin equivalents and are placed at the end of the gene symbol. Standardization for human gene mutation nomenclature became important as sequence information and human gene mutation databases became available. For example, specification is made for genomic DNA or cDNA and the A of the initiator methionine codon is designated as nucleotide +1. Nucleotide changes begin with the number and the change follows that number. For example, 1234delG indicates the deletion of G at nucleotide 1234, and 1234T>G indicates that at nucleotide 1234 of the specific sequence, T is replaced by G. A complete listing is beyond the scope of this book. The reader is referred to Antonarakis, Krawczak, and Cooper (2001).

CLASSIFICATION

No official nomenclature currently exists for the inherited biochemical errors. Thus, great variation is seen in schemes used for classification and description. Such schemes may be based on mode of inheritance (e.g., autosomal recessive-citrullinemia), the chief organ system affected (e.g., nervous system-Huntington disease), the biochemical pathway affected (e.g., urea cycle-argininemia), the general type of substance metabolized (e.g., amino acid-phenylketonuria), the specific cell type or tissue affected (e.g., red blood cell-adenylate kinase deficiency), the specific substance metabolized (e.g., branched chain amino acid-maple syrup urine disease), on a functional basis (e.g., active transport disorder-cystinuria), or by gene location (nuclear or mitochondrial).

Difficulties arise with any of these methods because in some disorders the basic defect is unknown, several organ systems can be involved (e.g., Holt-Oram syndrome, comprised of limb and heart defects), more than one type of inheritance has been identified for a disorder (e.g., retinitis pigmentosa), and so considerable overlap exists. For example, Tay-Sachs disease could be classified as a lysosomal storage disease, a neurologic disease, or an autosomal recessive disorder. The inborn errors of metabolism and specific subgroups within that group are discussed in this chapter, followed by other single gene defects.

HISTORICAL NOTE

The now classic association of certain familial biochemical disorders with Mendel's theories of inheritance was first made by Sir A. E. Garrod in the early 1900s. His detailing of the defect in alcaptonuria, his realization of its autosomal recessive inheritance, and his use of the term "inborn errors of metabolism" were so far ahead of his time that he was not fully appreciated until the formulation of the one gene-one enzyme hypothesis in 1941 for which Beadle and Tatum shared a Nobel Prize in 1958. Later this concept was modified to one gene-one polypeptide, but even this has proven somewhat simplistic as knowledge of the human genome has unfolded.

INBORN ERRORS OF METABOLISM

Most geneticists use the term "inborn error of metabolism" to describe a subgroup of inherited biochemical disorders that comprises those single-gene mutations affecting known enzymes and metabolism. With a few exceptions, these are inherited in an autosomal recessive manner. Enzymes catalyze most reactions in metabolic pathways by acting on substrates in sequence. Some enzymes are conjugated (holoenzymes); that is, they consist of a protein core (apoenzyme), and a cofactor (inorganic compound such as a metal ion), or a coenzyme (organic component such as vitamin) (see Figure 6.1). Interruption of any of the steps in forming a functional coenzyme can lead to a nonfunctional holoenzyme as well and can result in disease (e.g., methylmalonic acidemia can result from failure of coenzyme vitamin B_{12} to

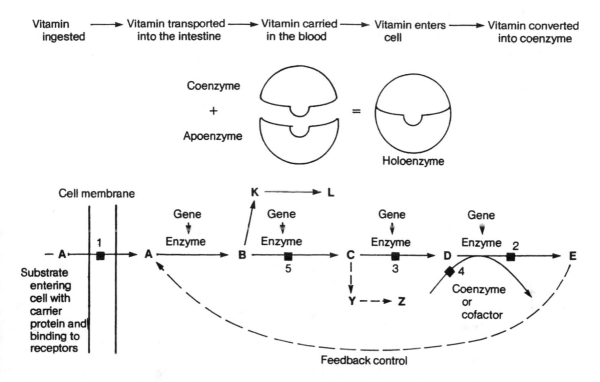

Vitamin ingested → Vitamin transported into the intestine → Vitamin carried in the blood → Vitamin enters cell → Vitamin converted into coenzyme

Coenzyme + Apoenzyme = Holoenzyme

FIGURE 6.1   *(Top)* Relationship between vitamins, coenzymes, apoenzymes, and holoenzymes. *(Bottom)* Hypothetical metabolic pathway illustrating consequences of metabolic blocks. *A,B,C,D,K,L,Y,Z* = substrates or precursors; ■ block, *E* = product (see text for explanation).

be either absorbed or utilized). Replacement of the defective coenzyme effectively treats these disorders (see chapter 15). Thus metabolic dysfunction can occur because of alterations in the substrate, apoenzyme, cofactor, transport proteins, membrane receptors, or holoenzymes. A defect or deficiency of the needed substance at any stage of a metabolic reaction is referred to as a "block" and may be partial or total.

Consequences of Blocks in Metabolic Pathways

Specific consequences of a metabolic block depend on the pathway of which it is a part, but some general statements apply. A schematic representation of a hypothetical metabolic pathway is shown in Figure 6.1. Using this diagram, it can be seen how a particular defect leads to various consequences or combination of consequences.

1. Lack of a functional transport carrier or membrane receptor protein means that a substance will not be able to get inside the cell (Block 1) and will be excreted, lost, or accumulated in the wrong place, leading to ill effects. It may also not then be available for participation in other reactions or pathways. For example, in cystinuria, the carrier responsible for transporting the amino acids cystine, lysine, ornithine, and arginine across the epithelial cell membrane in the renal tubules and in the intestinal wall is defective, excessive amounts are excreted, and renal calculi often occur. Hartnup disease is another example of a transport disorder. Familial hypercholesterolemia is a receptor disorder that is discussed in chapter 2).

2. The substrate (D) immediately before the block (Blocks 2 or 4) or a more distant precursor (A, B, or C) can accumulate. This substance may be toxic to the cell itself, interfere with other biochemical reactions, or give rise to systemic clinical manifestations. It may also be toxic because of the accumulation of the substrate or precursor itself (e.g., in Farber disease, ceramidase deficiency results in the accumulation of the lipid, ceramide, causing joint swelling, stiff joints, psychomotor retardation,

nodules, vomiting, hoarseness, and respiratory problems), or because such an accumulation (of substrate C) causes the opening of an alternate minor biochemical pathway (Y-Z) causing a product to be produced that normally is not, and it is this product that causes toxic signs and symptoms (e.g., in phenylketonuria [PKU] phenylpyruvic and phenylacetic acid are formed and excreted in the urine). In Figure 6.1, Block 4 would prevent the availability of a needed cofactor.

3. The usual product (E) of the metabolic pathway either cannot be produced (Blocks 1, 2, 3, 4, or 5), or it is produced in inadequate amounts or defective form. Clinical effects can be seen due to its direct lack (e.g., lack of melanin in albinism caused by lack of tyrosinase); if it is needed as a substrate for a subsequent reaction, then that reaction cannot occur and the clinical manifestations may be somewhat removed from the original defect (e.g, lack of phenylalanine hydroxylase in classic PKU prevents the conversion of phenylalanine to tyrosine to dopa, so melanin synthesis is diminished and persons with PKU have lighter hair and skin than their siblings).

4. Excess available substrate from the defective pathway (Block 5) may be channeled to another normal pathway (B-K-L), causing overproduction of its product, and this too may affect other reactions.

5. The usual product from the affected metabolic pathway may be functioning in a negative feedback loop or other control mechanism (dotted lines from E to A), and thus, when not produced, fails to control production of some precursor in its own or another pathway (e.g. in congenital adrenal hyperplasia caused by the lack of 21-hydroxylase, cortisol production is decreased, so the hypothalamus responds by secreting more corticotropin releasing factor, causing increased adrenocorticotropic hormone [ACTH] by the anterior pituitary).

CLINICAL MANIFESTATIONS OF INHERITED BIOCHEMICAL DISORDERS IN NEWBORNS AND INFANTS

In contrast to the chromosomal disorders and congenital malformations, most of the metabolic disorders show no gross anomalies at birth. Recognition of such disorders, and their ultimate diagnosis, are complicated by the fact that there are few precise clinical manifestations that can be considered diagnostic, and many defects of the same enzyme are due to alleles that take different clinical forms and may show a rapidly progressive severe infantile picture, a less severe later juvenile onset, and a milder adult form.

Clinical manifestations in the newborn and infant that should lead to further evaluation are shown in Table 6.1. Developmental assessment and signs and symptoms present in older children are discussed in chapter 9. Dietary history is particularly important, because infants with certain metabolic errors do not exhibit problems until the poorly tolerated food is introduced. Some infants develop symptoms of intolerance when they are switched from breast milk to formula because of changes in the nutrient composition. It is important to emphasize that early identification of an inherited biochemical disorder can allow for early treatment and eligibility for government funded programs, family studies, genetic counseling, reproductive decision making, life planning, and in subsequent pregnancies, prenatal detection, and even *in utero* treatment. Because few symptoms are pathognomonic of a disorder and can be used for diagnosis, most require biochemical or DNA testing for confirmation. Testing should be done for parents and sometimes other family members if appropriate.

Because the newborn can only respond to such illness in a limited variety of ways, any history of the death of a sibling in infancy, even if a diagnosis was established, should be an indication for heightened observation and an increased index of suspicion for the nurse working with newborns and infants. Oftentimes the initial presentation is nonspecific such as lethargy, poor feeding, failure to thrive, vomiting, irritability, and tachypnea. The major types of presentation may be thought of as: those that lead to intoxication and often neurologic deterioration from accumulation of toxic compounds, such as most of the organic acidemias; disorders that involve deficiency in energy production or utilization, often presenting with hypoglycemia, such as hyperinsulinism or fatty acid oxidation disorders; seizures, such as in vitamin responsive seizures of various types; jaundice/liver failure, such as fructose intolerance or tyrosinemia;

TABLE 6.1   Some Clinical Manifestations of Selected Inherited Biochemical Errors in Newborns and Early Infancy

Sign/symptom	Examples of disorders
Overwhelming illness, may resemble sepsis	Propionate metabolism defects, MSUD, glycemia
Lethargy	Urea cycle disorders, galactosemia, MSUD, GM_1 gangliosidosis, Gaucher disease, orotic aciduria, nonketotic hyperglycemia
Coma	Urea cycle disorders
Convulsions	PKU, Menkes disease, Krabbe disease, MSUD, urea cycle disorders, infantile hypophosphatasia
Exaggerated startle reflex	Tay-Sachs disease
Hypotonia	Urea cycle disorders, Tay-Sachs disease, Menkes disease, glycogen storage disease II, acid phosphatase deficiency
Poor feeding	Propionate metabolism defects, GM_1 gangliosidosis, Menkes disease
Failure to thrive	Propionate metabolism defects, galactosemia, glycogen storage disease I, Gaucher disease, hypophosphatasia, glycogen storage disease II, Andersen disease, orotic aciduria, Menkes disease, severe combined immune deficiency
Eczema	PKU
"Sand" in diapers	Lesch-Nyhan syndrome
Candidiasis	Severe combined immune deficiency, propionate metabolism defects
Jaundice	Galactosemia, G6PD deficiency, α-1-antitrypsin deficiency, Crigler-Najjar syndrome, erythropoietic porphyria, hypothyroidism, pyruvate kinase deficiency
Vomiting	Urea cycle disorders, galactosemia, propionate metabolism defects, isovalericacidemia, MSUD, PKU, fructosemia, Wolman disease, hypophosphatasia, Menkes disease, glycogen storage disease I
Cataract formation	Galactosemia, Hallermann-Strieff syndrome
Acidosis	Propionate metabolism defect, MSUD, isovaleric acidemia, oxoprolinuria, glutaric aciduria, pyruvate dehydrogenase deficiency
Enlarged abdomen	Propionate metabolism defect, MSUD, isovalericacidemia, oxoprolinuria, glutaric aciduria, pyruvate dehydrogenase deficiency
Diarrhea	Galactosemia, Wolman disease, severe combined immune deficiency
Characteristic odors of urine, sweat, etc.	
Musty, mousy	PKU, tyrosinemia
Burnt sugar	MSUD
Cheese, "sweaty feet"	Isovaleric acidemia
Hops, dried celery	Oasthouse urine disease (methionine malabsorption)
Hypoglycemia	Glycogen storage disease Ia, galactosemia, MSUD, propionate metabolism defects, isovaleric acidemia, galactosemia

Note: Urea cycle disorders mentioned above include carbamoyl phosphate synthetase I deficiency, citrullinemia, ornithine transcarbamylase deficiency, argininosuccinicaciduria, argininemia.
MSUD = maple syrup urine disease. Propionate metabolism defects = methylmalonic acidemia, propionic acidemia, multiple carboxylase deficiency. PKU = phenylketonuria.

and heartbeat disorders or cardiac failure suggesting mitochondrial fatty acid oxidation disorders.

An extreme example of a missed metabolic disorder was the Stallings case. Patricia Stallings brought her 3-month-old son to an emergency room in St. Louis with symptoms that included vomiting and lethargy. The laboratory reported finding ethylene glycol in this blood, suspicion of poisoning ensued, and the infant was placed in foster care. Another hospitalization for this infant occurred, and Patty Stallings was accused of feeding him antifreeze. The infant died. She was tried for his murder and found guilty. By this time she was pregnant again. When she had another son, a similar situation developed. Again, she was suspected of poisoning the second son. Alert geneticists read about the case and contacted legal counsel. This time the infant was diagnosed as having methylmalonic acidemia (MMA), a rare autosomal recessive biochemical disorder. After many twists and turns, Stallings was vindicated in the death of her first son, who was determined to have died from MMA, and she was released. Some cases of sudden infant death syndrome (SIDS) are known to be from inborn errors of metabolism, and increasingly this is investigated as a cause of death in these circumstances. In a study of unexpected early childhood deaths in Virginia, 1% had a postmortem screening result suggesting a metabolic disease—in some cases these were fatty acid oxidation disorders and organic acidemias (Centers for Disease Control and Prevention, 2003).

DISCUSSION OF SELECTED BIOCHEMICAL DISORDERS

Disorders following the inheritance patterns discussed in chapter 4 that are important because of frequency or because they illustrate an important point are discussed next. Other inherited biochemical disorders are discussed elsewhere in this book because of their suitability to other topics. Cystic fibrosis, hemophilia, achondroplasia, and osteogenesis imperfecta are discussed in chapter 8. See the index under the individual name of the disorder for detailed discussion of other disorders.

Hemoglobin and Its Inherited Variants

Hemoglobin (Hb) is important in genetics because (a) it was the source of the first molecular defect identified in a structural protein (Hb S by Pauling and co-workers, 1949), (b) its amino acid sequence has been completely determined, (c) it offers an easily accessible model system for studying structural and regulatory gene mutations, and (d) regulation of gene activation and inactivation in development can be studied.

The major normal adult hemoglobin (Hb A) is a tetramer composed of two alpha and two beta globin polypeptide chains that are associated with heme groups (see Table 6.2). Genes at different loci code for alpha (α) and beta (β) chains that contain 141 and 146 amino acids, respectively. The two pairs of genes that code for α chains are on chromosome 16, whereas the two pairs for gamma (γ) and one each for β and delta (δ) are all linked on chromosome 11.

During development, the embryo and fetus have different Hb chains present in order to meet their oxygenation needs. Zeta (ζ) and epsilon (ϵ) chains are the earliest synthesized and are usually found in embryos under 12 weeks. By 5 weeks of gestation, α, β, and γ synthesis begins. Major production of β chains coincides with the decrease in γ chain synthesis and does not reach its maximum rate until about 6 months after birth, when Hb F is less than 2% (Table 6.2). Therefore, any disorder that causes insufficient β-chain synthesis is not usually manifested clinically until the infant is 3 to 6 months of age. Delta chain synthesis begins just before birth.

More than 1,000 inherited hemoglobin variants have been identified, but only a relatively small number are clinically significant. There are two basic classes—those due to qualitative changes or structural changes, that is, an amino acid substitution or deletion in the globin part of the molecule, as in Hb S or Hb C; and those resulting from quantitative changes, such as deficient globin synthesis as in the thalassemias (see Table 6.3). This latter group includes the hereditary persistence of fetal hemoglobin. The substitution of one nucleotide base for another, resulting in a different amino acid in one of the chains, may change the charge of the Hb molecule and its electrophoretic mobility or it may be "silent." Changes can alter such qualities as oxygen affinity (Hb Kansas), solubility (Hb S), or stability (Hb Torino), resulting in cyanosis or hemolytic anemia, but the majority show no manifestations unless a stressor is encountered such as altered oxygenation, fever, or drug exposure (see chapter 18).

Hb S, Hb C, Hb E, and Sickle Cell Disease

The disorders of sickling include sickle cell anemia (SS), sickle cell trait (SA), or compound heterozygous states such as for an association of Hb S and Hb C (SC disease). Hb S and Hb C result from the substitution of valine and lysine, respectively, for glutamic acid at position 6 of the beta chain. Both

TABLE 6.2   Composition and Description of Normal Hemoglobin

Chain composition	Designation	Description	Percentage in normal adult
$\alpha_2\beta_2$	Hb A	Major normal adult hemoglobin	97–98.5
$\alpha_2\delta_2$	Hb A_2	Minor normal adult hemoglobin	1.5–3
$\alpha_2\gamma_2$	Hb F*	Fetal hemoglobin	1
$\zeta_2\epsilon_2$	Gower I	Embryonic hemoglobin	0
$\alpha_2\epsilon_2$	Gower II	Embryonic hemoglobin	0
$\zeta_2\gamma_2$	Portland Hb	Embryonic hemoglobin	0

*Hb F exists in 2 forms: $\alpha_2\gamma_2^{136\,ala}$ = alanine at position 136 in the gamma chain
$\alpha_2\gamma_2^{136\,gly}$ = glycine at position 136 in the gamma chain

of these Hbs can form various combinations with other mutant Hbs and thalassemia (e.g., Hb Sβ thalassemia). The combination of these two alleles, or SC disease, results in a milder degree of hemolysis but with greater maternal and fetal complications in pregnancy and a longer lifespan than is found in sickle cell disease. Hb SC disease occurs overall in about 1 in 833 persons. One parent of a person with SC will have Hb S trait (SA) and one will have Hb C trait (AC). The incidence of Hb C trait in American Blacks is 2% to 3% and 17%–28% in West Africa (see chapter 3). Hb C disease is often asymptomatic despite mild to moderate hemolytic anemia, but abdominal and joint pain may occur with splenomegaly. Hb E is most common in Southeast Asia, and the Hb E trait occurs in 15% to 30% of Southeast Asian immigrants to the United States, especially Cambodians and Laotians. It may also occur in American Blacks. Hb E disease is often asymptomatic except for mild anemia. Combinations of Hb E with thalassemias occur frequently in Southeast Asians, leading to more severe disease.

Sickle cell anemia or SS disease may be detected as part of newborn screening programs as discussed in chapter 11, or it may be diagnosed in childhood, and the genetics should be explained to families during genetic counseling. When diagnosis is confirmed, families should be taught about possible clinical manifestations that might occur and their complications. These can include overwhelming sepsis, painful sickle cell crises, splenic sequestration (abdominal distention with pallor and listlessness), dactylitis (hand-foot syndrome resulting from bone necrosis and manifesting with soft tissue swelling), leg sores and ulcers, symptoms

such as paresis that might indicate a stroke, other neurological symptoms, and respiratory distress. Parents should be taught about symptoms needing attention, such as those just mentioned, and signs of infection, jaundice, and fever. Usually penicillin prophylaxis will be begun by 2 months of age. The usual immunizations should add pneumococcal, meningococcal, influenza, and hepatitis B. Hydration is important, and folic acid supplementation may be useful. Newer therapies such as hydroxyurea hold promise, and a large multisite study has demonstrated reduced mortality (Steinberg et al., 2003). Other routine health examinations include electrocardiogram, dental care, ophthalmologic examination, teaching on pain managment, watching for gallstones, leg ulcers, and providing the appropriate care as indicated. Pain control protocols should be evaluated, and parents should be able to contact their primary care provider or the sickle cell center to be sure treatment is adequate, because emergency room care for SS is often not optimal. For the adolescent, sports activities, pregnancy possibilities and risks and contraception should be evaluated. For example, women with SS may be at higher risk for thrombosis when using oral contraception, and pregnancy may be riskier. The American Academy of Pediatrics (2002) has published health guidelines on sickle cell that have a list of resources for families. Increased survival of SS patients is thought to result from earlier diagnosis, better therapies and emphasis on patient education. McKerrell and colleagues (2004) in looking at patients with SS over 40 years of age found various differences in physiological parameters such as decreased hematopoietic potential and lower platelet counts as compared to younger patients.

TABLE 6.3 Examples of Selected Hemoglobin Variants

Designation	Chain composition	Comment
Hb S	$\alpha_2\beta_2^{6glu \to val}$	Point mutation in which valine is substituted for glutamic acid at beta chain position 6; reduced solubility of deoxy form
Hb C	$\alpha_2\beta_2^{6glu \to lys}$	Same as above but lysine is substituted for glutamic acid; trait (AC) found in 2% to 3% of American Blacks
Hb H	β_4	Tetramer of beta chains formed; impaired oxygen transport (see text)
Hb M Boston	$\alpha_2^{58his \to tyr}\beta_2$	Tyrosine substituted for histidine at alpha chain position 58; cyanosis, methemoglobinemia (see text)
Hb Barts	γ_4	Tetramer of beta chains formed; impaired oxygen transport (see text)
Hb Chesapeake	$\alpha_2^{92arg \to leu}\beta_2$	Leucine substituted for arginine at alpha chain position 92; high oxygen affinity, polycythemia
Hb Constant Spring	$\alpha_2^{+141-171}\beta_2$	Elongated alpha-chain due to alpha-chain termination mutation; has 31 extra amino acid residues, slow synthesis; may resemble a-thalassemia clinically
Hb Freiberg	$\alpha_2\beta_2^{23val \to del}$	Deletion of valine at beta chain position 23; increased Oxygen affinity; unstable Hb with mild hemolysis when exposed to sulfonamides
Hb Zurich	$\alpha_2\beta_2^{63his \to arg}$	Arginine substituted for histidine at beta chain position 63; mild hemolysis when exposed to sulfonamides, unstable Hb

Hb M and Methemoglobinemia

For Hb to fulfill its major function of carrying oxygen, the iron in the heme group must be in the ferrous (Fe^{++}) form. The tertiary structure or three-dimensional folding of the Hb molecule brings certain amino acids in both alpha and beta chains into close contact with the iron to maintain this form. Normal events allow about 3% of the iron to be oxidized to ferric form (Fe^{+++}), producing methemoglobin, which does not function well as an oxygen carrier. An enzyme, methemoglobin reductase, normally reduces the Fe^{+++} to Fe^{++}, so that Fe^{+++} is maintained at less than 1%. Methemoglobinemia can result from two genetic mechanisms—lack of methemoglobin reductase, a rare autosomal recessive condition (see chapter 18); or an amino acid substitution that alters the tertiary configuration and stabilizes the iron in the Fe^{+++} form. The latter group is known collectively as Hb M, and is designated individually by the place of discovery (e.g., Hb M Boston, Hb M Saskatoon, etc.), and are inherited as autosomal dominant disorders. If the Hb M substitution is in an alpha chain, then cyanosis is present from birth, but if it is in a beta chain, then it will not be seen until 3 to 6 months of age. The nurse should be aware that clinical problems depend on the percent of Hb M in the blood but are generally minimal for heterozygotes. Some problems may be iatrogenic, caused by invasive medical procedures to diagnose the cause of the cyanosis or by misguided restrictions due to suspected congenital heart problems. They are usually asymptomatic except for the cyanosis, although in some persons mild headache or exercise intolerance may occur and these are exacerbated by low oxygen conditions or stress. Hb M is frequent in Japan.

The Thalassemias

Normally, α and β globin chains are produced in equal amounts. The thalassemias are a group of disorders of Hb production that result from deficient or absent α or β globin chain synthesis. This change in the rate of synthesis of one or more globin chains creates an imbalance. Those with a deficiency in the alpha chain are α-thalassemias and are most prevalent in South East Asians, North Africans, and Blacks of African descent. The β-thalassemias result from a reduced rate of synthesis of β globin chain and are most prevalent in populations bordering the Mediterranean Sea, especially

Italy, Greece, Cyprus, and the Middle East. There are more than 200 possible mutations. Within a given population, a few mutations account for most defects. In Greece, five mutations account for 87% of defects, and in China, four mutations account for 91%. Classifications of thalassemia have been made at both the phenotypic and genotypic levels. There are many possible combinations. It is not unusual for a person to have thalassemia along with a structural Hb variant or more than one type of thalassemia. Genetic modifiers influence the phenotype and many are population specific. For a complete discussion of genotypic and phenotypic variants, see Weatherall and Clegg (2001). About 240 million people worldwide are heterozygotes for β-thalassemia.

The most severe alpha thalassemia is Hb Bart's hydrops fetalis, in which there is complete absence or inactivation of all four alpha genes, usually through deletion. This is often denoted as --/--. No alpha chain synthesis occurs, and Hb Barts tetramers and Hb H comprise most of the Hb present. Infants with the disorder are usually stillborn or die a few hours after birth. In Hb H disease, three of the four genes are absent (--/-α). Some normal Hb is produced, but the unstable Hb H causes hemolytic anemia, splenomegaly, microcytosis, and impaired oxygen transport. In alpha thalassemia trait, two of the four genes are absent (--/αα [called α⁰ thalassemia] or -α/-α [called α⁺ thalassemia]), and infants may have mild anemia with other hematologic findings. In silent gene carriers, one of the four genes are absent (-α/αα), and there may be no signs except for slight microcytosis. It is important to recognize the disorder to avoid mistreatment for iron deficiency anemia and for accurate genetic counseling.

In β-thalassemia, there may be a decreased synthesis of beta chains (β^+) or no production (β^0). In the homozygous state, β-thalassemia is known as "thalassemia major." Although the clinical course can vary, typically symptoms are not noticed right after birth because of the presence of Hb F in the normal newborn. It is not until Hb A synthesis should be dominant that the manifestations are noticed. Hb F may persist as a compensatory mechanism, but it is not sufficient to prevent symptom development. Infants are pale, jaundiced, fail to thrive, have hepatosplenomegaly, and show prominent bones in the skull, spine, and face as the marrow hypertrophies. Long bone fractures ensue and growth is retarded. The hemolytic anemia becomes so severe that transfusions are necessary, but unfortunately the frequent transfusions lead to iron deposition and therefore to cardiac and hepatic dysfunction and diabetes. Lung disease may also occur. Various approaches such as iron chelation with desferrioxamine and other agents have been used to remove the iron burden brought about by transfusion. One drawback is the need for injection and that discomfort and expense. Deferiprone is an oral agent often used with desferrioxamine, but there are questions about safety and efficacy. Other iron chelating agents such as ICL670A are being tested. More recently fetal hemoglobin augmentation has been used as a transfusion alternative. Most severely affected persons die during adolescence or young adulthood from complications of the iron overload, especially in the myocardium. Bone marrow transplantation is sometimes done, and gene therapy holds promise. Population screening is common in Mediterranean countries such as Greece and Italy. When blood is being screened, among the major findings suggesting thalassemia are mean cell volume (MCV) less than 72–75 fL and microcytic anemia. Among the many other nursing implications of this disorder is the need to provide genetic counseling including the option of prenatal diagnosis to the parents who are heterozygotes. They may function normally because one beta chain is normal while the other one is not. Nurses should be alert to the finding of an apparent anemia in persons of Mediterranean extraction for β-thalassemia and of southeast Asian extraction for α-thalassemia.

Lysosomal Storage Disorders

Lysosomal storage disorders is the terminology used to describe a heterogenous group of about 50 genetic diseases that have in common the accumulation of certain metabolites within the lysosome. This accumulation is the result of defective lysosomal enzyme activity or to a genetic defect in a receptor, activator protein, membrane protein, or transport molecule. The abnormal deposition and storage of the particular substance can result in effects on the central nervous system as well as systemic manifestations. The individual disorders vary from the mucopolysaccharidoses such as

Hurler disease; to the sphingolipidoses, which include the gangliosidoses such as Sandhoff disease and Tay-Sachs disease; glycogen storage disorders such as Pompe disease; as well as mucolipidosis IV, and Chediak-Higashi syndrome. Collectively the incidence is 1 in 7,000–8,000 live births. The majority are inherited in an autosomal recessive manner with the exception of Hunter disease and Fabry disease, which are X-linked recessive, and Danon disease (glycogen storage disease IIb), thought to be X-linked dominant. These disorders are generally progressive and may vary in severity and expression. Many of these disorders have variant forms that may differ in age of onset (often with a severe form with infantile onset and less severe juvenile or adult forms so that many patients first come to clinical attention as adults), clinical presentation or disease course. Those who present at adults are often not diagnosed promptly. For example, a 38-year-old man with Niemann-Pick disease type C was misdiagnosed as having schizophrenia for 8 years, and a late adolescent male with Tay-Sachs disease was misdiagnosed with catatonic schizophrenia. Adult onset Tay-Sachs disease can mimic Friedreich ataxia. Selected lysosomal storage disorders are summarized in Table 6.4, while the mucopolysaccharidoses are summarized in Table 6.5. The mucopolysaccharide disorders, Tay-Sachs disease, and Gaucher disease are discussed next as examples.

Mucopolysaccharide Disorders (Mucopolysaccharidoses)

The mucopolysaccharidoses (MPS) are a group of lysosomal storage disorders that are characterized by the accumulation of glycosaminoglycans (GAGs; the older term was "mucopolysaccharides"). GAGs are long-chain complex carbohydrates that may be linked to proteins to form proteoglycans. They are present in ground substances and tissues such as cell, nuclear, and mitochondrial membranes, cartilage, skin, bone, synovial fluid, umbilical cord, vitreous humor, and the cornea, where support is needed. They include chondroitin sulfate (SO_4), heparan SO_4, dermatan SO_4, keratan SO_4, and hyaluronan. When the specific lysosomal enzyme needed in degradation is defective, certain GAGs accumulate within lysosomes and are deposited, particularly in connective tissue, bone, viscera, the heart, the brain, and the spinal cord

giving rise to the particular symptom. There are distinct classification groups. Each has a pattern of deposition and urinary excretion of MPS that is valuable in diagnosis. These disorders are progressive and may show considerable variability in clinical severity. The major MPS are shown in Table 6.5. Affected persons need careful evaluation and management preoperatively for anesthesia. They are at risk because of upper airway problems often with respiratory infections, deposits in upper airway, cardiac pathology, rib cage restriction, and if developmentally delayed, they may have difficulty in understanding what is needed. Postsurgical mortality has been reported to range from 7% to 20%.

The combined incidence of all the MPS disorders is 1:25,000 newborns. MPS I is usually classified into Hurler syndrome (MPS IH, most severe), Scheie (MPS IS, mild), and Hurler/Scheie (MPS IH/S, intermediate). It is believed that these are actually points on a continuous spectrum of severity. Hurler syndrome is one of the most frequently seen. Clinically, it is not usually detected until 6–12 months of age, although infants may have umbilical or inguinal hernias, a large tongue, and may be unusually large. Usually, the syndrome does not develop fully until well into the second year. Cardiac disease is very common and cardiomyopathy may result in early death, even being a presenting symptom. Most affected children do not live past 14 years of age. The following case illustrates many typical features. A 22-month-old girl was referred to the genetic counseling center because of developmental delay and growth retardation. Examination revealed typical coarse facies, an enlarged tongue, kyphosis, hirsutism, and a protruding abdomen caused by an enlarged liver and spleen. Corneal clouding was noted. Her mother stated that the child had frequent colds and ear infections. The family history was negative; her 5-year-old brother was normal. Laboratory testing revealed findings characteristic of Hurler syndrome. Included in the usual genetic counseling of the family based on the AR inheritance was the information that prenatal diagnosis was available and could be used if another pregnancy was desired. A picture of a child with Hurler syndrome and characteristic features is shown in Figure 6.2. Efforts to predict phenotype on the basis of genotype are underway but currently it is only known that nonsense mutations will cause severe MPS I disease if

TABLE 6.4 Characteristics of Selected Lysosomal Storage Disorders

Disorder	Enzyme deficiency	Selected characteristics (infantile form unless noted)
Fabry disease (diffuse angiokeratoma)	α-galactosidase A	Onset in late childhood, adolescence, or adulthood; telangiectasia, pain attacks, autonomic dysfunction, angina, EKG changes, paresthesia, lymphedema, characteristic skin lesions, (angiokeratomas), corneal opacities, gastrointestinal disturbances, hypertension, renal failure, death by middle age usual.
Farber disease	Ceramidase	Psychomotor deterioration, subcutaneous nodules, failure to thrive, swollen joints, mental retardation, hepatosplenomegaly, hoarseness, death
Generalized gangliosidosis	β-galactosidase	Hepatosplenomegaly, skeletal abnormalities with dwarfism, joint stiffness, mental retardation, cerebral degeneration, decerebrate rigidity, death
Gaucher disease	Glucocerebrosidase	see text
Krabbe disease	Galactocerebroside β-galactosidase	Irritability, convulsions, mental and motor deterioration, deafness, blindness, death
Metachromatic leukodystrophy	Arylsulfatase A	Hypotonia, quadriplegia, blindness, leukodystrophy mental deterioration, megacolon, death
Niemann-Pick disease type A	Sphingomyelinase	Has many subforms; seizures, coronary artery disease, hepatosplenomegaly, failure to thrive, hypotonia, mental retardation, death
Pompe disease (glycogen storage disease type II)	α-glucosidase (acid maltase)	In infancy, hypotonia and hypertrophic cardiomyopathy with death usual by 1 year. Juvenile and adult forms feature progressive skeletal muscle weakness, respiratory involvement with little cardiac involvement.
Sandhoff disease	Hexosaminidase A&B	Muscle weakness and wasting, mental and motor deterioration, cerebellar ataxia, blindness, cardiomegaly, hepatosplenomegaly
Tay-Sachs	Hexosaminidase A	see text

Note: Each has one or more less-severe forms with later onset. All are autosomal recessive except Fabry disease, which is X-linked recessive.

found on both α-L-iduronidase alleles. Enzyme replacement therapy using recombinant human α-L-iduronidase (Aldurazyme laronidase) has been used in treatment in mucopolysaccharidosis I, as has hematopoetic stem cell transplantation and the combination of both. Cord blood transplantation as a source of stem cells shows promise for MPS I.

Tay-Sachs Disease

Tay-Sachs disease is the best known of the lysosomal storage diseases and is classified as a GM$_2$ gangliosidosis due to mutation of the *HEXA* gene encoding the α subunit of hexosaminidase A (Hex A), a lysosomal enzyme composed of alpha and beta polypeptides. At least 78 mutations in this gene have been identified. In the classic infantile form, the infant appears well except, perhaps, for an exaggerated Moro (startle) reflex. At 4 to 6 months of age, hypotonia, difficulty in feeding, and apathy begin. Motor weakness, developmental regression, and mental retardation follow. A cherry red spot is noticeable in the fundus on ophthalmic examination, and blindness occurs by 12 to 18 months. Neurologic deterioration follows. Seizures, decerebrate rigidity, and deafness occur with an eventual vegetative state. The head enlarges about 50% and hypothalamic involvement may cause precocious puberty. Death is inevitable and typically occurs by 2 to 4 years of age, although a few children have survived to 6 years. Tay-Sachs is most common in Askenazi Jews and in French Canadians from eastern Quebec. Both juvenile and adult forms have been described. Those with the juvenile form may develop symptoms between ages 1 and 9 years. Some patients with Hex A deficiency do not show onset until adolescence or adulthood, more commonly called adult GM$_2$ gangliosidosis. DNA testing is available. Screening for Tay-Sachs is described in chapter 11.

TABLE 6.5   Summary of Mucopolysaccharide (MPS) Disorders*

Disorder	Major clinical features	Enzyme deficiency
MPS I H Hurler	Mental retardation, coarse facies, skeletal and joint deformities, hepatosplenomegaly, deafness, dwarfism, corneal clouding; onset 6–12 months; fatal in childhood	α-L-iduronidase
MPS I S Scheie (formerly V)	Onset 5–15 years; normal height, normal intelligence, "claw" hands, stiffness and other joint problems, coarse facies, corneal clouding	α-L-iduronidase
MPS I H/S Hurler-Scheie compound	Intermediate between IH and IS	α-L-iduronidase
MPS II Hunter		
Severe	Like Hurler, but no corneal clouding; death usual in adolescence	Iduronidate 2-sulfatase
Mild	Survive to middle adulthood; intelligence not usually impaired	Iduronidate 2-sulfatase
MPS III Sanfilippo		
Type A	Clinically, both appear the same	Heparan-N-sulfatase (A)
Type B	Severe mental retardation, mild somatic effects; may include short stature, death usually occurs by 20 years of age; Types C and D have also been described	N-acetyl-a glucosaminidase (B)
MPS IV Morquio		
Type A	Severe skeletal effects (e.g., short trunk, prominent sternum, short neck, growth retardation, "knock-knees")	Galactosamine-α-sulfatase
Type B	May have corneal opacities and hearing loss; intelligence is usually normal	β galactosidase
MPS VI Maroteaux-Lamy Severe, intermediate, mild	Growth retardation and short stature; normal intelligence; skeletal deformities such as hip dysplasia, valvular heart disease, corneal changes, all to varying degrees	Arylsulfatase β
MPS VII Sly	Mild mental retardation, hepato-splenomegaly, skeletal deformities; may have cloudy corneas; few cases known	β glucuronidase

Note: Clinical features can vary from patient to patient.
*All are inherited in an autosomal recessive manner except Hunter syndrome, which is an X-linked recessive.

Gaucher Disease

Gaucher disease is a lysosomal storage disorder caused by deficiency of glucocerebrosidase and accumulation of glycosylceramide (glucocerebroside) that occurs in 3 forms: type 1, the visceral form that is usually chronic, often first appearing in adulthood; type 2, an acute neurological form often appearing in infancy; and Type 3, a subacute neurological type often appearing first in childhood. It affects 10,000 to 20,000 Americans. In contrast to many of the other disorders in this category, the adult form is the most prevalent, accounting for about 80% of cases. Inheritance is autosomal recessive and multiple alleles may cause mutations, with five mutations responsible for about 97% of the disease alleles among Ashkenazi Jews. A particular mutation, 1448C, occurs as a polymorphism in northern Sweden leading to type 3 disease. Another specific mutation, 1226G, leads to mild type 1 disease in homozygotes, and such individuals often are undetected unless revealed in the course of family or population studies. A rare perinatal-lethal type has been described, and is often associated with hydrops fetalis. In adult type 1, which is non-neuronopathic, Gaucher cells with

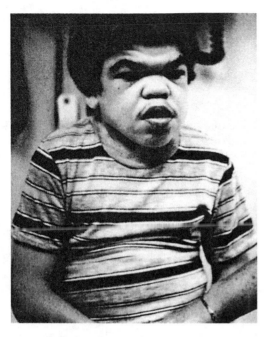

FIGURE 6.2   Boy with Hurler syndrome.

accumulated glucosylceramide infiltrate the spleen, liver, and bones. Patients may first experience nonspecific symptoms such as fatigue, easy bruisability, and enlarged abdomen with hepatosplenomegaly. Eventually, bone fractures, infarctions and necrosis, pain, thrombocytopenia, anemia, and infection occur. The pain may be nonspecific and migratory with episodes lasting 1 to 3 days. The age of onset is variable, ranging from birth to 80 years but commonly first presents in adulthood. Some may be asymptomatic entirely and others may not develop disease manifestations until they are in their 50s, in which case all of their children will already have inherited one mutant gene. Therapy for Gaucher disease can include treatment of symptoms, bone marrow transplantation with stem cells, enzyme therapy with alglucerase or imiglucerase, N-butyldeoxynojirimycin (OGT-918), and the potential of gene transfer and therapy. Treatment is expensive, however. Detection of carriers and prenatal diagnosis is possible. It has a high gene frequency in Ashkenazi Jews with a carrier frequency of about 7%, and population screening in this group for both carrier status and disease has been suggested, but accurate genetic counseling that includes prognosis can be difficult because of variability in expression.

Marfan Syndrome

Marfan syndrome is an autosomal dominant disorder that is extremely pleiotrophic (multiple phenotypic effects from a single gene). It is very variable in expression. While many persons with Marfan syndrome are detected in childhood or adolescence, often because of height, others remain undetected. One case in our genetic clinic came to light when a mother brought her son to the clinic for celiac disease follow-up (they were new to our clinic). When we looked at the mother, we believed she had Marfan syndrome, were able to follow-up on that suspicion, and referral to a cardiologist ultimately detected aortic dilatation requiring medication, perhaps preventing sudden cardiac complications. Marfan syndrome is believed present in about 1 in 10,000 persons but may be more frequent and underrecognized; 15%–30% represent new mutations.

The characteristic features include skeletal findings (tall stature compared to normal family members), pectus excavatum (hollow chest or pectus carnitum [pigeon chest]), reduced upper to lower segment ratio, arm span that may be greater than height, scoliosis, joint hypermobility, arachnodactyly (long spiderlike hands and long thumbs), and others; ectopia lentis and other ocular findings; aortic dilatation, dissecting aneurysms of the aorta, mitral valve prolapse, and other cardiovascular manifestations; and other findings. Marfan syndrome is the major reason for dissecting aortic aneurysms in persons under 40 years of age. A woman with Marfan syndrome is shown in Figure 6.3.

The major defect is a mutation of fibrillin, a glycoprotein in the microfibrils of the extracellular matrix. The defect is in the fibrillin gene, *FBN1* on chromosome 15q21.1. There is at least 1 other fibrillin gene on chromosome 5, *FBN2*, that is involved with congenital contractual arachnodactyly. Various mutations of the gene can occur leading to variable clinical variability, and some changes lead to related conditions such as familial ectopia lentis, familial tall stature, and others (see Pyeritz, 2002). It can be difficult to clinically distinguish Marfan syndrome from other conditions such as homocystinuria. De Paepe et al. (1996) updated the diagnostic criteria for Marfan syndrome in which detailed requirements for major and minor criteria are set forth and remain current.

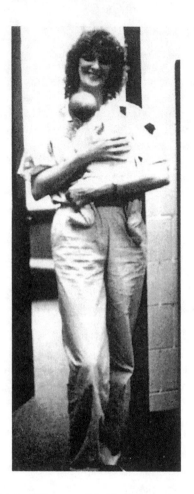

FIGURE 6.3   Woman with Marfan syndrome.

Because of their tall stature, it is not unusual for persons with Marfan syndrome to be athletes. Flo Hyman, the 6'5" Olympic volleyball team member, and various high school and university basketball stars have died suddenly due to ruptured aortas from Marfan syndrome. Thus it is important that the school nurse be sure that athletes have adequate sports physicals, and if Marfan syndrome is present that a full examination is done, including echocardiography, a slit lamp examination by an ophthalmologist, and others, depending on the symptoms. Often prophylactic β-adrenergic blockade such as propranolol or atenolol is prescribed. Activity needs modulation, and pregnancy poses increased risks needing close supervision depending on the person's cardiac status. Updated recommendations for physical activity and recreational sports have been issued (Maron et al., 2004).

Autosomal Dominant or Adult Polycystic Kidney Disease

Autosomal dominant polycystic kidney disease (ADPKD) is an autosomal dominant systemic disorder that has its manifestations usually noticed in adulthood, although renal cysts may begin in the fetus. Its frequency is 1:800–1,000. The renal cysts increase in both size and number and damage the kidney, but usually loss of function is not seen until the 30s or 40s. By age 50 years, about half of all patients develop renal failure, and about half have end-stage renal disease by 60 years of age. Penetrance is considered invariable by 70 years of age. Other symptoms and complications can be pain, infection, and hypertension. Polycystic liver disease may be manifested and affects women more severely than men. Hormonal influences such as pregnancy, birth control pills, and postmenopausal estrogen use are associated with more severe polycystic liver disease. Intracranial aneurysms occur more frequently in persons with ADPKD than in the general population, and the position of the *PKD1* mutation is of prognostic importance. An autosomal recessive form manifests in infancy or childhood. ADPKD accounts for approximately 5% of all cases of end-stage renal disease. There are at least three forms. Mutation of *PKD1* (on chromosome 16p13.3) coding for polycystin-1 found on renal tubular epithelium, is most common and accounts for 85%-95%. Mutation in *PKD2* accounts for most of the rest and maps to chromosome 4q22 coding for polycystin-2. There is at least one other rare form. There is some evidence that, in addition to the germline mutation, a second hit is needed for full manifestation. Identifying persons by linkage to markers such as KG8-CS is possible especially combined with renal ultrasonography. Direct genetic testing should be possible soon.

Huntington Disease

Described by George Huntington in 1872, Huntington disease (HD) was earlier known as "chorea." It is believed that some of the women burned as witches in Salem, Massachusetts, in the 1690s actually had HD. For many years, the famous folk singer Woody Guthrie was erroneously believed to be an alcoholic rather than a person who had HD.

This neurodegenerative disease is inherited in an autosomal dominant manner, but symptoms do not usually appear until age 35 years or over, although it can rarely occur in children. Until the age of 70 years, one could not be said to be absolutely free of the disorder. Bayes theorem has been used (especially before molecular diagnosis was possible) to take into account the symptom-free person's age to provide counseling. The story of the search for the gene causing HD is a very interesting one, involving large informative families in Venezuela. HD occurs in 1 in 10,000 persons.

The gene for HD, *IT15* (interesting transcript 15) located on chromosome 4p16.3, encodes the protein huntingtin whose function is still unknown. This gene, in the first exon, contains repeating triplets of CAG. CAG-repeat lengths of approximately 10 to 35 are normally seen. In HD, the unstable repeats expand. CAG-repeat lengths of 27 to 35 are considered mutable normal alleles, 36 to 39 are considered to have HD allele with reduced penetrance, and 40 or more are considered to be HD (ACMG/ASHG, 1998). Expansion is more frequent in paternal lineage. There is some overlap. When inherited from the father, in approximately one-third of cases the repeats expand to about two times the paternal repeat number, but in maternal transmission the allele changes by only a few repeats. This explains early observation of earlier onset and severity when the father was affected in contrast to the mother. Anticipation has been observed to be a feature of HD inheritance, and expansion is greatest in HD appearing in juveniles. There is a positive association between the number of CAG repeats and age of onset. More precise risk estimates can be determined by considering age and the number of CAG repeats in a particular person. The United States–Venezuela Collaborative Research project and Wexler (2004), suggest that other genes and environmental effects also influence age of onset. Presymptomatic or predictive testing for HD is available for affected families, but interestingly enough many have chosen not to avail themselves of this option. Issues relating to this are discussed in chapter 11.

HD is often not diagnosed until symptoms have progressed somewhat even though, in retrospect, it becomes apparent that signs were present earlier. HD encompasses motor, cognitive, or emotional impairment. It may begin with subtle behavioral changes such as forgetting things, inattention, irritability, impaired judgement, poor concentration, hypochondriasis, personality changes, and carelessness about hygiene. Symptoms such as slurred speech or unsteady gait can lead to arrest for alcoholism (known patients should wear medical identification). Promiscuity or an increased sexual drive may occur, resulting in increased numbers of descendants at risk. Over a period of as much as 10 to 20 years, the patient progressively deteriorates, showing increased tremor. Eventually, he or she becomes bedridden, develops swallowing difficulties, choking, and the loss of bladder and bowel control. Treatment options are largely symptomatic. A treatment approach in phase 1 clinical trials uses trehalose, a disaccharide, to ultimately inhibit polyglutamine induced protein aggregate formation and prevent associated brain pathology (Tanaka et al., 2004). These families are under great stress not only because of the condition of their family member, but also because of the uncertainty for others to develop it. Before identification by gene testing was possible, a counselee who was a member of a family at risk for HD stated that every time she forgot an item or spilled something, she wondered if this was the beginning of her own disease. Some persons have even changed their family name and relocated to avoid stigmatization because of HD in the family. Aspects of presymptomatic gene testing are considered in chapters 11 and 23.

Lesch-Nyhan Syndrome

Lesch-Nyhan syndrome is an X-linked recessive inherited disorder of purine metabolism caused by the virtual absence (less than 1.5%) of the enzyme hypoxanthine-guanine phosphoribosyltransferase (HPRT) with the mutant gene located at Xq26-27. More than 200 mutations in the gene are known. In the infant, the first sign may be the presence of orange "sand" (uric acid crystals) in the diaper. Parents often report retrospectively that the infant was irritable and "colicky," and hypotonicity may be seen. Developmental delay occurs by 3 to 6 months. It is characterized by a high rate of purine synthesis, hyperuricemia, increased uric acid excretion, spasticity, choreoathetosis, some degree of mental retardation and developmental delay (although often affected persons appear to be more intelligent than indicated by test scores), and behavioral abnormalities of compulsive self-mutilating and aggressive behavior. Some patients have tested with low normal IQs if the testing takes into account the motor and communication difficulties. Often the first diagnosis is a nonspecific "cerebral palsy." The compulsive self-mutilation includes chewing and biting the lips and fingers until tissue is destroyed, head banging, and teeth grinding. These children usually do not want to injure themselves and often welcome restraint from this behavior. The aggressive behavior may include hitting out at nearby persons. After such episodes they often apologize. The clear-cut association of a single-gene defect with specific behaviors has made Lesch-Nyhan syndrome of particular interest to behavioral geneticists. Two brothers with Lesch-Nyhan syndrome attended our genetics clinic. Both used wheelchairs to be mobile, were adept at getting around, and were quite charming despite the behavioral manifestations. This characteristic has been noted by others. Less severe deficiencies (8% or higher) of HPRT may result in excessive purine synthesis with gouty arthritis typically with onset in early adulthood, usually eventually resulting in kidney stones or a less severe syndrome characterized by little or no neurologic dysfunction. Persons with HPRT levels of 1.5% to 8% of HPRT may show uric acid overproduction symptoms as well as varying degrees of neurologic effects. Thus there is variation in clinical severity. Heterozygote detection of carrier mothers and prenatal diagnosis are possible. Treatment consists of drugs to decrease uric acid in the urine and blood, assuring high fluid intake and adequate nutrition, appropriate dental attention, and various approaches to treat the neurobehavioral manifestations, along with needed speech and physical therapy. In some cases, adequate nutrition reduces the self-mutilating behavior and spasticity.

Familial Dysautonomia (Riley-Day Syndrome, Hereditary Sensory and Autonomic Neuropathy [HSAN] Type III)

Familial dysautonomia is an autosomal recessive disorder that primarily affects the autonomic (central and peripheral) and sensory nervous systems.

It is most prevalent in Ashkenazi Jews (virtually 100%), in whom the incidence is 1:3,600 live births, with a carrier incidence of approximately 1 in 27–30. The gene has been located on the long arm of chromosome 9 (9q31). More than 99% of cases result from a single mutation in the gene IKBKAP. A mutation that causes familial dysautonomia in non-Jews has been identified. Familial dysautonomia is often noticed soon after birth because the infant has difficulty in sucking and swallowing with frequent choking. Tongue thrusting is a common mannerism, resulting in sores when teeth come in. The tongue is smooth and lacks fungiform papillae. Diagnosis may be made on a clinical basis consisting of alacrima, absent fungiform papillae of the tongue, depressed patellar reflexes, and lack of a red flare after intradermal injection of histamine. DNA testing can confirm the diagnosis. Carrier testing and prenatal diagnosis are possible.

Multiple systems are affected and clinical expression varies greatly from person to person even within families. Other symptoms include lack of overflow tears with crying; nondeliberate breath holding and cyanosis; poor bladder control, especially at night, with night wetting continuing into the teen years; excessive drooling; coordination problems; severe vomiting attacks and crises; progressive impairment of renal function with age; inability to distinguish tastes, heat, cold, and pain to varying degrees and in different body areas; small body size, with the average adult height of about five feet; and delayed puberty. Spinal curvature occurs in late childhood in most. Postural hypotension evidenced by weakness and dizziness occurs, especially if the patient rises quickly, and supine hypertension may be seen. Blood pressure lability, especially hypotension, becomes more problematic with age. Blotchy erythema can occur, evidencing the abnormal vasomotor control, and inappropriate temperature response to infection or the environment can result in episodes of fever or hypothermia. Respiratory problems can occur including lung disease secondary to frequent aspiration, and also to scoliosis and muscle weakness. Decreased chemoreceptor and baroreceptor sensitivity can result in abnormal responses to hypoxic and hypercapneic situations, including pressurized airplane cabins and high altitudes, as well as pneumonia. Neurological progression may also be seen with increasing age. Intelligence is generally normal but many may have problems in speech, executive planning, and organizational skills with some mildly impaired motor development. Cyclic dysautonomic crises can occur in about 40% with a pattern frequency that can be as frequent as daily, particularly following morning awakening, but which can result from stress. These crises may consist of abnormal gastrointestinal motility such as oropharyngeal incoordination, gastroesophageal reflux, and vomiting along with cardiovascular changes such as hypertension, tachycardia, and blotching. Secretions may be increased resulting in diaphoresis, gastrorrhea, bronchorrhea, and hypersalivation with drooling. Axelrod (2002, 2004) describes accompanying personality changes such as irritability, withdrawal, excitation, and/or picking at the skin. About 40% of surviving patients are over 20 years of age. There is a 50% probability for a newborn with familial dysautonomia to reach 40 years of age (Axelrod, 2004). As the affected person grows older, sensory abilities further decline; balance becomes worse; and disturbances such as depression, anxiety, and difficulties in concentration are seen. Nursing intervention and therapy is largely based on clinical manifestation and symptom control as well as family teaching and support. Major emphases include maintenance of nutrition and hydration, avoidance of aspiration, using drugs such as benzodiazepines and clonidine for crises, and managing blood pressure fluctuations. Ongoing care is a difficult and time-consuming task for parents, who need much support. Familial dysautonomia has been suggested for carrier testing in Ashkenazi Jews. Because mutation is known in non-Jews, familial dysautonomia should be considered in patients who meet clinical criteria but who are not of Ashkenazic Jewish descent.

Duchenne and Becker Muscular Dystrophy

The muscular dystrophies are a group of inherited muscle disorders for which the term "dystrophinopathies" is increasingly used. Duchenne muscular dystrophy (DMD) and Becker muscular dystrophy (BMD) are both X-linked recessive disorders that are allelic and result from different deletions in the dystrophin gene at Xp21.1. Mutation results in deficiency or defect of the functional gene protein product, dystrophin. This cytoskeletal protein is located as part of a dystrophin glycoprotein complex including dystroglycans and sarcoglycans in the muscle membrane. This complex is destabilized if dystophin is deficient or altered, resulting in lack of structural integrity of the muscle membrane. DMD is the most common (1 in 3,000–5,000 male births) and most severe. Initial common symptoms appear in early childhood, usually insidiously. These include abnormal gait, described as a ducklike waddle; toe walking; difficulty in climbing up steps; protruded abdomen; delayed walking; a tendency to fall; and the Gower's sign (climbing up oneself to get up from the floor by pressing on the thighs). In about one-third of affected patients, disease appears sporadically with no previously affected relative. Unless there has been a previously affected child in the family, the diagnosis is often delayed.

Boys with DMD usually lose the ability to walk between 7 and 13 years of age and may become wheelchair dependent. It is important to keep them ambulatory as long as possible to prevent deformities and degeneration. Muscle weakness is progressive with loss of function. The tendency for toe walking may lead to flexion contractures and forward hip tilt. Range of motion may help with these, but the child may benefit from braces. Death usually occurs in the 2nd decade of life because of respiratory infection and insufficiency, progressing from trivial to severe. A trend toward more aggressive support and new technologies available to manage respiratory problems in DMD has led to detailed guidelines and options (American Thoracic Society, 2004). Actual death may be sudden and caused by myocardial insufficiency. Dilative cardiomyopathy leading to arrhythmias may occur and can be treated with ACE inhibitors and beta-blockers if indicated. Congestive heart failure may occur. Boys with DMD are at increased risk for features of malignant hyperthermia when given anesthesia.

Once a child is diagnosed (in the past usually by serum creatine kinase levels, and today usually by DNA analysis and electromyography), female family members become concerned about their status as carriers. Females with an affected son and another affected male relative are obligate heterozygotes, but where there is only one affected male relative carrier status is more difficult to ascertain. Some carriers (about 10%) manifest mild symptoms such as pseudohypertrophy of the calves or muscle weakness. Carrier identification today is usually by DNA testing. DMD has been suggested as appropriate for newborn screening because, even though treatment is not available, further affected children in a family might be avoided. Corticosteroids have been used for some effects but the main hope lies in gene therapy.

BMD usually has its onset in adolescence. Ambulation is usual until about the age of 16 years. Affected males often survive into the 4th decade or later. Symptoms are similar and milder, often with exercise-related muscle pain. Usually the affected man eventually becomes dependent on a wheelchair. Dilated cardiomyopathy may occur that may necessitate heart transplantation. BMD usually shows the presence of muscle dystrophin but it is abnormal in size and quantity. Carrier detection is possible.

Neurofibromatosis 1 and 2

First characterized in 1882 by von Recklinghausen, neurofibromatosis attracted attention because of publicity resulting from the movie and play, *Elephant Man* (although Joseph Merrick did not actually have neurofibromatosis). There are two major types, neurofibromatosis type 1 (NF1), formerly called "von Recklinghausen disease," and neurofibromatosis type 2 (NF2), formerly called "bilateral acoustic neurofibromatosis." NF1 has a prevalence of approximately 1:2,500 to 1:5,000. Both are autosomal dominant (AD) disorders with one of the highest new mutation rates known, about 50%. It has been suggested that offspring of affected mothers are more severely affected than those of affected fathers but this has not been confirmed. The *NF1* gene was identified in 1990, is located at chromosome 17q11.2, and codes for neurofibromin, a protein product involved in control of cell growth and differentiation with a tumor suppressor function.

Despite widely variable clinical features and expression, a National Institutes of Health Consensus Development Conference (1988) established diagnostic criteria for NF1 that were reconfirmed by Gutmann et al. (1997). For diagnosis, a person must have two or more of the following: (1) six or more café-au-lait spots over 5 mm (0.5 cm) in prepuberty and over 15 mm (1.5 cm) in postpuberty (the normal population usually has none to three), (2) two or more neurofibromas of any type or one plexiform neurofibroma, (3) freckling in the axillary or inguinal regions, (4) optic glioma (tumor of the optic pathway), (5) two or more Lisch nodules (benign hamartomas of the iris), (6) a distinctive bony lesion such as dysplasia of the sphenoid bone or thinning of the long bone cortex, and (7) a first degree relative with NF1 by the previous criteria. Other features may develop. These include macrocephaly, short stature, spinal curvature (scoliosis or kyphosis), hemihypertrophy, neural crest malignancies (e.g., pheochromocytoma), hypertension, seizures, speech defects, and learning disabilities, especially visual–spatial learning problems. Knowledge of possible manifestations form the framework for diagnosis, treatment, and management. The café-au-lait spots are not usually seen at birth but develop around 1 year of age, and may fade in the elderly.

The severity of NF1 varies greatly. Even within a family one patient may have only café-au-lait spots, or axillary freckling, whereas another has macrocephaly, multiple neurofibromas, severe spinal curvature, learning disabilities, and hemihypertrophy. It is important to identify the person who has the gene mutation from someone who has an isolated physical characteristic. In my own practice I have seen several cases of NF1. One young woman sought genetic counseling regarding whether or not her 2-month-old son had inherited NF1. Her father had NF1 and had multiple neurofibromas on his body (see Figure 6.4). She had lost an eye to optic glioma and had macrocephaly, freckling, and hypertension. Interestingly, she did not regard herself as severely affected, believing that her father's manifestations would be harder to live with for her. Her son did show macrocephaly and one café-au-lait spot. Before all information was collected, she moved across the country and was followed by a genetic counseling center there. I later learned that her son was indeed affected. Nurses should also be aware of the worsening of symptoms that occurs in puberty and pregnancy. Patients should be advised to have a physical examination at least once a year because of the frequent progression to malignancy in the disease and to detect complications. The American Academy of Pediatrics' Committee on Genetics (1995) has published recommendations for health supervision

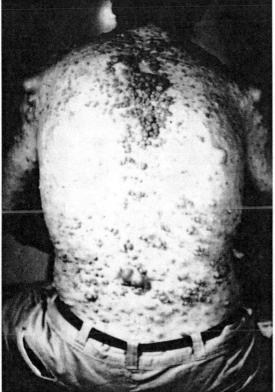

FIGURE 6.4   Multiple neurofibromas in man with neurofibromatosis.
Courtesy of Dr. Dorinda Shelley, Peoria, IL.

with anticipatory guidance for children with NF1. These recommendations include frequent ophthalmological examination, evaluation of speech, neurodevelopmental progress and learning needs, examination for neurologic pathology and skin lesions with changes, and others. A consensus statement on malignant peripheral nerve sheath tumors in NF1 has been issued (Ferner & Gutmann, 2002).

NF2 is less common, with a birth incidence of about 1 in 33,000 to 1 in 41,000. The gene for NF2 is located on chromosome 22q12.2 which codes for the protein merlin or schwannomin. It appears to be a tumor suppressor. There is considerable clinical and genetic heterogeneity. Onset is typically at age 15 years or older with a mean of 22 years, although 10% occur in childhood. A milder form may be present in adulthood after age 25 years. Clinical diagnostic criteria for NF2 (Gutmann et al., 1997) are: (1) bilateral vestibular schwannomas

(VS); (2) a parent, sibling, or child with NF2 plus (a) unilateral VS detected before 30 years of age, or (b) any two of the following: meningioma, glioma, schwannoma, or juvenile posterior subcapsular lenticular opacity. Others at risk who should have further monitoring and diagnosis include those below 30 years of age with a unilateral VS or meningioma and those with multiple spinal tumors who have a family history of NF2. Other indications for further evaluation may be found in Gutmann et al. The most consistent findings are vestibular schwannomas with related symptoms such as hearing loss, tinnitus, or vertigo. These are usually bilateral but may not develop simultaneously. Other cranial tumors such as meningiomas and gliomas may be seen and cataracts frequently occur. Various genotype–phenotype correlations have been noted. See Baser et al. (2004). Genetic testing is useful in some families but about half have no obvious family history. For those at risk where molecular testing is not possible, screening using MRI (usually recommended around age 15 years) and ophthalmologic assessment beginning in childhood is important. Treatment is usually surgical with radiation therapy done under certain circumstances. Treatment is most successful in specialty centers. Therapy targeted to molecules involved in merlin growth regulation is an area of current research. Counseling should include the fact that balance problems are often encountered and that there is a need for speech and hearing assessment and therapy.

Mitochondrial Diseases

Mitochondrial diseases can result from

- mutations in the mtDNA,
- defects in nuclear DNA that affect mitochondrial function such as defects of the Krebs cycle (these are becoming better understood and defined),
- defects in communication between mtDNA and nuclear DNA, and
- nonhereditary defects of mtDNA such as those resulting from zidovudine (an antiretroviral drug).

The number of known mitochondrial disorders has increased rapidly over the years. Gene mutations in the nucleus can also influence mitochondrial function and expression of mitochondrial mutations. Most nuclear gene defects resulting in mitochondrial disorders are associated with abnormalities of oxidative phosphorylation (OXPHOS). Deficiencies in mitochondrial ribosomal proteins are also thought to result in mitochondrial disease or to modify other involved genes.

In mitochondrial disease, every body tissue can be affected by mutations in mtDNA, and so diseases may be multisystemic. The major signs and symptoms traditionally involve skeletal muscle, the heart muscle, and the brain and nervous system but systemic manifestations may be seen, and certain constellations of features may occur. Unexplained hearing loss may be an early feature. Some symptoms that might alert the clinician to consider mitochondrial disorders include ataxia, weakness, seizures, respiratory insufficiency, failure to thrive, ophthalmoplegia, retinopathy, strokelike episodes, short stature, episodic vomiting, and sensorineural hearing loss. Phenotypic manifestation is wide ranging and some exhibit isolated deafness or diabetes. Symptoms may show wide clinical variability among patients and even within a family, and may worsen after exercise. In adults, exercise intolerance and generalized fatigue may be early indications. A review of major clinical features may be found in DiMauro, Tay, and Mancuso (2004). The athlete Greg Le Mond announced retirement from competitive cycling in December 1994 because of a mitochondrial myopathy. Laboratory results include abnormalities in serum lactate or pyruvate after exercise and ragged red fibres seen on muscle biopsy in certain disorders such as MERFF. Friedreich ataxia, a progressive neurodegenerative disease, is now known to be the result of mutation of a nuclear encoded mitochondrial protein known as frataxin which functions in some way to affect iron homeostasis in mitochondria and respiratory chain deficiency. The 1555A–>G mitochondrial mutation results in susceptibility to deafness after taking the aminoglycosides, and testing is available for this mutation which then has a very practical application in that another antibiotic can be used in treatment. Maternal transmission may be ascertained by family history. Probably because less is known about the trajectory of the mitochondrial diseases, a study by Read (2003) found that in contrast to children with PKU, mothers of children with mitochondrial diseases reported greater stress and worry, less satisfaction with social supports, greater difficulty in meeting their child's needs and greater impact on their lives including more missed work days. Mitochondrial inheritance is discussed in chapter 4.

Leber Hereditary Optic Neuropathy

Leber hereditary optic neuropathy (LHON) is an example of a disorder due to mitochondrial mutation and as such is maternally transmitted. At least 18 allelic variants are known but 3 are present in about 95% of families. Persons with LHON typically present in their 20s or 30s with sudden painless central visual loss and central scotoma. Other symptoms may include headache at onset, cardiac conduction defects, and dystonia with lesions in the basal ganglia. There appears to be incomplete penetrance, and a male bias in expression. There is a pediatric onset form. Environmental exposures such as exposure to tobacco smoke may play a role in expression.

BIBLIOGRAPHY

American Academy of Pediatrics. Committee on Genetics. (1995). Health supervision for children with neurofibromatosis. *Pediatrics, 96,* 368–372.

American Academy of Pediatrics. Committee on Genetics. Section on Hematology/Oncology. (2002). Health supervision for children with sickle cell disease. *Pediatrics,109,* 526–535.

American College of Medical Genetics. (1996). Statement on guidance for genetic counseling in advanced paternal age. *ACMG Newsletter, 6,* 13.

American College of Medical Genetics/American society of Human Genetics. Huntington Disease Genetic Testing Working Group. (1998). ACMG/ASHG statement. Laboratory guidelines for huntington disease genetic testing. *American Journal of Human Genetics, 62,* 1243–1247.

American Thoracic Society. (2004). Respiratory care of the patient with Duchenne muscular dystrophy. ATS consensus statement. *American Journal of Respiratory and Critical Care Medicine, 170,* 456–465.

Amrolia, P. J., Almeida, A., Davies, S. C., & Roberts, I. A. (2003). Therapeutic challenges in childhood sickle cell disease. Part 2: A problem-orientated approach. *British Journal of Haematology, 120,* 737–743.

Amrolia, P. J., Almeida, A., Halsey, C., & Roberts, I. A. (2003). Therapeutic challenges in childhood sickle cell disease. Part 1: Current and future treatment options. *British Journal of Haematology, 120,* 725–736.

Antonarakis, S. E., Krawczak, M., & Cooper, D. N. (2001). The nature and mechanisms of human gene mutation. In C. R. Scriver, A. L. Beaudet, W. S. Sly, & D. Valle (Eds.), *The metabolic and molecular bases of inherited disease* (8th ed., pp. 343–377). New York: McGraw-Hill.

Arun, D., & Gutmann, D. H. (2004). Recent advances in neurofibromatosis type 1. *Current Opinion in Neurology, 17,* 101–105.

Axelrod, F. B. (2002). Hereditary sensory and autonomic neuropathies. *Clinical Autonomic Research, 12*(Suppl. 1), 2–4.

Axelrod, F. B. (2004). Familial dysautonomia. *Muscle & Nerve, 29,* 352–363.

Bain, B. J. (2001). *Haemoglobinopathy diagnosis.* Oxford, England: Blackwell Science.

Bakanay, S. M., Dainer, E., Clair, B., Adekile, A., Daitch, L., Wells, L., et al. (2005). Mortality in sickle cell patients on hydroxyurea therapy. *Blood, 105,* 545–547.

Baser, M. E., Evans, D. G. R., & Gutmann, D. H. (2003). Neurofibromatosis 2. *Current Opinion in Neurology, 16,* 27–33.

Baser, M. E., Kuramoto, L., Joe, H., Friedman, J. M., Wallace, A. J., Gillespie, J. E., et al. (2004). Genotype-phenotype correlations for nervous system tumors in neurofibromatosis 2: A population-based study. *American Journal of Human Genetics, 75,* 231–239.

Beckerman, J., Wang, P., & Hlatky, M. (2004). Cardiovascular screening of athletes. *Clinical Journal of Sport Medicine, 14,* 127–133.

Beutler, E., Grabowski, G. A. (2001). Gaucher disease. In C. R. Scriver, A. L. Beaudet, W. S. Sly, & D. Valle (Eds.), *The metabolic and molecular bases of inherited disease* (8th ed., pp. 3635–3668). New York: McGraw-Hill.

Bonds, D. R. (2005). Three decades of innovation in the management of sickle cell disease: The road to understanding the sickle cell disease clinical phenotype. *Blood Reviews, 19,* 99–110.

Bonelli, R. M., & Hofmann, P. (2004). A review of the treatment options for Huntington's disease. *Expert Opinion in Pharmacotherapy, 5,* 767–776.

Boucher, C., & Sandford, R. (2004). Autosomal dominant polycystic kidney disease (ADPKD, MIM 173900, *PKD1* and *PKD2* genes, protein products known as polycystin-1 and polycystin-2). *European Journal of Human Genetics, 12,* 347–354.

Centers for Disease Control and Prevention. (2003). Contribution of selected metabolic diseases to early childhood deaths—Virginia, 1996–2001. *Morbidity and Mortality Weekly Report, 52,* 677–679.

Chinnery, P. F., DiMauro, S., Shanske, S., Schon, E. A., Zeviani, M., Mariotti, C., et al. (2004). Risk of developing a mitochondrial DNA deletion disorder. *Lancet, 364,* 592–596.

Clark, B. E., & Thein, S. L. (2004). Molecular diagnosis of haemoglobin disorders. *Clinical Laboratory Haematology, 26,* 159–176.

De Paepe, A., Devereux, R. B., Dietz, H. C., Hennekam, R. C., & Pyeritz, R. E. (1996). Revised diagnostic criteria for the Marfan syndrome. *American Journal of Medical Genetics, 62,* 417–426.

Desnick, R. J., & Brady, R. O. (2004). Fabry disease in childhood. *Journal of Pediatrics, 144,* S20–S26.

DiMauro, S., & Schon, E. A. (2003). Mitochondrial respiratory-chain diseases. *New England Journal of Medicine, 348,* 2656–2668.

DiMauro, S., Tay, S., & Mancuso, M. (2004). Mitochondrial encephalomyopathies: Diagnostic approach. *Annals of the New York Academy of Sciences, 1011,* 217–231.

Emery, A. E. H. (2002). The muscular dystrophies. *Lancet, 359,* 687–695.

Emery, A. E. H. (2002). Duchenne and other X-linked muscular dystrophies. In D. L. Rimoin, J. M. Connor, R. E. Pyeritz, & B. R. Korf (Eds.), *Emery and Rimoin's principles and practice of medical genetics* (4th ed., pp. 3266–3284). New York: Churchill Livingstone.

Ferner, R. E., & Gutmann, D. H. (2002). International consensus statement on malignant peripheral nerve sheath tumors in neurofibromatosis 1. *Cancer Research, 62,* 1573–1577.

Finsterer, J., & Stollberger, C. (2003). The heart in human dystrophinopathies. *Cardiology, 99,* 1–19.

Franchini, M., & Veneri, D. (2004). Iron-chelation therapy: An update. *Hematology Journal, 5,* 287–292.

Germino, G. G., & Chapman, A. B. (2001). Autosomal dominant polycystic kidney disease. In C. R. Scriver, A. L. Beaudet, W. S. Sly, & D. Valle (Eds.), *The metabolic and molecular bases of inherited disease* (8th ed., pp. 5467–5489). New York: McGraw-Hill.

Grabowski, G. A. (2004). Gaucher disease: Lessons from a decade of therapy. *Journal of Pediatrics, 144,* S15–S19.

Graff, C., Bui, T. H., & Larsson, N. G. (2002). Mitochondrial diseases. *Best Practices in Research and Clinical Obstetrics and Gynaecology, 16,* 715–728.

Gutmann, D. H., Aylsworth, A., Carey, J. C., Korf, B., Marks, J., Pyeritz, R. E., et al. (1997). The diagnostic evaluation and multidisciplinary management of neurofibromatosis 1 and neurofibromatosis 2. *Journal of the American Medical Association, 278,* 51–57.

Hayden, M. R., & Kremer, B. (2001). Huntington disease. In C. R. Scriver, A. L. Beaudet, W. S. Sly, & D. Valle (Eds.), *The metabolic and molecular bases of inherited disease* (8th ed., pp. 5677–5701). New York: McGraw-Hill.

Hillman, R. S., & Ault, K. A. (2002). *Hematology in clinical practice* (3rd ed.). New York: McGraw-Hill Medical Publishing Division.

Huntington's disease Collaborative Research Group. (1993). A novel gene containing a trinucleotide repeat that is expanded and unstable on Huntington's disease chromosomes. *Cell, 72,* 971–983.

Huson, S. M., & Korf, B. R. (2002). The phakomatoses. In D. L. Rimoin, J. M. Connor, R. E. Pyeritz, & B. R. Korf (Eds.), *Emery and Rimoin's principles and practice of medical genetics* (4th ed., pp. 3162–3202). New York: Churchill Livingstone.

Jinnah, H. A., & Friedmann, T. (2001). Lesch-Nyhan disease and its variants. In C. R. Scriver, A. L. Beaudet, W. S. Sly, & D. Valle (Eds.), *The metabolic and molecular bases of inherited disease* (8th ed., pp. 2537–2570). New York: McGraw-Hill.

Kakavanos, R., Turner, C. T., Hopwood, J. J.,

Kakkis, E. D., & Brooks, D. A. (2003). Immune tolerance after long-term enzyme-replacement therapy among patients who have mucopolysaccharidosis I. *The Lancet, 361,* 1608–1613.

Kishnani, P. S., & Howell, R. R. (2004). Pompe disease in infants and children. *Journal of Pediatrics, 144,* S35–S43.

Langbehn, D. R., Brinkman, R. R., Falush, D., Paulsen, J. S., Hayden, M. R. on behalf of an International Huntington's Disease Collaborative Group. (2004). A new model for prediction of the age of onset and penetrance for Huntington's disease based on CAG length. *Clinical Genetics, 65,* 267–277.

Leyne, M., Mull, J., Gill, S. P., Cuajungco, M. P., Oddoux, C., Blumenfeld, A., et al. (2003). Identification of the first non-Jewish mutation in familial dysautonomia. *American Journal of Medical Genetics, 118A,* 305–308.

Lo, L., & Singer, S. T. (2002). Thalassemia: Current approach to an old disease. *Pediatric Clinics of North America, 49,* 1165–1191.

Lynch, T. M., & Gutmann, D. H. (2002). Neurofibromatosis 1. *Neurologic Clinics of North America, 20,* 841–865.

Man, P. Y., Turnbull, D. M., & Chinnery P. F. (2002). Leber hereditary optic neuropathy. *Journal of Medical Genetics, 39,* 162–169.

Maron, B. J., Chaitman, B. R., Ackerman, M. J., Bayés de Luna, A., Corrado, D., Crosson, J. E., et al. (2004). Recommendations for physical activity and recreational sports participation for young patients with genetic cardiovascular diseases. *Circulation, 109,* 2807–2816.

McKerrell, T. D. H., Cohen, H. W., & Billett, H. H. (2004). The older sickle cell patient. *American Journal of Hematology, 76,* 101–106.

Midence, K., Fuggle, P., & Davies, S. C. (1993). Psychosocial aspects of sickle cell disease (SCD) in childhood and adolescence: A review. *British Journal of Clinical Psychology, 32,* 271–280.

Mignot, C., Gelot, A., Bessières, B., Daffos, F., Voyer, M., & Menez, F. (2003). Perinatal-lethal Gaucher disease. *American Journal of Medical Genetics, 120A,* 338–344.

Muenzer, J., & Fisher, A. (2004). Advances in the treatment of mucopolysaccharidosis type I. *New England Journal of Medicine, 350,* 1932–1934.

National Institutes of Health Consensus Development Conference. (1988). Neurofibromatosis.

Conference statement. *Archives of Neurology, 45,* 575–578.

Neufeld, E. F., & Muenzer, J. (2001). The mucopolysaccharidoses. In C. R. Scriver, A. L. Beaudet, W. S. Sly, & D. Valle (Eds.), *The metabolic and molecular bases of inherited disease* (8th ed., pp. 3421–3452). New York: McGraw-Hill.

Panepinto, J. A., Brousseau, D. C., Hillery, C. A., & Scott, J. P. (2005). Variation in hospitalizations and hospital length of stay in children with vaso-occulusive crises in sickle cell disease. *Pediatric Blood and Cancer, 44,* 182–186.

Percy, A. K. (2002). Gangliosidoses and related lipid storage diseases. In D. L. Rimoin, J. M. Connor, R. E. Pyeritz, & B. R. Korf (Eds.), *Emery and Rimoin's principles and practice of medical genetics* (4th ed., pp. 2712–2751). New York: Churchill Livingstone.

Pyeritz, R. E. (2002). Marfan syndrome and other disorders of fibrillin. In D. L. Rimoin, J. M. Connor, R. E. Pyeritz, & B. R. Korf (Eds.), *Emery and Rimoin's principles and practice of medical genetics* (4th ed., pp. 3977–4020). New York: Churchill Livingstone.

Read, C. Y. (2003). The demands of biochemical genetic disorders: A survey of mothers of children with mitochondrial disease or phenylketonuria. *Journal of Pediatric Nursing, 18,* 181–186.

Rees, D. C., Olujohungbe, A. D., Parker, N. E., Stephens, A. D., Telfer, P., Wright, J., et al. (2003). Guidelines for the management of the acute painful crisis in sickle cell disease. *British Journal of Haematology, 120,* 744–752.

Reynolds, R. M., Browning, G. G. P., Nawroz, I., & Campbell, I. W. (2003). Von Recklinghausen's neurofibromatosis: Neurofibromatosis type 1. *Lancet, 361,* 1552–1554.

Rodak, B. F. (Ed). (2002). *Hematology* (2nd ed.). Philadelphia: WB Saunders.

Rosebush, P. I., MacQueen, G. M., Clarke, J. T., Callahan, J. W., Strasberg, P. M., & M. F. Mazurek (1995). Late-onset Tay-Sachs disease presenting as catatonic schizophrenia: Diagnostic and treatment issues. *Journal of Clinical Psychiatry, 56,* 347–353.

Rosser, T. L., & Packer, R. J. (2003). Neurocognitive dysfunction in children with neurofibromatosis type 1. *Current Neurological and Neuroscience Reports, 3,* 129–136.

Rossetti, S., Chauveau, D., Kubly, V., Slezak, J. M.,

Saggar-Malik, A. K., & Pei, Y. (2003). Association of mutation position in polycystic kidney disease 1. *(PKD1)* gene and development of a vascular phenotype. *Lancet, 361,* 2196–2201.

Roush, W. (1997). Backup gene may help muscles help themselves. *Science, 276,* 35.

Saudubray, J. M., Nassogne, M. C., de Lonlay, P., & Touati, G. (2002). Clinical approach to inherited metabolic disorders in neonates: An overview. *Seminars in Neonatology, 7,* 3–15.

Scaglia, F., Towbin, J. A., Craigen, W. J., Belmont, J. W., Mith, E. O., Neish, S. R., et al. (2004). Clinical spectrum, morbidity, and mortality in 113 pediatric patients with mitochondrial disease. *Pediatrics, 114,* 925–931.

Schapira, A. H. (2002). Primary and secondary defects of the mitochondrial respiratory chain. *Journal of Inherited and Metabolic Diseases, 25,* 207–214.

Seegmiller, J. E., & Page, T. (2002). Purine and pyrimidine metabolism. In D. L. Rimoin, J. M. Connor, R. E. Pyeritz, & B. R. Korf (Eds.), *Emery and Rimoin's principles and practice of medical genetics* (4th ed., pp. 2468–2499). New York: Churchill Livingstone.

Shows, T. B., McAlpine, P. J., Boucheix, C., Collins, F. S., Conneally, P. M., Frezal, J., et al. (1987). Guidelines for human gene nomenclature. An international system for human gene nomenclature (ISGN, 1987). *Cytogenetics and Cell Genetics, 46,* 11–28.

Shulman, L. M., David, N. J., & Weiner, W. J. (1995). Psychosis as the initial manifestation of adult-onset Niemann-Pick disease type C. *Neurology, 45,* 1739–1743.

Slaugenhaupt, S. A. (2002). Genetics of familial dysautonomia. *Clinical Autonomic Research, 12*(Suppl. 1), 15–19.

Staba, S. L., Escolar, M. L., Poe, M., Kim, Y., Martin, P. L., Szabolcs, P., et al. (2004). Cord-blood transplants from unrelated donors in patients with Hurler's syndrome. *New England Journal of Medicine, 350,* 1960–1969.

Steinberg, M. H., Barton, F., Castro, O., Pegelow, C. H., Ballas, S. K., Kutlar, A., et al. (2003). Effect of hydroxyurea on mortality and morbidity in adult sickle cell anemia. *New England Journal of Medicine, 289,* 1645–1651.

Sutter, M., & Germino, G. G. (2003). Autosomal dominant polycystic kidney disease: Molecular genetics and pathophysiology. *Journal of Laboratory and Clinical Medicine, 141,* 91–101.

Sylvester, J. E., Fischel-Ghodsian, N., Mougey, E. B., & O'Brien, T. W. (2004). Mitochondrial ribosomal proteins: Candidate genes for mitochondrial disease. *Genetics in Medicine, 6,* 73–80.

Tanaka, M., Machida, Y., Niu, S., Ikeda, T., Jana, N. R., Doi, H., et al. (2004). Trehalose alleviates polyglutamine-mediated pathology in a mouse model of Huntington disease. *Nature Medicine, 10,* 148–154.

Taylor, S. D. (2004). Predictive genetic test decisions for Huntington's disease: Context apraisal and new moral imperatives. *Social Science & Medicine, 58,* 137–149.

Terlato, N. J., & Cox, G. F. (2003). Can mucopolypsaccharidosis type I disease severity be predicted based on a patient's genotype? A comprehensive review of the literature. *Genetics in Medicine, 5,* 286–294.

Thein, S. L. (2004). Genetic insights into the clinical diversity of b thalassaemia. *British Journal of Haematology, 124,* 264–274.

Thorburn, D. R. (2004). Mitochondrial disorders: Prevalence, myths and advances. *Journal of Inherited and Metabolic Diseases, 27,* 349–362.

The U.S.-Venezuela Collaborative Research Project, & Wexler, N. S. (2004). Venezuelan kindreds reveal that genetic and environmental factors modulate Huntington's disease age of onset. *Proceedings of the National Academy of Sciences USA, 101,* 3498–3503.

van Dellen, A., & Annan, A. J. (2004). Genetic and environmental factors in the pathogenesis of Huntington's disease. *Neurogenetics, 5,* 9–17.

Weatherall, D. (2004). The thalassemias: The role of molecular genetics in an evolving global health problem. *American Journal of Human Genetics, 74,* 385–392.

Weatherall, D. J., & Clegg, J. B. (2001). *The thalassaemia syndromes* (4th ed.). Oxford, England: Blackwell Publishing.

Wenger, D. A., Coppola, S., & Liu, S-L. (2003). Insights into the diagnosis and treatment of lysosomal storage diseases. *Archives of Neurology, 60,* 322–328.

Wilcox, W. R. (2004). Lysosomal storage disorders: The need for better pediatric recognition and comprehensive care. *Journal of Pediatrics, 144,* S3–S14.

Wilson, P. D. (2004). Polycystic kidney disease. *New England Journal of Medicine, 350,* 151–164.

Wong, C., & Richardson, D. R. (2003). β-thalassaemia: Emergence of new and improved iron chelators for treatment. *International Journal of Biochemistry & Cell Biology, 35,* 1144–1149.

Worton, R. G., Molnar, M. J., Brais, B., & Karpati, G. (2001). The muscular dystrophies. In C. R. Scriver, A. L. Beaudet, W. S. Sly, & D. Valle (Eds.), *The metabolic and molecular bases of inherited disease* (8th ed., pp. 5493–5523). New York: McGraw-Hill.

Young, A. B. (2003). Huntington in health and disease. *Journal of Clinical Investigation, 111,* 299–302.

Zeviani, M., Spinazzola, A., & Carelli, V. (2003). Nuclear genes in mitochondrial disorders. *Current Opinion in Genetics & Development, 13,* 262–270.

Zhao, H., Keddache, M., Bailey, L., Arnold, G. L., & Grabowski, G. (2003). Gaucher's disease: Identification of novel mutant alleles and genotype-phenotype relationships. *Clinical Genetics, 64,* 57–64.

Zlotogora, J. (2004). Parents of children with autosomal recessive diseases are not always carriers of the respective mutant alleles. *Human Genetics, 114,* 521–526.

7

Birth Defects and Congenital Anomalies

The term "birth defects" is a general one that was popularized by the March of Dimes. It encompasses the picture of an abnormal variation in form or structure without inferring a specific cause. Thus, it is with the infant born with a defect—appearance does not necessarily indicate etiology. For example, a cleft palate may be an isolated anomaly or part of a syndrome; it may be caused by a chromosome aberration, a single-gene disorder, an environmental insult, a combination of genetic and environmental factors, or unknown causes. The terms "birth defects" and "congenital anomalies" are essentially synonymous. Birth defects may be caused by chromosome disorders (e.g., trisomy 13), single-gene defects (e.g., Meckel syndrome), a combination of genetic and environmental factors (e.g., anencephaly), external physical constraints of the fetus in utero (e.g., torticollis), infectious agents (e.g., congenital rubella syndrome), drugs or chemicals (e.g., thalidomide embryopathy), radiation exposure in utero (e.g., microcephaly), or maternal metabolic factors (e.g., diabetes mellitus). Epstein (2004) estimates that 6% of birth defects are due to a chromosomal abnormality, 7.5% are due to a single gene defect, 20% are multifactorial and 6% to 7% are due to known environmental factors and teratogens. This chapter concentrates on single anomalies resulting from multifactorial causes and on deformations. Multifactorial inheritance is explained in chapter 4. Dysmorphology is concerned with prenatal abnormal structural development. Prenatal development is extremely complex involving cell proliferation, differentiation, migration, programmed cell death, fusion between adjacent tissues, proper chemical communication between tissues along with induction. The correct sequence and timing is crucial.

Recently, geneticists are identifying mutations in developmental genes such as homeobox genes, involved in specific steps in embryonic processes including patterning. An example is the *PAX3* gene, which is mutated in Waardenburg syndrome 1 (an autosomal dominant condition including patchy pigment abnormalities such as white forelock, deafness, and others). The deafness results from the need of the cochlea for melanocytes. Some developmental gene families may not be only patterning genes but oncogenes. *HOX* genes which play a role in hemopoiesis have been implicated in various cancers, especially leukemia. Recently there has been accelerated progress in understanding the basis of congenital malformations due to body patterning defects such as may occur in certain mutations of the sonic hedgehog gene and some cases of holoprosencephaly (a forebrain and midface congenital malformation with a range of severity and various degrees of mental retardation, seizures, and anomalies of other systems; when most severe there is cyclopia).

Various estimates have been made for the frequency of birth defects in the general population. Differences arise depending on the type of population surveyed, the criteria used to record an anomaly, and the age at which estimates are made. For example, neural tube defects have a high frequency in Ireland, and internal urinary tract anomalies are not usually detected at birth. The frequency of major congenital anomalies (defined as those that require surgery or interfere with normal livelihood) identified by 1 year of age is estimated to range from 4% to 7% and is about 3% at birth. The frequency of minor anomalies (e.g., a supernumerary nipple) is estimated at 10% to 12% or more depending on definition used. In active surveillance of malformations in newborns in Mainz, Germany from 1990 to 1998, major malformations and minor errors of morphogenesis were found to be 6.9% and 35.8% respectively. Risk factors significantly associated with malformations were: parents or siblings with malformations, parental consanguinity, more than three minor errors of morphogenesis in the proband, maternal diabetes mellitus, and using antiallergic drugs during the first trimester (Queisser-Luft, Stolz, Wiesel, & Schaefer, 2002). A higher incidence of congenital anomalies is found in twins. This chapter concentrates on those birth defects that are believed to be of multifactorial causation. The repercussions and impact of the birth of an infant with a congenital anomaly on the family are discussed in chapter 8.

TERMINOLOGY

The nomenclature associated with birth defects varies and can lead to improper conceptualization. Terms like malformations, anomalads, and complexes have not been used with consistent meaning in the literature. Definitions of the ones most likely to be encountered by the nurse and examples of each are given below:

- Malformation—A morphologic defect of an organ or part of an organ with poor tissue formation that results from an intrinsic abnormal developmental process (e.g., cleft lip)
- Disruption—The initial developmental process is normal, but a defective organ, or part of an organ or tissue, results from interference (usually external) with the process (e.g., limb defects resulting from thalidomide, amniotic band syndrome)
- Deformation—An abnormal form, shape, or position of a previously normal body part caused by mechanical forces (usually molding) on normal tissue (e.g., intrauterine restraint resulting in clubfoot)
- Syndrome—A recognized pattern of multiple anomalies presumed to have the same etiology (e.g., Down syndrome)
- Sequence—A pattern of multiple anomalies derived from a single prior anomaly; this replaces anomalad or complex (e.g., Robin sequence—micrognathia, large tongue, cleft palate)
- Association—Nonrandom occurrence together of a pattern of multiple anomalies, but that are not yet known to be a syndrome or sequence (e.g., VATER association—Vertebral defects, Anal atresia, Tracheo-esophageal fistula with esophageal atresia, Radial dysplasia, and Renal defects).

Other terms that describe various anomalies such as agenesis, aplasia, dysplasia, dyshistogenesis, hyperplasia, and hamartomas, are defined in the glossary.

REGISTRIES AND SURVEILLANCE SYSTEMS

Both registries and surveillance systems for birth defects exist. Registries, such as for congenital heart defects or immunodeficiency disorders, usually maintain a list of affected individuals along with clinical and genetic data. Surveillance systems monitor congenital anomalies and thus can provide an "early warning" system that may lead to detection of a new teratogen. The Centers for Disease Control and Prevention (CDC) monitor rates of birth defects in several geographic areas of the United States. Computerized, on-line information systems also exist to help in diagnosis and to identify new syndromes. The National Birth Defects Prevention Study is designed to conduct DNA testing and collect interviews and other information to further elucidate genetic and environmental factors involved in birth defects, especially those that are rarer. Problems common to registries are ascertainment, confidentiality, and privacy. In the United States, entry into them is voluntary, and patients should be asked to consent to entry or to any such recording of potentially identifiable data, although they often are not. Aspects of state and federal laws regarding genetic privacy and the Health Insurance Portability and Accountability Act of 1996 (HIPAA) impact on this use (see Cole and Fleisher, 2003; Sankar, 2003). Registries yield information about incidence and prevalence rates, serve as a source of research data, and allow the recall of clients for new or additional treatment or even preventive measures.

MULTIFACTORIAL CAUSATION AND INHERITANCE

The common congenital anomalies often have a familial basis, but they usually do not fit a Mendelian inheritance pattern or show an association with a chromosomal abnormality. While for the most part exact causes remain unknown, it is believed that many of the common congenital malformations and isolated birth defects are inherited in a multifactorial manner (involving the interaction of several genes and the environment). Some congenital anomalies show sex bias in their expression. Females seem to show tissue anomalies, while males often have more organ specific findings (see Table 7.1). The reasons for these are under investigation. In some cases, newer techniques have demonstrated non-multifactorial causes for congenital anomalies such as submicroscopic deletions and duplications. An example is DiGeorge or velocardiofacial syndrome (VCFS) where microdeletions of chromosome 22q11 are associated with ventricular septal and conotruncal heart defects in association with an absent thymus, facial abnormalities, hypoparathyroidism, immune deficiencies, and others. Thus even if a person had chromosomal or other testing that was negative years ago, it may be useful to repeat such testing in order to provide updated genetic counseling information. Multifactorial inheritance is explained in chapter 4.

DEFORMATIONS

Anomalies also result from mechanical factors causing constraint on the fetus. Such mechanical forces are commonly seen in mild form in the molding of the head during birth. They usually involve cartilage, bones, and joints. Often, as in congenital dislocation of the hip, the mechanical factors may be environmental ones that act on a susceptible constitution fitting the multifactorial model. Graham (1988) has identified some maternal and fetal factors leading to in utero fetal constraint and unusual position which are still current. They are as follows:

- Primigravida—The abdominal wall usually has more tone in the first pregnancy

- Breech presentation—This position is found in 3% to 4% of all pregnancies but is associated with 32% of all deformations
- Small size of the mother or pelvis
- Small or malformed uterus
- Uterine tumor
- Early engagement of the fetal head
- Unusual fetal position
- Large or malformed fetus
- Multiple pregnancy
- Oligohydramnios
- Unusual placental site

Sometimes deformations spontaneously return to normality. In other cases, such as severe clubfoot, corrective mechanical forces in the form of exercise, casts, or braces may be applied. It is important, if possible, to ascertain the cause leading to the deformation in order to provide accurate counseling to the parents.

DISRUPTIONS

Disruptions occur when previously normal tissues or organs are interfered with in some way. The most common type is due to early rupture of the amnion, causing a wide spectrum of possible abnormalities. As an example, shreds of amniotic membrane can adhere to the embryonic or fetal tissue, often encircling developing limbs producing constrictions or even amputation of a limb. The challenge is to distinguish these from other causes of malformation. For example, facial clefting from amniotic band disruption will usually not coincide with the usual cleft-lip sites. The recurrence risk for amniotic band disruption is extremely low.

CONGENITAL HEART DISEASE

The overall frequency of congenital heart disease (CHD) in the North American population is about 75 per 1,000 if trivial lesions are included, and 19 per 1,000 live births if only moderate and severe forms are included (Hoffman & Kaplan, 2002). Unlike most other congenital malformations, the sexes are about equally affected for the overall category of CHD. The etiology varies with about 1% to 2% being of environmental origin, often due to

TABLE 7.1   The Occurrence and Sex Distribution of Selected Congenital Anomalies*

Congenital anomaly	Incidence	Gender most frequently affected
Anencephaly	1:1,000	Female
Spina bifida	1:1,000	Female
Cleft lip with/without cleft palate	1:700–1,000—Caucasian 1.7:1,000—Japanese 0.7:1,000—Blacks	Male
Cleft palate alone	1:2,000-1:2,500	Female
Congenital heart defect	6–8:1,000	Equal
Developmental dysplasia of the hip	1:100–1:1,000	Female
Pyloric stenosis	5:1,000—males 1:1,000—females	Male
Clubfoot	1:1,000	Male
Hirschsprung disease	1:5,000	Male
Hypospadias	6:1,000—Caucasian males 2:1,000—Black males	Males only

*Frequency in U.S. unless stated otherwise.

teratogenic agents (e.g., lithium, alcohol, dilantin, retinoic acid, valproic acid), infection (congenital rubella), or maternal environment disturbances such as maternal PKU; about 5–10% are of chromosomal origin (e.g., Turner syndrome, trisomy 21); 5–10% resulting from a single-gene disorder (e.g., Holt Oram syndrome, an autosomal dominant disorder resulting from mutation of the *TBX5* gene that encodes a transcription factor, and consists of upper limb skeletal defects and cardiac anomalies); and the rest are believed to be accounted for by multifactorial inheritance mechanisms. There are some cases of CHD that do not fit traditional inheritance patterns. Some of these may be accounted for by mitochondrial inheritance, imprinting, germline mosaicism, or uniparental disomy (see chapter 4 for discussion of these mechanisms). Progress has also been made in identifying more single gene defects that result in CHD. One that has been recently identified is mutations in *TFAP2B*, which have been associated with Char syndrome, a familial form of patent ductus ateriosus. There appears to be a strong association between congenital complete heart blocks in the fetus and autoantibodies against Ro/SSA or La/SSB in their mothers, often associated with autoimmune disorders such as Sjögren's syndrome or systemic lupus erythematosus. Isolated ventricular septal defects are the most common CHD, and if tiny ones are included, the incidence can vary from 2% to 5% in newborns but 85% to 90% close spontaneously by a year of age.

An important consideration for nurses, especially those involved in routine physical examinations of infants and children, is that persons with CHD frequently have one or more extracardiac defects, ranging from 25% to 45% depending on the specific research report. Thus all children known to have CHD should be carefully evaluated in order to detect such other anomalies. Some anomalies, such as cleft palate, are readily apparent, but others, such as those of the urinary tract, are more difficult to detect. The most frequent extracardiac defects associated with CHD are those of the genitourinary tract, gastrointestinal tract, and musculoskeletal system. Nonimmune fetal hydrops is estimated to have a cardiac cause in as many as 25% of the cases. The most frequent congenital heart defects found in association with other anomalies are patent ductus arteriosus, atrial septal defects, atrioventricularis communis, tetralogy of Fallot, coarctation of the aorta, ventricular septal defects, and malposition defects. Some tend to be associated with specific syndromes (e.g., coarctation of the aorta and Turner syndrome). About 10% of all CHD are part of a syndrome. It is important to recognize these syndromes in order to provide accurate genetic counseling and management.

Recurrence risk figures vary for the type of defect as well as for other factors previously discussed. An overall risk to a sib of an affected individual is 2% to 4%. This increases to 6-12% if a second sib is affected. Harper (2004) gives the risk to offspring of an isolated case in an affected father and mother as 2–3% and about 5% respectively, while Allan and Baker (1993) list a risk of about 10% if there is an affected parent regardless of sex. Periconceptional multivitamin supplementation at levels recommended for routine prenatal use with at least 0.4 mg folic acid appears to be associated with a reduced risk for one group of severe heart defects (conotruncal defects), including tetralogy of Fallot and transposition of the great arteries. This is a simple measure that nurses can recommend. Because of effective early interventions, many persons with CHD survive into adulthood. There are clinicians who specialize in adult CHD, and it has been noted that some carry over from "precious" babies to "precious" adults, and may seek medical care accompanied by their parents even into their 30s. However, a European study following persons with CHD for 20 to 33 years generally showed them to be capable of leading normal lives, although they showed lower educational and occupational levels than comparative groups.

DEVELOPMENTAL DYSPLASIA OF THE HIP

Developmental dysplasia of the hip (DDH) was formerly known as congenital dislocation of the hip (CDH). The interaction of genetic and environmental factors in DDH is striking. It is now thought of by most as a deformation rather than a true congenital malformation, with an incidence of about 1% of all live births, depending on the criteria used and the age of assessment. A full range of severity from a lax dislocatable hip to a dislocated hip that cannot be reduced is possible. DDH is five to eight times more common in females, 60% are first-born children, and 30% to 50% are delivered in breech presentation. Environmental factors present after birth may contribute to DDH development. Cultures such as the Lapps and some Navajo Indian tribes in which infants are wrapped to a cradle board or swaddled, with legs in forced extension, show an incidence of DDH that is ten times greater than normal. A lower

than usual incidence is seen in societies that keep the infants in a "protective" position, in which the hips are partially abducted, as in the Hong Kong Chinese who carry infants on their back. Intrinsic factors leading to DDH have also been identified. These include the nature of the hip joint (e.g., a shallow-angled acetabulum is more susceptible to dislocation), or lax connective tissue either from heritable causes or hormones (e.g., inborn errors of estrogen or collagen metabolism, maternal estrogens, or hormones that may be given before delivery). Breech delivery is relatively common.

The nurse should carefully assess neonates and infants for clinical features of DDH by examining for shortening of the thigh with bunching up of tissue and skin fold accentuation, limitation of abduction, or other signs. The Ortolani or Barlow test may also be done. However, DDH may not be detected at birth, and surveillance should be maintained. Ultrasound screening of the neonatal hip has become more common and has a specificity and sensitivity of over 90%. Eastwood (2003) estimates that using risk figures alone for referred for ultrasound screening would miss 30% to 40%. DDH is relatively easy to treat early, but if it is discovered after 1 year of age it requires more complex management and complete correction may not be possible. Nurses should be especially alert in examining infants who are female, first-born, and delivered in a breech position. Health teaching should include information about optimum positioning. A still relevant retrospective study by David et al. (1983) found that the mean age at which parents noticed a problem was 11 months, but the mean age at diagnosis was 26 months. The reasons found for this delay in descending order of frequency are as follows: (1) failure of health professionals to follow up on symptoms reported by parents, (2) failure to routinely check hips after 3 months of age, (3) failure of parents to appreciate the significance of abnormalities, (4) failure of health professionals to examine the hips at birth, and (5) failure to follow up those congenital abnormalities that were found. The most common presenting signs and symptoms included limping, walking on tip-toe, unequal leg length, difficulty in crawling, delayed walking, noticeable short leg, asymmetric thigh creases, and uneven shoe wear. It appears that further education on DDH detection is needed for both professionals and parents.

NEURAL TUBE DEFECTS

One of the biggest success stories in prevention of genetic disorders has been the ability to prevent many neural tube defects by the periconceptual administration of folic acid as discussed later. In addition, a large proportion of neural tube defects (NTDs) can be detected prenatally by ultrasound, measurement of alpha fetoprotein in maternal serum and amniotic fluid, and measurement of acetylcholinesterase in amniotic fluid (see chapter 12). Spina bifida is estimated to have the third highest lifetime cost of any birth defect. The embryonic structure that gives rise to the central nervous system is the neural tube. Errors in its development encompass a group of malformations that include anencephaly, spina bifida, encephalocele, and hydrocephalus. In anencephaly, the vault of the skull is absent, with a rudimentary brain. It is not compatible with survival; affected infants are either stillborn or die shortly after birth. Spina bifida ranges in severity from spina bifida occulta, in which one vertebra is not fused and a tuft of hair may be present over the skin of the area, to meningocele, in which the meninges protrude or are herniated from the spinal canal but the cord is in its usual position, to myelomeningocele, in which both the meninges and the spinal cord protrude from the defective vertebrae. NTDs are considered to be open when neural tissue is either exposed or covered with a thin transparent membrane and closed when the neural tissue is covered with skin or a thick, opaque membrane (Figure 7.1). Closed lesions may not be detected by alpha fetoprotein determinations. Anencephaly and spina bifida are related etiologically and are generally discussed together. After having an infant with either anencephaly or spina bifida the recurrence risk is for either one, not just for the anomaly that was present in the affected infant.

Many epidemiological studies have been carried out, and many factors that are related to the occurrence of NTDs have been identified. It is now believed that at least four separate closures of the neural tube occur early in embryonic life. Each seems to be sensitive to different environmental agents and each has a different result when it fails to close. For example, "zipper" 1 is susceptible to folic acid deficiency while "zipper" 4 is susceptible to hyperthermia. The multiple closure theory helps

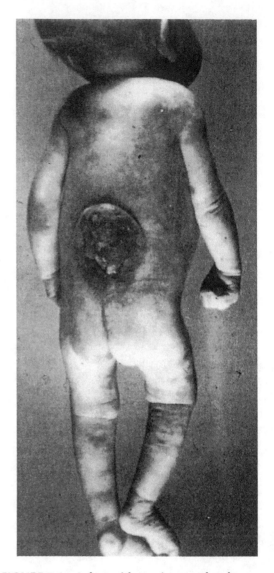

FIGURE 7.1   Infant with meningomyelocele.
Courtesy of Dr. John Murphy, Southern Illinois University School of Medicine, Springfield, IL.

to explain the varying epidemiological observations about neural tube defects. A consistent observation has been that NTDs are more frequent in poorer socioeconomic groups and after conditions that result in poor diets, especially folic acid deficiency but also possibly deficiency in ascorbic acid, zinc, and others. Some studies have found a higher risk of NTDs in obese women that is independent of folic acid intake.

The highest incidence is found among the Irish and in the United Kingdom, where the incidence is 4:1,000 to 5:1,000. It is also high among Sikhs and in parts of Egypt, Pakistan, and India, whereas the incidence is lowest in Blacks, Ashkenazic Jews, and most Asians. Females predominate, especially in anencephaly. In the United States, overall it is 2:1,000 with a higher rate in the eastern and southern United States, decreasing in the west. Hyperthermia (core body temperature over 100.4°F or 38°C), either from maternal illness with fever, or environmental, such as that with sauna or hot tub use, during early pregnancy has been shown by investigators such as Motulsky (1996) to be capable of causing NTD, especially anencephaly. Maternal hyperthermia has been suggested to also result in embryonic death, growth retardation and other developmental defects but evidence varies in research studies (Andersen et al., 2002; Edwards, Saunders, & Shiota, 2003). The effect of any environmental agent may be mediated by susceptible or non-susceptible maternal and fetal genotypes. A review of epidemiologic associations may be found in the reference by Tolmie (2002).

Morbidity and mortality are more severe in those with open lesions. Problems occur with morbidity in several areas; hydrocephalus (75%), impairment of sensation and paralysis below the level of the lesion, incontinence of urine and feces, and associated anomalies such as clubfoot and hip dislocation. There is a slight excess of mental retardation, but the full gamut of intelligence is seen. Mental impairment can result from hydrocephalus. Some learning and perceptual defects also occur. Short stature and central precocious puberty may occur. Adolescence is a particularly trying time for persons with spina bifida. Blum (1983) found that about 50% had no friends outside of school. In conducting a qualitative study on adults with NTDs, Nehring found that health concerns centered around bowel and bladder issues, skin and pressure ulcers, and joint pair and osteoarthritis. They also had concerns about ambulation and primary health care provision, but they were not depressed and indicated that they had a fairly good quality of life (Dr. Wendy Nehring, personal communication, January 2005). Prevention of the hydrocephalus can be accomplished surgically. By childhood, urinary incontinence is frequently managed by self-catheterization programs. Nonetheless, the burden on the family is an extreme one. Often the decision to selectively treat or nontreat these children is a difficult one

that has promoted much controversy, because many surgical procedures become necessary for survival and management.

Surgical repair may include the placement of a shunt. In some centers, fetal surgery is being performed to close myelomeningoceles to decrease shunting and improve motor function.

One professional of the author's acquaintance, who has spina bifida and would be regarded by most as successful, has said that he believes in euthanasia for such infants, and that he himself wished that he had not survived. Others feel differently. The Spina Bifida Association of America is a parents' group that provides support and leads for adoptive placement of children with spina bifida. Some couples decide on pregnancy termination if NTDs are diagnosed prenatally, while others decide to continue the pregnancy. The nurse should support the decision that the family believes is right for them. These issues are discussed further in chapters 8, 10, and 12.

The appearance of an infant with anencephaly is so shocking that often parents equate the severity of the infant's appearance with the risk of recurrence. In fact, it falls into the same general range of the other multifactorial disorders. Of course, recurrence risks must always be adjusted to the population incidence, ethnic background, number of affected relatives, epidemiological factors when known, and so on, but in general the risk of recurrence in the United States for a Caucasian couple after having one affected infant and no other affected relatives is believed to be 3% to 4%. The risk was formerly estimated at about 5%, but it has been adjusted downward after a large series of studies of actual recurrence rates observed among such couples. Interestingly enough, for aunts and uncles of the affected infant, the risk of one of their children to be affected is less than 1%, but it is higher for children of maternal relatives—6.7 per 1,000 for mothers' sisters and 2.2 per 1,000 for mothers' brothers, as opposed to 3.2 per 1,000 for fathers' sisters and 1.8 per 1000 for the fathers' brothers' children. After two affected siblings, the recurrence risk rises to 10% to 13%, but in Northern Ireland the risk may be as high as 20%. The risk for a woman with spina bifida to have an affected child is about 4%. Also see ACOG Practice Bulletin, "Neural tube defects," (2003), and Tolmie (2002). Management should include appropriate folic acid supplementation beginning preconceptionally, and expert management for the pregnancy, delivery, and pediatric aftercare. There is some indication that there is an increased risk for NTDs among siblings of children who have other birth defects, such as cleft lip and palate.

A couple seen for genetic counseling had one normal son and had just delivered a stillborn infant with anencephaly. The shock was so great that they were sure that the risk for recurrence of the defect was very high. In their minds, they only had a 50% chance of having a normal child. They were relieved to discover that it was only about 3% to 4%, and that prenatal diagnosis was available which could detect the majority of infants with NTDs, especially in women known to have previously had a child with NTD. Nurses should be sure to discuss the option of prenatal diagnosis with both members of such a couple, lest they disrupt their reproductive plans out of disproportionate fear of the recurrence of NTD. All such couples should be referred for genetic counseling in order to accurately determine their risk and to discuss with them the increased risk to other close relatives. Spina bifida can be part of many other syndromes, some of which are caused by single-gene defects or chromosomal aberrations, so all of the nursing actions listed in chapters 5 and 9 such as taking a picture of the aborted or stillborn infant, getting specimens for chromosome analysis, and so on are important in order to provide accurate genetic counseling for families. Hydrocephalus may be associated with 75% of the cases of spina bifida, but it may also be caused by an X-linked recessively inherited disorder (e.g., stenosis of the aqueduct of Sylvius) that can usually be distinguished.

The most important aspect of NTDs currently is prevention. From the early work of Smithells and others came the discovery first that recurrence of NTDs could be prevented by periconceptional supplementation of folic acid and vitamins followed by the discovery that the expansion of this supplementation could prevent first occurrences as well. The United States was behind many of the European countries in making widespread recommendations in this regard. Eventually, the CDC recommended 0.4 mg (400µg) of folic acid for all women of childbearing age. The American College of Medical Genetics supports that but also recommends that women with a previous history of NTDs take

4.0 mg of folic acid daily, optimally starting 3 months before conception. There has been recent discussion about increasing the level of this recommendation. Later, it was found that women with a polymorphic variation in the gene for the enzyme methylenetetrahydrofolate reductase, that led to low enzyme levels and increased plasma homocysteine (an amino acid) as a result, were at higher risk for children with NTDs. Folic acid supplementation lowers plasma homocysteine. Thus a relatively common polymorphism is one risk factor for NTDs. There is the possibility that interactions between certain allelelic variants of folate-related genes such as that for 5, 10 methylenetetrahydrofolate reductase (MTHFR) and cystathionine-β-synthase (CBS) may contribute to spina bifida risk. Some women who have had a pregnancy in which the fetus has an NTD have been found to have autoantibodies that bind to folate receptors and thus block folate uptake (Rothenberg et al., 2004).

Poor maternal nutrition, in general, may also contribute to NTD occurrence as well as to other birth defects such as imperforate anus, and dietary counseling that is ongoing and reinforced periodically should be done with females when they reach reproductive age. Ultimately, dietary education should be emphasized throughout school curricula. Cereal and bread enrichment with folic acid was debated in the United States before mandatory implementation in January 1998, partly because it was believed folic acid supplementation might mask pernicious anemia, allowing neurologic damage to progress (see chapter 3). A 23% decline in neural tube defects occurred in 2001 when compared with 1996 before food fortification. A study done by the Gallup organization (Centers for Disease Control and Prevention, 2002) indicated that 80% of reproductive-age women contacted had heard of folic acid but only 31% reported taking vitamins with folic acid before pregnancy. These findings and those in follow-up studies suggest the need for nurses to be more active in educating women of childbearing age about prevention.

OROFACIAL CLEFTS

The most common oral clefts are cleft lip with or without cleft palate (CLP), and cleft palate alone (CP). The incidence for CLP varies in the population (see Table 7.1) and is highest in Native Americans, Japanese, and Scandinavians. CP and CLP are considered to be genetically and etiologically distinct, and they may occur alone or with other anomalies. Over 340 syndromes that include CLP or CP have been recognized. About 70% of CLP cases, however, are nonsyndromic, and do not occur in association with other anomalies, whereas about 30% are syndromic and occur in association with abnormalities outside the region of the cleft (Cobourne, 2004). Thus, other anomalies should be looked for. Several chromosomal sites for susceptibility genes for nonsyndromic CLP have been identified at 2q37, 11p12-13, 12q13, and 16p13 (Blanton et al., 2004). Cleft uvula (1:80) and submucous cleft palates (1:1,000) are thought to represent incomplete forms of cleft palate. It also appears that congenital heart disease is prevalent in nearly 7% of all children with clefts, and so all children with clefts should be periodically evaluated with this in mind. It has been reported that children with CLP have short stature about four times more frequently than normal children when matched for age. Eventually catch-up growth should occur, particularly when nutrition is optimized and the cleft is repaired, unless the cleft is part of another syndrome. Growth velocity needs to be monitored. It has been suggested that parents of children with CP who either do not have overt CP or have an incomplete form may have a recognizable speech pattern defect. Such observations illustrate the importance of thorough family assessment before genetic counseling. It is important that the infant with a cleft be evaluated fully as previously described in order to exclude chromosomal disorders and single-gene defects such as van der Woude syndrome, in which the recurrence risk is high, or Gorlin-Goltz syndrome, in which the associated nevi may turn malignant. Van der Woude syndrome, illustrated in Figure 4.7, is the result of mutation in the interferon regulatory factor 6 (IRF6). Certin variations in this gene, specifically a single nucleotide polymorphism (SNP) at position 274 that codes for valine instead of isoleucine, appear responsible for a major contribution to CL with or without CP (Zucchero et al., 2004). Defects in another single gene, that of MSX1 (HOX7), has been associated with non-syndromic cleft lip and palate and may be responsible for as much as 2% of clefts (Jezewski et al., 2003).

Much research has been done in the elucidation of environmental and genetic interaction by using CP models in animals. The proper development of orofacial structures is complex and occurs early in embryonic life. Failure to achieve normal development can occur because: (1) neural crest cells fail to migrate to the craniofacial region, (2) an organ fails to reach the critical size or mass necessary to proceed with differentiation or to be in the right place at the right time to interact with another structure and therefore an inductive stimulus fails, (3) abnormal growth alters usual patterns and so abnormal anatomical relationships develop between structures, or (4) structures fail to meet and to fuse. For example, CP could occur because tissues that are supposed to fuse do not reach each other, or because such tissues meet but do not fuse. This may be because they are intrinsically incapable of fusing or because there is a delay of inductive mechanisms, interactions, and contact causing lost fusion competency. In the process of normal palate formation, such structural factors as a wide head can prevent shelves from meeting, cortisone can weaken the force of the shelves, and other teratogens can delay shelf movement and alter the growth rate of tissue. For development it is necessary for the palatine shelves to move from a vertical position alongside the tongue to a horizontal position and fusion. Some factors involved in this that must be in proper balance are tongue resistance, shelf force, head width, shelf width, mandible growth, tongue mobility, mucopolysaccharide synthesis, and the extension of the cranial base. Thus, a variety of mechanisms can disrupt the delicate balance of the process. Another contributor to the development of CL and CLP were maternal polymorphisms in the gene for methylenetetrahydrofolate reductase (especially 67TT and 1298CC genotypes), which were described above. Preconceptional multivitamins including B_{12} and folic acid supplementation, have been reported to reduce the recurrence risk of orofacial clefts by as much as 50%. On the other hand, cigarette smoking during pregnancy appears to be a risk factor. Maternal use of corticosteroids in the first trimester of pregnancy may be associated with an increased risk of CLP in the child (Edwards et al., 2003; Park-Wyllie et al., 2000).

The appearance of a child with a cleft is shocking to the parent who is expecting a normal baby.

They experience the same reactions most other parents experience for other birth defects: guilt, anger, denial, and concern (see chapter 8). Parents have also stated that an orofacial cleft was not an anomaly that could be hidden from others. They often feel that the appearance of such an infant is caused by some indiscretion on their part and that now everyone else will also know that. Great sensitivity and skill are needed on the part of the entire professional staff immediately after the birth of the infant and throughout the hospital stay. Before leaving the hospital, contact should be arranged for the parents with the cleft palate team, who will ultimately be involved in the lengthy treatment, and also with one of the cleft palate parent groups for support and in-hospital visitation. Referral may be made to the local home health care or community health agency for a home visit by a nurse.

An immediate challenge is that of feeding the newborn with a cleft. It is important for the nursing staff to spend time helping the mother to feel comfortable feeding her infant because she will soon be assuming this responsibility alone. Infants with CLP or CP often cannot create adequate suction and may need a different type of nipple or occasionally a small plastic "artificial palate." Breast-feeding may be possible, depending on the nature of the cleft. There are publications available to help the nurse assist the mother who wishes to do this, and mothers should not be discouraged. Infants should be held upright when fed to prevent choking and may need to be burped frequently, as they tend to swallow air. The infant may need 30 to 45 minutes or more to feed. Parents need to feel comfortable, the child needs nourishment, and both need to develop an emotional bond to one another. Many parent groups have individuals who come to the home and who have found various successful "tricks" for feeding. The American Cleft Palate Educational Foundation can supply addresses of the local chapter if this is not already known.

Early arrangements for genetic counseling are important because parents may hesitate to conceive a wanted subsequent child because of exaggerated fears of recurrence risk. Again, such risk depends on the extent of the defect and the number of individuals affected. Care must be taken to exclude the possibility of a syndrome. For example, when one child and no other family member has CP, the risk for recurrence is 2% and for CLP 2–6%. It is not uncommon for genetic counseling to be sought by an adult with CLP or CP. The risk for an affected parent and one sibling is about 1 in 10. Often such adults have experienced emotional trauma in their own life which they attribute to the anomaly, and they may require more in-depth counseling. Three-dimensional ultrasonography of the fetal face may have future use in prenatal detection.

The total habilitation of infants with oral clefts is complex, often requiring multiple surgical procedures and other therapies, and is generally agreed to be best accomplished by a team. The early involvement of the family with such a team provides ongoing family support as well as other optimal therapy. Team members usually consist of professionals with specialties in pediatrics, plastic surgery, audiology, speech pathology, nursing, genetics, dentistry, orthodontia, otolaryngology, social service, and general surgery. Other specialists may include psychologists, nutritionists, and radiologists. My former practice group, the Central Illinois Cleft Palate Team, planned for and discussed the scheduled patients prior to seeing them. After meeting with each patient and family, each member recorded their impressions and findings. These were shared, and the plans were then altered accordingly, finalized, discussed with the family, and evaluated. Comprehensive, coordinated, and integrated multidisciplinary services are essential.

The current trend is to repair cleft lips as early as possible, almost always before 3 months of age. Many surgeons allow an infant to resume nursing 24 hours after cleft repair. Mothers can manually express breast milk for feeding, during periods when the infant cannot nurse. A variety of procedures are used for CP closure, depending on the exact nature of the cleft and its extent.

During infancy and childhood, children with CLP have increased susceptibility to ear infections and frequently have hearing problems. Routine ear exams and testing should be done periodically, and their importance explained to the parents. Hearing loss can also be responsible for speech distortion, and hypernasality is a frequent finding. There is a tendency for the child with a cleft to develop speech later than usual, and therefore they may need some language stimulation, which can be carried out by parents in consultation with the speech pathologist. The hearing problems and discomfort may cause increased fussiness. Parents should be told that this may occur. The hearing and speech problems as well as appearance can contribute to psychological sequelae and problems needing counseling assistance for the client and family. A study in Norway (Turner, Thomas, Dowell, Rumsey, & Sandy, 1997) found few differences in educational and job attainment for people with CLP, but earning power was lower. Fewer people with CLP married and, if they did, it was later in life. In another study of health-related quality of life in children with craniofacial anomalies, many interrelated outcomes were seen—children with lower health quality of life ratings also had lower behavioral and mental health ratings which were associated with family functioning, and parents believed that their child's self esteem was tied to their physical health and function (Warchausky, Kay, Buchman, Halberg & Berger, 2002). It has been found that some adults with CLP have certain structural brain anomalies that can lead to mild cognitive impairment or seizures (Nopoulos, 2002). Christensen and colleagues (2004) found that persons with CLP had an increased risk of mortality not only in infancy and early childhood but also in later life, up to age 55 years, a finding that has implications for health care support throughout the lifespan. Thus, thorough assessment is necessary for accurate immediate and longterm guidance, interventions, and treatment and for accurate genetic counseling.

Because closure of the palate may be done in stages, and may require surgery on the nose or lips as well, correction in full may depend on waiting for the attainment of certain growth stages for optimum results. This is often difficult to accept when both the child and parents are concerned with achieving a good cosmetic appearance. Research indicates that school experiences may not always be positive, as educators may possess inadequate knowledge and inaccurate information. Parents should be encouraged to involve appropriate school personnel in the restoration process, and it may be beneficial for there to be contact between members of the cleft palate team and the school. Many adults who had clefts are less verbal and less social than control groups, with a lower rate of marriage and children. It is never too late for such persons to receive genetic counseling. One client seen by us was a women in her 50s who had an unrepaired cleft palate. She was extremely concerned

about the risk of clefting in her potential grandchildren. Nurses should also realize that the relatively slow habilitation process of some individuals with clefts can lead to feelings of dissatisfaction with professionals that parents may hesitate to openly express. Booklets designed for parents of children with clefts at various age groups can be obtained from the American Cleft Palate Educational Foundation. See Appendix B.

BIBLIOGRAPHY

ACOG Practice Bulletin, Neural Tube Defects. No. 44. (2003). *International Journal of Gynecology & Obstetrics*, 123–133.

Allan, L., & Baker, E. J. (1993). Prenatal diagnosis and correction of congenital heart defects. *British Journal of Hospital Medicine, 50*, 513–522.

American College of Medical Genetics. (1994). *Folic acid and pregnancy*. Retrieved from http://www.faseb.org/genetics/acmg/po.1-27.htm

American College of Medical Genetics. (1997). *Statement on folic acid: Fortification and supplementation*. Retrieved from http://www.faseb.org/genetics/acmg/po.1-23.htm

Andersen, A. M., Vastrup, P., Wohlfahrt, J., Andersen, P. K., Olsen, J., & Melbye, M. (2002). Fever in pregnancy and risk of fetal death: A cohort study. *Lancet, 360*, 1552–1556.

Bender, P. L. (2000). Genetics of cleft lip and palate. *Journal of Pediatric Nursing, 15*, 242–249.

Benirschke, K., Lowry, R., Opitz, J. M., Schwarzacher, H. G., & Spranger, J. W. (1979). Developmental terms—some proposals: First report of an international working group. *American Journal of Medical Genetics, 3*, 297–302.

Blanton, S. H., Bertin, T., Patel, S., Stal, S., Mulliken, J. B., & Hecht, J. T. (2004). Nonsyndromic cleft lip and palate: Four chromosomal regions of interest. *American Journal of Medical Genetics, 125A*, 28–37.

Blum, R. W. (1983). The adolescent with spina bifida. *Clinical Pediatrics, 22*, 331–335.

Botto, L. D., Olney, R. S., & Ericson, J. D. (2004). Vitamin supplements and the risk for congenital anomalies other than neural tube defects. *American Journal of Medical Genetics, 125C*, 12–21.

Brucato, A., Jonzon, A., Friedman, D., Allan, L. D., Vignati, G., Gasparini, M., et al. (2003). Proposal for a new definition of congenital complete atrioventricular block. *Lupus, 12,* 427–435.

Carlisle, D. (1998). Feeding babies with cleft lip and palate. *Nursing Times, 94*(4), 59–60.

Centers for Disease Control and Prevention (2002). Folic acid and prevention of spina bifida and anencephaly. *Morbidity and Mortality Weekly Report, 51*(No. RR-13), 1–19.

Centers for Disease Control and Prevention. (1996). Prevalence of spina bifida at birth— United States, 1983–1990: A comparison of two surveillance systems. *Morbidity and Mortality Weekly Report, 45*(No. SS-2), 15–26.

Centers for Disease Control and Prevention. (1998). Use of folic acid-containing supplements among women of childbearing age— United States, 1997. *Morbidity and Mortality Weekly Report, 47*(7), 131–134.

Chakravarti, A. (2004). Finding needles in haystacks—*IRF6* gene variants in isolated cleft lip or cleft palate. *New England Journal of Medicine, 351,* 822–824.

Christensen, K., Juel, K., Herskind, A. M., & Murray, J. C. (2004). Long term follow up study of survival associated with cleft lip and palate at birth. *British Medical Journal, 325,* 1405–1414.

Cobourne, M. T. (2004). The complex genetics of cleft lip and palate. *European Journal of Orthodontics, 26,* 7–16.

Cohen, M. M., Jr. (2002). Malformations of the craniofacial region: Evolutionary, embryonic, genetic, and clinical perspectives. *American Journal of Medical Genetics (Semin. Med. Genet.), 115,* 245–268.

Cole, L. J., & Fleisher, L. D. (2003). Update on HIPAA privacy: Are you ready? *Genetics in Medicine, 5,* 183–186.

Czeizel, A. E., & Dudás, I. (1992). Prevention of the first occurrence of neural tube defects by periconceptional vitamin supplementation. *New England Journal of Medicine, 327,* 1832–1835.

David, T. J., Parris, M. R., Poynor, M. U., Hawhaur, J., Simm, S., Rigg, E., et al. (1983). Reasons for late detection of hip dislocation in childhood. *Lancet, 2,* 147–148.

Deanfield, J., Thaulow, E., Warnes, C., Webb, G., Kolbel, F., Hoffman, A., et al. (2003). Management of grown-up congenital heart disease. *European Heart Journal, 24,* 1035–1084.

de Franchis, R., Botto, L. D., Sebastio, G., Ricci, R., Iolascon, A., Capra, V., et al. (2002). Spina bifida and folate-related genes: A study of gene-gene interactions. *Genetics in Medicine, 4,* 126–130.

Eastwood, D. (2003). Neonatal hip screening. *Lancet, 361,* 595–597.

Edwards, M. G., Agho, K., Attia, J., Diaz, P., Hayes, T., Illingworth, A., et al. (2003). Case-control study of cleft lip or palate after maternal use of topical corticosteroids during pregnancy. *American Journal of Medical Genetics, 120A,* 459–463.

Epstein, C. J. (2004). Human malformations and their genetic basis. In C. J. Epstein, R. P. Erickson, & A. Wynshaw-Boris (Eds.), *Inborn errors of development: The molecular basis of clinical disorders of morphogenesis* (pp. 3–9). New York: Oxford University Press.

Epstein, C. J., Erickson, R. P., & Wynshaw-Boris, A. (Eds.). (2004). *Inborn errors of development: The molecular basis of clinical disorders of morphogenesis.* New York: Oxford University Press.

Finnell, R. H., Gould, A., & Spiegelstein, O. (2003). Pathobiology and genetics of neural tube defects. *Epilepsia, 44*(Suppl. 3), 14–23.

Gelb, B. D. (2004). Genetic basis of congenital heart disease. *Current Opinion in Cardiology, 19,* 110–115.

Goodman, F. R. (2003). Congenital abnormalities of body patterning: Embryology revisited. *Lancet, 362,* 651–662.

Gore, A. I., & Spencer, J. P. (2004). The newborn foot. *American Family Physician, 69,* 865–872.

Gorlin, R. J., Cohen, M. M., & Hennekam, R. C. M. (2001). *Syndromes of the head and neck* (4th ed.). London, England: Oxford University Press.

Graham, J. M. (1988). *Smith's recognizable patterns of human deformation* (2nd ed.). Philadelphia: W.B. Saunders.

Hague, W. M. (2003). Homocysteine and pregnancy. *Best Practice & Research Clinical Obstetrics & Gynaecology, 17,* 459–469.

Harper, P. S. (2004). *Practical genetic counselling* (6th ed.). Oxford, England: Oxford University Press.

Hoffman, J. I. E., & Kaplan, S. (2002). The incidence of congenital heart disease. *Journal of the American College of Cardiology, 39,* 1890–1900.

Huang, T. (2002). Current advances in Holt-Oram syndrome. *Current Opinion in Pediatrics, 14,* 691–695.

Jezeweski, P. A., Vieira, A. R., Nishimura, C., Ludwig, B., Johnson, M., O'Brien, S. E., et al. (2003). Complete sequencing shows a role for *MSX1* in non-syndromic cleft lip and palate. *Journal of Medical Genetics, 40,* 399–407.

Jones, K. L. (1997). *Smith's recognizable patterns of human malformation* (5th ed.). Philadelphia: W.B. Saunders.

Kaufman, B. A. (2004). Neural tube defects. *Pediatric Clinics of North America, 51,* 389–419.

Lammer, E. J., Shaw, G. M., Iovannisci, D. M., Van Waes, J., & Finnell, R. H. (2004). Maternal smoking and the risk of orofacial clefts: Susceptibility with *NAT1* and *NAT2* polymorphisms. *Epidemiology, 15,* 150–156.

Lee, J., Nunn, J., & Wright, C. (1997). Height and weight achievement in cleft lip and palate. [corrected and republished article originally printed in *Arch Dis Child* 1996 Oct; 75(4):327-9]. *Archives of Disease in Childhood, 76,* 70–72.

McDonald, S. D., Ferguson, S., Tam, L., Lougheed, J., & Walker, M. C. (2003). The prevention of congenital anomalies with periconceptional folic acid supplementation. *Journal of Obstetrics and Gynaecology Canada, 25,* 115–121.

Morcuende, J. A., & Weinstein, S. L. (2003). Developmental skeletal anomalies. *Birth Defects Research (Part C), 69,* 197–207.

Motulsky, A. G. (1996). Nutritional ecogenetics: Homocysteine-related arteriosclerotic vascular disease, neural tube defects, and folic acid. *American Journal of Human Genetics, 58,* 17–20.

Mulliken, J. B. (2004). The changing faces of children with cleft lip and palate. *New England Journal of Medicine, 351,* 745–747.

Murray, J. C. (2002). Gene/environment causes of cleft lip and/or palate. *Clinical Genetics, 61,* 248–256.

Park-Wyllie, L., Mazzotta, P., Pastuszak, A., Moretti, M. E., Beique, L., Hunnisett, L., et al. (2000). Birth defects after maternal exposure to corticosteroids: Prospective cohort study and meta-analysis of epidemiological studies. *Teratology, 62,* 385–392.

Queisser-Luft, A., Stolz, G., Wiesel, A., & Schaefer, K. (2002). Malformations in newborn: Results based on 30,940 infants and fetuses from the Mainz congenital birth defect monitoring system (1990–1998). *Archives of Gynecology and Obstetrics, 266,* 163–167.

Ramstad, T., Ottem, E., & Shaw, W. C. (1995). Psychosocial adjustment in Norwegian adults who had undergone standardised treatment of complete cleft lip and palate. I. Education, employment and marriage. *Scandanavian Journal of Plastic Reconstructive Surgery, Hand Surgery, 29,* 251–257.

Reinhard, W., Fischer, M., & Hengstenberg, C. (2005). Grown-up congenital heart disease: A "problem" to take care of. *European Heart Journal, 26,* 8–10.

Rietberg, C. C. Th., & Lindhout, D. (1993). Adult patients with spina bifida cystica: Genetic counselling, pregnancy and delivery. *European Journal of Obstetrics & Gynecology and Reproductive Biology, 52,* 63–70.

Rintoul, N. E., Sutton, L. N., Hubbard, A. M., Cohen, B., Melchionni, J., Pasquariello, P. S., et al. (2002). A new look at myelomeningoceles: Functional level, vertebral level, shunting, and the implications for fetal intervention. *Pediatrics, 109,* 409–413.

Rizos, M., & Spyropoulos, M. N. (2004). Van der Woude syndrome: A review. *European Journal of Orthodontics, 26,* 17–24.

Roovers, E. A., Boere-Boonekamp, M. M., Castelein, R. M., Zielhuis, G. A., & Kerkhoff, T. H. (2005). Effectiveness of ultrasound screening for developmental dysplasia of the hip. *Archives of Diseases of Childhood Fetal Neonatal Edition, 90,* F25–F30.

Rothenberg, S. P., da Costa, M. P., Sequeira, J. M., Cracco, J., Roberts, J. L., Weedon, J., et al. (2004). Autoantibodies against folate receptors in women with a pregnancy complicated by a neural tube defect. *New England Journal of Medicine, 350,* 134–142.

Roye, B. D., Hyman, J., & Roye, D. P., Jr. (2004). Congenital idiopathic talipes equinovarus. *Pediatrics in Review, 25,* 124–130.

Sadove, A. M., van Aalst, J. A., & Culp, J. A. (2004). Cleft palate repair: Art and issues. *Clinics in Plastic Surgery, 31,* 231–241.

Sankar, P. (2003). Genetic privacy. *Annual Review of Medicine, 54,* 393–407.

Scherl, S. A. (2004). Common lower extremity problems in children. *Pediatrics in Review, 25,* 52–62.

Shaw, G. M., Carmichael, S. L., Yang, W., Harris, J. A., & Lammer, E. J. (2004). Congenital malformations in births with orofacial clefts among 3.6 million California births, 1983–1997. *American Journal of Medical Genetics, 125A,* 250–256.

Shaw, G. M., Lammer, E. J., Wasserman, C. R., O'Malley, C. D., & Tolarova, M. M. (1995). Risks of orofacial clefts in children born to women using multivitamins containing folic acid periconceptionally. *Lancet, 346,* 393–396.

Smithells, R. W., Sheppard, S., Schorah, C. J., Sellers, M. J., Nevin, N. C., Harris, R., et al. (1980). Possible prevention of neural-tube defects by periconceptional vitamin supplementation. *Lancet, 1,* 339–340.

Spina bifida. Key primary issues. (2002). *Australian Family Physician, 31,* 66–69.

Spranger, J., Benirschke, K., Hall, J. G. (1982). Errors of morphogenesis: Concepts and terms. Recommendations of an international working group. *Journal of Pediatrics, 100,* 160–165.

Spritz, R. A. (2001). The genetics and epigenetics of orofacial clefts. *Current Opinion in Pediatrics, 13,* 556–560.

Sykes, J. M., & Tollefson, T. T. (2005). Management of the cleft lip deformity. *Facial and Plastic Surgery Clinics of North America, 13,* 157–167.

Tolmie, J. L. (2002). Clinical genetics of neural tube defects and other congenital central nervous system malformations. In D. L. Rimoin, J. M. Connor, R. E. Pyeritz, & B. R. Korf (Eds.), *Emery and Rimoin's principles and practice of medical genetics* (4th ed., pp. 2975–3011). New York: Churchill Livingstone.

Trollmann, R., Strehl, E., & Dorr, H. G. (1998). Precocious puberty in children with myelomeningocele: Treatment with gonadotropin-releasing hormone analogues. *Developmental Medicine and Child Neurology, 40,* 38–43.

Turner, S. R., Thomas, P. W., Dowell, T., Rumsey, N. & Sandy, J. R. (1997). Psychological outcomes amongst cleft patients and their families. *British Journal of Plastic Surgery, 50,* 1–9.

Ulman, C., Taneli, F., Oksel, F., & Hakerlerler, H. (2005). Zinc-deficient sprouting blight potatoes and their possible relation with neural tube defects. *Cell Biochemistry and Function, 23,* 69–72.

van Rijen, E. H. M., Utens, E. M. W. J., Roos-Hesselink, J. W., Meijboom, F. J., van Domburg, R. T., Roelandt, J. R. T. C., et al. (2003). Psychosocial functioning of the adult with congenital heart disease: A 20–33 years follow-up. *European Heart Journal,* 1–12.

van Rooij, I. A. L. M., Vermeij-Keers, C., Kluijtmans, L. A. J., Ocké, M. C., Zielhuis, G. A., Goorhuis-Brouwer, S. M., et al. (2003). Does the interaction between maternal folate intake and the methylenetetrahydrofolate reductase polymorphisms affect the risk of cleft lip with or without cleft palate? *American Journal of Epidemiology, 157,* 583–591.

Wald, N. J. (2004). Folic acid and the prevention of neural-tube defects. *New England Journal of Medicine, 350,* 101–103.

Walker, F. (2003). Precious adults: A lesson in grown-up congenital heart disease. *Lancet, 362,* 241–242.

Waller, D. K., Keddie, A. M., Canfield, M. A., & Scheurele, A. E. (2002). Sex ratios in infants with congenital anomalies. *Teratology, 66,* 60.

Warchausky, S., Kay, J. B., Buchman, S., Halberg, A., & Berger, M. (2002). Health-related quality of life in children with craniofacial anomalies. *Plastic and Reconstructive Surgery, 110,* 409–414.

Weinfeld, A. B., Hollier, L. H., Spira, M., & Stal, S. (2005). International trends in the treatment of cleft lip and palate. *Clinics in Plastic Surgery, 32,* 19–23.

Witt, C. (2003). Detecting developmental dysplasia of the hip. *Advances in Neonatal Care 3*(2), 65–75.

Yoon, P. W., Rasmussen, S. A., Lynberg, M. C., Moore, C. A., Anderka, M., Carmichael, S. L. (2001). The National Birth Defects Prevention Study. *Public Health Reports, 116*(Suppl. 1), 32–40.

Zucchero, T. M., Cooper, M. E., Maher, B. S., Daack-Hirsch, S., Nepomuceno, B., Ribeiro, L., et al. (2004). Interferon regulatory factor 6 *(IRF6)* gene variants and the risk of isolated cleft lip or palate. *New England Journal of Medicine, 351,* 769–780.

III

Assessing and Intervening with Clients and Families at Genetic Risk

8

Impact of Genetic Diseases on the Family Unit: Factors Influencing Impact

Many factors influence the impact of a congenital anomaly, genetic disease, mental retardation, or other disability on the family and the way in which they respond and cope. (In this chapter, "disability" and "genetic disorder" are used in the broadest sense.) Due to space limitations, a brief description of the impact will be presented here with a few specific examples. Most of the material contained in this chapter should be modified in light of such factors for individual families. Some of them are as follows:

- The size, structure, and stage of the developmental cycle of the family. Families in which there is only one other child function differently from those in which the affected child is the last of seven or eight normal ones. In the latter case, researchers speculate that life may be less disrupted because there are more hands to help with all that needs to be done, and also because parental investment in each child is less. In general, the most successful in coping are homes in which two parents are present and they have matured in their marriage or relationship. Parents who have an affected first child early in their marriage have not yet developed their own interrelationships before having to cope with an additional burden. The age of other children also determines family function. The sex of the affected child is also relevant. It appears that families with one sib near in age and of the same sex as the affected child are at the greatest risk. There is some evidence to show that fathers may have more

difficulty in coping with severely affected sons. Thus all the above knowledge should be obtained when planning care.

- Religious, ethnic, and cultural beliefs and practices. Some couples believe that a child who is mentally retarded or physically affected has been sent to them as a "special gift from God." Others, on such a discovery, curse God and lose faith. If strong faith is present, it can be used to provide support and comfort to the family. It is important to understand who within the cultural or ethnic group are the authority figures. They may be helpful in easing integration into the larger family and community. It is also useful to know the cultural views of disease, disability, healing, the body, and death, and how the individual is believed to influence, or be influenced by, life events.
- Availability of and relationship with extended family members or close friends. Having many relatives available may mean more helping hands and loving support if the relationships are positive ones. Lack of an extended family means that there will be less relatives to call on, but friends may fill the gap.
- The prior status of the relationship between parents. It appears that those who had a satisfactory relationship prior to the genetic problem have the best chance of remaining intact.
- Coping resources both tangible and intangible. Some communities or neighborhoods are able to form a network that provides loving support for families. Some individuals learn to draw on deep

resources that they did not realize they possessed. The nurse should make every effort to identify and mobilize support from parent groups, private, public, and governmental agencies and foundations.

• The visibility and severity of the disorder and its meaning to the family and religious, ethnic, cultural, and other groups with which they identify. In certain groups, superstitions associated with particular defects may cause the avoidance and rejection of the individual and family. Certain disorders have become more acceptable than others, through the media and through the appearance of the affected person. Society may have more tolerance for a cute little girl with braces on her legs than for an 18-year-old adolescent who is mentally retarded and cannot control motion or drooling. Hidden disorders such as congenital heart defects may cause burdens in the way of finances, care, and concern but not in appearance. Craniofacial anomalies, until they can be corrected, may cause suffering that is related to the reaction of others. Many societies equate beauty with goodness and ugliness with evil. Other disorders, although manageable and not very evident physically, can cause tiredness, stress, and worry through constant attention to diet, medication, and treatment protocols. The meaning of the disorder to each parent should be explored, often separately.

• Variables relating to individual family members include personalities, past experiences, views of roles, attitudes toward child rearing, education, etc.

• How the family functions together and has dealt with previous crises. This ability may be assessed by observation, interview, or the use of tools such as the Family APGAR or Parenting Stress Index.

• The lifestyle and plans of the family. A family who travels and camps extensively may have to modify such plans if they now have a child who cannot walk or who requires special food that cannot last for a long time on trips. They can be helped to plan and modify activities in a way that may include everyone.

• Other attributes of the disorder. This includes the severity of the disease, its natural history, age of onset, types and frequency of treatment, the necessity for surgery or repeated hospitalizations, and the long-term outlook so that future planning can occur.

INITIAL IMPACT—LOSS OF A DREAM

There is no appropriate time for the birth of a child with a congenital anomaly, disability, or genetic disorder. Such an event is a devastating crisis for the parents and also for the hospital staff. During pregnancy, the parents dream of having a perfect child who is invested heavily with the parents' self-image and future hopes. They have envisioned a happy event, expecting to receive praise and compliments and expecting the opportunity to "show off" the ideal infant who was to be the physical proof of their love. Instead, their worst fears have materialized—they have lost their wished-for, perfect child and instead have been presented with a child who may be threatening, anger-evoking, anxiety-producing, unattractive, and who may appear unlovable. In order to form an attachment to the child they actually have, parents must mourn the loss of their ideal child and reconcile their expectations with reality. The parents may pass through emotions akin to those usually discussed in relationship to death and dying as they mourn their loss. A major difference, however, is that they may not have the luxury of time in which to mourn the loss of their ideal child, because there is the urgency of the need to take care of the living, severely affected infant who is the reality. Reactions to the birth of an affected infant or to later diagnosis include shock, disbelief, denial, guilt, grieving, mourning, hostility, anger, anxiety, bargaining, resentment, shame, sorrow, self-pity, and eventually adaptation and adjustment, although this may not always occur. Similar feelings may occur if a diagnosis is made prenatally. It is, however, important for the nurse to realize that these phases are not timebound and, in addition, parents may return to any of these emotions in any order and at any time, not only within a short time period but throughout the life of the affected individual. In the case of long-term and lifelong problems, the very presence of the child over the years can be enough to retrigger earlier emotions. Families tend to periodically go through repeated sadness or "chronic sorrow" as classically described by Olshansky (1962), in which case intense grieving is reinvoked and reexperienced. Members of families may be at different stages at different times.

Some disorders are obvious because of their severe manifestations or their visibility. These are diagnosed at or soon after birth. In others, signs and symptoms are more subtle or do not appear until later in life, and diagnosis may only come after months of suspicions, anxiety, and worry, or diagnosis may come like a "bolt from the blue". Nevertheless, parents of all may experience the previously discussed reactions. In any case, most clinicians are in agreement that the parents should be informed of the possibility of a problem in an honest and straightforward manner as soon as suspicion is sufficient to warrant confirmatory testing and diagnostic procedures. Attempts to hide the suspicion of a problem are rarely successful. Parents sense the averted gaze, changed behavior, and the embarrassment or avoidance of the staff whether it be in a hospital, clinic, or office setting. They may respond with increased anxiety and even hostility that leads to the failure of formation of a trusting, therapeutic relationship. Parents who have initiated discussion of the possibility of some abnormality in their child because they are "slow" or because "something is just not right" cannot be dismissed with vague reassurances and the admonition "not to worry" or with the response that the parents are overly concerned about nothing. Whether or not their suspicions can be confirmed, the parents' observations should be respected and responded to honestly and respectfully. Even if nothing is wrong with the infant, something may be wrong within the relationship within the family, and further counseling may be needed. Parents who are fobbed off in a superficial way become adversarial and believe information is being suppressed. They will not be able to fully reestablish a comfortable relationship with the involved practitioners. It is not uncommon for parents who have felt that something was wrong with their child to experience sudden crystallization of their feelings that spark such urgency that they may arrive at the emergency room. Staff there may regard their appearance as unreasonable and unnecessary, adding to the burden and to misunderstandings.

Telling the Family

Unless the unavoidable situation occurs in which the mother alone sees a visibly affected infant in the delivery room, the parents should be told together as soon as possible. A quiet, private room should be found for this purpose, so that the parents can react unrestrainedly and ventilate their feelings freely. Ideally, the physician should be the one to give the initial news. It is appropriate for the primary nurse or clinical nurse specialist to also be present. Hospital policy should cover what is to be done if no physician is present. The professionals should choose a time when they are not in a hurry so that there is time to listen to and console the parents. Explanations should be short, simple, and repeated in slightly different ways. In this initial period when parents feel shock, numbness, and disbelief, they need to feel that their reactions are okay and legitimate. They should not feel abandoned, isolated, and alone with their problem. The nurse can use touch to show caring and provide some comfort. Before the end of this initial discussion, definite arrangements should be made for a second discussion within a day or two. The clinician should try to return any phone calls to parents promptly and make himself or herself available to talk further with them. The way in which parents are first told about their child's disorder will long be remembered by them and influence their adjustment. This applies to those receiving news of a problem after prenatal diagnosis. Yet researchers have found, depending on the study, that in about half the cases, one parent was first told alone, often in a public place such as the hospital corridor or waiting room or even by telephone. One mother recalled waiting at home for news of preliminary tests on her five-year-old child and receiving a telephone call to pack a bag for him and come to the hospital because he had leukemia and further tests were needed. It later turned out that the initial diagnosis was in error, but the memory, bitterness, and distrust remain, even though that child is now an adult. Nurses, particularly in obstetric and pediatric settings, should assert some leadership for planning how such news will be handled if no plan exists, or for modifying it if it is not a sensitive one. Even a small demonstration of concern, such as the offer of a cup of coffee, can be meaningful and remembered by the family years later.

The staff may feel uneasy, helpless, and may be inexperienced in handling their feelings. They may feel revulsion for a grossly malformed infant, inadequate in meeting the needs of the family or in lack of knowledge to respond to questions. This can result in patterns of avoidance that contribute to the parents' aloneness. They may resent the parents for arousing these feelings. Parents are extremely sensitive to the reactions of those around them at this time. The acceptance and positive attitude of the staff toward the infant and family can foster the development of positive feelings. The staff, therefore, should have the opportunity to talk about such problems before they arise in the work setting and, especially at the time of such an event, to air concerns, feelings, and emotions, and to discuss positive plans and approaches for the family. Such discussions may be led by someone experienced in counseling or group work. Some institutions have instituted psychosocial and/or ethical rounds. Other consultants could be available for the staff to call if needed. Recently, an unfortunate situation occurred in an obstetric setting at a hospital. The mother of an infant born with a cleft palate was told by the nursing staff that she could not breast-feed her infant. Lack of knowledge led to a crisis that could have been prevented by prior discussion and staff planning to try to meet the needs of an already extra-vulnerable mother. Information on breast-feeding that can be used for infants with clefts can be obtained through cleft lip and palate parent groups, La Leche League, as well as through local expert consultants. In my practice, lists of such experts or organizations were maintained, as they are in many genetic centers. Isolation of another sort can result because the mother of an affected infant feels cut off from the joy of the other mothers around her in the obstetrics unit, even in the era of early discharge.

The parents of a newborn with an anomaly usually need to see the child as soon as possible, because their fantasies are often worse than the reality. However, parents should not be forced to see the infant if they are not ready to do so. They may fear attaching themselves emotionally to an infant who may not live or whom they are not ready to accept. It is often reassuring and helpful for the nurse to remain with them for at least part of the time when they first see their affected baby. The nurse's calmness can help to stabilize some of their own anxieties and fears and begin a positive relationship. Thus, the nurse should work out his or her feelings before this time. The nurse may also need to show the parents how to touch, hold, or move the infant, especially in cases such as

osteogenesis imperfecta or spina bifida. The nurse can also use this opportunity to point out relevant positive features about the infant in the same manner that would be appropriate with an unaffected infant. At an appropriate moment, the nurse can allow the parents to have some time alone with their baby. Parents of an infant born with anencephaly 2 years previously told this geneticist that their daughter did not look as bad as they had expected. Their being able to touch and hold her before she died was still an important memory to them. For infants with a lethal perinatal disorder, nurses should be aware that it is harder for parents to work through their grief if they have not been able to see, touch, hold the infant, and say goodbye in their own way. Appropriate arrangements to do this can still be made even if the infant has already been taken to the morgue. Many hospitals routinely take photographs of the deceased newborn, both for future genetic counseling purposes and because the parents may wish to have these later. Some parents are reluctant to form an attachment with an infant who may not be taken home then or ever. These feelings should be respected and understood. The feelings probably will require further exploration and the basis for them need to be ascertained so that appropriate helping interventions can be used.

Because of the severity of illness, some infants may have to be transferred to a hospital with facilities for the high-risk infant. This may require their location to be more than fifty miles away from home or the local hospital, combining physical and emotional separation Every effort should be made by the nursing staff to facilitate parent-child bonding and interaction. For example, obtaining breast milk or saving the mother's milk may allow the continuation of breast-feeding when it is later feasible. Volunteer efforts can be used to transport the parents if this is a problem. If, for some reason, parents cannot be with their infant, the need for cuddling should be met by the nurses or by the use of soft materials and other substitutes. The parents should be able to get clear, honest information about the infant's progress, and facilitation of this should begin before transfer.

The initial impact of a newly discovered genetic disorder in the adolescent or the adult has different ramifications. In the case of Huntington disease, they may have already completed their own family while unaware of their own status, thus placing their children at risk. Much of both the initial and long-term impact depend on those factors discussed earlier, and also on how disruptive the disorder is to the daily life and long-range plans of the person. Some of the feelings that may accompany such a discovery are similar to those in which the individual discovers that he/she is a carrier for a deleterious recessive gene, as discussed in chapter 11.

Emotional Responses

Parents

As parents experience the emotions mentioned previously, various feelings and responses occur. During denial and disbelief, parents may raise the possibility of diagnostic error and seek a diagnosis with a more favorable prognosis. This can result in "shopping around" behavior or a frantic search for a miracle. The competent professional conveys willingness to reaccept the family without hard feelings. The family may also question the competency of the professional staff or even insist that their baby was switched with another in the nursery. During denial, the professionals may have to explain the disorder over and over without losing patience. The explanation should still be short and simple. The parents actually know the truth but have not yet accepted it. Various authors recommend saying something like, "I realize it must be hard to realize that your baby has Down syndrome when you were expecting a normal baby during the pregnancy," which acknowledges the normality of their reaction but also presents reality. When experiencing anger and hostility, families may project these feelings onto the professional staff, as described in chapter 10. This can be particularly trying, and it is tempting for the staff, who may already feel the burden of having been through so much with the family, to reject them as being ungrateful rather than to recognize the normality of this response. The nurse can listen supportively, remembering that it is useless either to agree or to offer a defense of a fellow professional under such attack, but permit expression and verbalization of such feelings so that they can be resolved. The questions, "Why is God punishing me? " or "What did I do to deserve this?" may dissolve into self-guilt, blame, and feelings of failure. Imagined and real transgressions, events, and sins may be brought up and examined. Some of these may include practicing contraception, not wanting the pregnancy, having an abortion previously, riding in a car in late pregnancy, strenuous exercise, taking a medication during pregnancy, the enjoyment of sexual relationships in late pregnancy, and other events that are often culturally significant. It is important for the nurse to have some awareness of the explanations for congenital malformations that are common in various cultures and belief systems, such as the "evil eye," the placing of a curse as evidence of being punished by God, for consorting with the devil, or because of seeing a horrifying sight during pregnancy. It may be necessary in a later session with clinicians to ask the parents what they think may be explanations for the disorder in order to dispel misinformation. Other clues may be obtained from the clients' history. It may also be necessary to raise some issues by saying something like, "Sometimes parents blame themselves when their infant is born with [anomaly] . . .," and await a response so that such thoughts can be brought to the surface and examined. Each parent may blame the other, "I shouldn't have married you; your family has bad genes." The failure to have a healthy child may be seen as evidence of weakness on the part of the parent, or of "bad blood." It is a major threat to the parents' self-esteem. Sometimes these feelings carry over and affect other decisions in years to come. A young unmarried couple who had a son with trisomy 13 came for counseling 2 years later. Their son had died soon after birth. They had decided to marry, but the man's family was fighting the marriage with the argument that it was "her bad blood" that had caused their child to be malformed, and that all their future children would be so affected. The couple was referred to counseling because his family wanted medical proof of their point. Clearly, deeper issues here had never been resolved. Interestingly, it was the father who had a chromosome defect.

Grief, sorrow, and depression are prominent emotions. The normality of these emotions should be recognized. Parents should be allowed to freely express these emotions, and nurses should encourage open expression. Remaining silently with the parents, and perhaps putting an arm around them, helps to show them that they are not alone and that someone cares. It also helps to build an atmosphere of trust.

Parents may feel emotions that they fear are unacceptable to the staff and to society at large. They may wish for their child to die, consider abandonment, or even contemplate killing the child. One nurse, who was later seen for genetic counseling, told the author that after having an infant with trisomy 18, all she could do was wish for the baby to die. "All the time I was having these feelings, the staff kept telling me how they were doing everything they could to save my baby. I knew that I couldn't tell them how I really felt. I worked with many of them, and I knew they would never understand." This state of events persisted for more than a week while the infant was transferred to a high-risk center, where he finally died. Both the emotional and financial cost were high, but she felt that she had maintained her image in a place that was important to her. Such feelings are very common and need wider understanding of their naturalness among professionals, so that parents can express such feelings and work them out.

There may be some differences in reactions between fathers and mothers. An affected infant may be a threat to the manhood of the father. He may wish to abandon both his mate and the child and, in fact, often does, although not always immediately. The rate of marital dissension and dissolution among such families is very high. The father often remarries in an effort to prove that he can father a normal child. Interventions should be aimed at fostering understanding, sharing feelings with a trained listener, and finding ways in which the father and mother can let the other know that he or she is appreciating each other's efforts and thinking of them, even when they are not physically present. Stress, tension, fatigue, and unspoken guilt or blame may result in disintegration of sexual relations. Parents should be informed that this often happens and should be referred for specific therapy if needed. The mother may feel that she has failed as a woman. This can result in attempts to give her mate another "normal" child, no matter what the cost. The father may also feel helpless and useless with the infant or child, and spend more time at work in an effort to feel useful somewhere. At the same time, the mother may feel trapped, abandoned, and even more alone. A father may also feel a loss of attention from his mate. Finances are now a critical problem and both may feel overwhelmed. Joint decision-making should

be encouraged. During later counseling, when the parents are ready, the concept of pregnancy as a joint endeavor should be emphasized. When true, the joint responsibility for genetic transmission should be emphasized. Parents may experience a breakdown in communications because of each unconsciously blaming the other.

Other Relatives

Other relatives can either create tensions or help to ease them. Grandparents may be as shocked and emotionally devastated as the parents. Sometimes, however, grandparents can be very free with advice and accusations or stir up old feelings, further driving a wedge between the parents. They may be the source of "old wives' tales." The parents of an affected child may already feel that they have failed their own parents. Sometimes the grandparents expect the parents to comfort them, further draining the parents' emotional resources and energy. On the other hand, if the grandparents can set aside some of their own grieving, they can be very supportive. They should recognize the limits of what they can provide, however. No matter how much they may wish to do so, they should not be turned into full-time babysitters for a long-term period, or into substitute parents. They may need some suggestions of some tangible ways in which they can help. This can include the provision of transportation, babysitting, visiting, or providing special activities for the other children, helping with household chores or repairs, and running errands. They should not be forgotten when counseling is being provided for the family because they, too, need to express and resolve their feelings. Relatives such as aunts, uncles, and cousins may also be helpful, particularly if there are one or two key family members who can "organize" how this will be accomplished.

Siblings

It is imperative that the parents think through ways in which it will be most appropriate to tell their other children about the birth of the affected infant. Children are very perceptive and will quickly realize that something is wrong. The nurse can suggest ways to tell them (e.g., while doing a "buffer" activity together such as gardening or walking). Failure to explain may result in their imagining things that are worse than the reality.

Explanations should be kept short and simple and be in keeping with the age and development of the other children. An important issue to keep in mind is that normal sibling rivalry and jealousy may have existed previously. The unaffected child may have wished that the new baby would never come home, or that his or her older sib would get sick and die. It may now seem that these thoughts have come true. Parents should be made aware of these kinds of feelings and helped to identify ways in which they can be addressed and resolved.

Decisions and Options

At a time after the initial session with the family, depending on the degree of readiness and the magnitude of decisions that must be made, the disorder should be explained and discussed in simple, understandable language, as well as what the implications are for care, immediate and long-term treatment, prognosis, and the long-range outlook that includes a realistic presentation of both the burdens and resources available. The urgent decisions should be separated from the long-term ones. For example, the parents of a child born with Down syndrome who has esophageal atresia need to make an immediate decision about surgery. The moral and ethical questions of whether or not to treat or institute intensive care measures for infants with severe congenital anomalies are unresolved ones. In a still relevant study by Shaw, Randolph, and Manard (1977), physicians responded to questions about repairing duodenal atresia in various conditions if the parents did not wish it to be done. Some of the issues revolve around questions of who should decide on such options—the professionals, the parents, or both; who represents the infant in such decisions; can the parents be responsible for decision-making given the emotional shocks sustained; whether or not passive nontreatment is preferable to active euthanasia (which is not legal in most societies); whether quality of life is as important as living or dying, and again who decides; whether all infants with severe disease should receive "extraordinary" treatment and, indeed, what constitutes extraordinary treatment; how the professional staff can reconcile their own beliefs and feelings with that of the family, and to what degree they should be obligated to participate in decisions that run counter to their own value systems, whether they be sustaining or terminating lives. Increasingly, society has seemed to place more emphasis on quality of life rather than prolongation. It should be clear to the parents at this time that any short-term care decisions are not bound to any long-term care options, and that these are not irrevocable. The practitioner may need to raise options available for future care such as home care, foster care, adoption, and placement in a residential setting or rarely, institutionalization. Parents often hesitate to raise such options if they believe that others perceive them as unacceptable. Some clinicians believe that parents should not take home children who are born with lethal disorders such as anencephaly. The complex issue of selective nontreatment of infants with handicaps has engendered both feelings and various pieces of legislation. One set of these was the so-called "Baby Doe" legislation, which no longer is in place. Baby Doe was an infant born with Down syndrome and esophageal atresia in Bloomington, Indiana. Both the parents and physician chose to delay surgical repair, parenteral nutrition was not given, and Baby Doe died 6 days later. This provoked heated debate in regard to withholding treatment and feeding from the affected infant.

Special Nursing Points

Other points important to nurses include the following:

- Remember that the discovery of a genetic disorder or anomaly is a shattering experience.
- It can permanently and abruptly alter the life plans of a family in ways that the professional staff may not begin to understand or be able to relate to. For example, a mother may have been planning to enter college or establish a career, or a father may have been planning to take a financial risk by changing jobs.
- Recognize that different people cope with such a shock in different ways. Resist labeling parents as noncaring, rejecting, etc.
- Do not inject personal biases.
- Build a trusting and permissive atmosphere.
- Emphasize the legitimacy of the parents' feelings.
- Work with the family in identifying family strengths, supports, limitations, and other concerns,

such as time, financial obligations, and other children.

- Build on family strengths.
- Raise the issue of prebirth expectations and how these may be related to present feelings. The mother may need to verbally relive the pregnancy before she can go on.
- Gauge willingness and ability of parents to cope.
- Parents are not cheered by knowing that events could have been worse. For them, this is as bad as things can get, even if the anomaly appears minor to the staff (e.g., an extra digit or a cleft lip).
- Special care procedures, such a moving the child with osteogenesis imperfecta or feeding the infant with cleft palate, should be taught, demonstrated, and redemonstrated to the parents, with return demonstration by the parents. Support needs to be available the first times the parents attempt such care. Success in such endeavors helps bolster parental self-confidence, shows them that they can cope, and gives them some sense of self-worth.
- Recognize that the emotions they are experiencing are exhausting and disorganizing. Decision making may be difficult and may need to be postponed.
- Observe and record the interactions of parents with each other and with their child, family communication patterns, their concerns, their needs, and what issues have been explored and discussed, so that nursing plans and interventions are not repeated but are built on what has occurred previously.
- Help the father and mother maintain open communication and plan for their roles at home. Before discharge, help parents plan for what supplies and equipment will be needed and where they can be obtained. Plan for preparations that are needed, including the time and person designated to undertake care of this child and others, do the laundry, etc. Help them explore whether a period of job absence will be necessary and whether additional help at home from a relative, friend, or professional is needed. Home care services providing professional nurses or aides can be useful. Some states offer stipends to families for home care.
- Ascertain the support systems available to the family.
- Contact parent groups of persons with similarly affected children. These provide various types of assistance, from financial to equipment, to tele- phone crisis lines, to friendly listening and sharing, to sharing coping measures, to hospital visiting, and more.

- Work with parents to plan a timetable that includes needs of normal siblings and time alone for the parents; tension-reducing activities.
- Help parents sort long-term monumental problems into manageable daily tasks and short-term goals so that parents are not overwhelmed immediately.
- Offer opportunities to ask questions and voice concerns.
- Remember that the state of crisis will continue at home as well.
- Follow-up care and regularly scheduled sessions with the care coordinator is essential to arrange before parents leave the hospital.
- Obtain information on, and refer parents to, respite care facilities and programs.
- Nurses should be involved in the establishment of groups that meet on evenings or weekends so that fathers, siblings, and other relatives can be included, if such groups do not already exist.
- Plan for follow-up should include counseling for grief resolution, marital and family relationships, reproductive options discussion, and genetic counseling.
- Nurses should be aware of factors that put a child with an anomaly at a higher risk for child abuse such as parental isolation from support, friends, and community; fatigue; failure to establish bonding with the infant; persons who are poor problem solvers and who are disorganized; those who feel inadequate; and adolescent parents.
- The nurse can talk individually to each parent to ascertain any special concerns that may not have been elicited. Parents may need to understand that each can react to the crisis in different ways, and that each may have a deep degree of feeling but react and cope differently. Promote mutual awareness of each parent's feelings.
- The infant with an anomaly is still an infant with basic needs, and the child who now has a diagnosis of a genetic disorder is still the same child he or she was before the diagnosis. The nurse should encourage the parents to define the child in this way rather than as a defective individual.
- Help parents and family to rebuild self-esteem and feel that they are human beings worthy of being liked.

- Make it clear to the family that you are willing to listen and talk, and be sure that you are willing when called on.
- If the parents have not raised the issue, the nurse should ask the parents if they have considered discussing the newly diagnosed disorder with siblings, grandparents, neighbors, other relatives, and friends. The nurse should help them to think through possible approaches.
- Some family crises are less apparent. For example, the birth of an unaffected child to a family whose other children all have galactosemia may be a crisis for them.
- Be aware of some of the signs of successful adjustment—an intact family unit, the resumption of sexual relationships between partners, appropriate plans for future reproduction in light of genetic counseling and family goals, ability to help other parents, realistic plans for management of the affected child, retention of the family health practitioner, and ability to relate to others are some measures that can be used.
- Remember to ask the parents, ". . . And how are you doing?"

LIVING WITH A GENETIC DISORDER OR DISABILITY

Meaning and Impact

The crisis of a child with a genetic disorder is not limited to birth or initial diagnosis, but is present when the family is home again with the affected infant or the child whose status has been altered. Genetic disorders or defects are (a) chronic or long-lasting; (b) permanent, even if repaired, because the genetic material has been altered in some way; (c) familial, because it affects the genetic material of others, reproductive plans, risks for others to have affected children, and also because it impacts on the family in social, economic, physical, and psychological ways; (d) threatening, because the person's self-identity is altered and threatened, and this may extend to the rest of the family; and (e) labeling, as the person and family may now see themselves in terms of the disorder, that is, "we are a PKU family," "I am handicapped." This also results in a new way of identifying oneself.

The practice of hiding away the malformed or retarded child has not left our society. In October 1982, a 14-year-old was found in Geneva, Illinois, who had never left the house or attended school. The father, a mechanical engineer, told the press that his son was kept secluded because he didn't want the other children stigmatized first by his being "cross-eyed" and later because of "retardation." Other more recent instances occasionally come to light.

The burden of a genetic disorder is more than just the financial costs. A disorder such as trisomy 13, which is usually lethal before the age of 1 year, carries an intense but short impact. One such as hemophilia is less intense, has periods of acuteness, and is a long-term burden but can be a greater one. Organization of health care is such that it may be difficult to provide the continuity that families need. Bureaucracy may mean wasted energy in locating services and resources which are separated in different agencies. The family and household with an affected child undergoes major changes. The familiar and usual are gone. The ramifications can be great and people differ in their ability to cope. Some of the ways that genetic disorders impact on the family and community are listed in Table 8.1.

Financial costs to the family may occur in subtle ways. These include costs of special diets, day care, household help, housing adaptations, buying special equipment and clothing, and travel. If the family is not in a large city, travel to major medical centers means more than just the expense of transportation. It may mean the need for more than one person to accompany the child, lost work time, arrangements for the other children in the family, an overnight stay, and eating in a restaurant. The need to remain near a major or specialized treatment center may cause a loss of geographic mobility for the family and also lost career opportunities and job changes leading to loss of both promotion and higher pay. Even routine mobility is not simple. Shopping, clinic visits, going to church or synagogue, movies, or the laundromat may involve elaborate preparations. Everyday kinds of items, such as finding a primary care practitioner, may be fraught with unexpected problems. Some alterations in the family life and living arrangements may be readily apparent, but others are not so obvious. These include the need to adapt the

TABLE 8.1   Burden of Genetic Disease to Family and Community

Financial cost to family
Decrease in planned family size
Loss of geographic mobility
Decreased opportunities for siblings
Loss of family integrity
Loss of career opportunities and job flexibility
Social isolation
Life-style alterations
Reduction in contributions to their community by families
Disruption of husband-wife or partner relationship
Threatened family self-concept
Coping with intolerant public attitudes
Psychological affects
Stresses and uncertainty of treatment
Physical health problems
Loss of dreams and aspirations
Cost to society of institutionalization or home or community care
Cost to society because of additional problems and needs of other family members
Cost of long-term care
Housing and living arrangement changes

household for optimal care, which may include physical remodeling; altering sleeping arrangements so that the affected child sleeps with the parents, not alone, causing two siblings to now share rooms, or causing an unaffected sibling to share a room with the affected person; therapeutic measures such as medical treatment, developmental stimulation, special dental attention; extra routine work such as special food preparation, longer feeding times, longer bathing and dressing times with extra work; and difficulties in locating special equipment, from car seats to eating utensils to wheelchairs. There is less time and money for leisure. Along with all of this, the parents may find themselves becoming more and more fatigued. They may rarely get an uninterrupted night's sleep or rarely sleep late for years. The fatigue, the feelings discussed earlier, concerns about the future, the sheer frustrations, the fear of having another affected child, altered sleeping arrangements, the strain of repeated hospitalization, and the lack of finding time away from the household for relaxation impact greatly on the relationship between the father and mother and cause additional stress. As these stresses and tensions grow, the partners'

sexual relationship may be disrupted, leading to further stresses and tensions. Parents may choose reproductive plans based on their desire to show their normality by producing a normal child, the belief that they owe their partner or family a normal child, or they may refrain from having another child because of inappropriate fears or perception of risks. Each partner may isolate himself or herself from the other, and from other family members. Helping the partners to reestablish contact and grow within the marriage is important for the entire family. It is also important for society because those families that ultimately cope the best are those with two parents in the home.

Feelings described earlier are particularly prone to occur at times of normal developmental milestones and times when the child attains an age at which a certain activity is commonly associated (e.g., kindergarten entry) and which is not possible because of the child's condition. Such feelings may also occur when a neighbor's child joins Little League baseball, begins dancing lessons, or has his or her first date. Wikler, Wasow, and Hatfield (1981) call this a "normal response to an abnormal situation" in which a sense of renewed loss is felt.

The recognition of this response should help the nurse to anticipate and deal with ongoing and exacerbated times of stress and provide appropriate coping measures and support services at times when they may be most needed. For many parents, difficulties increased rather than decreased in adolescent and young adult years.

Parents need reassurance as to the normality of their feelings. At some time in their lives all parents occasionally wish that their normal child did not exist or are angry at him/her. These feelings are not abnormal merely because the child has a defect.

Reactions of Society and Stigmatization

Disabilities may be visible and obvious (e.g., cleft lip), visible but concealable (e.g., mild spina bifida), or invisible (e.g., type 1 diabetes mellitus). The latter two may "pass" as normal. Each of these presents its own problems. Society as a whole values normality, physical wholeness, and attractiveness. Impairments can elicit attitudes, reactions, and behaviors that erect barriers and may provoke public curiosity, avoidance, or withdrawal. Such attitudinal barriers are those that, according to Cornelius (1980), "limit the potential of disabled people to be independent individuals." These include avoidance, fear, insensitivity, stereotyping, misconception, discrimination, invisibility, insecurity, and intolerance. An example of such stereotyping may be seen in the case of a person who sees a blind skier and does not question the stereotype of the blind as not capable, but thinks of that individual skier as an exception. Affected individuals are often treated as though they are invisible. One family with three teenagers, one of whom was blind, was in a restaurant. The waitress asked each in turn what they would like to order. When she reached the blind teen, she asked the mother, "And what will he have?"

Researchers have demonstrated cultural uniformity in aversion to the handicapped. Bone disorders seem to elicit pity, whereas mental retardation and neurological problems elicit revulsion and fear. Those seen as less than perfect are stigmatized. Those associated with the affected person receive what Goffman calls a "courtesy stigma." This extends to parents, siblings, and marital partners. By association these individuals are perceived as contaminated and viewed less favorably. Such a courtesy stigma may also be extended to professionals who work with persons with disabilities.

Affected persons may see themselves in the framework of the reaction of others—as forever different. Through this they develop their self concept. They may become what others expect, defining themselves by their disability, seeing themselves as "special," and impairing their personality development. Those with invisible disabilities may have even greater problems with self identity. Gliedman and Roth (1980) refer to the handicapped as a minority. As such, they share prejudice and powerlessness in society with older adults, women, poor, homeless, and mentally ill. The media may perpetuate negative images and portray disabilities as demeaning. Strangely enough, organizations trying to help may use images that evoke pity and play on stereotypes in order to collect funds. Other societal attitudes may characterize the disabled as more noble than others. Thus children who try to engage in normal activities because it is something they want to do may be seen as trying to do them because they are super-brave. As citizens, nurses can help to see that citizens who are disabled are included in decision-making bodies such as community planning groups, and in decision-making where they work; become active in attempts to make facilities acceptable to all or understandable to all (e.g., signing for the deaf at school functions); ask persons who are disabled how they can best be assisted if they look as if they need help; do not support the portrayal of disabled in demeaning, negative, or condescending ways; voice objections to such portrayal in writing or verbally, depending on the setting and situation; help channel compassion into constructive and realistic channels; and participate in programs on how to interact with individuals who are disabled.

Report after report documents that some of the greatest problems families and individuals face are in handling the negative attitudes and behaviors of other individuals, communities, and society. Disabilities may confront observers with their own discomfort, fears, and vulnerability, causing such behavior. Parents may feel further devalued. Already having been shattered, some parents relate how they lose confidence, shrink inside, and eventually cannot cope with outside attitudes. This may result in their isolation and further removal from potential support systems. Parents' groups may insulate individuals against stigmatization. They show families that there are others like them. They are not alone. Parents themselves can help by taking such situations, discussing how members feel about them, and learning some ways in which they can be handled. Role-playing may be done. Depending on the situation encountered, parents may matter-of-factly be able to give a simple explanation. Children are naturally curious and ask questions. Accurate, simple information can be given in a nonjudgmental way. When children are told to be quiet or not "to ask that," or are taken quickly away, they suspect something is taboo and develop negative feelings. Some parents of affected children either do not find it worthwhile to, or cannot, cope, responding to a question like, "What a cute little girl. Is she about three?" with an affirmative answer, although the short-statured child is 6 years of age. One potential danger exists if parents become only comfortable with parents in similar situations, becoming self-ostracized and bitter.

Affected children and their siblings also need help in order to explain their problem to others. For example one little boy who was asked in preschool why he had no arms replied, "I just came that way." The other 4-year-old children accepted this explanation. Older children may need more information to respond, and parents and professionals should help them get it. Sibling groups are often helpful in this regard. For all age groups, explanations to children about the disability should be preceded by ascertaining how the child views the illness. This, then, should be considered in the explanations.

Support and Problems

Some support should be available for the family when they return home from the hospital. A very important aspect is to focus on the present for the time being. The nurse can help the family to prepare a daily schedule for the parents and the rest of the family that allows a reasonable sharing of family responsibilities and aims at maintaining as normal a life as is possible. Time alone for some enjoyable activity should be planned, even if it is for 15 minutes a day. Leisure time for the marital partners and for the family should be included. Eventually, long-term plans can incorporate necessary changes

and planned activities within the progression of the disorder, but they should not be done too early (e.g., major home construction, anticipating the need for entrances that allow wheelchair passage for persons with muscular dystrophy). Relatives, neighbors, and friends should know the basic needs, abilities, limitations, and plans for coping. The nurse can help to locate needed resources.

A major need is respite care. There are several models and types. These include group day care, community group residences that keep a few beds open or are totally for respite care, programs within group care or residential treatment facilities, hospitals or pediatric nursing homes, private respite providers that take a few children in private homes, camping facilities, some trained persons who come to the home, and sometimes state institutions. They may provide care for a few hours, overnight, or longer periods of time such as 2 or 3 weeks. They are valuable as backup for emergencies or for vacations. Some take affected individuals weekly for short periods of time on an ongoing basis, allowing parents to have a night out alone, or to devote themselves to an activity involving the normal children that they would not be able to do otherwise. Nurses should check the availability in their communities. Respite can provide relief from what one of McKeever's (1981) fathers describes as "like being in a war that never ended."

Parents should have some person whom they can contact if they cannot cope with a procedure when they are home. Parents may feel inadequate at first, but they usually quickly grow into their new responsibilities if support is provided. Marshalling financial assistance should be an early priority, before resources are exhausted.

Much has been written about the maladaptation of parents. The typical parents of affected children are like the typical parents of normal children. They vary in their ability to cope with stress. Like anyone else, they can take a certain amount, but if it is severe and ongoing, they can develop problems. Reactions to stress and the desire to lead normal lives are not rejection but a normal response. What they need is recognition of their difficulties and pressures, reassurance of their normality, access to supportive others and parents' groups, and realistic help. Parents who are tired and fatigued do not need tranquilizers but physical relief from their burden in the form of respite care.

The labeling of parents is not helpful, nor is the victim-blaming approach. Other helpful measures include the availability and arrangement for counseling services in the home community, the opportunity for the family to share feelings together and with a trained professional, the opportunity for the father and mother to individually redefine feelings about themselves and the family, the provision of factual knowledge about the disease at intervals, and the assurance that no question is not worth asking or stupid. Factual knowledge can relieve some uncertainty and allow the family to feel in control. Some parents have difficulty in relating to parents' groups because they want to be with "normal" people. Both parents and children have the potential to develop chronic health problems of their own if stress is not relieved, and the nurse should be alert for such development. These can include menstrual difficulties, impotency, headaches, ulcers, hypertension, obesity, and so on.

Nurses should carefully review the plan of care with families and evaluate coping before adding to it, and families should be an integral part of the decision-making. Even the addition of one more 15-minute routine by a well-meaning nurse can be the straw that breaks the camel's back. Parents should not be made to feel guilty if they skip one treatment, and praise should be given for what they are doing well. Many families become the "experts" on the care of their child, and it is tiring for them to have yet another professional take a history and advise them on what should be done. Realistic goals should be set for the child. The nurse and parents should review these. Parents may have false hopes or unrealistic expectations for progress and may be discouraged, whereas the professional views progress as rapid.

Professionals can help parents develop realistic assertiveness. The parents should be able to communicate effectively, relate to professionals as partners, but be able to express their needs and "stick up" for their rights. They should learn to document their needs. It will be necessary for them to learn to keep their own records. Both parents and professionals should become comfortable with such behavior. Professionals bring attitudes from both their education and their culture to the relationship. Parents who are "nice" and well-behaved may not get the help that is actually needed. In a type of bargaining phase, parents may secretly expect that if they are "good," they will be rewarded with improvement to normality. Professionals can all too easily go along with the assumption that if the parents do everything they are told, the child will improve. This can lead to overly intense efforts and parent burnout. Every effort must be made to support and help the parents. If the family disintegrates, both normal and affected members are lost.

The affected child and the rest of the family should be periodically assessed and reevaluated for problems. The nurse should be aware that an adolescent with Down syndrome who is depressed may be so for reasons other than Down syndrome, and this needs to be kept in mind. Progression should be discussed. Parents may find that they were encouraged by relatively rapid responses and progress during infancy, but that progress has slowed down. Drooling that was cute in infancy may be viewed as repulsive in the adolescent. A more realistic appraisal of ultimate potential may be possible by the school years. Coping with physical needs and care may become more of a strain as the parent ages and as the affected person becomes larger and heavier. The option of residential care should be discussed periodically. Parents who rejected the idea years before may welcome it at another time. They may not be able to raise the issue themselves, however. After years of home care, they may be able to relinquish the child more easily knowing that they tried their best.

Siblings—Feelings and Effects

The effect of having a disabled sibling varies with the type and severity of the disability as well as other factors previously discussed. Those siblings that have been identified as being at greatest risk for the most negative impact are the normal sibling in a two-child family, the oldest female sibling who may assume or be expected to assume the role of "little mother," the sibling closest in age and of the same sex as the affected sibling, younger siblings who no longer receive much parental attention, and siblings in families where the parents remain unable to accept and adapt to their situation, although each family may be different. How the sibling perceives the parents' reaction toward the affected sibling is important in ultimate adjustment. There are many small but cumulative stresses for the unaffected sibling. They may worry about whether or not to invite a friend to the house, what to tell their friends, whether or not to take the affected sibling with them on some outings, whether they will be stigmatized because of their association with their affected sibling, what to do if others tease their sibling, and so on. They may not know whether to defend their sibling from the teasing of others, remove him or her from the situation, or remain quiet. Often the normal sibling may end up angry and frustrated with him or herself, the affected sibling, and friends. Parents may add to these feelings by insisting that the normal child include the affected sibling in his or her activities. Parents sometimes resist the provision of counseling for the normal sibling because they are afraid that family "secrets" will be revealed. If the unaffected sibling's needs go unrecognized, he or she may feel that they are not important. The nurse should periodically ask the parents about the other children in the family—if they appear affected, what kinds of questions they ask, how the parents have answered them, and so on. The nurse can also indicate that the siblings may have various concerns and needs appropriate to their ages, and suggest ways in which the parents can meet or deal with them. Alternatives should be suggested so that the parents can vary their approach. It may be necessary for the nurse to ask about the parents' involvement in school and extracurricular activities of the unaffected sibling, and suggest ways that the parents can find time for participation on some level. In some communities, volunteers from Project Help or FISH or similar groups from religious or service organizations are on call to provide transportation or shopping services for those who need them. If the affected sibling dies, parents may idealize him or her, and the unaffected sibling can never "live up" to the image. Other effects and concerns of siblings are as follows:

• They may be concerned about their own vulnerability. They may find it difficult to directly ask their parents about their concerns.
• Siblings may feel guilty about being born "normal" and occasionally resent the affected sibling.
• Sometimes siblings are jealous because the affected sibling takes so much of the parents' time and then they feel guilty for this emotion.
• They may be embarrassed at the affected sibling's disorder.

• They may feel deprived of their own childhood and free time.
• They may feel that they do not measure up to society's expectations that they love their affected sibling, and thus feel guilty.
• They may be pushed into overcompensating for affected siblings. Parents may have unrealistically high expectations that the normal sibling struggles to achieve.
• They may be repressed in their abilities if they are younger than the affected sibling, so that they do not pass the affected sibling.
• They may feel emotionally neglected with no one to tell their problems to.
• They may be deprived of childhood "extras" such as dancing lessons, music lessons, participation in community sports, or scouting because of inadequate finances or lack of transportation.
• They may experience difficulty in having friends over to their house.
• They may not have their parents at school functions because of the need to stay with the other sibling.
• The unaffected sibling may have feelings of hostility, anger, and aggression toward the affected sibling, just as he or she might toward any other sibling. It should be emphasized that such feelings are normal, and some suitable mechanism for expression should be found. Naturally, the normal sibling cannot be allowed to punch a sibling with hemophilia, but the aggression can be expressed in another way.
• Children normally interpret events differently at different stages of development. They may develop fantasies about the affected sibling.
• They may have feelings of isolation and separation from rest of society.
• In early adolescence, a major concern may be how not to identify with the affected sibling, and they often try to maximize their differences.
• The disabled sibling may be envious of the nondisabled sibling and may be quite capable of manipulating situations and provoking anger.
• Unaffected siblings may particularly resent compromises in their life if the disability is an invisible one and they cannot understand why so much attention is focused on the affected sibling.
• They question their essential normality—If John is retarded, how can I be normal?

• Siblings (and/or their mates) often fear that they will have similarly affected children. When they reach the middle or late teens, the siblings themselves should receive genetic counseling.

• They may feel a loss of privacy.

• Unaffected siblings are often more embarrassed by same-sex affected siblings.

Groups for siblings, even if not of the same disorder, can help siblings realize that they are not the only one with a disabled sibling. Parents should be encouraged to provide activities for the normal sibling, perhaps by arranging for a grandparent to financially aid with extracurricular lessons or by arranging transportation with a relative, friend, or neighbor. Unaffected siblings may want to participate in care of the affected sibling, and this can increase feelings of self-worth and self-esteem, but they should not feel responsible for the sibling. Another concern of unaffected siblings is what will happen to their affected sibling when their parents can no longer care for him or her. They may believe that their parents expect them to assume responsibility (and the parents may). They may worry about how they can ever find a marriage partner who will be willing to assume this task. Some effects may be beneficial. In families who have made a successful accommodation, siblings may gain compassion, a greater understanding of people, more sensitivity to issues such as prejudice, and more tolerance toward other people in general. Issues for siblings may continue into adulthood as their parents age, and the issue of responsibility and who will be the caregiver once the parents die begin to surface. These issues then affect the sib's partner and other family members.

PROBLEMS AT VARIOUS STAGES OF THE LIFE CYCLE

Infancy and Preschool

The affected infant is a baby with the same needs as all infants plus some additional ones. If infants are loved and accepted within their family, they will believe others can also love and accept them. Therefore, the nurse can apply many of the techniques used with other infants to the disabled one. Parents should be encouraged to cuddle, talk to, smile at, and generally interact with their infant. The parents may need help to recognize the times of greatest receptivity. The nurse may need to help them find ways in which this will be most effective, depending on the basic problem. For example, the blind infant can be helped to "see" his or her parents by moving his or her hands over the parents' faces and by verbalizing who is present. Emphasis should be placed on the maximum development of the child's potential. This should include the provision of an enriched environment, the development of independent mobility, and special exercises or experiences that are individually designed. This may be accomplished through infant stimulation programs in which a professional comes to the home once or twice a week to teach the parent techniques and to assess progress, or it may be one in which the parent comes to a daily or weekly parent-infant program at a clinic, school, or children's center. There is a variety of opinion on the effectiveness of the programs that varies with the type, but in general the nurse should encourage opportunities to maximize potential. At the home visit or at the clinic, the nurse can also keep track of physical development and developmental milestones using appropriate instruments, and can inquire about the kinds of attention span, moods, reactions, responses to new events, etc., so that parents can be made aware of such assessment. Social contact should be developed and encouraged. Sometimes parents have a hard time finding such activities for the child who is a preschooler. The nurse may be able to assist in locating appropriate resources or to encourage the parents to develop their own. The nurse may need to explain to parents that developmental delay is expected in certain conditions and may be able to provide estimates of ages at which children with specific disorders may acquire such skills.

Childhood

In childhood the child can begin to assume responsibility for some of his or her own needs if feasible. For example, the child with cystic fibrosis can hold his or her own nebulizer. The emphasis should be on what they can do rather than what they cannot do. Opportunities for independence should be maximized, and ways to compensate for or circumvent problems should be found. Wherever possible, self-activity regulation should be encouraged. Realistic skills and talents should be developed and strengthened. For example, a boy with hemophilia might join the band, dramatics, or become the team manager for the football team rather than play the game. One such boy developed skills and became a magician, fascinating his classmates and providing after-school jobs in adolescence. Success in school depends in part on the establishment of a positive relationship with the school—with the teachers, nurse, and administration. Before enrolling in school, the family, and perhaps the physician and nurse who have been involved, should meet with school officials to explain the disorder, what it means in terms of events likely to be encountered in the school setting, what constitutes the need for serious medical concern, and what effects the disability may or may not have on performance. It may often be necessary to reiterate such points during a school year. Such advocacy becomes a never-ending job. The school nurse can assist teachers in working out daily problems or discussing their insecurities. When problems arise, parents should first try to solve them informally, at the lowest level. Before school entry, they should know the school system and its administrative structure and know their rights. Various pieces of legislation have addressed educational rights for the disabled such as the Individuals with Disabilities Education Act, termed IDEA. Before the age of 3 years, most communities provide an individualized family service plan, usually through early intervention agencies; and later an individualized education plan is developed. Information can also be obtained from advocacy organizations or the state department of education. Inclusion should not mean nonprovision of needed special services. If concerns about the nonprovision of services occurs, the parents should be encouraged to seek the help of state advocacy or human rights groups. If at all possible, parents, on the birth of a child who will need special educational services, should actively involve themselves in their school districts, either by seeking election to the school board or by becoming active in the PTA or in a parent advisory group. The appearance of the child can influence the teacher's expectations. One set of parents, with a child with Down syndrome who had borderline intelligence, had plastic surgery performed on her face to remove stigmata of Down syndrome because she was being judged on expectations of retardation rather than on her real abilities.

Decisions about main-streaming versus special education classes are beyond the scope of this chapter. Some believe that many special education programs do not prepare or try to prepare mentally normal children for pursuing higher education or careers above the unskilled or semi-skilled level but aim for sheltered workshop situations. However, others believe that "contained" classrooms do offer opportunity in some cases. More advocacy on the part of affected individuals is needed in the elementary as well as the high school setting.

In late childhood the need to be like one's peers asserts itself. As much as possible, the child's appearance and clothing should be like those of their peers. This can be a very difficult period for parents. Information about the illness should be given to the child so that he/she can respond factually when needed. Throughout this period, parents should let them know that illness is not caused by something they did, thought, or were being punished for. Household tasks and responsibilities can be given that are realistic for them and can be attained. They should be able to achieve success but not be given superfluous work. In schools with an open-minded attitude, real strides can be made for inclusion. In one elementary school that I am familiar with, a girl in a wheelchair was one of the cheerleaders. It may be that the parents, a friend, or a professional may need to suggest ways for inclusion that are practical.

Adolescence and Adulthood

Adolescence is a difficult period for the family of children without disabilities. For the parents of the disabled child, it may present additional challenges. Needs include the desire to be like one's peers, establishment of identity, self-determination, independence, a need for respect, and the establishment of satisfactory, intimate, or sexual relationships. Future education, employment, and independent living should be considered. There may be a tendency to treat affected children like Peter Pan who never grew up. Therefore, topics of sexuality, appropriate behavior, information about menstruation and hygiene routines, contraception, family life, and self-stimulatory behaviors are never discussed. Sexuality is still an area that families may find difficult to deal with, although schools and independent living centers are more inclusive of this kind of information. Sexual success is related to the development of productive personalities and the ability to relate to others. Yet society often attempts to deny the sexuality of the disabled. To partially address this issue, various groups are providing packaged sex education programs to schools or sexual counseling that is aimed at special needs of the disabled. Marriage and parenthood should be presented as real options.

The need to be like one's peers and physical appearance are very important. Other adolescents who were friends of the affected person may form new attachments. Adolescents also habitually engage in risk-taking behaviors. For persons with hemophilia, or osteogenesis imperfecta, this period can have serious consequences. Because suicide rates have also been observed to be higher in adolescents with chronic illnesses and visible defects, this may be an appropriate time to provide counseling and support. The opportunity for social interaction should also be provided, perhaps through groups of persons with disabilities or through normal school or church activities, depending on which is most comfortable for the adolescent. Adolescents find it difficult to maintain special diets or wear special clothing at this time.

This is also a period to reevaluate and design future goals, to estimate future functional capacities, and to help the family begin thinking about independent living. At this time, options such as small group homes for young adults with disabilities should be explored. This may be very difficult for parents who have provided care for so many years. Indeed, the disabled person may have difficulty in exchanging the passive role of receiver for an active one, if this has not been a goal he or she has worked toward. It is important that personal independence skills to the degree possible be attained in areas of personal needs, household activities, responsibility, and others. If the affected person wishes to go to college, then living arrangements should be explored at the colleges of interest. Ongoing counseling to support separation is needed for the affected person and also for the parents. As barriers, both architectural and those that discriminate in employment, begin to fall,

less-apparent ones may become evident. For example, the workplace may be accessible, but public transportation may limit free mobility. Many cities have developed apartment complexes of disabled and nondisabled persons with architectural adaptations and easily available transportation. Familiarity with the Americans With Disabilities Act may prove useful.

During adolescence and adulthood, and sometimes in late childhood, parents report that they often feel more concerns and fears about the ultimate future for their child. They may state that they feel more isolated and alone. The physical needs for children with severe disabilities may be a strain as the child weighs more and the parents may have less strength or may be experiencing their own physical limitations. Sometimes, behaviors become more problematic such as inappropriate laughter, tantrums, uncontrollable movements, or loud vocalizations. Thus, outside assistance may be needed at this time even if it was not necessary earlier. Future planning may need to take place as adulthood approaches. Parents begin to realize their own mortality and may want a sibling to agree to assume care for the affected person when they can no longer provide care or when they die. This brings to the fore old and new family strains, as the sibling and his or her family may or may not desire or be able to assume this care. In one study by Krauss, Seltzer, Gordon, and Friedman (1996), only about 1/3 of siblings planned to co-reside with their adult sibs who had mental retardation.

Although most genetic disorders are diagnosed early, others are not manifested or identified until adulthood. Depending upon the age of diagnosis, the impact may be on the person's educational plans, work and career aspirations and trajectory, and on plans for selecting a mate and having a family. If the person already has a family, concerns may revolve around the burden of illness for the family, the financial impact or future planning, effects on the job, possible role reversal as the mate or children may need to take over responsibilities, and the perceived burden on the family and friends. For many, the identification of genetic disease in adulthood, such as Gaucher disease, may significantly alter plans. The need for frequent treatment or therapy or a poor prognosis may impact upon insurance coverage, causing the individual to compromise career plans to stay within a particular company's health plan. Alternatively, knowledge of a genetic disorder in an adult can result in not being considered for raises and promotions. Such discrimination may be subtle or overt. This attitude could be seen as experienced by Tom Hank's character in the movie, *Philadelphia,* although the disease in question was acquired immunodeficiency syndrome (AIDS). The prospect of enduring a chronic illness over time may represent a perceived care burden. Issues that the nurse might raise for the person and/or family to consider include durable power of attorney and living will. For a single person or single-parent family, the financial impact and problem of care is quite different than in a two-parent family. Role reversal, the children caring for the parent, may be a distressing component. If physical care is involved, the older person may feel embarrassed at the loss of privacy and need for physical care. Of special concern has been the need to provide age and condition appropriate care for the adult who has what is considered to be a pediatric genetic disorder. Many health care providers who specialize in adults are not readily familiar with disorders such as cystic fibrosis, whereas pediatric specialists are not readily familiar with concerns and conditions of the adult such as normal aging processes and common disorders such as hypertension. The medical or health care home concept has evolved that includes comprehensive family-centered health care that centralizes the patient information needed.

PROBLEMS ENCOUNTERED IN SPECIFIC GENETIC DISORDERS

With all that has been discussed in this chapter, some disorders present unique sets of problems. A few of these are discussed below.

Osteogenesis Imperfecta

Osteogenesis imperfecta (OI) is a genetic disorder of the connective tissue, with an incidence in the West of about 1:20,000 live births. Types I through IV result from mutation in either the *COL1A1* or *COL1A2* gene that encode both chains in Type I collagen. The mutations can be varied including point mutations, exon splicing defects, deletions, and others. There are four major classes of OI (see

Table 8.2), types V through VII have been suggested but are not yet universally accepted. These types are not thought to be caused by type I collagen gene mutations. Basically, OI is characterized by connective tissue and bone defects including one or more of the following: bone fragility and osteoporosis leading to fractures, blue sclerae, progressive bone deformities (including long bone curvature), presenile hearing loss, and dentinogenesis imperfecta (a dentin abnormality of the teeth showing opalescence and blue or brown discoloration). Other features may include hernias, joint hyperlaxity, elevated body temperature of 1 or 2°F, heat intolerance, varying degrees of short stature, triangular face, and large "tam o'shanter" shaped skulls. Variability in clinical expression is common, and Type I may be mild enough so that it is missed altogether. Some individuals may suffer hundreds of fractures in a lifetime, whereas others suffer only one or a few and still others have little bone fragility; some have little height effect, others are two to three standard deviations below the mean, and others are six or more deviations below the mean. Kyphosis and scoliosis are very common as the individual gets older. OI is considered to be inherited in an autosomal dominant manner although in some cases autosomal recessive transmission apparently occurs. OI may occur sporadically. Complicating the usual findings, cases of parental mosaicism have been described in 5% to 7% of clinically unaffected couples. To rule out parental mosaicism or a mildly affected parent in cases where only one family member is affected, a leukocyte DNA analysis can be done in order to provide accurate genetic counseling. It should be noted that patients in any of the 4 major classifications can have their first fracture at birth. Persons in types I, III, and IV can have their first fracture at any time of life. Further heterogeneity may exist within these classes, and although subdivision can be done, this is not uniformly accepted. Although the reason for growth deficiency is not fully understood, growth hormone for treating the short stature has been used in clinical trials. Bone marrow transplant to produce normal cells, stem cell manipulation and transplantation, and gene therapy to suppress the dominant mutant allele may hold future treatment promise. Because of the severe burden of OI, prenatal diagnosis should be offered both to parents who have OI and to those

TABLE 8.2   Classification of Osteogenesis Imperfecta

Type	Inheritance	Characteristics
IA	AD	Bone fragility (mild to moderate severity), blue sclerae, progressive hearing loss in about 50%, mild bruising, short stature (average for population, but shorter than family), normal teeth.
IB	AD	Essentially same as IA but have dentinogenesis imperfecta (opalescent teeth). About two thirds of the total cases are Type I.
II	AD (possible heterogeneity) May be AR form	Lethal perinatal type: affected persons are either stillborn or die in early infancy; multiple fractures are present at birth; infants have short, curved, deformed limbs, broad thighs, and are small for age; crumpled femurs, and beaded ribs are characteristic radiological findings; occasionally because of poor skull bone ossification they are erroneously believed to be in breech position during pregnancy; comprise about 10% of total osteogenesis imperfecta cases.
III	AD May be AR in some	Severe bone fragility leads to severe progressive deformities; some infants have numerous fractures at birth; sclerae are usually pale blue fading to white with increasing age. There is marked postnatal growth failure; the skull is less poorly ossified than Type II; severe short stature may not be seen until 2 or 3 years of age. These are the shortest of osteogenesis imperfecta patients. Dentinogenesis imperfecta is usually present. Possible basilar invagination leading to compression. May have scoliosis, chest deformities and progressive limb deformities. Faces may be flat, macrocephaly present, and hearing loss is common.
IVA	AD	Similar to type IA except that sclerae are normal, and is usually more severe. Bone fragility (mild to moderate severity); postnatal short stature common, +/- skeletal deformities. Teeth usually normal.
IVB	AD	Similar to type IB but more severe and with normal sclerae. Dentinogenesis imperfecta may be found.
V	AD probable	Moderate severity, normal sclerae, mild to moderate short stature, radial head dislocation common, teeth usually normal, tendency to form hypertrophic calluses at fracture sites.
VI	? AD probable	Moderate to severe skeletal deformities, normal sclerae, normal teeth, scoliosis, fish scale-like appearance of bone lamellation, osteoid accumulation, moderate short stature.
VII	AR	Moderate to severe deformity and fragility, rhizomelia of humerus and femur, mild short stature.

who have had an affected child. In those choosing to continue the pregnancy, a cesarean section to minimize fetal trauma can be done, and arrangements for delivery in a specialty hospital should be made.

Those who are diagnosed in infancy present immediate problems and challenges to the new parents and to the nursing staff. The simple act of lifting the child may cause bones to break. In diapering, the infant should never be lifted by the ankles but supported carefully in good alignment. The crib, and later the playpen, should be mesh and padded. All treatment tables should also be padded. The infant can be most easily held or transported in an infant seat, on a padded piece of plywood, or on a pillow so that support is provided. Because of the ongoing body temperature elevation, light clothing should be used and water, or later juice, should be offered frequently. Infants with OI have the same need for physical contact and stimulation as other infants, but parents and others may be afraid to handle them because of fragility. The nurse should help the parents to learn to be secure in handling and help promote bonding as well as using stroking and touching. Those children with severe disease will have many hospitalizations. Nurses should be willing to listen to both the parents and the child who usually have become quite expert by early childhood in how movement can be best accomplished. At the time of diagnosis, one of the most helpful things that the nurse can do is to refer the family to one of the organizations for OI. Some Web sites include Osteogenesis Imperfecta Foundation (http://www.oif.org), and NIH Osteoporosis and Related Bone Disease National Resource Center (http://www.osteo.org). Many local chapters have persons who are experienced in handling and other problems of these children, and also hotlines that give the parents someone to call who understands when they have just broken one of their child's bones, perhaps with something as simple as a hug. Children with ultimate short stature can be referred to a group aimed at that problem. See Appendix B. Other nursing points include the following:

• Before a diagnosis of OI is made, the parents of the infant who is sustaining fractures may be suspected of child abuse. Such an experience can be a very traumatic one for the parents. Radiologic confirmation of OI due to the presence of Wormian bones, the types of fractures, the presence of blue sclera, or dentinogenesis imperfecta, and a family history of OI or its signs and symptoms may all help in establishing the true diagnosis, as will DNA testing.

• Many normal infants have blue sclera, and so use of this feature as a sign is not usually an effective one in infancy, unless the infant is very deeply colored. Often more severe disease is associated with normal sclera.

• Selecting infant clothing with Velcro(r) or ties instead of buttons can minimize trauma in severe disease.

• Small frequent feedings may be necessary in infants and children whose chest deformities are such that the stomach is impinged on. If the teeth are severely damaged, adjustments may be necessary. Plastic bottles should be used.

• Careful assessment of motor skills with a standardized scale such as the Peabody scale is necessary to ascertain status and monitor progress.

• A major need is to treat fractures present to prevent deformities, and to prevent further fractures. Parents will need to learn emergency care for fractures as well as cast care.

• Strengthening programs can be planned so the person can eventually lift limbs against gravity. Various orthotic devices and water activities can be developed by physical and occupational therapists and referral should be made for these services.

• The potential for respiratory insufficiency due to instability of the ribs and infections is present. Coughing can result in rib fracture, and each fracture episode can increase deformity, further decreasing respiratory capabilities.

• Respiratory infections can be life-threatening in infants and children with severe disease, and so measures should be directed at prevention and prompt treatment.

• Children may experience delay of developmental milestones, such as standing and walking, because of fear of fractures and pain.

• Various types of equipment, such as mobiles, padded platforms on casters, caster carts, standing A-frames, and weight-relieving walkers are available to allow the child to achieve normal mobility and exploration and to facilitate development.

• As the child grows older, in severe OI, both surgical and nonsurgical management that includes various orthopedic procedures such as extensible rodding and bracing may be necessary. There have been many improvements in surgical procedure and technology.

• With the risk of each surgery there is also the risk of anesthesia. Of particular concern is the ease of fractures of both bones and teeth, thoracic deformities, and possible presence of airway anomalies, and the tendency to develop hyperthermia during the administration of anesthesia.

• Newer approaches to therapy include using bisphosphonates to improve bone mass, and pamidronate may be used intravenously in severe forms and appears particularly useful when begun early. Long-term efficacy and safety is not known. Oral bisphosphonates may be used in later therapy. Another approach is the transplantation of mesenchymal stromal cells into bone marrow. Somatic gene therapy is another avenue of interest.

• Rather than use a blood pressure cuff or a tourniquet, gentle manual pressure is often recommended when drawing blood in order to prevent fractures.

• Those who have dentinogenesis imperfecta should be advised to maintain good dental care because such teeth tend to wear more easily.

• Children with OI generally have normal to superior intelligence, and if at all possible should be kept in regular school classrooms. This means careful planning and discussion with school administrators, teachers, and nurses to alleviate their fears and call attention to special needs (i.e., thirst and need for access to fluids).

• Children with OI should be observed for, and periodically tested for, hearing loss.

• Children born to a parent with opalescent teeth and OI who develop opalescent teeth should be carefully watched for fractures.

• By late childhood, scoliosis should be observed for, because 80% to 90% of all OI patients may develop this complication. Pain from these or from vertebral collapse needs to be watched for. About 25% are said to have basilar invagination which can progress to complications requiring neurosurgery.

• Children with OI often dislike milk, so that normal calcium intake should be provided in other ways (e.g., milk in puddings, cheese, cereals).

• In general, restrictions regarding lifestyle should be individually tailored. In the mildly affected individual, even such activities as skiing may be appropriate.

• By puberty, skeletal stability seems to increase, and the number of fractures usually lessen. At the same time, adolescent rebellion may occur, and activity may increase to an unrealistic extent (e.g., motorcycle racing) and actually result in increased injury.

• At any time, persons with OI may be prone to develop hernias because of the effects on collagen.

• Depending on the ultimate height achieved, the severity of disease and the presence of deformity, the person with OI may or may not have difficulty with sexual relationships because of limited hip motion and the ease of fracture. Mildly affected patients often reproduce. Pregnancy problems may include respiratory problems, increased spontaneous fractures, increased awkwardness, and an increased susceptibility to hernias. Careful monitoring of the pregnancy is necessary, and cesarean section may be necessary due to the possibility of fractures in labor and delivery. Genetic counseling and prenatal diagnosis should be provided.

Although it might be thought that quality of life in people with OI would be severely impacted, a 2002 paper (Widmann, Laplaza, Bitan, Brooks, & Root) found that while the SF-36 self-assessment questionnaires were significantly lower in physical function compared to U. S. adult norms, the mental component scores were similar to the norms. High levels of employment and education were achieved although ambulation was a major limitation. Anecdotal studies have indicated low levels of depression and social success in this population.

Cystic Fibrosis

"Woe to that child which when kissed on the forehead tastes salty. He is bewitched and soon must die." This folksaying from northern Europe as quoted by Welsh & Smith (1995) was an early reference to cystic fibrosis (CF). Today, the picture is brighter. The median age for a person with CF to live is more than 30 years. CF is the most common semilethal genetic disease in Caucasians, with an incidence of about 1:2,000 to 1:2,500 live Caucasian births. It is especially frequent in certain ethnic groups such as the Hutterites in Alberta, Canada where the frequency is 1:313. It is less frequent in American blacks and Asian populations. It is transmitted in an autosomal recessive manner. The frequency of heterozygote carriers in white populations is about 1:25; in Ashkenazi Jews about 1:29; in Hispanics, 1:48, in American blacks, 1:65; and in Asians about 1:150. The basic defect is a mutation in the *CFTR* gene on chromosome 7q31.2 whose product is the cystic fibrosis transmembrane conductance regulator. This protein is expressed in the membrane of epithelial cells which line such structures as the pancreas, intestines, sweat ducts, vas deferens and lungs, influencing water balance and sodium transport. This protein is involved in chloride ion channel function (an ion channel is essentially a protein tunnel that crosses the cell membrane and changes conformation as it opens and closes in response to various signals), regulating and participating in transport of chloride and probably other electrolytes across epithelial cell membranes. Some *CFTR* mutations cause an abnormal protein to be produced or no protein production, but others cause defective regulators of, or conductors through, the CFTR ion channel or defective regulation of other channels. McKone, Emerson, Edwards, and Aitken (2003) functionally classify *CFTR* alleles into five classes according to whether the mutation results in defective protein production, processing, regulation, conductance, or reduced amounts of functioning CFTR protein. More than 1,000 *CFTR* mutations are known. The most common mutation (accounting for about 2/3 across populations) is ΔF508del, a deletion of phenylalanine at position 508, that results in abnormal protein folding and lack of CFTR at the cell membrane. There are three other mutations that are particularly common—G551D, G542X and R553X, all of which act in various ways to cause deficiency of CFTR. There can be some complexities. For example, those with CF due to ΔF508, may have an ameliorating mutation also, as normal sweat electrolyte concentrations may occur if they also have the R553Q mutation. The degree of deficiency can vary. When *CFTR* function is 10% or greater, usually abnormalities are not seen. Thus the specific mutation a person has can influence the clinical expression and course and can be useful in counseling within a family. Genotype-phenotype correlations are of interest in predicting both mortality and morbidity. Those who are most severe, with less than 1%, usually have the full spectrum of involvement, including pancreatic exocrine deficiency, progressive pulmonary infection, and congenital absence of the vas deferens. Genetic testing is complicated because of the large number of *CFTR* mutations known. Most commercial tests look for 70, which should identify most of the common mutations. About 1% of persons with CF do not demonstrate known gene mutations, and about 18% only show one mutated gene despite symptoms. Because of variability in pulmonary disease among those with the same *CFTR* genotype, a search has been done for other influences, both genetic and environmental. Environmental factors that were postulated to influence variability of phenotype included *P. aeroginosa, Burkholderia cepacia,* tobacco use, and nutrition. CF modifier genes have also been suggested and most associations to date require more investigation. Various approaches such as twin and sibling pair designs, microarray analysis of respiratory epithelium, and other approaches are being used. Clearly more is to be learned about severity and variability in phenotype.

Generally, a child will have the same mutation as his/her carrier parents, so that prenatal testing for the mutations known to be carried by the parents is accurate. Diagnosis is still done sometimes, but not usually, by sweat testing, but genotyping, tests of pancreatic function, and using nasal potential-difference measurements are more common.

Because of the frequency of carriers in the Caucasian population, a White person with cystic fibrosis who plans reproduction has a risk of 1:50 that his or her children will be affected, if his or her partner is unaffected and has no family history of cystic fibrosis [1 (the affected person can only pass on a mutant gene) × 1:25 (the carrier rate in the population) × 1/2 (chance of carrier passing on the mutant gene)]. Other estimates would similarly apply for other ethnic groups depending on the frequency of the mutant allele in that ethnic population.

Many of the symptoms of CF result from the fact that in CF, mucus and serous secretions are abnormally concentrated, sticky, or dry, allowing blockage of ducts and other structures to occur. The most obvious systems affected are the respiratory and gastrointestinal and give rise to the most common symptoms including progressive lung disease, sinusitis, pancreatic exocrine insufficiency (found in about 90% to some degree) which can lead to diabetes mellitus, and infertility in males. More about how the mutant gene actually manifests effects is being elucidated. It is believed that because of abnormal thickening, mucin from the lung pools in the lungs, perhaps stimulated by the bacteria *Pseudomonas aeruginosa* protects that bacteria from the body's immune system. The salty secretions may also influence body defense. This may partly explain why people with CF are so susceptible to infections with *P. aeruginosa*. A common presentation is in childhood with a persistent cough, often with colonization, and perhaps loose bulky stools and failure to thrive. There is extreme variability in the severity of clinical illness and in the system involved. About 50% are diagnosed before 1 year of age. Those with milder disease or less common manifestations may not be diagnosed until adolescence or adulthood and frequently have previously been misdiagnosed as having asthma, chronic sinusitis, pancreatitis, celiac disease, or chronic bronchitis. Because aspermia is present in 95% to 98% of males with cystic fibrosis, infertility with azoospermia should lead the practitioner to include cystic fibrosis as a diagnostic possibility. Certain *CFTR* gene mutations result in congenital bilateral absence of the bas deferens without necessarily showing other effects of CF such as lung manifestations. One way this can occur is due to TG dinucleotide repeats (see chapters 4 and 6) in the *CFTR* gene affecting RNA splicing resulting in reduction of the transcript leading to male infertility and in some cases, nonclassic CF. Men seeking assisted reproduction by such techniques as intracytoplasmic sperm injection are now usually tested for CF status before the procedure is done, and depending on results, further testing of their partner and counseling would be done. Females may have delayed puberty as well as decreased fertility. Various presenting manifestations may be seen in different age groups, as shown in Table 8.3.

Advances in cystic fibrosis care and experience at specialized centers have allowed survival with good life quality into adulthood, with a median age of survival of over 30 years presently. For those persons with CF born in the 1990s, the median survival is predicted to be more than 40 years of age. Management is dependent on the severity of disease, age of diagnosis, and degree of involvement of body systems. It is aimed at controlling and preventing respiratory infections, maintaining nutrition, minimizing unpleasant gastrointestinal effects, preventing and treating complications, and providing support, teaching, and counseling to the client and the family. Treatment may include postural drainage with chest percussion, antimicrobial therapy, diet therapy including determining a diet to result in stabilization of pulmonary function and optimal growth, paying attention to energy expenditure, pancreatic enzymes and fat-soluble vitamins, antiinflammatory therapy, use of

TABLE 8.3   Various Presenting Signs and Symptoms of Cystic Fibrosis in Various Age Groups

Newborn

Meconium ileus	Intestinal atresia
Melconium plug syndrome	"Salty" taste

Infancy

Failure to thrive	Steatorrhea
"Salty" taste	Hypoproteinemia, anemia, edema
Rectal prolapse	Hypoprothrombinemia, hemorrhage
Heat prostration/dehydration	Rapid finger wrinkling in water
Frequent, bulky stools	Abdominal distention

Childhood

Frequent, bulky, offensive stools	Heat prostration/dehydration
Chronic secretory otitis media	Inguinal hernia
Intussusception	Hydrocele
Biliary cirrhosis, jaundice	Type 1 diabetes mellitus
Rectal prolapse	

Adolescent/young adult

Aspermia (males)	Chronic cough
Infertility	Bronchiectasis
Chronic cervicitis (females)	Glucose intolerance
Thick cervical mucus (females)	Type 1 diabetes mellitus
Cervical polyps (females)	Intestinal obstruction
Delayed secondary sexual development	Reactive airway disease, asthma
Poor growth/small for age	Acute pancreatitis

All ages

Chronic cough	Sinusitis
Elevated sweat electrolytes	Clubbed fingers
Nasal polyps (especially below 16 years of age)	Recurrent pneumonia, bronchitis
Absence of vas deferens (males)	Bronchiectasis
Cor pulmonale	Sputum culture showing *Staphylococcus aureus* or *Pseudomonas aeruginosa*
Pancreatic insufficiency and malabsorption	
Presence of hard fecal masses in right lower quadrant of abdomen	Family history of similar symptoms, infant deaths, diarrhea

bronchodilators and aerosolized substances such as recombinant human deoxyribonuclease (rhDNase I, dornase alfa, Pulmozyme), and more drastic measures such as lung transplantation. Because use of high-dose pancreatic enzyme supplements can cause the complication of fibrosing colonopathy, it has been recommended that the daily dose should be below 10,000 units of lipase per kg. Detailed recommendations for adult care for CF are found in Yankaskas et al. (2004). Gene therapy appears to hold great promise. One theory holds that intrauterine gene therapy would be preferred because the *CFTR* gene is needed in development. Testing for status as a CF carrier in couples planning pregnancy, in those with a family history of CF, partners of persons with CF, and as a part of prenatal screening programs has been recommended by an NIH consensus panel but is not yet universally endorsed. Newborn screening and widespread population carrier screening are becoming more widespread and CDC in 2004 stated that newborn screening for CF was justified (see chapter 11). Specific nursing points include the following:

• Be alert for common presenting signs and symptoms of CF when assessing clients and refer them for further testing if appropriate.

• Nurses working with clients with CF should have an understanding of the pathogenesis, genetics, treatment principles, and common problems faced by the CF client and family at different stages.

• The child (when appropriate) and the family should be educated regarding the natural history of CF at multiple points in culturally competent and educationally appropriate ways. Anticipatory guidance can be useful.

• Help newly diagnosed families to locate CF centers for comprehensive treatment.

• Help families locate private, state, and federal financial and other aid resources such as Maternal Child Health Services, Division of Crippled Childrens Service's, Supplemental Security Income, Medicaid, and the Cystic Fibrosis Foundation as well as lay organizations and support groups.

• Be sure that the family is referred to and obtains genetic counseling.

• Anticipate that in severe involvement of the gastrointestinal tract, there may be problems associated with toilet training, so provide help and guidance for the parents.

• The nurse should be alert for and teach the parents to be alert for subtle signs of respiratory infection such as decreased weight gain and loss of appetite, so that prompt treatment can be instituted to prevent permanent damage. Appropriate infection control procedures are important (see Saiman & Siegel, 2003).

• Promote feelings of independence and control—let the child hold his or her own nebulizer; when the child is old enough, he or she may do his or her own bronchial drainage and percussion; allow the assumption of some responsibility for medications and diet.

• Help the family find easy ways to keep track of the medications that must be taken at various times, such as a labeled sectioned plastic box or egg container, since the client may take 40 to 60 pills per day.

• After optimum physical activity has been determined by the treatment team, work with the parents toward specific plans so that inappropriate limitations are not set.

• Advise both the client and family not to self-medicate. This is particularly important in regard to any preparations that suppress coughing.

• Problems may arise with self-esteem due to small size for his or her age, coughing with sputum production, and offensive flatus and stools if not well controlled. Provision for counseling may be needed.

• Help the client and family to realize the connection between the control of objectionable symptoms and compliance with medications and treatments.

• Help older children and teenagers to plan their diets so that fatty foods are avoided, but avoid over restriction that leads to noncompliance. Most clients can find a balance because they want to avoid symptoms such as offensive flatus and stools and abdominal pain.

• Nutrition planning in children should include adequate calories, low but adequate fat, and attention to the need for the supplementation of fat-soluble vitamins. Nutritional supplements may be needed. Help the family with understanding of why the child may have a large appetite and still not gain weight rapidly.

• Before the child enters school a conference should be held with the teacher, principal, and school nurse. This should include basic information about CF, the fact that the cough is not infectious, the need for physical activity and sports participation within tolerance, the possible need for extra food during the day, the medication program and the need for privacy in taking them, and the fact that the child's intelligence is unimpaired. Information suitable for school personnel can be obtained from the Cystic Fibrosis Foundation.

• Help parents to work around special events when carrying out the treatment regimen so as to maximize compliance.

• Provide hobby and career guidance that includes information on avoiding inhaled respiratory irritants.

• Be alert to new treatment trends such as the possibility of substituting certain physical exercise programs for postural drainage.

• Growth retardation and late physical development may allow others to think of the child as younger than he/she really is and must be periodically assessed. Again, counseling may be needed for client or family.

• Help the family cope with cycles of illness, health, treatment regimens, and the ongoing fear of death. Be alert for the older child or adolescent who may covertly attempt suicide by abandoning therapy. Be able to refer family to appropriate mental health services.

• Although there is no known impairment of sexual performance or desire, most males with cystic fibrosis are sterile, and decreased fertility may be present in females due to thick cervical mucus. Menstrual problems and vaginal yeast infections due to antibiotic therapy are common, and the client should be referred to a gynecologist experienced in the care of CF patients. Encourage both females and males to consider alternative reproductive plans and options such as contraception, sterilization, adoption, and assisted reproductive options (see chapter 27). Preconception counseling and family planning information is important in adolescence, and genetic counseling may also need to be provided. Pregnancy in cystic fibrosis women may be complicated because of pulmonary function changes and the increased cardiac work load. Couples contemplating having children should also be encouraged to consider the necessary increase in everyday work and activities.

• Remain alert for symptoms of glucose intolerance and diabetes mellitus, because this is a relatively common complication.

• Reassure adolescents who have delayed menarche, puberty, or secondary sexual characteristics that these will ultimately occur.

Hemophilia

Hemophilia A (classical hemophilia) and hemophilia B (Christmas disease) are caused by deficiencies of coagulation factor VIII (antihemophilic factor) and coagulation factor IX, respectively. Their incidence is 1:4,400 to 1:7,500 male births. Hemophilia A results from a mutation on the gene located on Xq28, while hemophilia B results from mutations at Xq27 of which more than 2,100 are known. Both are transmitted in an X-linked recessive manner, and about one third result from a new mutation with no prior family history. In such isolated cases, without prior positive family history, it is important to determine if the mother is a carrier. Females at risk can have a determination of relevant factor activity, and those below the normal range can confirm carrier status, but in those falling within the normal range, the possibility of the mother being a carrier is not excluded. DNA testing may be useful in certain cases to detect carriers. Information from these tests and information from the family history, such as the number of unaffected sons in the family, are used in Bayesian calculations to provide more precise genetic counseling in the absence of DNA testing. Prenatal diagnosis for women who are known carriers has been accomplished.

The severity of clinical disease varies with the percent of the blood level of factor present, ranging from those with little factor present and severe disease (50–70%), to essentially normal coagulation efficiency at levels of 50% or higher. The availability of concentrated factor preparations such as cryoprecipitates, comprehensive care programs, and the use of therapeutic and prophylactic home infusions radically altered treatment, complications, and prognosis, allowing less disruption of family plans. However, those with hemophilia suffered a setback when human immunodeficiency virus (HIV) entered the blood supply, infecting thousands with hemophilia. The use of recombinant factor VIII and factor IX concentrates for home infusion is now the recommended type. Desmopressin, an antidiuretic hormone analogue, can be used to raise the factor VIIIC concentration in persons with mild hemophilia A. In addition to treatment, prophylaxis may be used several times a week through infusion to prevent bleeds. While long-term information is not yet available, this approach may be an option for some, permitting even a young child with severe hemophilia to have a normal life with few or no bleeds and few restrictions. Gene therapy is under investigation.

The major problem in hemophilia is hemorrhage into the joints and muscles that, if not stopped, can result in prolonged bleeding leading to deformities and immobilization. These often occur spontaneously, that is, where no recallable injury has occurred but which probably result from normal physiologic strains that are usually unnoticed. The most common sites are ankles, knees, wrists, and elbows. For parents of boys with hemophilia, in the past, these were a constant overhanging concern, because their occurrence usually meant hospitalization and carried the risk of loss of function, nerve damage, deformity, the wearing of various orthopedic appliances, long school absences, and high costs. Often parents were overprotective, but such spontaneous bleeds were not really presently preventable until the advent of prophylaxis. Some boys notice a "bubbly" feeling at the site of the bleed before it is otherwise noticed. Most infants with hemophilia develop symptoms in the 1st year of life. They may first be noticed in the form of subcutaneous hematomas, easy bruising, or even at circumcision, and may follow intramuscular injections or mouth injury. Often the parents are suspected of child abuse. Some specific points for nurses include the following:

- The nurse should understand the type of bleeding that occurs—slow, steady, internal bleeding as opposed to gushing from superficial cuts—as well as the program therapy and genetics. Thus the child with hemophilia is not usually going to "bleed all over the neighbor's carpet."
- Families with members who have hemophilia should be referred to comprehensive care centers and to hemophilia organizations. See Appendix B.
- In infancy and early childhood, the same precautions should be taken that are used for all such children, for example, safety-approved car seats,

seat belts, a gate at the head of the stairs, high chairs with belts, etc. It is usually not necessary to pad the child's clothes, the furniture, or have the baby wear a helmet.

- At early ages, parents need to become familiar with manifestations of bleeding, because they may be inexperienced with the disorder and the infant is not yet able to tell them. Some of these are irritability, lumps, a limb that is not being moved, and warmth.
- Intramuscular injections should be avoided, but immunizations are essential. Most necessary injections can be given into deep subcutaneous tissue.
- No aspirin or aspirin-containing medications should be given. A list of over-the-counter medications that contain aspirin should be given to the parents, as well as safe substitutes for common problems.
- Prophylactic dental care is essential because dental problems can cause severe problems later. A dentist experienced in caring for hemophiliacs is desirable.
- The child should be allowed to play normally, but obvious contact sports such as football and hockey should be discouraged. Sports encouraged should be reviewed. In general, swimming, biking, and running are all good. However, it is normal for children to try such things for themselves at some point. Some risks are normal, but those such as motorcycle racing that may be taken up by a teenager may be considered self-destructive and need counseling services.
- Fear of bleeding and pain can interfere with normal strivings toward independence and assertiveness. Parents should try to avoid overprotectiveness and help the child develop independence. Such concerns are usually part of the counseling component at hemophilia comprehensive care centers.
- Parents should know first-aid measures and what to do in emergencies and for head injuries.
- Parents should be advised not to probe child's ears for deep cleaning.
- When the child enters school, the teacher, principal, and school nurse should be thoroughly briefed on hemophilia, emergency procedures, and any activity limitations. If this is not monitored, the child may be unnecessarily restricted and overprotected. Teachers should be taught how to handle superficial cuts (with a Band-Aid, as for

others). In any complaint of headache, throat pain, severe fall, or blow, parents should be notified and prompt treatment should be instituted.

- Children should wear some type of identification disc with their diagnosis. These may be obtained from the National Hemophilia Foundation, Medic Alert, or a similar group.
- The family should realize that stress may initiate a bleed, and this should be observed for if such situations are encountered. If this becomes frequent, special counseling may be needed.
- By later childhood usually the child with hemophilia can "be in control," mix their concentrate, do their own venipunctures, etc.
- Eventually, the child with hemophilia and his parents become experts in the disorder, and nurses may be able to learn from them. An inexperienced practitioner should never be sent to start an infusion or give an injection to a hospitalized person with hemophilia.
- Another time of family stress may be in adolescence. It is not unusual for boys with X-linked disorders to verbally blame their mothers for their condition. This reactivates guilt feelings, and professional help may be needed.
- In adolescence, the person with hemophilia and his sisters should receive genetic counseling and family planning information. The potential carrier may have psychological problems that have not been attended to, and the nurse should be aware of this possibility.
- Financial resources may be strained, even with home therapy. States differ in their benefits, and nurses should help the family find resources.

Short Stature and Achondroplasia

There are several ways of defining short stature. One of the most common is a height of two standard deviations below the mean or the 3rd percentile for height adjusted for parental height. The Little People of America (LPA), an organization founded by the actor Billy Barty, uses 4'10" or below as an adult to define short stature. The lay public has often used "dwarf" to describe disproportionate short stature and "midget" for proportionate short stature. The LPA notes that the term "midget" is offensive to many. There are many ways to classify short stature—by prenatal and postnatal onset, by normal variant and pathologic, and by

proportionate and disproportionate. Under normal variant short stature are included familial short stature, in which the parents are short and the offspring is healthy with normal skeletal maturity, and constitutional growth delay, in which growth is distributed over longer periods of time and, in effect, the child is genetically programmed to take longer to mature. Such children are healthy but have delayed bone age and may have delayed puberty with the potential to develop emotional problems. Pathologic short stature includes certain types of intrauterine growth retardation, including those caused by infection, chromosome disorders, certain syndromes, hormonal disturbances, developmental anomalies, psychosocial disturbances, malnutrition, chronic diseases, and skeletal dysplasias including disorders such as achondroplasia and OI.

Society generally values tallness and equates it with power. The social and psychological effects of short stature are profound. For some types of short stature, final adult height can be predicted. For some of the disorders with short stature, growth hormone has been used to increase final height, but this is not effective for achondroplasia which is the most common cause of disproportionate short stature. In achondroplasia, surgical procedures to lengthen the legs may be a consideration. Achondroplasia is due to mutation in the fibroblast growth factor receptor-3 gene *(FGFR3)* on chromosome 4p16.3. It can be recognized at birth but is not always. The limbs are short and the head is large with a prominent forehead and mandible, a flattened area at the base of the nose, "trident" hands, and marked hypotonicity. Later, kyphosis and lordosis may develop. It is important to remember that there is no intellectual impairment. It is transmitted in an autosomal dominant manner with complete penetrance and often occurs as a sporadic mutation (in about 7/8 of new cases), related to increased paternal age. In a study by Stoll and Feingold (2004) paternal grandparents of people with achondroplasia had significantly higher cancer rates than maternal grandparents, which they suggest might be due to mutation in a mutator gene leading to cancer in one ancestor and to germ cell mutation in that ancestor's offspring. The mean height for females and males with achondroplasia is about 48 in. and 52 in., respectively. More than 10,000 persons with achondroplasia live in the U. S. The American Academy of Pediatrics (1995) has developed health supervision recommendations for persons with achondroplasia at various age ranges. Some special points for nurses include the following:

- In achondroplasia, total development is eventually achieved, but there is some degree of delayed developmental milestones in achondroplasia such as head control and walking. Parents should be made aware of this. The use of backpack carriers and walkers is not recommended.
- The need to control weight is lifelong. On smaller persons, a small amount of weight gain is more evident than on others, and skeletal pressure should be minimized. The relationship of weight to height, and growth progress, should be monitored through growth charts specifically developed for achondroplasia [(see Hunter, Hecht, and Scott (1996) and American Academy of Pediatrics (1995)].
- Persons with achondroplasia are particularly prone to middle ear infections because of abnormal placement angle of the eustachian tube. All treatment should be prompt to preserve hearing. Hearing tests should be done at frequent intervals, and speech evaluation should be done.
- Persons with achondroplasia may be prone to snoring and may need evaluation for sleep apnea.
- Prophylactic dental care and good oral hygiene are essential because dental problems are frequent. Orthodontic braces are usually necessary.
- Watch for complaints of numbness or pains in the back and thighs due to the narrowness of spinal column in achondroplasia.
- In small-statured individuals, emotional maturation can be slow. It is tempting for parents and other relatives to overprotect the short-statured person and shield him or her from the world.
- In the early years, the short-statured person may be the mascot or the center of attention. Later, popularity may diminish, friends may drop away, and isolation may occur. Counseling and the provision of social contacts through interests and hobbies and through organizations such as the LPA should be facilitated. In one study of quality of life, persons with achondroplasia were found to have significantly lower mean scores overall and in the domains of health and functioning, social and economic, psychological and spiritual, and family

when compared with controls. They also had lower self-esteem (Gollust, Thompson, Gooding, & Biesecker, 2003). Thus, they may need counseling or assistance in dealing with non-medical issues.

- Some short-statured children are so busy in early years trying to overcome size-related problems that skills for learning readiness are neglected. This should be watched for and prevented.
- The short-statured person may assume the role of mascot or court jester in school. Eventually this can result in the indignity of being lifted or carried involuntarily.
- Parents, relatives, neighbors, and friends should orient themselves to the age of the short-statured person, not their height, as an index of maturity.
- Nurses should always treat the short-statured person with dignity.
- Independence should be encouraged. Ways should be found for children to do things for themselves, not to have things done for them. Many companies and organizations provide suggestions and equipment for modifications of clothing, cars, etc. Tricycles can be adapted, for example. Devices are available for reaching light switches if they cannot be lowered, and for wiping oneself after using the toilet.
- In sports, the short-statured person may not be able to compete. Activities in which success may be enjoyed should be encouraged. The person may enjoy music or art, or may wish to be scorekeeper, etc.
- Parents and professionals should be alert for the tendency of short-statured persons to isolate themselves or seek very young or old friends, and try to provide other opportunities for peer contact.
- School can be very traumatic for little people. They need help in ways to handle teasing and taunting. Some suggest an aggressive verbal approach. Others suggest developing an alliance with a large-sized classmate. It should be kept in mind that most children have nicknames and most go through a period of cruelty, but teasing and bullying can be extremely detrimental. LPA may also be able to supply support.
- When giving medications to the short-statured person, it should be remembered that size must be considered and dosage may need to be altered.
- The adolescent should be helped to obtain clothes appropriate to his or her age.

- Short-statured persons can and do hold a variety of jobs such as in entertainment, music, hairdressing, welding, teaching, etc. They should be free to pursue jobs of their choice.
- In the job market, they may face prejudice, self-doubt, and embarrassment. Some companies attempt to pay less for the same jobs.
- One major difficulty is that public transport may not be possible to use and this may limit career selection. Devices such as those to assist in reaching the car accelerator and brake are available to make driving possible.
- Short-statured persons may have difficulty in many routine tasks—doing laundry, shopping, banking, using public telephones, etc., because of high counters and shelves.
- When taking histories or interviewing short-statured persons, one should ask, "What is your job?" not "Do you work?"
- The early adult years may be ones of identity crisis, despondency, or anger over their perceived imperfect body. They may have difficulty forming close friendships and relationships with those of the opposite sex. Counseling services can be provided.
- Adult short-statured individuals can be helped when difficulties are noticed, but no issue should be made of it.
- Skeletal problems can influence sexual relationships and sex counseling may be needed.
- Pregnancy, particularly in women with achondroplasia, may present problems and cesarean section may be necessary.
- The LPA has an adoption committee that works with agencies to help two short-statured persons adopt short-statured children, particularly if they both have the same type of genetic defect or are afraid of having a normal-sized child.
- Both parents and short-statured children on growth hormone therapy may have unrealistic expectations of results or expect to grow like Jack's beanstalk—overnight They need to know what to realistically expect.

CONCLUSIONS

The occurrence of genetic disease in a family presents many challenges to all members, close and extended. This chapter has discussed some general effects with applications to specific illnesses as examples of what the nurse can do. Families will eventually normalize in regard to their routines to some extent after the initial diagnosis. Successful adaptation should be a goal. Literature from many of the chronic diseases including cancer, specific genetic diseases, and HIV can be helpful to the nurse in finding applications to rarer genetic disorders. See Appendix B for support organizations.

BIBLIOGRAPHY

American Academy of Pediatrics. Committee on Children with Disabilities. (1997). General principles in the care of children and adolescents with genetic disorders and other chronic health conditions. *Pediatrics, 99,* 643–644.

American Academy of Pediatrics. Committee on Genetics. (1995). Health supervision for children with achondroplasia. *Pediatrics, 95,* 443–451.

American Academy of Pediatrics. (2004). Policy statement. The medical home. *Pediatrics, 113,* 1545–1548.

American College of Medical Genetics. (1998, Winter). Statement on genetic testing for cystic fibrosis. *American College of Medical Genetics College Newsletter, 10,* 9.

Austin, J. (1991). Family adaptation to a child's chronic illness. *Annual Review of Nursing Research, 9,* 103–120.

Baine, S., Rosenbaum, P., & King, S. (1995). Chronic childhood illnesses: What aspects of caregiving do parents value? *Child Care, Health and Development, 21,* 291–304.

Baumann, S. L., Dyches, T. T., & Braddick, M. (2005). Being a sibling. *Nursing Science Quarterly, 19,* 51–58.

Bolton-Maggs, P. H. B., & Pasi, K. J. (2003). Haemophilias A and B. *Lancet, 361,* 1801–1809.

Bregman, A. M. (1980). Living with progressive childhood illness: Parental management of neuromuscular disease. *Social Work and Health Care, 5,* 387–408.

Breslau, N., & Prabucki, K. (1987). Siblings of disabled children. Effects of chronic stress in the family. *Archives of General Psychiatry, 44,* 1040–1046.

Bullinger, M., & von Mackensen, S. (2004). Quality of life assessment in haemophilia. *Haemophilia, 10*(Suppl. 1), 9–16.

Centers for Disease Control and Prevention. (1997). Newborn screening for cystic fibrosis: A paradigm for public health genetics policy development. *Morbidity and Mortality Weekly Report, 46, (RR-16),* 1–24.

Centers for Disease Control and Prevention. (2004). Newborn screening for cystic fibrosis. *Morbidity and Mortality Weekly Report, 53*(RR-13), 1–36.

Chamberlain, J. R., Schwarze, U., Wang, P-R., Hirata, R. K., Hankerson, K. D., Pace, J. M., et al. (2004). Gene targeting in stem cells from individuals with osteogenesis imperfecta. *Science, 303,* 1198–1201.

Cohen, F. L. (1994). Research on families and pediatric human immunodeficiency virus disease: A review and needed directions. *Journal of Behavioral and Developmental Pediatrics, 15*(3), S34–S42.

Cornelius, D. A. (1980). *Barrier awareness.* Washington, DC: Regional Rehabilitation Research Institute on Attitudinal, Legal, and Leisure Barriers.

Cuppens, H., & Cassiman, J. J. (2004). CFTR mutations and polymorphisms in male infertility. *International Journal of Andrology, 27,* 251–256.

Dray, X., Kanaan, R., Bienvenu, T., Desmazes-Dufeu, N., Dusser, D., Marteau, P., et al. (2005). Malnutrition in adults with cystic fibrosis. *European Journal of Clinical Nutrition, 59,* 152–154.

Driskell, R. A., & Engelhardt, J. F. (2003). Current status of gene therapy for inherited lung diseases. *Annual Review of Physiology, 65,* 585–612.

Eggers, S., & Zatz, M. (1998). Social adjustment in adult males affected with progressive muscular dystrophy. *American Journal of Medical Genetics (Neuropsychiatric Genetics), 81,* 4–12.

Englebert, R. H., Uiterwaal, C. S., Gerver, W-J., van der Net, J-J., Pruijs, H. E., & Helders, P. J. (2004). Osteogenesis imperfecta in childhood: Impairment and disability. A prospective study with 4-year follow-up. *Archives of Physical Medicine and Rehabilitation, 85,* 772–778.

Fanos, J. H., & Johnson, J. P. (1992). Still living with cystic fibrosis: the well sibling revisited. *Pediatric Pulmonology, 8*(Suppl.), 228–229.

Fanos, J. H., & Wiener, L. (1994). Tomorrow's survivors: Siblings of human immunodeficiency virus-infected children. *Journal of Behavioral and Developmental Pediatrics, 15*(3), S43–S48.

Fear of stigma drives father to seclude son. (1982, October 9). Bloomington, IL: *Pantagraph,* p. 3.

Featherstone H. (1980). *A difference in the family.* New York: Penguin.

Gliedman, J., & Roth, W. (1980). *The unexpected minority.* New York: Harcourt Brace Jovanovich.

Goffman, E. (1965). *Stigma: Notes on the management of spoiled identity.* Englewood Cliffs, NJ: Prentice Hall.

Goldberg, R. T. (1974). Adjustment of children with invisible and visible handicaps: Congenital heart disease and facial burns. *Journal of Counsulting Psychology, 21,* 428–432.

Golden, S. (1975). A new city, a new doctor. *Exceptional Parent, 5*(6), 25–27.

Gollust, S. E., Thompson, R. E., Gooding, H. C., & Biesecker, B. B. (2003). Living with achondroplasia in an average-sized world: An assessment of quality of life. *American Journal of Medicial Genetics, 120A,* 447–458.

Green, S. E. (2004). The impact of stigma on maternal attitudes toward placement of children with disabilities in residential care facilities. *Social Science & Medicine, 59,* 799–812.

Gupta, V. B., O'Connor, K. G., & Quezada-Gomez, C. (2004). Care coordination services in pediatric practices. *Pediatrics, 113,* 1517–1521.

Haga, N. (2004). Management of disabilities associated with achondroplasia. *Journal of Orthopedic Sciences, 9,* 103–107.

Hallum, A. (1995). Disability and the transition to adulthood: Issues for the disabled child, the family, and the pediatrician. *Current Problems in Pediatrics, 25,* 12–50.

Hefferon, T. W., Groman, J. D., Yurk, C. E., & Cutting, G. R. (2004). A variable dinucleotide repeat in the *CFTR* gene contributes to phenotype diversity by forming RNA secondary structures that alter splicing. *Proceedings of the National Academy of Sciences USA, 101,* 3504–3509.

Hilman, B. C., Aitken, M. L., & Constantinescu, M. (1996). Pregnancy in patients with cystic fibrosis. *Clinical Obstetrics and Gynecology, 39,* 70–86.

Hunter, A. G. W., Hecht, J. T., & Scott, C. I., Jr. (1996). Standard weight for height curves in achondroplasia. *American Journal of Medical Genetics, 62,* 255–261.

Knafl, K., Breitmayer, B., Gallo, A., & Zoeller, L. (1996). Family response to childhood chronic illness: Description of management styles. *Journal of Pediatric Nursing, 11,* 315–326.

Krauss, M. W., Seltzer, M. M., Gordon, R., & Friedman, D. H. (1996). Binding ties: The roles of adult siblings of persons with mental retardation. *Mental Retardation, 34,* 83–93.

Kushner, H. S. (1983). *When bad things happen to good people.* New York: Avon.

McKeever, P. T. (1981). Parent-child relationships: Fathering the chronically ill child. *MCN. American Journal of Maternal Child Nursing, 6,* 114–124.

McKeever, P., & Miller, K-K. (2004). Mothering children who have disabilities: A Bourdieusian interpretation of maternal practices. *Social Science & Medicine, 59,* 1177–1191.

McKone, E. F., Emerson, S. S., Edwards, K. L., & Aitken, M. L. (2003). Effect of genotype on phenotype and mortality in cystic fibrosis: A retrospective cohort study. *Lancet, 361,* 1671–1676.

McLean, K. R. (2004). Osteogenesis imperfecta. *Neonatal Network, 23*(2), 7–14.

McPherson, M., Weissman, G., Strickland, B., van Dyck, P. C., Blumberg, S. J., & Newacheck, P. W. (2004). Implementing community-based systems of services for children and youths with special health care needs: How well are we doing? *Pediatrics, 113,* 1538–1544.

Mercer, R. T. (1977). Crisis: A baby is born with a defect. *Nursing, 7*(11), 45–47.

Merlo, C. A., & Boyle, M. P. (2003). Modifier genes in cystic fibrosis lung disease. *Journal of Laboratory and Clinical Laboratory Medicine, 141,* 237–241.

Michaud, L., and the Committee on Children with Disabilities. (2004). Prescribing therapy services for children with motor disabilities. *Pediatrics, 113,* 1836–1838.

Midathada, M. V., Mehta, P. J., Waner, M., & Fink, L. M. (2004). Recombinant factor VIIa in the treatment of bleeding. *American Journal of Clinical Pathology, 121,* 124–137.

Muñoz-Furlong, A. (2003). Daily coping strategies for patients and their families. *Pediatrics, 111,* 1654–1661.

Olshansky, S. (1962). Chronic sorrow: A response to having a mentally defective child. *Social Casework, 43,* 190–193.

Pho, L. T., Zinberg, R. E., Hopkins-Boomer, T. A., Wallenstein, S., & McGovern, M. M. (2004). Attitudes and psychosocial adjustment of unaffected siblings of patients with phenylketonuria. *American Journal of Medical Genetics, 126A,* 156–160.

Prockop, D. J. (2004). Targeting gene therapy for osteogenesis imperfecta. *New England Journal of Medicine, 350,* 2302–2304.

Ratjen, F., & Döring, G. (2003). Cystic fibrosis. *Lancet, 361,* 681–689.

Rauch, F., & Glorieux, F. H. (2004). Osteogenesis imperfecta. *Lancet, 363,* 1377-1385.

Resnick, M. D., Bearman, P. S., Blum, R. W., Bauman, K. E., Harris, K. M., Jones, J., et al. (1997). Protecting adolescents from harm: Findings from the National Longitudinal Study on Adolescent Health. *Journal of the American Medical Association, 278,* 823–832.

Roth, S. P., & Morse, J. S. (Eds.). (1994). *A life-span approach to nursing care for individuals with developmental disabilities.* Baltimore: Paul H. Brookes Publishing.

Saiman, L., & Siegel, J. (2003). Infection control recommendations for patients with cystic fibrosis: Microbiology, important pathogens, and infection control practices to prevent patient-to-patient transmission. *American Journal of Infection Control, 31*(Suppl. 3), S1–S62.

Shapiro, A. D., Paola, J. D., Cohen, A., Pasi, K. J., Heisel, M. A., Blanchette, V. S., et al. (2005). The safety and efficacy of recombinant human blood coagulation factor IX in previously untreated patients with severe or moderately severe hemophilia B. *Blood, 105,* 518-525.

Sloper, P., & Turner, S. (1996). Progress in social-independent functioning of young people with Down's syndrome. *Journal of Intellectual Disability Research, 40*(Part 1), 39–48.

Solnit, A. J., & Stark, M. H. (1961). Mourning and the birth of a defective child. *Psychoanalytic Study of the Child, 16,* 523–537.

Starke, M., Wikland, K. A., & Möller, A. (2002). Parents' experiences of receiving the diagnosis of Turner syndrome: An explorative and retrospective study. *Patient Education and Counseling, 47,* 347–354.

Stoll, C., & Feingold, J. (2004). Do parents and grandparents of patients with achondroplasia have a higher cancer risk? *American Journal of Medical Genetics, 130A,* 165–168.

Stoneman, Z., & Berman, P. W. (Eds.). (1993). *The*

effects of mental retardation, disability, and illness on sibling relationships. Baltimore: Paul H. Brookes Publishing.

Strawhacker, M. T., & Wellendort, J. (2004). Caring for children with cystic fibrosis: A collaborative clinical and school approach. *Journal of School Nursing, 20,* 5–15.

Suskauer, S. J., Cintas, H. L., Marini, J. C., & Gerber, L. H. (2003). Temperament and physical performance in children with osteogenesis imperfecta. *Pediatrics, 111,* e152–e161.

Teitel, J. M., Barnard, D., Israels, S., Lillicrap, D., Poon, M. C., & Sek, J. (2004). Home management of haemophilia. *Haemophilia, 10,* 118–133.

Thorin, E., Yovanoff, P., & Irvin, L. (1996). Dilemmas faced by families during their young adults' transitions to adulthood: A brief report. *Mental Retardation, 34,* 117–120.

Upham, M., & Medoff-Cooper, B. (2005). What are the responses and needs of mothers of infants diagnosed with congenital heart disease? *MCN American Journal of Maternal Child Nursing, 30,* 24–29.

Ward, L. M., Rauch, F., Travers, R., Chabot, G., Azouz, E. M., Lalic, L., et al. (2002). Osteogenesis imperfecta type VII: An autosomal recessive form of brittle bone disease. *Bone, 31,* 12–18.

Welsh, M. J., & Smith, A. E. (1995, December). Cystic fibrosis. *Scientific American, 273*(6), 52–59.

Widmann, R. F., Laplaza, F. J., Bitan, F. D., Brooks, C. E., & Root, L. (2002). Quality of life in osteogenesis imperfecta. *International Orthopaedics, 26,* 3–6.

Wikler, L., Wasow, M., & Hatfield, E. (1981). Chronic sorrow revisited: Parent vs. professional depiction of the adjustment of parents of mentally retarded children. *American Journal of Orthopsychiatry, 5,* 63–70.

Wind, W. M., Schwend, R. M., & Larson, J. (2004). Sports for the physically challenged child. *Journal of the American Academy of Orthopedic Surgery, 12,* 126–137.

Yankaska, J. R., Marshall, B. C., Sufian, B., Simon, R. H., & Rodman, D. (2004). Cystic fibrosis adult care. Consensus conference report. *Chest, 125*(Suppl.), 1S–39S.

9

Assessment of Genetic Disorders

The collection of information from the histories, physical assessment, and observation, with the available laboratory results, allows integration of the important components into a data base that can be used for deciding on and gathering of further needed information, additional tests, counseling, and decision making. For clients who come for genetic services and counseling, it is typical to begin with history taking and interview. However, the initial recognition of the need for genetic evaluation may arise in another setting, when an alert practitioner suspects a genetic problem because of family history, physical findings, observation, discussion with the family, or knowledge of a related problem in a known relative. For example, the nurse may notice that the mother of a child being evaluated because of multiple anomalies has a minor malformation such as clinodactyly. Such an observation in a family being seen at our cleft palate center led to the uncovering of a four-generation history of an autosomal dominant disorder with mild expression in most members but severe expression in the child.

HISTORY

Specific questions to be asked depend on the reason for the evaluation, the client's responses to questions asked, previous information, and on information from observation, laboratory data, or physical assessment. Therefore, it is difficult to prescribe exact questions to be asked when taking the history, except for standard baseline data. Sometimes printed forms that can be filled in by the client or the client's parents are mailed before the counseling visit, then further questions are designed on the basis of these responses. Other counselors prefer to collect history information through interview. This can be time consuming, but it does allow the counselor to observe family interactions that later will help in the formulation of effective approaches in counseling. The incorporation of the history and pedigree into general medical practice could result in the identification of genetic risk factors not otherwise identified. In a report by Frezzo, Rubinstein, Dunham, and Ormond (2003), approximately 20% of the enrolled patients were at an increased risk for disease with a genetic component that was not uncovered by chart review. Family history assessment is a valuable tool that is underused in clinical practice. Further development of risk assessment instruments and algorithms are needed. Some family history instruments may be found on the Web site for the National Coalition for Health Professional Education in Genetics (http://www.nchpeg.org) and the American Medical Association (http://www.ama.org).

Family and Health Histories

The importance of family histories to identify conditions in families that may be inherited and that require further follow-up as well as assisting in risk assessment is enjoying a resurgence. The nature of the problem and the answers to questions asked of the family seeking counseling determines the extent of information needed. Both members of a couple should be present, if possible, in order to get accurate information about both sides of the family. Even if one partner has consulted with the other, the relevant questions may not have been asked. A history should cover at least three generations, including the grandparents, siblings, half-siblings, parents, offspring, aunts, uncles, and cousins. Thus first-, second-, and third-degree relatives should be considered, and more if warranted. Information to be gathered in taking the family history includes (1) the correct legal name of the counselees, including the maiden names of the female members (the same or even very similar names may indicate consanguinity, which the counselor can then pursue); (2) racial, ethnic, and country of origin information (many genetic disorders are more frequent among certain groups); (3) place of birth (certain possible environmental exposures or the suggestion of consanguinity); (4) baseline information, such as address and telephone number; (5) occupation (certain ones suggest the possibility of genotoxic exposures, see Occupational History discussed next, and chapter 14); (6) date of birth, can be used in determining risk for development of disorder. For example, if the brother of an affected person with Huntington disease is the grandfather of the counselee and is 75 years of age and unaffected, the chances of his having the gene mutation are essentially nil, which means that the grandchild will not be at risk; and (7) for each individual in the pedigree, the current and past health status should be ascertained and verified when necessary for the problem. Specific health problems known to have a heritable component should be asked about when ascertaining the status of the family members. Information gathered from the history is used to prepare the pedigree. All information should be confirmed by medical records, laboratory data, photographs, autopsy reports, and other objective methods whenever possible. Other information that should be sought for each individual in the family includes: (1) current and past health status; (2) age and cause of death of deceased individuals; (3) the presence of birth defects, retardation, familial traits, or similarly affected family members; and (4) specific inquiries should be made about offspring, miscarriages, stillbirths, severe infant and childhood illnesses, and deaths for each eligible member, even if the inquiries do not appear related to the problem at hand. For example, two generations of a family seen at our counseling center came because the brother of the counselee had spina bifida. In taking the family history, I noted that there seemed to be a large number of miscarriages and stillbirths in the family. In the end, the investigation revealed the presence of a rare inherited chromosomal translocation in the family of which the young couple had not been aware. Counseling eventually extended to family members in Scotland with the sending of blood specimens for final diagnosis and counseling. This is another reason for detail—the uncovering of an unrecognized problem.

Other questions may depend on the replies and on observation. For example, if the index case has osteogenesis imperfecta type III, then when taking the history the counselor should inquire specifically about blue sclera, fractures, deafness, discolored teeth, and "loose" joints in other family members. Some questions might be age dependent. One might ask whether at a certain age any family member showed a specific symptom that relates to the problem at hand. The age of onset of any health problem should also be recorded. For example, such information is useful in determining whether a person may be at risk for an inherited type of cancer (see chapter 23). The counselor should ask if anyone in the family was a twin; if all the children are the natural children of both parents; and if any prior matings occurred. Further questions are based on answers to initial questions. The family history may be useful in devising health prevention. Men with a family history of prostate cancer should have earlier screenings more often than others, for example. Family history is discussed further in this chapter under Pedigrees.

Reasons for obtaining a negative family history when one child is affected in a family can include any of the following: (1) disorder is a new mutation; (2) artificial insemination; (3) donated ovum; (4) adoption; (5) very small family size; (6) nonpaternity; (7) nonpenetrance in a parent; (8) minimal expression of trait in a relative that was missed; (9) rare trait; (10) lack of knowledge of person giving the history; (11) deliberate withholding of information by informant; (12) failure of the interviewer to ask the critical questions; (13) presence of a chromosome abnormality such as a deletion in the affected person, allowing the expression of a mutant gene present on the other chromosome; (14) germline mosaicism; (15) uniparental disomy; and (16) epigenetic events. Therefore, a negative family history does not rule out a genetic component.

Environmental, Occupational, Social Histories

Environmental exposures can result from the person's primary occupation, second job, residence location, volunteer activities (e.g., firefighting), recreational activities, and hobbies. Information can be gathered in a written form, with follow-up on interview or by interview directly, depending on the information collected or the problem at hand. Information should be gathered for both the client and the other persons living in the household because, for example, the person doing the laundry may be exposed to fibers on the clothing of the worker. Information to be gathered includes name of the employing company, job title, kind of work done, work schedule, and number of a hours worked. The interviewer should ask the kinds of materials that the person is exposed to on the job. It may be more productive to ask about specific materials such as radiation, chemicals, fumes, dust, fibers, tobacco, gasses, temperature extremes, microorganisms, and vibrations. If the person is not sure, then it may be necessary to get data sheets from the employer about specific substances, depending on how critical the information is to the problem at hand.

The same type of information should be ascertained for secondary jobs, schools, hobbies, and so on. Sometimes the job itself can alert the interviewer to possibilities of toxic exposures. The person should be asked about any specific safety measures or protective devices that are used and also about his or her own smoking history. Clients should also be asked about contact with domestic animals, for example, cats, dogs, birds, and about the proximity to any farm animals on the job or at home. If it is not clear what the job or hobby entails, then the interviewer can ask exactly what a person with that job title does or ask them to describe a typical workday, either verbally or in writing. Any affirmative answers about exposure should be followed up to determine the duration of exposure, the frequency, and the last time the person was exposed, whether they were eating, drinking, or smoking at the time, and the concentration of exposure, if possible. Ill effects, such as skin reactions, should be asked about specifically. If a worker has been noncompliant in the use of protective devices, they may not wish to tell the

interviewer about it, and skill may be needed to elicit needed information. The person should be asked how long they have been at this job and what kind of work they did on their last job, if pertinent. Someone who is not currently working should be asked what kind of job they had last, or what kinds of work they have done for the longest period, in order to obtain the needed information. Positive answers to any questions should be followed up. For example, a woman who is considering pregnancy and works in a pet-boarding kennel can be advised on safe methods of disposal of excreta and handling the animals to minimize her own exposure without jeopardizing the job. Information to be obtained regarding the place of residence should include its location, the composition of the household, the source of drinking water or food (especially in rural areas), type of community, the proximity of any factories, knowledge of any chemical spills or waste exposure, noticeable air pollution, the type of insulation and heating, insecticide or pesticide exposure, what is used to clean the home, and other data, as relevant. Social data should be obtained as appropriate. Because exposure to various agents has detrimental effects on reproduction, the client should be specifically asked if he or she or his or her mate have had any problems in this area including difficulty in conception, changes in libido or menses, spontaneous abortions, stillbirths, infertility, intrauterine growth retardation, infants with birth defects or mental retardation, and children with developmental disabilities or childhood malignancies. If a problem appears to be job or environmentally related, then the client should be asked if anyone at work or in his/her neighborhood has had similar problems (see chapter 14). Persons should also be asked about any military service and what it entailed.

Medication and Drug Use

It is helpful to ask the client to bring a list of drugs that have been taken in the time period that is relevant. If the interview is after the birth of an affected child, then this period should include a few months before pregnancy in both the male and female partner and then during the pregnancy in the female. In some cases, the client can bring in his or her medications and containers. Clients should be asked about prescription drugs, over-the-counter medications, home remedies, botanicals, and "folk" medications. Specific medications can be asked about, if they are known to be popular among persons of the client's ethnic group or geographic location. Another method to ascertain drug use is to have a checklist of common types of drugs and ask the client to indicate the ones that which have been used. If responses are negative, then the interviewer can ask about vitamins, mineral supplements, or what the client does for headache, stomach ache, menstrual cramps, and so on. Many clients may omit items that they do not consider to be drugs or medications. There is also reluctance to discuss "street" or illicit drug use. Use of social drugs such as caffeine, alcohol, or cigarette smoking must also be explored. For each drug taken, the dose, frequency of use, reason for use, duration, and approximate dates should be obtained. Facilitation of accurate assessment of drug and medication use can be accomplished by teaching and encouraging clients to keep an accurate list of all those taken. The practitioner should also keep a record of prescription and recommended drugs. Cigarette smoking, alcohol, and drug use in pregnancy and prevention of ill effects from such use are discussed in chapter 13. Questions that can be asked of the client after receiving a positive response to a question about alcohol use, such as "Do you ever drink any wine, beer, or mixed drinks?" are discussed in chapter 13. A nutritional diary that represents what the person has eaten for a week can be used to suggest nutritional concerns. Any past drug or food allergies or reactions should be asked about, both in the client and in other family members. This may elicit a genetic susceptibility or predisposition that can be used to prevent problems in the individual or other relatives as well as to provide information about the current problem (see chapter 18). The client should also be asked whether he or she has ever been told not to take a certain medication or eat a certain food.

Reproductive, Pregnancy, and Birth History

There is some overlap between the reproductive and family history, as all stillbirths, miscarriages, abortions, infant deaths, or offspring should be noted when discussing the family. Information should be obtained for all pregnancies, but one resulting in an affected child should be considered in depth. Such information should include: (1) age at each pregnancy for both parents; (2) weight gain; (3) exposure to radiation, drugs and medications, alcohol, as well as smoking habits for both parents; (4) outcome of each pregnancy including miscarriages, stillbirths, or infant deaths; (5) contraceptive use immediately prior to pregnancy; (6) vaginal bleeding or discharge during the pregnancy; (7) the occurrence of any accidents, illnesses, fevers, rashes, etc. during pregnancy; (8) work, hobbies, or travel of both parents that might have led to any toxic exposures; (9) any medical treatments during pregnancy; (10) nutrition and food habits including pica; (11) type of delivery; (12) presence of blood group incompatibilities; (13) health of all infants previously born, including low birth weight and prematurity; (14) if all offspring had the same parents; (15) medical history of chronic disease, infections, or venereal disease; (16) information about fetal movement, uterine size, details of labor and delivery, that is, complications, the amount (scarce or excess) of amniotic fluid present, length of labor, type of anesthetic and perinatal medications (if any); (17) Apgar score, birth weight, and head circumference; (18) whether the client has had any difficulty becoming pregnant; and (19) whether there is any other relevant information that the client feels should be known. Answers to these questions determine the direction of further questions. One of the reasons for asking this type of information is to try to determine whether a problem such as mental retardation could have been caused by environmental factors during the perinatal period. If this seems a likely possibility, then this must be followed further. This information should be recorded in detail, for example: for radiation, the time of pregnancy during which exposure occurred, part of the body X-rayed, reason for the X-ray, and so on. Confirmation through records would then be necessary for accuracy. Detailed prenatal risk assessment forms have been devised. However, in general, those persons at greatest risk for a poor pregnancy outcome related to birth defects and genetic disorders include increased maternal age (35 years and above); increased paternal age (40 years and above); decreased maternal or paternal age (especially below 15 and 20 years, respectively, which is believed in part to be due to nutritional needs of the young mother vs. the fetus); rapid consecutive pregnancies; poor reproductive history; history of alcohol abuse, drug intake, or smoking; underweight or overweight; poor nutrition; multiple gestation; oligohydramnios; polyhydramnios; previous unfavorable pregnancy outcome; maternal metabolic or genetic disease; maternal-fetal incompatibility; previous infant weighing 10 pounds or over or with growth retardation; maternal chronic disease, especially seizure disorders; infectious or sexually transmitted disease in pregnancy; as well as those factors listed as indications for prenatal diagnosis (see chapter 12) and those in the prevention of mental retardation (see chapter 20).

If the woman is currently pregnant, then the date of the last menstrual period and the expected date of delivery should be obtained. Large prenatal or prepregnancy clinics may have little time to take detailed histories or conduct in-depth interviews with every client. Various clinics have attempted to devise a short questionnaire that acts as a screening device for potential genetic problems for the pregnancy. When clients answer affirmatively to any of the specific questions, then the chart is flagged for an in-depth interview with a geneticist, counselor, or nurse. The interview may need to be immediate if the need for prenatal diagnosis appears possible, or else it can be scheduled at the next prenatal visit. Information needing follow-up that can be ascertained on such screening tools are maternal age of 35 or over; paternal age of 40 or over; specific ethnic groups with higher risk of known detectable disorders; previous stillbirth, infant death, two or more miscarriages; the birth of a previous child or member of the family who has a birth defect or genetic disorder; previous prenatal diagnosis; drug or alcohol use; maternal disease such as diabetes mellitus or maternal phenylketonuria; family history of retardation or anemia; or any particular problem or concern that the mother identifies. These questionnaires are usually set up in a simple yes/no format using simple language. They may need to be in the native language of the client.

Women who are determined to be at high risk for unfavorable pregnancy outcome may be eligible for prenatal diagnosis (see chapter 12). If this is not feasible or the mother elects to continue the pregnancy after learning that the fetus is affected,

arrangements can be made for the best possible care in a hospital center that is equipped with facilities for the high-risk mother and infant.

Not infrequently, the taking of a pregnancy history follows the birth of a child with a defect of some type or a stillbirth. Thus retrospective information about the pregnancy is apt to be influenced not only by the same factors responsible for obtaining a negative family history, but also by feelings of guilt (real or imagined) or any other emotions surrounding this type of event (see chapter 8).

PEDIGREES

A pedigree is essentially a pictorial representation or diagram of the family history. By clearly laying out the information obtained from the family histories it can (1) allow the geneticist to visualize relationships of affected individuals to the family at-hand seeking counseling; (2) pinpoint any vital persons who should be examined or tested; (3) elucidate the pattern of inheritance in a specific family; (4) allow for various types of complex pedigree analysis and linkage studies if needed and applicable; (5) allow other professionals working with the family to quickly see what information has been collected on which family members, thus saving unnecessary repetition and facilitating the collection of further data; (6) facilitate the brief notation of other data relevant to effective counseling, such as family interactions.

Modifications of the pedigree as "genograms" are sometimes used in mental health settings for diagraming family systems, interactions, and events with significant emotional impact. The widespread use of pedigrees requires the nurse to understand their meaning and to be able to construct one from a family history. With experience, the counselor can construct a pedigree directly while interviewing the family, thereby saving time. Computer programs specifically for pedigree construction are available. Symbols commonly used in pedigree construction are illustrated in Figure 9.1. There may be some variation in the use of some symbols because there is no formal standard, although one has been proposed, and American and European systems differ somewhat. Any use of symbols that deviate from those in common use should be spelled out in a key placed at the top of

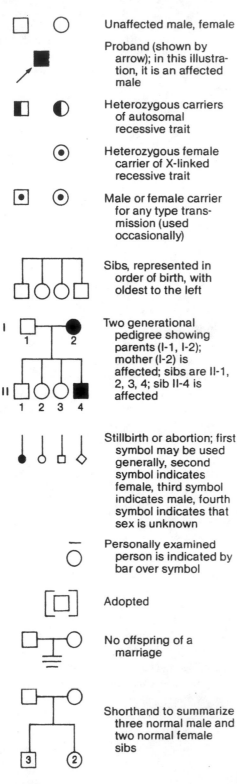

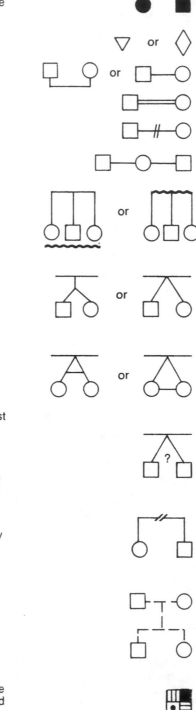

□ ○ Unaffected male, female

Proband (shown by arrow); in this illustration, it is an affected male

Heterozygous carriers of autosomal recessive trait

Heterozygous female carrier of X-linked recessive trait

Male or female carrier for any type transmission (used occasionally)

Sibs, represented in order of birth, with oldest to the left

Two generational pedigree showing parents (I-1, I-2); mother (I-2) is affected; sibs are II-1, 2, 3, 4; sib II-4 is affected

Stillbirth or abortion; first symbol may be used generally, second symbol indicates female, third symbol indicates male, fourth symbol indicates that sex is unknown

Personally examined person is indicated by bar over symbol

Adopted

No offspring of a marriage

Shorthand to summarize three normal male and two normal female sibs

Affected female, affected male

Sex unknown or unspecified

Mating or marriage

Consanguinous mating or marriage

Divorce

Multiple marriage (as shown, woman has had two husbands)

Sibs, birth order unknown

Twins, dizygotic (male and female illustrated)

Twins, monozygotic (females illustrated)

Twins, zygosity unknown (males illustrated)

Shorthand for half-sibs

Illegitimate offspring indicated by dashed line

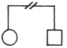

Ways to show four different manifestations of a disorder that would then be explained in an accompanying key

FIGURE 9.1   Commonly used pedigree symbols.

the pedigree. The family names and/or initials should be on the pedigree along with the date, the person who is giving the family history, the name and title of the pedigree recorder, the date of the pedigree, and dates for any subsequent additions. Some "rules" for pedigree construction and interpretation are as follows:

1. Pedigree construction usually begins in the middle of the sheet of paper to allow enough room.
2. Males are represented by a square and females by a circle (if the person is affected with the disorder in question, the symbol is shaded in).
3. An arrow, sometimes with a "P" at the shaft end, represents the proband or propositus, and the pedigree drawing usually begins with this person (if the counselee is different, sometimes a "C" is placed under that person's symbol).
4. For a mating or marriage, a horizontal line is drawn between a square and a circle (sometimes a diagonal line is used for convenience; traditionally, males in a couple are drawn on the left).
5. Offspring are suspended vertically from the mating line and are drawn in order of birth.
6. Generations are symbolized by Roman numerals.
7. The order of birth of sibs within a family is indicated by the use of Arabic numbers (the sibship line is sometimes drawn more thickly than the mating line; if birth order is unknown, a wavy line is used).
8. The name of each person (maiden names in cases of married women) and their date of birth should be included.
9. In general, to be adequate, a pedigree should include at least the parents, offspring, siblings, aunts, uncles, grandparents, and first cousins of the person seeking counseling (accurate data are not always available for each of these and may need to be added after the counselee gets further information).
10. Pedigrees may indicate unmentioned consanguinity or suggest it because of the occurrence of the same name on both sides of the family or because of the same place of birth of an ancestor that is revealed by the history or pedigree.
11. When the rough pedigree is redrawn, a mate's family history may be omitted if it adds nothing to the elucidation of the family study, but it should be retained in the file.
12. The pedigree should be dated and signed with the name, credentials, and position of the person drawing it.
13. Pedigrees can be shortened by grouping large numbers of similar-sexed normal children in one symbol.
14. Causes of death or health problems should be noted.
15. Adoptions are shown by brackets.
16. For assisted reproduction, the donor (D) is drawn to the right of the female partner with a diagonal line to the pregnancy symbol or child. For a surrogate, a straight line is suggested to the pregnancy symbol and a diagonal line follows from the couple. Other variants exist (see Bennett et al., 1995).
17. For evaluation, both clinical and laboratory data may be listed as an E, E_1, E_2, etc. to denote each individual evaluation which is defined in the key. A "?" is used if results are not documented or available and an asterisk is used next to the pedigree symbol to denote a documented evaluation. If the exam is negative, a "–" sign is used, a "+" sign is used for a positive examination, and if uninformative, a "u" is used.

As part of the examination of the pedigree, one should look for consanguinity, male-to-male transmission, female-to-male transmission, the ratio of male to female sibs, whether males and females are affected in equal numbers, the birth order of affected persons, and other characteristics of the patterns of inheritance as discussed in chapter 4. Sometimes the mode of inheritance cannot be determined from the history and pedigree because of small family sizes or because there are no instances of certain types of transmission (there may not be the presence of a critical transmission). Distinctions between autosomal dominant and X-linked dominant inheritance may be difficult to make if there is no opportunity to observe critical transmissions (all daughters of affected males and none of his sons normally inherit his X chromosome) (see inheritance patterns in chapter 4). Sample pedigrees for different modes of inheritance are shown in Figure 9.2.

CLINICAL, DEVELOPMENTAL, AND PHYSICAL ASSESSMENT

Data from the history can suggest specific areas for comprehensive physical assessment. Also, certain findings should suggest the possibility of a genetic component and the need for further evaluation. Clinical clues that suggest the need for further evaluation and testing also depend on the age of the person. A newborn girl who has lymphedema should have a chromosome analysis because of the possibility of Turner syndrome (see chapter 5); however, the lymphedema rapidly disappears, and the next time of suspicion may be when menstruation and the development of secondary sex characteristics are delayed. Likewise, Wilson disease should be considered in the child or adolescent who experiences acute liver failure. The appearance of certain features may be considered normal at a certain age, and deviant at another. Wrinkled skin in a 65-year-old is unremarkable. In a one-year-old infant, it might suggest the possibility of progeria. An early age of onset of an adult-type tumor or a common disease such as coronary heart disease should suggest the possibility of a strong genetic influence in this family and should be investigated. The cry of the newborn may reflect nervous system pathology. Certain odors are associated with specific biochemical abnormalities (see chapter 6), especially in the infant or child. Other signs and symptoms of metabolic errors in infants are discussed in chapter 6.

Between 13% and about 40% of otherwise normal newborns will have one minor anomaly; less than 1% will have two. Most newborns with three or more may not be normal. The occurrence of two, and especially, three minor malformations in an otherwise normal infant should alert the practitioner to search carefully for one or more major defects and consider chromosome studies (see chapter 5). In the early study by Marden, Smith, and McDonald (1964), of the infants with two or more minor defects, 90% had one or more major ones. Other studies, for example by Méhes,

Mestyan, Knoch, and Vinceller (1973) and Leppig, Werler, Cann, Cook, and Holmes (1987), showed the same association but to a much lesser degree. Sometimes the major anomalies were not visible (e.g., congenital heart disease) or not yet apparent (e.g., mental retardation). In active surveillance of malformations in newborns in Mainz, Germany from 1990 to 1998, major malformations and minor errors of morphogenesis were found to be 6.9% and 35.8% respectively. Risk factors significantly associated with malformations were: parents or siblings with malformations, parental consanguinity, more than three minor errors of morphogenesis in the proband, maternal diabetes mellitus, and using antiallergic drugs during the first trimester (Queisser-Luft, Stolz, Wiesel, & Schaefer, 2002). Chromosome studies also should be initiated as discussed in chapter 5. Computerized and Internet data bases, such as POSSUM, and dysmorphology books with photos as well as photo libraries are available to assist in identification of syndromes.

Physical examinations of children and adolescents can provide an opportunity for detection of those disorders making their appearance around puberty and even provide a forum for preconceptual counseling for adolescent girls. For girls or women with significant menorrhagia, it is recommended that they be screened for von Willebrand disease (a hereditary bleeding disorder characterized by deficiency of von Willebrand factor needed for optimum platelet adhesiveness), since about one-third of adolescent girls presenting with menorrhagia at menarche were found to have this. It is important to screen before initiation of oral contraceptive therapy since this may mask the diagnosis. Sometimes these examinations take place in a "sports physical" setting, where screening is rushed and there is pressure to approve a child for sports. It is important, however, to assess the child for such conditions as Marfan syndrome (see chapter 6), and for other potential causes of genetically based potential impairment.

The objective of this section is to discuss those measures and observations that are of particular importance in genetic disorders, rather than physical assessment in general.

Measurements

Measurements used in the detection or confirmation of genetic disorders and congenital anomalies

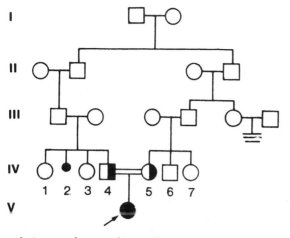

Autosomal recessive pedigree of T family
illustrating consanguinity; the diagnosis
indicates that the parents, IV-4 and IV-5,
are obligate heterozygotes

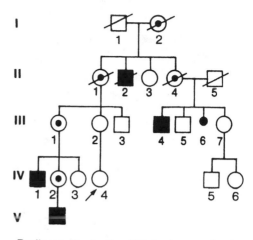

Pedigree illustrating X-linked recessive inheritance; the status of III-2 and IV-4 are
not yet know and cannot be determined
from the pedigree, although IV-2 must be a
carrier because both her brother and son
are affected, and retrospectively, this
marks III-1 and II-1 as carriers.

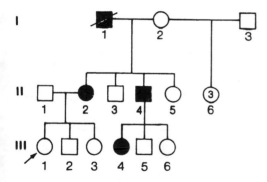

Pedigree illustrating autosomal dominant
inheritance in Huntington disease; the
age of III-1 must be taken into account
when risk is determined

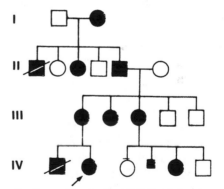

Pedigree illustrating X-linked dominant
inheritance; note that all daughters of the
affected father are affected, and no sons
of the affected father are affected; all
affected males have affected mothers

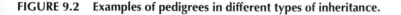

FIGURE 9.2   Examples of pedigrees in different types of inheritance.

include many that are too complicated or too time consuming to be practical in the routine examination of the normal infant and child, but that are useful when an abnormality is suspected. The extent to which the nurse uses such measurements depends on his or her area of practice. For the normal infant and child, height, weight, and head cir-

cumference is usual. Other measurements, such as inter-inner canthal distance, inter-outer canthal distance, interpupillary distances, upper and lower body segment ratios (U/L), arm span, chest circumference, internipple distance, ear measurements, philtrum measures, palpebral fissure slant, and various craniofacial measures are only done

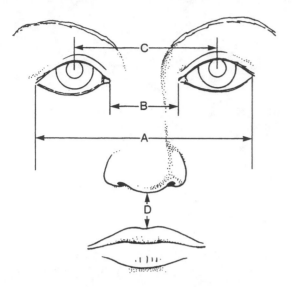

FIGURE 9.3   Identification of facial parameters used in measurement. *A* = Outer canthal distance. *B* = Inner canthal distance. *C* = Inter pupillary distance. *D* = Philtrum length.

(After Feingold, M., Bossert, W. B.: Normal values for selected physical parameters. An aid to syndrome delineation. Bergsma, D. (Ed.). White Plains, The National Foundation—March of Dimes, BD: OAS X(13): 1974). Used with permission.

when suspicion so dictates. See Figure 9.3 for illustration of what is measured for some of the above. Measurements should also be done of a stillborn infant, including foot length, crown-rump, crown-heel and weight. Parameters and directions for many general and specialized measurements can be found in the references by Feingold and Bossert (1974), Jones (1997), Salinas (1980), Ward, Jamison, and Allanson (2000), and Gorlin, Cohen, and Hennekam (2001). Craniofacial examinations today are often evaluated by cephalometrics, three-dimensional craniofacial surface imaging from CT scans, magnetic resonance imaging, and computer-driven techniques. Serial photographs using digital and other technology across age are also used.

Usually the practitioner begins with the height and weight. The same technique should always be used, as well as the same standardized tables. Measurements should ideally be made at the same time of day. One unusual result should not cause immediate concern, but serial measurements should be kept so that growth velocity can be examined.

Growth velocity is greatest in infants, falling until puberty when a growth spurt occurs. A growth rate of 5 cm per year has been recommended as the lower limit of normal. Children below the 3rd percentile in height who are growing at a rate below 5 cm per year require further investigation. When using charts for the comparison of a given child's measurements to standardized tables, it is important to remember that they must be derived from data obtained from the same ethnic group and country and not be based on outdated standards. Parental stature and measurements, the child's birth weight, and maturity should always be considered when evaluating unusual results. Isolated measurements should not be completely relied on, but rather the overall rate and pattern should be considered. Various studies have demonstrated that correlation still persists between birth weight and height and current parameters even in late adolescence and early adulthood. If it appears that height is abnormal, then the ratio of upper body segment to lower body segment, limb lengths, and the arm span should be determined to ascertain whether disproportionate growth is present and, if so, of what type. It is important for diagnosis, treatment, and counseling to determine the type of growth disorder. Many chromosome and metabolic disorders have failure to thrive or altered growth as a component. These merit full investigation.

Other growth disorders may be noted. Macrosomia may be seen in the offspring of diabetic mothers. Unusual obesity, associated with hypotonia, and later hypogonadism, is a feature of Prader-Willi syndrome (see chapter 4). Failure to thrive may be organic or nonorganic, and the cause should be determined. The failure of needed substances to be utilized results in failure to thrive in many inherited biochemical disorders. It is important to inquire about feeding practices, gastrointestinal symptoms, and food intolerance. Fatty, foul-smelling stools can indicate cystic fibrosis; whereas bulky, foul stools after weaning from breast milk may indicate acrodermatitis enteropathica. Delayed or precocious puberty can be assessed by means of criteria for pubertal stage attainment. Hypogonadism and delayed puberty are frequent components of many genetic disorders and must always be fully investigated.

Head size depends in part on, and reflects, the growth of the brain, and therefore relates to ultimate intelligence. In measuring head circumference, an accurate, nonstretchable tape measure should be used. The child's head must be held still, and the tape is placed over the most prominent part of the occiput, posteriorly, and just above the supraorbital ridges, or eyebrows, anteriorly. The tape is held snugly and the measurement is read over the forehead. At birth, the average value is about 35 cm, with a variation of 1.2 cm above or below in over half of normal full-term infants. There is about a 5 cm increase in the next 4 months, and an increase of 5 more cm by 1 year of age. Head size should always be evaluated within the context of other factors such as body size, weight, and chest circumference. These should approximate each other in percentile position. For example, an otherwise very small child whose head circumference is above the 50th percentile could actually have hydrocephalus. Variation in size can be caused by familial characteristics and racial or ethnic group, as well as from other causes. A large head size can result from hydrocephalus, Tay-Sachs disease, a tumor, megaloencephaly, or a large-sized infant. A small head size (microcephaly) can result from idiopathic causes, inadequate brain growth, craniostenosis, or be due to a small-sized infant. Any deviation in size can be reassessed in a short period of time by serial measurements. The earlier in development that brain growth deficiency occurs, the greater the potential for developmental delay and usually the more marked the microcephaly. Because microcephaly is a relatively common finding after intrauterine infection, this would alert the clinician to particularly look for other common symptoms or signs of congenital infection, such as chorioretinitis.

Appraisal and Assessment

One should always begin with a general appraisal and observation before conducting a systematic assessment. The photographing of any unusual features provides a permanent record, allows for consultation, and permits later study. Attention should be paid to any concerns of the parents about "slow" development. Attention should also be paid to the child who is so quiet that his or her parents "hardly know they have a baby." Children with xeroderma pigmentosa often cry on sun exposure, an event that occurs before any other signs

and symptoms. Parents' recall of developmental milestones, except for walking, is generally thought to be unreliable. Therefore, it may be a good idea for hospitals or offices to give the parents a book in which to record important developmental milestones. Many developmental screening tools and techniques are available for such assessment. Among the most commonly used are the Denver Developmental Screening Test, the Brazelton Neonatal Behavioral Assessment Scale, the Bayley Scales of Infant Development, the Developmental Profile, and the Kansas Infant Developmental Scale (KIDS) test. There are others that are more specialized. During assessment, particular attention should be paid to the head and face area, the skin, and the limbs, because the majority of deviant development has some reflection in these areas. Clinical findings seen in some genetic disorders are organized by region in Table 9.1. This is not an all-inclusive list.

Indications suggesting specific disorders (e.g., unusual infections in childhood in immune disorders), and those that should suggest the need for further evaluation, are given throughout the book and at the end of this chapter. The frequency of syndrome association in blindness, deafness, cleft lip/palate, failure to thrive, and mental retardation preclude their discussion here, but mandates their full evaluation.

Head, Neck, and Face

In looking at the head and face, the shape should be observed. Variation can be due to normal factors or pathology. Mild asymmetry may be present in the newborn because of intrauterine factors and birth. In microcephaly, a tapering is noted from the forehead to the vertex. Premature closure of the cranial sutures (craniostenosis) can result in abnormal shape if there is compensatory growth toward sutures that remain open. Palpating a bony ridge suggests premature closure. This is serious either alone or as part of a syndrome. Delayed closure of the fontanels can result from hydrocephalus or from hypothyroidism, whereas premature closure might result from microcephaly, craniostenosis, or hyperthyroidism. A third fontanel located between the anterior and posterior is found in 5% to 15% of normal infants, but according to the classic by Goodman and Gorlin (1977), it is found in about 60% of infants with Down syndrome and

TABLE 9.1   Selected Minor/Moderate Clinical Findings Suggesting Genetic Disorders*

Location and finding	Examples of genetic disorders/syndromes in which found
Head, neck, face	
Macroglossia	Beckwith-Wiedemann syndrome
Lip pits	Van der Woude syndrome
Smooth tongue	Familial dysautonomia
"Tongue thrusting"	Familial dysautonomia
Short philtrum	DiGeorge syndrome, orofaciodigital syndrome
Smooth philtrum	Fetal alcohol syndrome
Long philtrum	Robinow syndrome
Micrognathia	Cornelia de Lange syndrome, Robin sequence
Broad nose	Fetal hydantoin syndrome
Low nasal bridge	Achondroplasia, Down syndrome, Kniest dysplasia
Prominent nose	Rubenstein-Taybi syndrome, trichorhinophalangeal syndrome
Malar hypoplasia	Bloom syndrome
Low-set ears	Potter syndrome
Facial asymmetry	Klippel-Feil syndrome
Frontal bossing	Achondroplasia
Coarse facies	Mucopolysaccharide disorders
Lip pigmentation	Peutz-Jeghers syndrome
Teeth	
Natal teeth	Ellis-van Creveld syndrome, Hallermann-Strieff syndrome
Large teeth	47,XYY
Conical teeth	Ellis-van Creveld syndrome
Hyperdontia (supernumerary)	Gardner syndrome, orofaciodigital syndrome
Reddish or purple teeth	Some porphyrias
Opalescent, brownish teeth	Osteogenesis imperfecta (some types)
Hypodontia	Hypohydrotic ectodermal dysplasia
Eyes, ocular region	
Nystagmus	Chediak-Higashi syndrome, albinism
Cataract (infancy)	Galactosemia
Cherry-red spot (macula)	Tay-Sachs disease (infantile)
Setting sun sign	Hydrocephalus
Blue sclera	Osteogenesis imperfecta, Roberts syndrome
Aniridia	Wilms tumor
Glaucoma	Lowe syndrome
Retinal detachment	Ehlers-Danlos syndrome, Stickler syndrome
Hypertelorism	Aarskog syndrome
Hypotelorism	Trisomy 13
Ptosis	Aarskog syndrome, Smith-Lemli-Opitz syndrome, Steinert myotonic dystrophy
Up-slanted palpebral fissure	Down syndrome, Pfeiffer syndrome
Down-slanted palpebral fissure	Aarskog syndrome, Coffin-Lowry syndrome
Short palpebral fissure	Fetal alcohol syndrome
Night blindness	Refsum syndrome
Epicanthal folds	Down syndrome
Kayser-Fleischer ring	Wilson disease
Iris coloboma	Cat-eye syndrome
Arcus corneae (child)	Familial hypercholesterolemia IIA
Synophrys	Cornelia de Lange syndrome
Lens dislocation	Marfan syndrome
Limbs, hands, feet, trunk	
Arachnodactyly	Marfan syndrome, homocystinuria
Polydactyly	Ellis-van Creveld syndrome, trisomy 13
Broad thumb/toe	Rubenstein-Taybi syndrome
Syndactyly	Apert syndrome, Poland syndrome
Joint hyperextensibility	Marfan syndrome, Ehlers-Danlos syndrome
Asymmetric shortening	Conradi-Hunermann syndrome
Clenched hand	Trisomy 13

TABLE 9.1   *(Continued)*

Location and finding	Examples of genetic disorders/syndromes in which found
Clinodactyly	Down syndrome, Silver Russell syndrome
Brachydactyly	Turner syndrome, Smith-Magenis syndrome
Crusted lesions on fingertips	Richner-Hanhart syndrome
Broad, shieldlike chest	Turner syndrome
Pectus excavatum	Marfan syndrome, homocystinuria
Skin, hair, nails	
Hirsutism	Cornelia de Lange syndrome, leprechaunism, Hurler syndrome
Widow's peak	Optiz syndrome
Upswept, crewlike hair	Microcephaly
Sparse hair	Ellis-van Creveld syndrome, Menkes syndrome
White streak	Waardenburg syndrome
White hair	Albinism
Low hairline	Turner syndrome, Noonan syndrome
Stubby, wiry, coarse hair	Menkes syndrome
Xanthomas	Hypercholesterolemia IIa
Café-au-lait spots	Neurofibromatosis I
Photosensitivity	Bloom syndrome, the porphyrias, xeroderma pigmentosum
Hyperelastic skin	Ehlers-Danlos syndrome
Loose skin	Cutis laxa, Ehlers-Danlos syndrome
Brownish yellow skin	Gaucher disease (adult)
Shagreen patch	Tuberous sclerosis
Leaf-shaped white macules	Tuberous sclerosis
"Marble swirls"	Incontinentia pigmenti
Large pores (orange-peel)	Conradi-Hunermann syndrome
Thick skin	Hurler syndrome
Telangiectasia	Ataxia-telangiectasia
Port wine hemangioma	Sturge-Weber syndrome, von Hippel-Lindau disease
Nail hypoplasia	Ellis-van Creveld syndrome
Transverse crease	Down syndrome, Seckel syndrome
Blisters	Epidermolysis bullosa
Growth disorders	
Macrosomia	Beckwith-Wiedemann syndrome
Obesity	Prader-Willi syndrome, Laurence-Moon syndrome
Cry (infant)	
Hoarse, weak	Farber disease
Catlike, mewing	Cri-du-chat syndrome (5p-)
Low-pitched, growling	Cornelia de Lange syndrome
Genitalia	
Hypogonadism	Klinefelter syndrome, Prader-Willi syndrome
Pigmented areas on penis	Bannayan-Riley-Ruvalcaba syndrome
Cryptorchidism	Aarskog syndrome, Rubinstein-Taybi syndrome, Noonan syndrome
Macro-orchidism	Fragile X syndrome
Ambiguous genitalia	Congenital adrenal hyperplasia
Bifid scrotum	Fryns syndrome
Labia majora hypoplasia	Prader-Willi syndrome, 18q- syndrome
Double vagina	18q- syndrome
Micropenis	Klinefelter syndrome, 48,XXXY syndrome
Enlarged clitoris	Fraser syndrome
Other	
Omphalocele	Beckwith-Wiedemann syndrome
Hernia	Hurler syndrome, Beckwith-Wiedemann syndrome
Seizures	Menkes syndrome, Sturge-Weber syndrome
Single umbilical artery	Sirenomelia, VATER association
Photophobia	Acrodermatitis enteropathica, Richner-Hanhart syndrome

*Reflexes are not included.

85% of those with congenital rubella syndrome. The finding of a large fontanel for age without increased intracranial pressure can be found in many skeletal disorders such as achondroplasia, Apert syndrome, osteogenesis imperfecta, various chromosome abnormalities, progeria, and congenital rubella syndrome.

Various facies have been described in syndromes. Coarse facies develop in most of the mucopolysaccharide disorders because of the deposition of mucopolysaccharide in the tissue. These are not seen until late infancy or early childhood when enough accumulation occurs. Not too long ago, the expression "funny-looking kid" was used to describe patients with unidentified dysmorphic features. This is not acceptable terminology; any dysmorphic features should be defined by measurement and photographs should be taken if acceptable to the counselee. Identification using online databases and publications on syndromes can aid in diagnosis. Observation of the nose and lips should be made. A saddle nose may be a minor variant that is not an anomaly, but a wide nasal bridge can be seen with hypertelorism and a low nasal bridge with such disorders as achondroplasia. The philtrum is the vertical groove from the columnella of the nose to the carmine border of the upper lip. It is smooth in patients with fetal alcohol syndrome. Cleft lip and palate may occur as single defects or as part of a syndrome (see chapter 7). A bifid uvula may be dismissed by the practitioner, but it is important because of its frequent association with submucous cleft palate. The teeth provide another accessible location for examination, as many genetic disorders are reflected here. Hypodontia is found in 2% to 9% of normal persons (excluding third molars) and also in Witkop syndrome, focal dermal hypoplasia, Rieger syndrome, and Ellis van Creveld syndrome. Hyperdontia is found in 0.1% to 3.6% of normal persons and neonatal teeth in less than 1 in 2,000.

Eyes and Ocular Region

Congenital cataract is the most frequent cause of remedial childhood blindness. To prevent the effects of visual deprivation, it is important to perform surgery by the time the infant is 2 months of age. Both unilateral and bilateral cataracts may be manifested by the appearance of a milky, hazy, or white pupil with absence of the red reflex when examined with the ophthalmoscope from about a foot away. Unilateral cataracts may also be noticed because one eye may appear larger than the other, the eye may just "not look right," or a unilateral squint may be present. In bilateral cataracts, parents may report that the infant "does not seem to look at them," or by 3 months of age, nystagmus and squinting may be seen. Prompt referral to an ophthalmologist is essential. Cataracts may be inherited, sporadic, part of a syndrome, or a single anomaly. They are often the first abnormality noticed in congenital rubella and some biochemical errors. Different colored (heterochromic) irises are often seen in Waardenburg syndrome type I, but some families have isochromic pale blue eyes instead. Brushfield spots (see chapter 5) are speckled areas in the iris that are seen in about 20% of normal children, especially those with very clear eyes, and about 50% of those with Down syndrome. Hypertelorism represents an actual increase in distance between the orbits. Sometimes this distance appears wide because of a low nasal bridge, increased space between the two inner corners of the eye (telecanthus), or because of short palpebral fissures. The palpebral fissure is from the inner to the outer corner of the eye. It is normally horizontal. Up-slanting palpebral fissures are found in about 4% of normal individuals. The distance between the inner corners of both eyes (inter-inner canthal distance) is usually the same as the distance from the inner to the outer corner of one eye. Parry (1981) defines as an anomaly, widely spaced eyes with an inter-inner canthal distance above 3 cm between 1 year of age and 2 years of age and above 3.5 cm between 2 years of age and 10 years of age. Epicanthial folds can be present in about one third of all newborns, but it is unusual in a normal Caucasian child after age 10 years. It is often present in children with Down syndrome. Curly, long eyelashes and thick eyebrows that meet in the middle (synophrys) are frequently found in the Brachmann de Lange syndrome. Abnormal eyebrow patterns may be seen in Waardenburg syndrome type I.

Ears

Much variation exists in the external ear. It should be looked at for symmetry, position, type of insertion, and size. Low-set ears is a descriptor commonly used. It can be easy for ears to appear to be low set because of other features such as a short or extended neck, tilted ear, small chin, or high cranial vault, any of which can be present alone or in conjunction with another syndrome. Various researchers have demonstrated that subjective impressions may be due to an optical illusion. Assessment of the position of the ear should ultimately be done by objective measurements. One assessment that is easy to do clinically is to consider that a line (or piece of straight-edged paper) drawn from the lateral corner of the eye normally should intersect the upper point of attachment of the external ear to the head. Another measure is to consider that a line from the midpoint of the eyebrow should approximate the upper edge of the external ear, and a line from the base of the columnella of the nose should approximate the lower insertion of the external ear.

Various degrees of malformation of the ear occur. Besides cosmetic considerations, their importance lies in their association with hidden middle ear anomalies, resulting in deafness, and their association with renal disease (e.g., Potter syndrome), which was as high as 22.5% in Bergstrom's (1980) series. Infants or children (even as young as 1 week old) with even a minor ear malformation should have their hearing tested and renal status evaluated. Early detection of hearing problems may allow either surgical correction or prevention of the development of speech, language, and behavior problems by prompt therapy. Very minor malformations (e.g., preauricular pits or ear tags) may be important in syndrome recognition.

Those infants and children who will be at high risk for hearing impairment, and who should be very carefully assessed, include the following: (1) family history of hearing loss in early childhood, particularly in parent or sibling; (2) maternal illness during pregnancy, especially rubella, cytomegalovirus; (3) known prenatal exposure to a drug known to be ototoxic; (4) prematurity; (5) neonatal icterus (severe); (6) presence of certain congenital anomalies, especially ear malformations as discussed, cleft lip, cleft palate, head or neck malformations; (7) anoxia at birth; (8) neurologic abnormalities, including neonatal seizures; (9) parental reports of failure to respond appropriately to sounds; (10) delayed or poor speech; and (11)

those having chronic ear infections. Parents are most likely to be the ones who first suspect hearing loss, and their concerns should be followed up.

Skin, Hair, and Nails

The skin should be inspected for pigmentation, lesions, texture, and hair distribution. Many skin lesions are genetic in origin or are a reflection of other genetic disorders, as the skin is derived from all three embryological layers. It is estimated that 7% of newborns have a skin lesion at birth. A normal variant is the Mongolian spot, which is present in 90% of infants of Black and Asian origin and also occurs frequently in those of Mediterranean origin. The Mongolian spot is a blue or bluish-gray nevus that usually occurs on the back or buttocks. Although it occasionally persists into adulthood, it usually disappears in early childhood. Its importance lies in the fact that it has been mistaken as a sign of child abuse when seen in the emergency room, and it should be realized that this is a benign normal variation. Another benign lesion is the "stork bite" or salmon patch, which is a capillary hemangioma on the eyelids, the forehead, or the back of neck that usually fades within a few months. Port wine stains are intradermal capillary hemangiomas that discolor the skin and range from faint pink to deep purple. They are permanent unless surgically removed. Certain cosmetic products are available to conceal them. They may be associated with deeper hemangiomas such as those of the nervous system in Sturge-Weber syndrome. The finding of depigmented spots that are present at birth in 90% of infants with tuberous sclerosis means that the practitioner should examine the newborn carefully. An ultraviolet light may be necessary to do this in infants with light skin. A butterfly rash that may appear later in childhood is also seen in Bloom disease (see chapter 23) and lupus erythematosus. Sometimes the dysfunction of other systems is not seen until later in life.

Abnormal hair patterning and development may reflect abnormal brain development or other developmental deviation. Variations such as double whorls may be familial in some cases and not abnormal. A widow's peak may be a normal variant or may suggest hypertelorism and deviant migration of embryonic structures. Hair pigmentation may be altered in a variety of syndromes. Hair is lighter than normal for the particular family in children with phenylketonuria. A patch of white hair may indicate Waardenburg syndrome and should prompt a hearing test. Facial and body hirsutism may be due to ethnic and racial variation, occurring normally in Native Americans, Latinos, and persons of Mediterranean background. It also may occur in syndromes such as Brachmann de Lange syndrome. Photosensitivity is frequent in such diverse disorders as albinism, porphyria (chapter 18), and chromosomal instability syndromes (chapter 23). Abnormalities of hair texture, such as the "steel wool type" hair found in Menkes disease (a defect in copper metabolism with retardation), may represent pathology or again be a family variant (e.g., woolly hair, dominantly inherited in certain Caucasian families). The nails also may reflect genetic disorders. Hypoplastic nails may be seen in nail-patella syndrome and the ectodermal dysplasias. They should alert one to look further.

Limbs, Hands, Feet, Skeleton, and Trunk

The hands also may reflect a variety of single malformations or more complex disorders. Polydactyly is one of the more common single malformations, especially in Blacks, but should alert the practitioner to rule out other anomalies. Clinodactyly, or the incurving of the fifth digit, is a variation that is often a component of syndromes that might be missed, but it can also be a general population variation. Syndactyly denotes webbing of the digits. In some cases, hand positioning may give a clue to other problems or help in diagnosis. Typical of this is the overlapping hand position seen in trisomy 13, and "hitchhikers thumb" seen in Marfan syndrome. Palmar crease variation, such as the transverse crease, may be found in about 5% to 10% of normal infants but is more frequent in children with other abnormalities, especially with Down syndrome. Dermatoglyphics is the study of the patterning of dermal ridges, but it has fallen into disuse. Alterations in these are frequent in many syndromes, but they are rarely pathognomonic for any one. Dermatoglyphic alterations of both the hands and feet may contribute additional data and provide a permanent record for later study.

The feet may reflect the same anomalies as the hands. In addition, wide separation of the toes may be easier to notice. "Rocker-bottom" feet are a frequent accompaniment of several chromosome disorders including trisomies 13 and 18. Equinus varus (clubfoot) is discussed in chapter 7. During the first 2 years of life, it is important to be alert for developmental dysplasia of the hip. In the newborn and infant, the Ortolani and Barlow tests as well as ultrasound can be used for detection. In the older infant and child, extra skin folds can be seen on the side; if the child is supine with the knees flexed, they will not be at the same level. When the child walks, limping may be seen, especially when the infant is tired, and when the child stands on the leg of the affected side only, the pelvis droops on the opposite side. Developmental dysplasia of the hip and its assessment are discussed in chapter 7. Typical signs and symptoms are not present in cases of bilateral developmental dysplasia of the hip.

When looking at the trunk, supernumerary nipples and widely spaced nipples should be observed. Internipple measurement standards are available to confirm such suspicions. Examination for sacral dimpling and for a tuft of hair in the lower back area should be performed. The latter may represent occult spina bifida, which may not be present in such a mild form in other family members. Particularly in later childhood and adolescence, observation should be made for scoliosis, which may occur in about 10% to 13% of early adolescents. Although mild curvature may be of no consequence, that which is progressive needs attention. A history of poor posture, observation of awkward gait, apparent unequal arm lengths, unequal shoulders, one prominent hip, one prominent shoulder blade, and unequal hemlines may provide the clue. It is common for scoliosis to develop in children with prior muscle disease or prior irradiation for malignancy. All school children should be evaluated for scoliosis either in the school or the clinic. The skeleton, chest, and trunk should also be examined for conditions such as pectus excavatum (hollow chest) and pectus carinatum ("pigeon" breast) often seen in Marfan syndrome and homocystinuria. Observation should be made for lordosis and kyphosis, and upper and lower-body-segment ratios should be observed.

Neuromuscular

The practitioner should test the infant for the usual reflexes. The Moro or startle reflex is exaggerated in the infant with Tay-Sachs disease. In the newborn, poor sucking, reduced activity, and unequal or altered reflexes may provide clues about disorders. The "floppy" infant may demonstrate lack of active movement and unusual posturing. Later, delays in achieving motor milestones is seen. The floppy infant may assume the "frog" position when he/she is lying on the back and also demonstrate head lag. Assessment must be related to gestational maturity, because preterm infants may be normally somewhat hypotonic. In the traction response, the infant's hands are grasped and he/she is pulled to a sitting position. More than minimal head lag and full arm extension indicates postural hypotonia in the full-term newborn. A protruding ear auricle as well as ptosis of the eyelid may indicate hypotonia or a neuromuscular disorder. Delay in motor milestones, clumsiness, frequent falling, the inability to climb stairs, and unusual gaits such as waddling and toe walking may be seen in muscle disease. An important aspect of assessment is observation during which the practitioner can assess the child's gait, posture, and play activity. The answers to certain questions determine further direction. Is weakness intermittent? Is it accompanied by atrophy? Muscle cramps during exercise have a different meaning from those that occur at rest. The improvement of fatigue with exercise is different from that in which effort results in fatigue. The enlargement of specific muscle groups, especially in the calves, should be noted in children. Dubowitz (1995) provides a history form for use in cases of suspected muscle disorders.

Changes in gait, tremors, seizures, personality changes, and cognitive degeneration all may be features of different genetic disorders and may require investigation, the nature of which depends on the symptom and the age of the client. Seizure activity in the newborn and infant is often associated with inborn errors of metabolism (see chapter 6). Seizures can be difficult to detect in neonates and may be manifested as minimal aberrations such as nystagmus, "rowing" or "swimming" motions of extremities, eyelid flutter, abnormal cry, abnormal positioning of limbs, or apneic periods, as well as overt clonic or tonic movements.

Genitalia

The genitalia are a frequent site of congenital anomalies, and are easier to observe in males than females. These anomalies may result from many etiologies including teratogenesis, and show great variability in expression. Abnormalities tend to be more frequently observed in males than in females. Sexual development in relation to age may be assessed by use of the Tanner criteria. At birth, an important condition to identify is ambiguous genitalia so that further genetic studies can be done to identify the genetic sex.

SUSPECTING A GENETIC COMPONENT AND REFERRAL TO THE GENETICIST

When a genetic component is suspected because of findings from physical or developmental assessment, family history, or observation, referral to a geneticist should be initiated. Genetic concerns may be sharpened when a couple is contemplating marriage or a family. Development of the nurse's mind-set to "think genetically" may result in suspicions of genetic factors that may otherwise be ignored. For example, the early age of onset of a common disease such as coronary heart disease or a common cancer may indicate a heritable component and should be evaluated further. Situations in which genetic evaluation or counseling are indicated include the recent occurrence, discovery, or known presence in the client, his or her mate, or a blood relative of any of the following:

1. presence of disease in the family known or believed to have a genetic component, including chromosome, single gene, or multifactorial disorders;
2. any abnormality affecting more than one member of a family;
3. single or multiple congenital abnormalities;
4. delayed or abnormal development;
5. mental retardation;
6. failure to thrive in infancy or childhood;
7. short or extremely tall stature;
8. any apparent abnormalities or delays in physical growth or unusual body proportions;
9. abnormal or delayed development of secondary sex characteristics or sex organs;
10. cataracts, leukocoria or cherry-red spot in retinas of infants or children, and/or blindness;
11. deafness;

12. familial occurrence of neoplasms;
13. the occurrence of multiple primary neoplasms, bilateral neoplasms in paired organs, or the occurrence of adult-type tumors in a child;
14. the early onset of common disorders such as coronary heart disease or cancer;
15. hypotonia in an infant or child;
16. seizures in a newborn or infant;
17. skin lesions that may have a genetic component such as café'-au-lait spots in neurofibromatosis I;
18. infertility;
19. repeated spontaneous abortions (usually two to three or more);
20. stillbirths or infant deaths due to unknown or genetic causes;
21. consideration of mating or marriage to a blood relative;
22. females exposed to radiation, infectious diseases, toxic agents, or certain drugs immediately before or during pregnancy;
23. males exposed to radiation, toxic agents, or certain drugs who are contemplating immediate paternity;
24. females 35 years of age and older who are considering pregnancy or are already pregnant;
25. males 40 years of age and older who are considering paternity;
26. members of ethnic groups in which certain genetic disorders are frequent and appropriate testing, screening, or prenatal diagnosis is available;
27. unexpected drug or anesthesia reactions; and
28. any other suspicious sign or symptom suggestive of genetic disease that the nurse believes needs further evaluation. When in doubt, the practitioner can contact the geneticist to discuss concerns.

Referral of a person with a suspected genetic problem to a geneticist or genetic clinic is an appropriate and important nursing responsibility.

BIBLIOGRAPHY

Aarskog, D. (1992). Syndromes and genital dysmorphology. *Hormone Research, 38*(Suppl. 2), 82–85.

Aase, J. M. (1990). *Diagnostic dysmorphology.* New York: Plenum.

Aase, J. M. (1992). Dysmorphologic diagnosis for the pediatric practitioner. *Pediatric Clinics of North America, 39,* 135–156.

Acheson, L. (2003). Fostering applications of genetics in primary care: What will it take? *Genetics In Medicine, 5,* 63–65.

Allanson, J. E. (1997). Objective techniques for craniofacial assessment: What are the choices? *American Journal of Medical Genetics, 70,* 1–5.

Allanson, J. E. (2002). Pitfalls of genetic diagnosis in the adolescent: The changing face. *Adolescent Medicine, 13,* 257–268.

American College of Obstetricians and Gynecologists. (1996, November). Committee Opinion. *Genetic evaluation of stillbirths and neonatal deaths.* No. 178, 1-3.

Audrain-McGovern, J., Hughes, C., & Patterson, F. (2003). Effecting behavior change: Awareness of family history. *American Journal of Preventive Medicine, 24,* 183–189.

Bennett, R. L., Steinhaus, K. A., Uhrich, S. B., O'Sullivan, C. K., Resta, R. G., Lochner-Doyle, D., et al. (1995). Recommendations for standardized human pedigree nomenclature. *Journal of Genetic Counseling, 4,* 267–279.

Bergstrom, L. (1980). Assessment and consequence of malformation of the middle ear. *Birth Defects Original Article Series, 16*(4), 217–241.

Boere-Boonekamp, M. M., Kerkhoff, T. H., Schull, P. B., & Zielhuis, G. A. (1998). Early detection of developmental dysplasia of the hip in The Netherlands: The validity of a standardized assessment protocol in infants. *American Journal of Public Health, 88,* 285–288.

Cassidy, S. B., Allanson, J. E. (Eds.). (2001). *Management of genetic syndromes.* New York: John Wiley.

Dosen, A. (2005). Applying the developmental perspective in the psychiatric assessment and diagnosis of persons with intellectual disability: Part I—Assessment. *Journal of Intellectual and Developmental Disabilities Research, 49*(Pt. 1), 1–8.

Dubowitz, V. (1995). *Muscle disorders in childhood* (2nd ed.). Philadelphia: W.B. Saunders.

Dudley-Brown, S. (2004). The genetic family history assessment in gastroenterology nursing practice. *Gastroenterology Nursing, 27,* 107–110.

Evans, C. D. (1995). Computer systems in dysmorphology. *Clinical Dysmorphology, 4,* 185–201.

Evans, D., & Levene, M. (1998). Neonatal seizures. *Archives of Disease in Childhood Fetal & Neonatal Edition, 78,* F70–F75.

Feingold, M., & Bossert, W. H. (1974). Normal values for selected physical parameters. *Birth Defects, 10*(13), 1–16.

Frezzo, T. M., Rubinstein, W. S., Dunham, D., & Ormond, K. E. (2003). The genetic family history as a risk assessment tool in internal medicine. *Genetics in Medicine, 5,* 84–91.

Friedlander, Y., Siscovick, D. S., Weinmann, S., Austin, M. A., Psaty, B. M., Lemaitre, R. N., et al. (1998). Family history as a risk factor for primary cardiac arrest. *Circulation, 97,* 155–160.

Gardosi, J. (1997). Customized growth curves. *Clinics in Obstetrics and Gynecology, 40*(4), 715–722.

Georgieff, M. K. (1995). Assessment of large and small for gestational age newborn infants using growth curves. *Pediatric Annals, 24,* 599–607.

Goodman, R. M., & Gorlin, R. J. (1977). *Atlas of the face in genetic disorders* (2nd ed.). St. Louis: CV Mosby.

Goodman, S. I., & Greene, C. L. (1994). Metabolic disorders of the newborn. *Pediatrics in Review, 15,* 359–365.

Gore, A. I., & Spencer, J. P. (2004). The newborn foot. *American Family Physician, 69,* 865–872.

Gorlin, R. J., Cohen, M. M., Jr., & Hennekam, R. C. M. (Eds.). (2001). *Syndromes of the head and neck* (4th ed.). New York: Oxford University Press.

Graham, J. M., Jr., & Rimoin, D. L. (2002). Abnormal body size and proportion. In D. L. Rimoin, J. M. Connor, R. E. Pyeritz, & B. R. Korf (Eds.), *Emery and Rimoin's principles and practice of medical genetics* (4th ed., pp. 1066–1082). New York: Churchill Livingstone.

Grover, S., Stoffel, E. M., Bussone, L., Tschoegl, E., & Syngal, S. (2004). Physician assessment of family cancer history and referral for genetic evaluation in colorectal cancer patients. *Clinical Gastroenterology and Hepatology, 2,* 813–819.

Halac, I., & Zimmerman, D. (2004). Evaluating short stature in children. *Pediatric Annals, 33,* 170–176.

Harrison, T. A., Hindorff, L. A., Kim, H., Wines, R. C. M., Bowen, D. J., McGrath, B. B., et al. (2003). Family history of diabetes as a potential public health tool. *American Journal of Preventive Medicine, 24,* 152–159.

Hunt, S. C., Gwinn, M., & Adams, T. D. (2003). Family history assessment. *American Journal of Preventive Medicine, 24,* 136–142.

Hunter, A. C. W. (2002). Medical genetics: 2. The diagnostic approach to the child with dysmorphic signs. *Canadian Medical Association Journal, 167,* 367–372.

Hyer, W., Cotterill, A. M., & Savage, M. O. (1995). Common causes of short stature detectable by a height surveillance programme. *Journal of Medical Screening, 2,* 150–153.

Irvine, A. D., & McLean, W. H. I. (2003). The molecular genetics of the genodermatoses: Progress to date and future directions. *British Journal of Dermatology, 148,* 1–13.

Johnson, C. F., & Opitz, E. (1973). Unusual palm creases and unusual children. *Clinical Pediatrics, 12*(2), 101–112.

Jones, K. L. (1997). *Smith's recognizable patterns of human malformation* (5th ed.). Philadelphia: W.B. Saunders.

Jones, K. L., & Jones, M. C. (2002). A clinical approach to the dysmorphic child. In D. L. Rimoin, J. M. Connor, R. E. Pyeritz, & B. R. Korf (Eds.), *Emery and Rimoin's principles and practice of medical genetics* (4th ed., pp. 998–1010). New York: Churchill Livingstone.

Kelly, T. E. (1980). *Clinical genetics and genetic counseling.* Chicago: Year Book Pub.

Koster, E. L., McIntire, D. D., & Leveno, K. J. (2003). Recurrence of mild malformations and dysplasias. *Obstetrics & Gynecology, 102,* 363–366.

Kuhnert, B., & Nieschlag, E. (2004). Reproductive functions of the aging male. *Human Reproductive Update, 10,* 327–339.

Leppig, K. A., Werler, M. M., Cann, C. I., Cook, C. A., & Holmes, L. B. (1987). Predictive value of minor anomalies. I. Association with major malformations. *Journal of Pediatrics, 110,* 530–537.

Marden, P. M., Smith, D. W., & McDonald, M. J. (1964). Congenital anomalies in the newborn infant, including minor variations. *Journal of Pediatrics, 64,* 357–371.

Méhes, K., Mestyan, J., Knoch, V., & Vinceller, M. (1973). Minor malformations in the neonate. *Helvitica Pediatrica Acta, 28,* 477.

Parry, T. (1981). Recognition and early detection of birth problems. *Australian Family Physician, 10*, 389–396.

Popich, G. A., & Smith, D. W. (1972). Fontanels: Range of normal size. *Journal of Pediatrics, 80*, 749–752.

Pyeritz, R. (1997). Family history and genetic risk factors. *Journal of the American Medical Association, 278*, 1284–1285.

Queisser-Luft, A., Stolz, G., Wiesel, A., & Schaefer, K. (2002). Malformations in newborn: Results based on 30940 infants and fetuses from the Mainz congenital birth defect monitoring system (1990–1998). *Archives of Gynecology and Obstetrics, 266*, 163–167.

Raymond, G. V., & Holmes, L. B. (1994). Head circumference standards in neonates. *Journal of Child Neurology, 9*, 63–66.

Rich, E. C., Burke, W., Heaton, C. J., Haga, S., Pinsky, L., Short, M. P., et al. (2004). Reconsidering the family history in primary care. *Journal of General Internal Medicine, 19*, 273–280.

Rimoin, D. L., Lachman, R., & Unger, S. (2002). Chondrodysplasias. In D. L. Rimoin, J. M. Connor, R. E. Pyeritz, & B. R. Korf (Eds.), *Emery and Rimoin's principles and practice of medical genetics* (4th ed., pp. 4071–4115). New York: Churchill Livingstone.

Rogers, M. (1996). MJA Practice essentials. 4. The significance of birthmarks. *Medical Journal of Australia, 164*, 618–623.

Roye, B. D., Hyman, J., & Roye, D. P., Jr. (2004). Congenital idiopathic talipes equinovarus. *Pediatrics in Review, 25*, 124–130.

Rubeiz, N., & Kibbi, A-G. (2002). Disorders of pigmentation in infants and children. *Clinics in Dermatology, 20*, 4–10.

Salinas, C. F. (1980). An approach to an objective evaluation of the craniofacies. *Birth Defects, 16*(5), 47–74.

Scherl, S. A. (2004). Common lower extremity problems in children. *Pediatrics in Review, 25*, 52–62.

Scheuner, M. T. (2003). Family history: Where to go from here. *Genetics In Medicine, 5*, 66–67.

Silengo, M., Valenzise, M., Sorasio, L., & Ferrero, G. B. (2002). Hair as a diagnostic tool in dysmorphology. *Clinical Genetics, 62*, 270–272.

Sivan, Y., Merlob, P., & Reisner, S. H. (1983). Philtrum length and intercommissural distance in newborn infants. *Journal of Medical Genetics, 20*, 130–131.

Tanner, J. M., & Davies, P. S. W. (1985). Clinical longitudinal standards for height and height velocity for North American children. *Journal of Pediatrics, 107*, 317–329.

Thacker, P. D. (2004). Biological clock ticks for men, too. *Journal of the American Medical Association, 291*, 1683–1685.

Tolmie, J. L., McNay, M., Stephenson, J. B. P., Doyle, D., & Connor, J. M. (1987). Microcephaly: Genetic counseling and antenatal diagnosis after the birth of an affected child. *American Journal of Medical Genetics, 27*, 583–594.

Tyagi, A., & Morris, J. (2003). Using decision analytic methods to assess the utility of family history tools. *American Journal of Preventive Medicine, 24*, 199–207.

Ulijaszek, S. J. (1994). Between-population variation in pre-adolescent growth. *European Journal of Clinical Nutrition, 48*(Suppl. 1), S5–S14.

Wade, M. S., & Sinclair, R. D. (2002). Disorders of hair in infants and children other than alopecia. *Clinics in Dermatology, 20*, 16–28.

Ward, R. E., Jamison, P. L., & Allanson, J. E. (2000). Quantitative approach to identifying abnormal variation in the human face exemplified by a study of 278 individuals with five craniofacial syndromes. *American Journal of Medicial Genetics, 91*, 8–17.

Warne, G. L. (1982). The assessment of growth in children. *Australian Family Physician, 11, 422*, 425–427.

WHO. (1987). *Birth weight surrogates—the relationship between birth weight, arm and chest circumference.* Programme on maternal and child health. Geneva, Switzerland: WHO.

Yoon, P. W., Scheuner, M. T., & Khoury, M. J. (2003). Research priorities for evaluating family history in the prevention of common chronic diseases. *American Journal of Preventive Medicine, 24*, 128–135.

10

Genetic Counseling

HISTORICAL BACKGROUND

In response to increasing knowledge of the role of genetics in health and disease, Reed proposed the term "genetic counseling" in 1947, although the giving of genetic advice and the transmission of certain traits were not new ideas. Crude pedigrees were found among ancient peoples in relation to animal breeding. During the Middle Ages in Scotland, an adult male who developed "falling sickness" was castrated, and his children were killed. One African tribe valued polydactyly as evidence of superiority; children born with five digits were decapitated, as was their mother, who was suspected of infidelity. In the Talmud (collected Jewish law) there is a provision for not performing ritual circumcision on newborn males born to mothers whose brothers showed bleeding tendencies. Originally, genetic counseling was based largely on family histories and pedigrees, and consisted of estimating and explaining the risk of occurrence or recurrence of a trait or disease. Today, advances in knowledge and techniques have expanded the scope of information, allowed great precision in diagnosis and meaningful risk determination, and resulted in viable alternative treatments and options. However, genetic counseling also should continue to emphasize the human elements of education, communication, counseling, anticipatory guidance, and support.

DEFINITION

In response to increased demand for genetic counseling and the realization that little was known about the best ways to offer such services, a committee of

the American Society of Human Genetics developed the following definition, which is still accepted today. It was agreed that:

> ". . . genetic counseling is a communication process which deals with the human problems associated with the occurrence, or the risk of occurrence, of a genetic disorder in a family. This process involves an attempt by one or more appropriately trained persons to help the individual or family (1) comprehend the medical facts, including the diagnosis, the probable course of the disorder and the available management; (2) appreciate the way heredity contributes to the disorder, and the risk of recurrence in specified relatives; (3) understand the options for dealing with the risk of recurrence; (4) choose the course of action which seems appropriate to them in view of their risk and their family goals and act in accordance with that decision; and (5) make the best possible adjustment to the disorder in an affected family member and/or to the risk of recurrence of that disorder." ("Genetic Counseling," pp. 240–241)

WHO PROVIDES GENETIC COUNSELING SERVICES?

Until 1981, there was no accreditation, certification, minimum standards, or practice levels established for the practice of medical genetics or genetic counseling. This led to varying ability levels of individuals in practice and to uneven qualitative outcomes of counseling, a situation that became of great concern. Controversy about the ideal person to provide genetic counseling services became evident, with particular territorial disputes between MDs in varying specialties and PhD human geneticists, and to a lesser degree among social workers, nurses, genetic associates, and others. The American Board of Medical Genetics was incorporated for the certification of those providing medical genetic services that included clinical evaluation, genetic counseling, biochemical and cytogenetic laboratory work, prenatal diagnosis and counseling, and the coordination of services and resources. After review of educational credentials, experience, summaries of cases in which the applicants played a role, references, and examinations, the first group of professionals was board certified in 1982. They included clinical geneticists, PhD medical geneticists, genetic counselors, clinical cytogeneticists, and clinical biochemists. Recertification is required for those certified in 1993 or after, and certification is now limited to 10 years before recertification is necessary for those people. In 1992, the American Board of Genetic Counselors began certification of genetic counselors. The Genetic Nursing Credentialing Commission, an affiliate of ISONG, allowed nurses with a baccalaureate or master's degree, respectively to be recognized as a Baccalaureate Genetics Clinical Nurse or an Advanced Practice Nurse in Genetics but this is not certification for counseling. Some states have enacted laws requiring genetic counselors to be licensed.

In larger centers, genetic services are often offered by a team of professionals that may include any of the following as core individuals: physician, geneticist, genetic counselor, genetic associate, nurse, nurse practitioner, social worker, psychologist, or pastoral counselor. In many settings, the role of genetic counselor is assumed by a physician or a geneticist, and in satellite or outreach programs, by nurses who receive specific education in clinical genetics. In other areas outside major metropolitan areas, a geneticist may both coordinate and provide genetic counseling, using other professionals as they are appropriate for the specific counselee. In some clinics, nurses coordinate genetic services, particularly in the community. Today, many applications of genetics are becoming part of primary care practices. For example, in smaller communities, physicians and certified nurse midwives may provide genetic counseling prior to prenatal diagnosis. Physicians or advanced practice nurses may explain genetic tests for familial cancers in some settings. Thus across the United States there is much variation in the way in which counseling is provided and where it is located, some of which is related to the complexity of the individual counseling situation and the needs of the client.

THE SETTING

Genetic counseling is done in a variety of settings—genetic counseling centers or clinics, specialty clinics (e.g., cleft palate), general clinics, offices, agencies, laboratories, and other sites. In larger cities geneticists are often affiliated with hospitals and medical centers, whereas in smaller communities they may be located in individual offices or at a university, and in rural areas they may be part of a regional outreach program or located at an agency, clinic, or office. While recognizing the need for health professionals' education in genetic counseling, the counselee is entitled to privacy. One or two others may be allowed at a session, but a roomful of observers is not a proper or effective way to provide this service. If the counselee consents, use of a two-way mirror or a tape recorder may allow less obtrusive educational involvement.

REFERRAL OF CLIENTS

The major sources of referrals are physicians, nurses, self-referrals, social service agencies (e.g., planned parenthood and mental health departments), adoption agencies, speech and hearing clinics, health departments, and teachers. Although health practitioners in the clinical specialties of obstetrics and pediatrics still dominate referrals, an increasing number originate from family practice, community health, and medical and surgical practitioners of all types. Nurses wishing to locate genetic services in their communities or regions can usually find them either by checking the phone book, the nearest medical school, the biology department of a university, through the local or national March of Dimes, the Internet, the American Board of Medical Genetics, or the American Board of Genetic Counselors.

Any persons with the referral indications given in chapter 9 are candidates for genetic counseling referral. Those persons most likely to be referred for genetic counseling are the following:

- persons or couples who have had a child with a birth defect or known genetic disorder,
- persons or couples who are known to be heterozygous carriers of a specific genetic disease,
- persons affected by a trait or disorder known or suspected to be inherited,
- persons who have a known or suspected inherited disorder in the family and are contemplating either marriage or starting a family,
- persons who are experiencing reproductive problems such as infertility, multiple miscarriages, or stillbirths,
- persons who are contemplating marriage to a relative or entering an interracial marrage,
- members of ethnic groups with a high frequency of specific known genetic disorders to detect carrier status,
- those with possible exposure to toxic agents, illnesses, or mutagens during pregnancy,
- women 35 years of age and older who are considering prenatal diagnosis, and
- persons seeking risk assessment prior to genetic testing and/or interpretation of genetic tests for certain complex disorders, such as cancer or heart disease.

Genetic counseling is also offered in conjunction with testing and screening programs, and for those considering adoption or various reproductive technologies, as discussed in chapter 11. About 90% of those who should be so referred are not. Indications that nurses can use as a guide for referral are given in chapter 9. If a formal referral is initiated, the counselees should bring all relevant records, family data, and even photographs with them, or have it sent before they have their first appointment. The genetic counselor should be notified of the referral by phone or letter. The nurse or the referring professional should also check with the counselee to see that follow- through has actually occurred.

The person who is seeking genetic counseling may be called the consultant or counselee. The term "proband" or "propositus" refers to the index case or to the person who first brought the family to the attention of the geneticist, for example, the affected child. In practice the actual counselee may be more than one person, for example, mother, father, and child.

Some clients are very self-directed and motivated to seek counseling. Others may be there because "the doctor told me I should come." Elements of the Health Belief Model are relevant here in that the client must perceive that a serious situation exists, there is some personal vulnerability, and that the benefits derived from the indicated action will outweigh the barriers or risks. Other factors such as denial and guilt are also operative. In one still relevant study by Fraser and co-workers (1974), parents who were referred for counseling waited 2 years or more after having a child with a birth defect before seeking help. This kind of delay on the part of the clients still occurs. This example points out that the referring professional's role does not end with providing the information that genetic counseling is available, but that they should follow up on their initial referral.

TIMING

Because many emotions are involved in a genetic disorder, it is not always helpful to provide genetic counseling immediately after the birth of an affected child or the unexpected diagnosis of a genetic disease in an adult. These events can precipitate a family crisis. Genetic disease is often perceived as permanent and untreatable. Shock followed by denial is often the first part of the coping process. When counselees are seen in this phase, which may be present 3 to 6 months after the crisis, they do not know what they want to know, and they may not hear what is said to them. Anxiety and anger follow and this may be directed outwardly as hostility or inwardly as guilt. At this point, the counselee may be ready to intellectually understand and adjust only on an intellectual level. Depression occurs next, and if the counselee can achieve behavioral adjustment, successful accommodation can occur. Obviously, counselees may cycle between phases. Covert anger and avoidance behavior may lead to clients canceling, not keeping, or arriving late for their appointments. Staff who do not understand the basis for this behavior may demonstrate anger and hostility towards the client, which obviously will act to negate efforts to establish a good client-counselor relationship. However, an initial early interview can be used to assess the degree of negative feelings and to use intervention techniques or to provide support services for ongoing counseling if it appears indicated. Usually a family history can be obtained and may provide the clients with the feeling that they are taking some positive action. A second appointment is then scheduled. These feelings are further described in Chapter 8.

COMPONENTS OF GENETIC COUNSELING

As the setting, the professionals providing services, and the reasons for seeking counseling vary, so too does the counseling process. Nevertheless, all genetic counseling has some common elements. The usual components of the genetic counseling process are shown in Table 10.1. Their application and sequence also vary because the geneticist does not always know what additional information is needed until after the assessment process, the interview, and the histories are completed (e.g., chromosome analysis may need to be done, past records obtained, an illness in another family member confirmed). Usually there is more than one session anticipated, with information gathered and a relationship established first, and plans made to collect other needed data on which to formulate diagnoses or recurrence risks. The first session usually may take at least 1 hour. It is hard to know how this will change, as the time spent with clients for any health-related condition continues to be related to cost-benefit and maximizing profits.

Initial Interview

Some services mail a family history questionnaire and wait for its return before scheduling an appointment, whereas others collect the information at the first interview. The initial interview is often conducted by the nurse. In a smaller center, the counselor or coordinator may conduct it. At this time one can (1) obtain an initial appraisal of any interaction or dynamics; (2) get the reason they are seeking counseling; (3) elicit preliminary concerns; (4) find out their expectations of genetic counseling; (5) discuss the usual elements and procedures involved; (6) ascertain the counselee's educational, cultural, and ethnic background; and (7) orient them to the clinic if appropriate. These are

important steps because clients often state that they "don't know why they are there" or that they came because "my doctor told me I should," but they do not believe that they need services. Those feeling this way often express dissatisfaction with the entire process and outcome. Formality and the manner and order of greeting the counselees is important in many cultures. For example, among traditional Koreans, men are expected to be greeted before women.

Obtaining a History and Preparing a Pedigree

Most information regarding the taking of the history is discussed in chapter 9. There are, however, some points that should be considered here. The taking of the family history also gives the counselor a chance to observe family interactions and to provide clues for effective approaches when discussing risks and options. It is very helpful to have both members of a couple present when the history is taken, because one person rarely has the precise information necessary about both sides of the family or, if they have attempted to gather it beforehand, they may not have asked the relevant questions indicated by the suspected genetic disorder (e.g., in neurofibromatosis in the family, it may be helpful to know if axillary freckling is present in any relatives who cannot be personally examined). If all agree, it may be helpful to have an older relative present for part of the information gathering because they may have detailed information about the family. Taking the history is time consuming because one cannot just ask a general question such as: "Does anyone in your family have a birth defect, mental retardation, or genetic disease?" The concepts of disease, disability, and retardation may be culturally defined. Many counselees do not even know what constitutes a genetic disease, and they may not equate "slowness" with mental retardation. Thus questions must be specifically tailored for the individual, at their level of understanding, and within their sociocultural context. The history-taking must result in the preparation of a pedigree which may be helpful in determining the mode of transmission operating in a given family, even in the absence of a definite diagnosis, that will allow a basis for counseling (see chapter 9).

TABLE 10.1   Components of Genetic Counseling*

- Initial interview
- Family history, pedigree preparation and analysis, other histories
- Assessment of counselee—physical examination, etc.
- Considering potential diagnoses
- Confirmatory or supplementary tests or procedures such as:

Chromosome analysis	Developmental testing
Biochemical tests	Dermatoglyphics
Molecular DNA testing or analysis	Electromyography
X-ray films	Prenatal diagnosis
Biopsy	Immunological tests
Linkage analysis	

- Establishment of an accurate diagnosis
- Literature search and review
- Use of Internet resources and registries
- Consultation with other experts
- Compiling of information and determination of recurrence risk
- Communication of the results and risks to the counselee and to the family, if appropriate
- Discussion of natural history, current treatment options, and anticipatory guidance, if relevant
- Discussion of options
- Review and questions
- Assessment of understanding and clarification
- Referrals—for example, prenatal diagnosis and specialists
- Support of decisions made by counselee
- Follow-up
- Evaluation

*Order may vary depending on the reason for initial referral; psychosocial support should be provided throughout the process; all explanations should be culturally appropriate for counselees and appropriate to their educational level.

Anyone who has done such a history is aware of some of the problems and pitfalls that may be encountered. One couple came for counseling in which one of the issues was whether or not the disorder, which had incomplete penetrance, was a sporadic event, or was caused by an autosomal dominant gene in that family. I was told that "Aunt Mary had something wrong with her. She was never allowed to marry, and they mostly kept her in her room." This could or could not be relevant to the situation at hand and needed to be further explored and documented. Sometimes this is difficult because people are reluctant to talk about defects and mental retardation in their families.

Often additional family information needs to be obtained and sent to the counselor. Some families do not wish to let other members know that they are seeking counseling and this greatly complicates the obtaining of accurate information. A negative family history can have several meanings. If a couple has come for counseling, it is important to talk to the mother alone at some point in the interview. In such privacy, it is possible to ascertain the possibility of nonpaternity of the present mate, of sperm donation, or of adoption that has not yet been revealed to the child who may be accompanying his/her parents. Thus a negative family history may mean that this mutation is a sporadic or new one, or may be due to other reasons (see chapter 9 for a complete list) including failure of the interviewer to ask the critical questions, conduct a thorough assessment or the withholding of information by the client.

Another sensitive area is that of consanguinity. By asking the names of all the relatives in the family history, the counselor can ask about those with the same last name on both sides of the family. Another way to ascertain this is by determining where both families have lived at various points in time, of what ethnic origin they are, and where they came from when they came to this country. Occasionally couples who did not realize they were related discover that they indeed have a common ancestor. A counselee whose child had Ellis-van Creveld syndrome (dwarfism with polydactyly and heart disease, which is common in the Pennsylvania Dutch) turned out to be married to a cousin. Both had Pennsylvania Dutch ancestors. One can also lead into the subject by asking if there is any chance at all that the two partners are related.

Deaths of siblings or stillbirths should be pursued. A parent may initially say that a child died of heart disease (which he or she did), and not think it relevant to mention that the child had Holt-Oram syndrome. It is particularly important, especially in the case of parents who have had a child with a visible malformation, that in concluding the history of the pregnancy the counselor raise issues that the couple may otherwise leave unspoken but not necessarily unthought, such as "Many times, parents who have had a baby with anencephaly feel that some event in their pregnancy (like a long car trip taken against advice) caused or contributed to it." It is important to get them to verbalize any feelings on this issue so that they can be dealt with. The client may feel that they are being punished for an indiscretion or sin that is real or imagined. They may, aloud or silently ask, "Why me? What did I do to be punished like this?" In many cultures (e.g., Italian and other Mediterranean, some African, Caribbean, and Latin), there may be the belief that the malformation was the result of a curse or of the "evil eye" (el mal ojo). Thus the counselor must adjust the tone and content of the counseling toward the cultural group of the counselee. It is also important to know how the culture views not only the occurrence of a genetic condition but also beliefs about healing and the body. Who are the authority figures in the culture? How can they be included in facilitating adjustment? What is the decision-making power of the individual and couple, or are there others who will have a major influence? What are the concepts of privacy and stigma or shame in this culture? The occurrence of a genetic disorder can also be used to accentuate family difficulties that may have been latently present before the event, such as "I told you not to marry her; her family is no good." The history taking can be concluded by asking, "Is there anything else you think I should know about you or your family, or that you would like to tell me?" It is not infrequent that even after a long initial counseling session, a counselee has telephoned to supply information that he or she "forgot" to tell me and that turns out to be quite relevant.

Establishing a Diagnosis

The family history is a first step in the establishment of a diagnosis, if it has not been made before the client seeks genetic counseling. Diagnoses should be confirmed where possible. When no diagnosis has been established, then one of the roles of the geneticist is to recommend appropriate testing in order that one can be made. This may include chromosome analysis, molecular testing, or biochemical testing that is appropriate to the possible disorder, symptomatology, or ethnic group of the counselee; X-ray films; skin or muscle biopsy; electromyography; or others. Carrier status should be established if it is relevant and possible. If the syndrome is unknown, then referral to specialists may be indicated. For example, photographs, laboratory records, histories, physical examination data, and specimens may all need to be sent to an expert in a rare disorder or entered into a computerized system for an opinion. Sometimes the establishment of a diagnosis is not possible. The affected person may be deceased and essential information or autopsy results were not obtained, all testing and examination results are inconclusive, or a syndrome may not have been previously identified. This points up the need for the nurse to be alert for the need to obtain pictures, specialized measurements, and tissue specimens in cases of spontaneous abortions and stillbirths (see American College of Obstetricians and Gynecologists, 1996). The genetic counselor should know his or her own limitations in diagnosis and be able to provide referral to get answers. For example, the client's eyes may need examination by an expert in ophthalmology. The affected persons should be carefully examined, if feasible. Family members who are at a risk for the disorder should be meticulously examined, especially when they are asymptomatic, in order to detect minimal signs of disease. An example is the case of a 30-year-old man who was at risk for facioscapulohumeral muscular dystrophy IA, (an autosomal dominant disorder with muscle weakness and retinal anomalies) and showed no obvious symptoms of muscle dysfunction, but when seen by a neurologist was found to have a "forme fruste" or minimal manifestation of the disorder, a finding which considerably changed the risk for his transmitting the gene. Sometimes, despite the best of efforts and for a variety of reasons, no diagnosis can be established. In one case a woman in her mid-20s was contemplating having children. The problem was that she had a 22-year-old brother who had a muscle disorder, and she sought counseling to determine the risk of one of her children having the disorder. Unfortunately, her brother's diagnosis was made years before, when all muscle weaknesses of that variety were lumped into a single category and named accordingly. In more recent years, they had been found to be heterogenous and transmitted by different modes of inheritance. Her brother was severely physically incapacitated but unaffected as far as intelligence was concerned—he had graduated from college. The counselor suggested that he be re-diagnosed in order to accurately determine her risk, as the family history was unhelpful in this regard. The counselee felt very strongly that she did not want him to know she was concerned about a child of hers having the disorder, but after all the years she had watched him grow and develop, she felt that she could not assume this responsibility in her own child. She therefore refused any communication with him in regard to diagnosis by herself, another family member, a physician, or the counselor. The only options at that time were to review with her the risks for the two types of inheritance then known to be involved and refer her for some psychological counseling in hopes that she might modify her feelings. She subsequently moved out of state, so follow-up was not achieved. Sometimes when a precise diagnosis cannot be made, the history and pedigree clearly reveals the mode of inheritance operating in that particular family, and counseling can then proceed on that basis. Searches of the literature may be valuable in locating case reports with similar features and contacting the author, or in locating experts who are using new techniques for rare disorders.

Inaccurate diagnosis can result from failure to recognize mild expression of a disorder. In another situation, young adults who learned that their institutionalized sibling had tuberous sclerosis, and that this could be inherited, sought counseling.

Examination included using a Woods lamp to look at the skin for white, leaf-shaped macules and expert ophthalmological evaluation. Neither sibling had mental retardation or seizures, which are often part of the disorder. One was ultimately found to have characteristic skin lesions, and therefore could be presumed to be affected. Counseling could proceed on the basis of the risk of transmitting this autosomal dominant disorder and the unpredictability of its severity in any children he might have. Sometimes the counselee may deliberately conceal stigmata of a disorder. In chapter 6, a woman with Waardenburg syndrome type I who only had the white forelock of hair, was described. When speaking to the counselor privately, she revealed that she dyed her hair to conceal it. However, she did not want the counselor to tell her husband (this was a second marriage) that she, in fact, had the gene that was present in its full blown form in her child, because she felt that she could not handle the guilt or blame she believed would be forthcoming.

Another type of diagnostic problem is exemplified by the case of a couple who was referred to a counselor for infertility. A chromosome analysis was done that revealed that the wife had a male karyotype of 46,XY. She had testicular feminization syndrome. It is important to emphasize that she was not a male in non-genetic ways. She was raised as a female, believed she was a female, and looked phenotypically like a female, but could not conceive. She was married to a normal man. Some counselors believe that the counselor should not give them a specific diagnosis, but just tell them generally that there is a chromosome problem causing the infertility and recommend adoption. Others believe that full disclosure is necessary and can be accomplished if handled in a sensitive way, with provision for back-up ongoing psychological counseling. No matter which course of action is chosen, there will certainly be many problems to be faced.

Determining and Communicating Recurrence Risks and Discussing the Disorder

After the initial visit there may be a considerable lapse of time during which all of the information is assembled. If the counselee is not aware that this is a usual occurrence, there may be considerable concern generated, so this information should be included at the conclusion of the initial visit. When the process of information gathering is completed, the geneticist must use all of the information collected to determine the risk of recurrence of a disorder for a child of the counselee, or for the counselees themselves to be either a carrier or to develop the disorder in question. When planning the process of sharing the acquired information with the counselee, the geneticist takes into account the educational level and the ethnic, socioeconomic, and cultural background of the couple. Genetics is a very complex area, and most high school graduates have little comprehension of the subject matter. Sometimes pretests are used to assess information about a specific technique or disorder, such as before deciding on testing for cystic fibrosis or deciding whether or not to have amniocentesis. Many counselees are reluctant to acknowledge that they do not understand the counselor, and so they may come away from the session with misinformation and confusion. Therefore, the counselor must take care to explain things in simple terms and repeat the content in different ways. The use of pictures, videotapes, computer programs, audiotapes, charts, photographs, and diagrams is helpful. In some Native American cultures, storytelling is an appropriate way to communicate the information. Understanding may also be assessed by asking the client to repeat the information in his/her own words as the session proceeds. Clients can also be asked to discuss the meaning of this information to them so that misconceptions can be addressed. Most counselees already have formed an idea about recurrence risks before genetic counseling, which is usually higher than the real risks. Some counselors also form ideas about risks in which they arbitrarily label those above 10% as high and below 10% as low. This pre-interpretation of material in order to present material simply is not acceptable.

Recurrence risks can be presented in different ways. The meaning of probability or odds can sometimes be clarified by the use of special color-coded dice appropriate to the mode of inheritance. Coin flipping is another method used. Risks can be phrased in more than one way, and the manner of their presentation is important. For example, one can say, "For each pregnancy, there is a one in four

chance that the infant will have Hurler disease;" or one can say, "For each pregnancy, there is a three in four chance that the baby will *not* have Hurler disease." In the Mendelian disorders, it is important to clarify that this risk is true for each pregnancy, that "chance has no memory," and so although they may have one affected child already, this does not influence the outcome of future pregnancies (aside from the possibility of gonadal mosaicism). In any case, the counselee must process the information relative to the risk of recurrence and make it personally meaningful as each views it in terms of his/her own life experience. The meaning of a high risk of having male children with genetic disease may be different to a Mexican-American couple where a higher cultural value is placed on a male infant than to one of different ethnic origin. For some Bedouin populations, among whom about 60% of marriages are consanguineous, childbearing has a very high value. Women attain a higher status when they become mothers. Therefore, for example, some families prefer to take a 25% risk of a child affected with an AR disorder, and have the child die soon after birth, than not have children or practice selective pregnancy termination.

Unfortunately, few actual cases are straightforward, in which the entire picture is clear. For example, a couple may come for counseling where the wife has a sister with a given AR disorder, and the question they are asking is, "What is the risk that we would have a child with the same disorder as the sister?" Because this is an AR disorder, the logical step would be to determine the carrier status of each of the counselees. In some cases this is not yet possible with reliability for carrier detection or for prenatal diagnosis. Theoretically, the wife has a prior risk for being a carrier of 2/3. Because her parents were both obligate carriers, out of the normal appearing children, 2/3 would be expected to be carriers, and 1/3 would not possess the mutant gene (see chapter 6). In the absence of any family history or evidence to the contrary, the husband's risk is assumed to be that of the population at large. If the disorder was a common one such as for cystic fibrosis, the risk would be greater than for most other genetic disorders—in the nature of about 1/25. Since only 1/4 of their children would have a chance of being affected if they were both carriers (as each has a 50% chance of passing on the mutant gene to any one offspring), then the final risk in the case of cystic fibrosis without further data as to carrier status is $2/3 \times 1/25 \times 1/4 = 1/150$. If the disorder is very rare, then the risk of the other mate having the same gene in the absence of any family history or similar ethnic background is negligible. Individuals regard the risk given in terms of their life situation and personal values. Such a couple should be urged to consider the risk in light of what the disorder means to them, as one of them has had a different experience by living with an affected person than has the other one. It is important that such a couple keep in close touch with the geneticist because many more disorders are becoming amenable to molecular DNA testing approaches.

Sometimes the counselee's perception of the risk is quite different from that of the counselor's. Some see a risk of 50% for an affected child as "having a chance to break even" and do not view it as high. Others find a 2% risk unacceptable. Risks are also seen in light of what they are for. Some can accept a high risk for a child to be born with a cleft lip, whereas for others even a minimal risk of mental retardation cannot be borne. Sometimes the counselor can be surprised by the client's response. A couple who both have achondroplasia were told that their chances of conceiving a child of normal stature are only one in four. This was good news to them, as they believed they would have difficulty in adjusting to raising a child of normal stature. Pearn (1973) gives an opposite example. A woman who had two children with celiac disease was given a risk of 10% for the next pregnancy to be similarly affected. This estimate was too low for her because she believed that the adjustment of the whole family to a gluten-free diet would be compromised by the birth of a normal child. Sometimes it is difficult for the counselor to remain neutral when parents with a genetic disorder choose to have a child who has a high risk for having the same disorder; however, most believe that the genetic counselors need to support their clients in their decisions or refer them to someone who can. Risk figures may also be looked at by the clients in terms of what else is going on in their lives. For example, women who are illegal immigrants, in an abusive relationship, struggling with poverty, dangerous and unsanitary living conditions, and other issues may not regard genetic risks for a pregnancy as a pressing life issue regardless of the extent of that risk.

Along with risk figures, the natural history and impact of the disorder in question should be discussed, as the burden may not be appreciated or else it may be exaggerated. Then, options appropriate to the individual counselee's problem can be discussed. These include prenatal diagnosis, a treatment plan, and reproductive options available. Alternatives such as "taking a chance," adoption, sterilization, sperm and egg donation, embryo transfer, and in vitro fertilization can be presented if they are relevant. Weaver & Escobar (1987) list 24 ways to have or obtain children. Although the couple should make the ultimate decision for options, the counselor may encourage them to think it over for a period of time, if time is not a critical factor in their situation. In some cultures the counselees may need to consult the entire family or certain respected members such as elders. Then the counselor should support their decision and help to make arrangements to facilitate it regardless of the personal opinion of the counselor. If that is not possible, they should be sure that another staff member meets with the clients to do that. If the family has sought genetic services because of the need to ascertain what the problem is in a family member, then decision-making centers around the need to plan for the resources necessary for coping. To do this, they must have some ideas of what types of problems and what degree of disability and deterioration may be realistically expected, what treatments and resources are available, what living adjustments need to be made, and what kinds of ultimate outcomes are possible. What is considered a disability varies from culture to culture. Arrangements may be made with persons who have made various types of decisions in this regard. In the case of deciding on reproductive alternatives, it may be useful to have them meet with parents of a child with the disorder in question, and perhaps both with parents who have chosen pregnancy termination and those who have not. Long-term help with coping may be provided by the same genetic group during the counseling sessions or referrals and arrangements may be made by the coordinator for comprehensive ongoing care. The counselees may need to have their self-worth affirmed and perhaps mourn the loss of their "normal" child, if they have not already done so. The issues involved in the birth of an infant with a defect, effects on the family, and living with a genetic disorder in the family are discussed in chapter 8.

In some disorders it is desirable to notify extended family members that they are at risk for a detrimental gene, chromosomal aberration, or of an adverse outcome because of their possible condition. The counselee's permission for this, and for a release of information, should be obtained. Discussion of this might occur before testing for the particular disorder, and on receipt of results, and this can be complicated. The siblings of an affected person may need to be tested or examined and the extent of this could depend on their age. If a couple is seeking counseling after birth of an affected infant, it may be appropriate to inform the parents that genetic counseling would be important in the future for other family members, such as other children in the family, at the appropriate age. In cultures such as the Japanese, privacy may be quite valued.

After risks and options have been discussed, understanding can be assessed. Counselees should be able to tell the counselor in their own words what they understand about the disorder, how it was caused, what the risk is for recurrence, and what kinds of options are available and should be considered. Counselees should always be asked if there is anything else they want to know or if there are any other questions.

Directive vs. Non-Directive Genetic Counseling

Traditionally, the trend in counseling was for non-directive style in the presentation of the above information, perhaps largely in reaction to some of the negative practices of eugenics and "genetic hygiene." However, some counselors now advocate the directive approach. They believe that when a client asks what to do or "What would you do, if you were in my place?," an honest answer can be given with the modifier of "I lean toward doing . . ., but I do not know for certain how I would act if I were you." Many believe that the counselor's role is to clarify issues and options and to be helpful to the client in reaching a decision. Some counselors employ non-directiveness for reproductive decisions but are more directive for treatments such as diet in PKU. Clients should always be supported in the decisions that they reach.

The use of a directive approach without modifiers may reflect traditional paternalistic/ maternalistic views of counseling. An approach reflecting an omnipotent or a one-sided relationship can be accentuated by the sometimes intimidating physical setting of a hospital or clinic, particularly if the genetic counseling is taking place in the context of a clinical trial. The use of a non-directive approach implies that both decision-making and chosen courses of action become primarily the responsibility of the counselees and not the counselor. This allows the counselee to maintain autonomy and control and to play an active role in decision-making. It also provides some feelings of security for the counselor by relieving him or her of any decision-making burden. Another reason for using a value-neutral non-directive approach in genetic counseling is that the counselor often does not know the client well, or does not have an ongoing relationship with them because the counselor is usually not the regular health care giver. Therefore, the counselor may not be aware of the counselee's resources, coping abilities, family and financial circumstances, values or belief systems, or understand the impact of the genetic problem at hand on this particular counselee. The counselees possess some information that is not necessarily shared with the counselor but contributes to their ultimate decision. However, the non-directive approach contrasts with traditional medical practice. Therefore, some counselees expect to be told what to do as one counseling outcome, and they are confused when expected to make their own decisions. Yarborough, Scott, and Dixon (1989) point out that clients may expect that the counselor should give expert advice because of their professional skills and knowledge. They may expect that as part of duty fulfillment and "getting their money's worth." On the other hand, even this recognition may make the client "susceptible." Clarke (1991) questions whether any counselor can be value neutral. For example, does an offer for prenatal diagnosis imply a recommendation to accept that offer or a tacit recommendation to terminate an abnormal pregnancy? Does respect for a client's decisions and autonomy ever conflict with the principle of avoiding harm? Michie, Bron, Bobrow, and Marteau (1997) analyzed counseling transcripts of 131 counselees and found a mean of 5.8 advice statements, 5.8 evaluative statements and 1.7

reinforcing statements per consultation. However, Kessler (1997) distinguishes coercion as a defining aspect of directiveness, as do Baumiller et al. (1996) and the National Society of Genetic Counselors (1992). Bartels, LeRoy, McCarthy, and Caplan (1997) reported that 72% of the genetic counselors in their study reported that they were sometimes directive. There seems to be a need to re-evaluate communication processes in genetic counseling and conduct research on the interaction between the client and the counselor. Non-geneticists providing counseling, such as physicians, may tend to be more directive. In the evaluation of my own counseling service, and in that of others in which I have participated, many families have expressed the wish that more direction be given to them, that is, "If I were you, I would do . . . ." The use of the modified approach discussed earlier, may give more direction without being coercive.

Probably few genetic counselors can always use a completely directive or non-directive approach. For one thing, it can be almost impossible for the counselor not to communicate some of their own feelings and opinions by nonverbal cues or voice tones. Probably today, most genetic counselors believe that their role lies chiefly in the clarification of issues and options once the material necessary has been presented in a way that can be understood. When counselees have reached a decision, every effort should be made to facilitate and support that decision.

Group vs. Individual Genetic Counseling

Group, rather than individual, genetic counseling, is a relatively new consideration for those in similar circumstances, such as carrier screening for Tay-Sachs disease, or for those who are considering prenatal diagnosis because of advanced maternal age. Advantages include verbalization of questions by some participants that other participants may have hesitated to ask, feelings of a shared group experience, realizing that they were not alone with their problem, maximizing cost effectiveness, and widening access to a busy professional. Disadvantages include the loss of privacy and confidentiality, reluctance to expose sensitive or private issues and concerns that may result in their never being aired, unintentional coercion to accept feelings, values, or decisions of the majority of the group,

and a sense of feeling pressured. Much thought should be given to these issues, and careful evaluation accomplished when they are being tried. Sometimes group counseling is used for discussing general material and assessing risk, followed by individual counseling for those at increased risk.

Preconception or Prepregnancy Genetic Counseling

Preconception or prepregnancy genetic counseling may be considered to identify couples at increased risk for less than desirable pregnancy outcome. Good assessment, family, health, social, occupational, and environmental histories, physical examination, and knowledge of genetic risk factors can help to identify such individuals who are often seen in the primary care setting (also see chapters 9, 12, 13, and 14). Today, all women considering pregnancy should be counseled to be on an appropriate diet, have rubella and varicella titers determined, have appropriate folic acid and multivitamin supplementation, review any medications and drugs they may be using, discuss alcohol, drug, and cigarette use, be told to avoid hot tubs, discuss potential risks based on ethnic origin, and the like (see chapter 13). Important is the information that women should take 0.4 mg of folic acid daily prior to conception, and if they have a previous history of neural tube defects, they should take 4.0 mg of folic acid daily, starting optimally at 3 months before conception. Their male partner should also be counseled, for example, to avoid environmental chemicals, cigarette smoking, certain drugs, and radiation. Carrier screening for certain genetic diseases, particularly in certain ethnic groups may be appropriate as pregnancy is considered. ACOG, for example, has developed guidelines for carrier screening in persons of Eastern European Jewish descent (2004). Some may have concerns or be at a risk that prompted them to seek counseling. Identification of such individuals, coupled with appropriate action, can result in a more favorable pregnancy outcome. For example, women with altered maternal metabolism such as those with diabetes mellitus or PKU can benefit from strict control and diet therapy before pregnancy. Someone who had a corrected congenital anomaly themselves might have anxiety reduced by knowing the actual risk. For women with genetic disorders, such as

Ehlers-Danlos disease type IV, a connective tissue disorder, the problem to be considered may be the effect of the disorder on the pregnancy that does not include heritability and also the effect of the pregnancy on the disorder. Parents may not be aware that relatively minor problems in themselves may, in fact, mean that they are at increased risk for a more severe outcome in their children, such as in the case of a mother with spina bifida occulta and the possibility of a more full-blown neural tube defect in a subsequent child. In cases of disabilities arising from unknown or non-genetic causes, such counseling can still be useful in terms of optimum pregnancy management in a setting best able to cope with any anticipated problems, and also for aspects of identifying the most common hazards likely to be encountered so that they can be prevented, rather than treated, which might involve increased risk to the fetus. An example would be, in the case of the potential of urinary tract infection, the avoidance of factors that might contribute to infection and proactive measures such as adequate fluid intake could reduce the chance that medication would be necessary. Women should be asked about any bleeding tendencies in themselves or menorrhagia, especially at menarche, which could prompt evaluation for von Willebrand disease, an inherited bleeding disorder (see chapter 9).

Persons at risk thus need to consider their chances of conception, the effect of a pregnancy on their own health, the effect on the developing fetus in the uterus, how it impacts on any pregnancy complications, and also their chances of having a child with a similar disorder if they are themselves affected. They can then consider reproductive options, therapeutic options, and the possibility of prenatal diagnosis, if available and desired, before embarking on the pregnancy.

Follow-up

After counseling is completed, a post-counseling follow-up letter should be sent to the counselee and the referring professional, reiterating the essential information that was covered in the counseling session. This gives them something tangible to refer to when needed. A follow-up phone call is used to see if there are any additional questions. A home visit can be arranged through the community health nurse or genetic clinic nurse to assess coping, to identify problems, and to answer questions.

Evaluation

Like the mythical Greek bearers of bad news who were beheaded, hostility and covert anger are often directed at the bearer of "bad" genetic news—the counselor. This is particularly true in cases in which the disorder in question is of unknown etiology, the recurrence risk cannot be determined with reliability, or when the client comes to the genetic counseling service reluctantly or with misconceptions and unrealistic expectations. One case I recall was a couple who were referred by their rural physician for possible Down syndrome in their 11-month-old infant. The evaluation determined that the child was normal. However, the parents later called the counselor to complain that all their time and money were wasted because nothing was wrong! Sometimes clients who participate in non-directive counseling are more likely to feel that nothing was done for them, as they may want someone else to take the responsibility for making decisions. Members of some ethnic groups by virtue of their cultural norms, for example, some Asian groups, may expect a more directive approach from the counselor who is considered an authority.

Conducting an evaluation is difficult. One needs to know whether knowledge of the disorder was increased, relief of psychological distress was achieved, or whether or not subsequent actions taken by the client were appropriate. To do this, one needs to have an assessment of the knowledge before counseling, and an optimal time period at which to measure the psychological parameter. To decide on the appropriateness of the counselee's actions requires many value judgments by the counselor. Over the years, it has been documented that a substantial percentage of genetic counseling clients do not remember accurately what was discussed with them during the counseling session. There has been some debate over what counts as success in genetic counseling, and who makes those decisions. As concepts of cost and time have entered primary health care, they are entering genetic counseling as well. One study by Surh et al. (1995) evaluated the time spent in delivering counseling, which included counseling, case review, phone calls, follow-up letters, specimen gathering, and the laboratory report, and analyzed them by professional and condition. For cystic fibrosis, the median time spent was 93 minutes (range 65 to 273); and for fragile X, 185 minutes (range 85 to 625). A study by Rowley, Loader, Sutera, and Kozyra (1995) looked at counseling for hemoglobinopathy carriers by primary providers and genetic counselors. While similar on most parameters, significantly fewer clients seen by the primary provider referred the partner for testing. Other suggestions for evaluation of services include audit. The question is what is to be audited. Is it time spent, such as discussed previously, is it whether or not a client has chosen a certain option, or is it something else? This gets into various ethical issues.

THE NURSE IN THE GENETIC COUNSELING PROCESS

As discussed previously, nurses may play a variety of roles in genetic counseling that reflect their preparation, area of practice, primary functions, and setting. These roles will involve collaboration with other disciplines. One of the prime ways in which the nurse who is not involved in the offering of direct genetic services can help is by recognizing and referring those clients and families in need of such services to the appropriate professionals. If the nurse is not sure, he or she should find out from another knowledgeable person. It may be a reasonable standard of practice to know which patients to refer to genetic specialists or counselors. Whether or not genetic counseling has been offered to hospitalized patients and their families for whom it would be appropriate can be noted on the chart and discharge summary, along with the results. Nurses also need to assess clients' understanding of any treatments to be carried out, such as for prophylactic penicillin in children with sickle cell anemia to prevent infection, and help the clients plan how they will implement the therapy, especially over the long term.

If not providing the direct counseling or education, other ways in which nurses may assist clients or families with genetic or potential genetic problems are listed below:

- Become familiar with terminology and concepts used in genetics.
- Become involved with public education about genetic disorders and their prevention.
- Help increase public awareness of availability of genetic services.
- After providing a referral or information about genetic counseling, follow up on the action that was taken.
- May tell clients what they can expect from the genetic counseling session.
- May accompany clients to the session if, for example, the nurse has a close professional relationship with them, and all parties involved agree.
- Identify meaning of the genetic problem involved for this client and family.
- Clarify misinterpretations and misunderstandings including information about presymptomatic or cancer risk assessment.
- Reinforce the information given by the geneticist.
- Help in alleviating guilt of family.
- Encourage the family or client to voice fears about issues such as acceptance, stigmatization, dependency, and uncertainties.
- Assess the coping mechanisms of the client or family and build upon strengths.
- Be able to explain meanings of results of commonly used genetic tests in the practice area of the nurse.
- Help in identifying and getting external supports needed—friends, agencies, financial aid sources, equipment resources, and others.
- Help the family identify ways to cope with the reactions of family, relatives, friends, and others.
- Refer client or family to community resources, schools, parent groups, and so on.
- Act as a liaison between the client or family and the resources and sources they will need.
- If the nurse identifies a significant degree of misunderstanding and misinterpretation, he or she may notify the geneticist so that the family may be recontacted immediately.
- Assess the client and family's ability to carry out the treatment plan or long-range goals.
- Be sensitive to common potential problems, such as strains within the mate relationship and problems arising in siblings (see chapter 8).

- Help the individual or family to reaffirm self-worth and value.
- Refer the family for further psychotherapeutic counseling if it appears necessary.
- Assist the family in decision-making by clarifying and identifying viable options.
- Clarify the available options related to reproductive planning and assist clients in obtaining necessary information.
- Be alert for crises in parenting if it is the child who has a genetic disorder.
- It may be appropriate for nurses to found and lead a group of parents if none exists in the area.
- Support decisions of client or family.
- Maintain contact and follow-up.
- Apprise counselor of any special information about the counselee that may assist him or her (e.g., cultural beliefs of the community).
- Assist in placing the genetic counseling information in the client's cultural context.
- Act as advocate for the family.

SOCIAL, LEGAL, AND ETHICAL ISSUES IN GENETIC COUNSELING

Some of the issues in this area overlap with those that are covered in the discussions of genetic screening, prenatal diagnosis, and genes and future generations (see chapters 11, 12, and 27), because counseling is a component of other programs. These include the issues of privacy; confidentiality; disclosure; sharing results with others, including family members, spouse, and outside persons such as insurance companies or employers; whether the counselor has a major responsibility to the counselee, to others, or to society; access to information, handling sensitive information such as uncovering misattributed parenthood; duty to recontact; and the issues of directive vs. nondirective counseling. Some of these issues have been discussed previously. Issues more specific to genetic counseling per se are discussed in this chapter. Whether the primary responsibility is to the counselee as an individual or to society is discussed in chapter 27 and is also addressed in the discussion of modes of counseling.

Most genetic counselors consider themselves responsible to the counselee. However, during the genetic counseling process, the counselor may encounter information that is important to relatives of the counselee. By knowledge of the disorder and its pattern of transmission, and by examining the pedigree of the family, other relatives at risk may be identified. Sometimes, the counselee will not wish for such relatives to be contacted for several reasons—fear of stigmatization, a desire not to be in contact with certain relatives, a belief that the relative will not want the information obtained, and others. This is a very delicate situation that deals with sensitive information. The President's Commission for the Study of Ethical Problems in Medicine and Biomedical and Behavioral Research (1983) recommended that under certain circumstances, the professional genetic counselor's primary obligation to a client may be subsumed. Their report states:

> "A professional's ethical duty of confidentiality to an immediate patient or client can be overridden only if several conditions are satisfied: 1) reasonable efforts to elicit voluntary consent to disclosure have failed; 2) there is a high probability both that harm will occur if the information is withheld and that the disclosed information will actually be used to avert harm; 3) the harm that identifiable individuals would suffer would be serious; and 4) appropriate precautions are taken to ensure that only the genetic information needed for diagnosis and/or treatment of the disease in question is disclosed."

Because of the complexity of breaching professional confidentiality, even in the context of the "duty to warn," it has been suggested that the person contemplating such action seek review by "an appropriate third party." Sometimes, the genetic counselor may be in a position to act as mediator between the counselee and other relatives in order to communicate information. The President's Commission has also recommended that changes be sought in adoption laws that will ensure that genetic risk information can be communicated to adoptees or biological relatives at risk. The Committee on Assessing Genetic Risk of the Institute of Medicine (1994) has also commented. They believe that patients should be encouraged to share genetic status information with their spouse. This, however, can have later consequences. For example, in a case in South Carolina, the husband of a woman known to be at risk for Huntington disease sought to terminate her parental rights, and she was ordered by the court to undergo genetic testing. The Committee also stated that while patients should share genetic information that would avert risk with relatives, that

> confidentiality be breached and relatives informed about genetic risks only when attempts to elicit voluntary disclosure fail, there is a high probability of irreversible or fatal harm to the relative, the disclosure of the information will prevent harm, the disclosure is limited to the information necessary for diagnosis or treatment of the relative, and there is no other reasonable way to avert the harm. (Institute of Medicine, Committee on Assessing Genetic Risks, p. 278)

For example, a relative at risk for malignant hyperthermia (see chapter 18) could have his or her life endangered by exposure to certain anesthetic agents if they possessed the mutant gene. In another situation, Tassicker et al. (2003) describe the situation where a pregnant woman whose male partner has a 50% chance for having Huntington disease wants to have prenatal diagnsosis but the male partner does not want to know his status. They pose the question of whether the right of the pregnant mother to know the status of her fetus outweighs the right of the father at risk to not know his genetic status. Leung (2000) presents the case in which one adult sibling is diagnosed with Wilson disease and does not wish to inform the other siblings who are patients of the same physician. The choices are to inform the siblings with appropriate education and counseling and refer them for testing, perform testing for Wilson disease when other blood tests are being done without informing them of the reason, or not inform them. The author concludes that the physician has an overriding duty to warn them, but discussants share other conclusions. There are many such examples of ethical issues that advances in genetics engender.

Another more recent statement on disclosure is by the American Society of Human Genetics (1998). Their discussion includes the point that genetic information is both personal and familial, and they provide a discussion of legal, and ethical considerations as well as international perspectives. Confidentiality is generally applied to genetic information like other medical information. They state however that ". . . confidentiality is not absolute, and, in exceptional cases, ethical, legal, and statutory obligations may permit health-care professionals to disclose otherwise confidential information" (p. 474). They outline exceptional circumstances that permit disclosure:

> (1) Disclosure should be permissible where attempts to encourage disclosure on the part of the patient have failed; where the harm is likely to occur and is serious and foreseeable; where the at-risk relative(s) is identifiable; and where either the disease is preventable/treatable or medically accepted standards indicate that early monitoring will reduce the genetic risk. (2) The harm that may result from failure to disclose should outweigh the harm that may result from disclosure. (p. 474)

Finally health-care professionals are said to have a duty to inform counselees that information obtained may have familial implications. They further state that the patient should be informed about the implications of their genetic test results and about potential risks to their family members. It is suggested that this be done both before genetic testing and when results are communicated. The American Society of Clinical Oncology (2003) also has a prepared statement in regard to disclosure and duty to warn family members who are at risk for genetically susceptible cancers, which is discussed in chapter 23. It is expected that the recent HIPAA regulations will have some impact in the area of disclosure.

Another issue is "duty to recontact." This refers to the possible obligation of the provider to contact a person who has previously sought counseling about advances in care that might benefit them. Examples of this include an ambiguous diagnosis or no diagnosis where a new test is now available, or those in which advances alter prognosis or estimates of the risk of reoccurrence. Many believe that while this is ethically desirable, it may be difficult to actually accomplish in regard to feasibility.

Areas of legal obligation in genetic counseling remain somewhat unclear, although some standards of care exist, particularly in regard to prenatal diagnosis. Those who are at known risk, however, are to be identified, receive appropriate information so that they can make choices, and be referred for services that may not be locally available. For example, an Ashkenazi Jewish couple contemplating pregnancy should be told about the availability of Tay-Sachs carrier testing, and what their risks would be to have a child with this disorder.

BIBLIOGRAPHY

Aalfs, C. M., Mollema, E. D., Oort, F. J., de Haes, J. C., Leschot, N. J., & Smets, E. M. (2004). Genetic counseling for familial conditions during pregnancy: An analysis of patient characteristics. *Clinical Genetics, 66,* 112–121.

Abramovsky, I., Godmilow, L., Hirschhorn, K., & Smith, H. (1980). Analysis of a follow-up study of genetic counseling. *Clinical Genetics, 17,* 1–12.

Agan, N., & Gregg, A. R. (2002). Elements of a genetics counseling service. *Obstetrics & Gynecology, 29,* 255–263.

American College of Obstetricians and Gynecologists. Committee Opinion. (1996, November). *Genetic evaluation of stillbirths and neonatal deaths.* (No. 178).

American College of Obstetricians and Gynecologists. ACOG Committee Opinion. (2001). Genetic evaluation of stillbirths and neonatal deaths. No. 257. *Obstetrics and Gynecology, 97*(5 Pt. 1), Suppl. 1–3.

American College of Obstetricians and Gynecologists. (2004). Prenatal and preconceptional carrier screening for genetic diseases in individuals of Eastern European Jewish descent. Committee Opinion, No. 298. *Obstetrics & Gynecology, 104,* 425–428.

American Society of Clinical Oncology. (2003). American Society of Clinical Oncology policy statement update: Genetic testing for cancer susceptibility. *Journal of Clinical Oncolgy, 21,* 2397–2406.

American Society of Human Genetics Social Issues Subcommittee on Familial Disclosure. (1998). Professional disclosure of familial genetic information. *American Journal of Human Genetics, 62,* 474–483.

Andrews, L. (1997). Body science. *American Bar Association Journal, 83,* 44–49.

Bartels, D., LeRoy, B. S., McCarthy, P., & Caplan, A. L. (1997). Nondirectiveness in genetic counseling: A survey of practitioners. *American Journal of Medical Genetics, 72,* 172–179.

Baumiller, R. C., Cunningham, G., Fisher, N., Fox, L., Henderson, M., Lebel, R., et al. (1996). Code of ethical principles for genetics professionals. An explication. *American Journal of Medical Genetics, 65,* 179–183.

Bernhardt, B. A. (1997). Empirical evidence that genetic counseling is directive: Where do we go from here? American *Journal of Human Genetics, 60,* 17–20.

Braithwaite, D., Emery, J., Walter, F., Prevost, A. T., & Sutton, S. (2004). Psychological impact of genetic counseling for familial cancer: A systematic review and meta-analysis. *Journal of the National Cancer Institute, 96,* 122–133.

Brundage, S. C. (2002). Preconception health care. *American Family Physician, 65,* 2507–2514.

Chadwick, R. F. (1993). What counts as success in genetic counseling? *Journal of Medical Ethics, 19,* 43–46.

Clarke, A. (1991). Is non-directive genetic counseling possible? Lancet, 338, 998-1001.

Clarke, A. (1993). Response to: What counts as success in genetic counseling? *Journal of Medical Ethics, 19,* 47–49.

Clayton, E. W., Hannig, V. L., Pfotenhauer, J. P., Parker, R. A., Campbell, P. W., III, & Phillips, J. A., III. (1995). Teaching about cystic fibrosis carrier screening by using written and video information. *American Journal of Human Genetics, 57,* 171–181.

Cole, L. J., & Fleisher, L. D. (2003). Update on HIPAA privacy: Are you ready? *Genetics in Medicine, 5,* 183–186.

Conti, A., Delbon, P., & Sirignaano, A. (2004). Informed consent when making genetic decisions. *Medical Law, 23,* 337–353.

Cutillo, D., Weinblatt, V., Nakata, N., Cronister, A., Wang, F., & Donnenfeld, A. E. (2003). Comparison of face to face and telephone genetic counseling. *xxxx101*(Suppl.), 19S–20S.

Donnai, D. (2002). Genetic services. Clinical Genetics, 61, 1-6.

Dugan, R. B., Wiesner, G. L., Juengst, E. T., O'Riordan, M. A., Matthews, A. L., & Robin, N. H. (2003). Duty to warn at-risk relatives for genetic disease: Genetic counselors' clinical experiences. *American Journal of Medical Genetics, Part C (Seminars in Medical Genetics), 119C,* 27–34.

Falk, M. J., Dugan, R. B., O'Riordan, M. A., Matthews, A. L., & Robin, N. H. (2003). Medical geneticists' duty to warn at-risk relatives for genetic disease. *American Journal of Medical Genetics, 120A,* 374–380.

Fisher, N. L. (Ed). (1996). *Cultural and ethnic diversity. A guide for genetics professionals.* Baltimore: Johns Hopkins University Press.

Fraser, F. C. (1974). Genetic counseling. *American Journal of Human Genetics, 26,* 636–661.

Genetic counseling. (1975). *American Journal of Human Genetics, 27,* 240–24.

Hallowell, N., Foster, C., Eeles, R., Ardern-Jones, A., Murday, V., & Watson, M. (2003). Balancing autonomy and responsibility: The ethics of generating and disclosing genetic information. *Journal of Medical Ethics, 29,* 74–83.

Hanoch, Y., & Pachur, T. (2004). Nurses as information providers: Facilitating understanding and communication of statistical information. *Nurse Educator Today, 24,* 236–243.

Institute of Medicine. (1994). *Assessing genetic risks. Implications for health and social policy.* Washington, DC: National Academy Press.

Kessler, S. (1992). Process issues in genetic counseling. *Birth Defects: Original Article Series, 28*(1), 1–10.

Kessler, S. (1997). Psychological aspects of genetic counseling. XI. Nondirectiveness revisited. *American Journal of Medical Genetics, 72,* 164–171.

Koch, L., & Nordahl Svendsen, M. (2005). Providing solutions—defining problems: The imperative of disease prevention in genetic counseling. *Social Science & Medicine, 60,* 823–832.

Leung, W-C. (2000). Results of genetic testing: When confidentiality conflicts with a duty to warn relatives. *British Medical Journal, 321,* 1464–1465.

Leuzzi, R. A., & Scoles, K. S. (1996). Preconception counseling for the primary care physician. *Medical Clinics of North America, 80*(2), 337–369.

Liu, W., Icitovic, N., Shaffer, M. L., & Chase, G. A. (2004). The impact of population heterogeneity on risk estimation in genetic counseling. *BMC Medical Genetics, 5,* 18–24.

Mariman, E. C. M. (2000). Act to resolve conflict. *British Medical Journal, 321,* 1465.

Lucassen, A., & Parker, M. (2001). Revealing false paternity: Some ethical considerations. *Lancet, 357,* 1033–1035.

Lucassen, A., & Parker, M. (2004). Confidentiality and serious harm in genetics—preserving the confidentiality of one patient and preventing harm to relatives. *European Journal of Human Genetics, 12,* 93–97.

Mehlman, M. J., Kodish, E. D., Whitehouse, P., Zinn, A. B., Sollitto, S., Berger, J., et al. (1996). The need for anonymous genetic counseling and testing. *American Journal of Human Genetics, 58,* 393–397.

Michie, S. (1994). Genetic counseling. *Journal of Medical Ethics, 20,* 268–271.

Michie, S., Bron, F., Bobrow, M. & Marteau, T. M. (1997). Non-directiveness in genetic counseling: An empirical study. *American Journal of Human Genetics, 60,* 40–47.

National Society of Genetic Counselors. (1992). National Society of Genetic counselors code of ethics. *Journal of Genetic Counseling, 1,* 41–43.

Offit, K., Groeger, E., Turner, S., Wadsworth, E. A., & Weiser, M. A. (2004). The "duty to warn" a patient's family members about hereditary disease risks. *Journal of the American Medical Association, 292,* 1469–1473.

Parker, M., & Luckassen, A. (2003). Concern for families and individuals in clinical genetics. *Journal of Medical Ethics, 29,* 70–73.

Pearn, J. H. (1973). Patients' subjective interpretation of risks offered in genetic counseling. *Journal of Medical Genetics, 10,* 129–134.

Plantinga, L., Natowicz, M. R., Kass, N. E., Hull, S. C., Gostin, L. O., & Faden, R. R. (2003). Disclosure, confidentiality, and families: Experiences and attitudes of those with genetic versus non-genetic medical conditions. *American Journal of Medical Genetics Part C (Seminars in Medical Genetics), 119C,* 51–59.

Plunkett, K. S., & Simpson, J. L. (2002). A general approach to genetic counseling. *Obstetrics and Gynecology Clinics of North America, 29,* 269–276.

Port, K. E., Mountain, H., Nelson, J., & Bittles, A. H. (2005). Changing profile of couples seeking genetic counseling for consanguinity in Australia. *American Journal of Medical Genetics, A, 132A,* 159–163.

President's Commission for the Study of Ethical Problems in Medicine and Biomedical and Behavioral Research: Screening and Counseling for Genetic Conditions. (1983). Washington DC: GPO.

Puñales-Morejon, D. (1997). Genetic counseling and prenatal diagnosis: A multicultural perspective. *Journal of the American Medical Women's Association, 52*(1), 30–32.

Puñales-Morejon, D., & Penchaszadeh, V. B. (1992). Psychosocial aspects of genetic counseling: Cross-cultural issues. *Birth Defects: Original Article Series, 28*(1), 11–15.

Rapp, R. (1997). Communicating about chromosomes: Patients, providers, and cultural assumptions. *Journal of the American Medical Women's Association, 52*(1), 28–29, 32.

Reed, S. (1980). *Counseling in medical genetics* (3rd ed.). New York: Alan R. Liss.

Rowley, P. T., Loader, S., Sutera, C. J., & Kozyra, A. (1995). Prenatal genetic counseling for hemoglobinopathy carriers: A comparison of primary providers of prenatal care and professional genetic counselors. *American Journal of Human Genetics, 56*, 769–776.

Sankar, P. (2003). Genetic privacy. *Annual Review of Medicine, 54*, 393–407.

Sharpe, N. F. (1994). Psychological aspects of genetic counseling: A legal perspective. *American Journal of Medical Genetics, 50*, 234-238.

Surh, L. C., Wright, P. G., Cappelli, M., Kasaboski, A., Hastings, V. A., Hunter, A. G., et al. (1995). Delivery of molecular genetic services within a health care system: Time analysis of the clinical workload. *American Journal of Human Genetics, 56*, 760–768.

Swan, L. L., & Apgar, B. S. (1995). Preconceptual obstetric risk assessment and health promotion. *American Family Physician, 51*, 1875–1885.

Tassicker, R., Savulescu, J., Skene, L., Marshall, P., Fitzgerald, L., & Delatycki, M. B. (2003). Prenatal diagnosis requests for Huntington's disease when the father is at risk and does not want to know his genetic status: Clinical, legal, and ethical viewpoints. *British Medical Journal, 326*, 331–333.

Uhlmann, W. R., Ginsburg, D., Gelehrter, D., Nicholson, J., & Petty, E. M. (1996). Questioning the need for anonymous genetic counseling and testing. *American Journal of Human Genetics, 59*, 968–970.

Wachbroit, R., & Wasserman, D. (1995). Clarifying the goals of non-directive genetic counseling. *Philosophy & Public Policy, 15*(2&3), 1–6.

Weaver, D. D., & Escobar, L. F. (1987). Twenty-four ways to have children. *American Journal of Medical Genetics, 26*, 737–740.

Wille, M. C., Weitz, B., Kerper, P., & Frazier, S. (2004). Advances in preconception genetic counseling. *Journal of Perinatal and Neonatal Nursing, 18*, 28–40.

Wolff, G., & Jung, C. (1995). Non-directiveness and genetic counseling. *Journal of Genetic Counseling, 4*, 3–25.

Yarborough, M., Scott, J. A., & Dixon, L. K. (1989). The role of beneficence in clinical genetics. Non-directive counseling reconsidered. *Theoretical Medicine, 10*, 139–140.

11

Genetic Testing and Screening

Genetic testing may be offered or conducted within the context of general or targeted population screening programs or be offered to specific at-risk individuals and families, but the term "genetic testing" commonly refers to the use of specific tests for individuals who are believed to be at increased risk for a specific genetic condition because of their family history or symptom manifestations. The Task Force on Genetic Testing defined a genetic test as "The analysis of human DNA, RNA, chromosomes, proteins and certain metabolites in order to detect heritable disease-related genotypes, mutations, phenotypes, or karyotypes for clinical purposes" (Holtzman & Watson, 1997, p. 6). This can be a very inclusive definition and others look towards a narrower one. Their definition excludes testing solely for research, for somatic mutations, and for forensic purposes. They subdivide predictive testing performed in apparently healthy people into presymptomatic tests and predispositional tests. Genetic testing can include laboratory assays and other tests performed on blood, urine, fibroblasts, amniotic fluid or cells, chorionic villi, hair bulbs, squamous cells from the buccal mucosa or other tissue samples. Genetic screening involves testing of populations or groups that is independent of a positive family history or symptom manifestations and includes some predictive genetic testing. Screening may include population-based programs that are commonly sponsored by hospitals, health centers, community groups, or governmental agencies such as heterozygote (carrier) and newborn screening, those aimed at all pregnant women for detection of fetal anomalies, such as maternal serum screening for alpha-fetoprotein and other markers, or those conducted in the context of a specific industry or workplace for predictive screening. The concept of testing is aimed at individuals or families for specific reasons such as family history that may include carrier, presymptomatic, or predictive testing for traditional genetic disorders or for diseases such as certain breast cancers that may be called "cascade" screening when offered to extended family members. Genetic tests may be done for:

- detecting or diagnosing a present disease state,
- determining carrier status,
- detecting disease susceptibility,
- detecting abnormalities in the fetus, and
- the prediction of diseases in usually asymptomatic persons that may include late-onset or adult disorders.

Although there can be differences in the use of the term "screening," an acceptable definition is the presumptive identification of an unrecognized disease or defect in an apparently healthy individual. Genetic screening was more specifically defined by the Committee for the Study of Inborn Errors of Metabolism (1975) of the National Academy of Sciences, and this is still the accepted definition. Essentially it is a search in a population for:

1. persons who possess genotypes that are associated with the development of genetic disease. The usual purpose is so that treatment can be instituted or the natural course of the disease altered. An example of this is screening newborns for PKU in order to restrict their diet to prevent mental retardation.

2. persons with certain genotypes that are known to predispose the individual to illness. An

example of this is the identification of individuals with G6PD deficiency who, after being identified, can avoid the precipitation of hemolytic anemia by avoiding certain foods and drugs, as discussed in chapter 18.

3. persons who are the heterozygous carriers of recessively inherited genes that, in autosomal recessive disorders (in double dose), can cause genetic disease in their descendants. An example of this would be screening programs for the detection of Tay-Sachs carriers. This type of screening provides information to an individual so that he or she can make reproductive plans for the future. Genetic counseling, including the discussion of reproductive options and the availability of prenatal diagnosis, is an essential component of this type of screening;

4. persons with polymorphisms (variations) not now known to be associated with a disease state. This allows for the gathering of information relative to the genetic makeup of the population. This may begin as research and later have therapeutic value. A common example is in the observed variation of the human blood groups.

Screening may be whole-population based or may be more specifically directed, for example to a particular ethnic group. Genetic testing is usually directed at specific persons at elevated risk.

As further technical advances in disease detection and diagnosis occur, the potential for the expansion of genetic testing and screening programs will grow. Therefore, nurses will be increasingly involved in such programs and in different practice settings. In the community, program emphasis may be on the identification of individuals who are carriers of a deleterious gene but are not ill themselves, or screening may involve the identification of individuals who are potentially susceptible to exposure to certain chemicals used in the workplace. Nurses working with newborns and infants will certainly be part of neonatal screening whether it is in the hospital or community. School nurses in some areas may be involved in screening programs or in the results of genetic tests for a specific child. Nurses may be responsible for or involved in planning for such a program, implementing it, and evaluating the outcomes. As genetic testing and screening become integral parts of primary care, health professionals themselves

will need to understand the tests, the meaning of the results, the emotional and psychological impact of both positive and negative results, the potential for impact on insurability and employment and what options are available, and be able to provide education and interpretation of the results to clients and family members.

The previous definition(s) lead to the major acceptable reasons for genetic testing and screening—treatment, supportive management, successful adaptation, education, the provision of reproductive information, the offering of prenatal diagnosis and reproductive options, genetic counseling, implementation of preventive strategies often to modify risk or disease severity, the description of the natural history of a genetic disease when no treatment is available, and the gathering of information for research purposes such as enumeration. The use of genetic screening for political or eugenic ends is never acceptable, and is discussed later in this chapter. Genetic testing of gamete donors and for presymptomatic or predictive reasons such as for Huntington disease are discussed later in this chapter. Genetic testing related to prenatal diagnosis, cancer, and Alzheimer disease are discussed in chapters 12, 23, and 21, respectively.

INFORMATION BEFORE CHOOSING GENETIC TESTING/SCREENING

Genetic testing and screening should take place within the context of adequate and appropriate education provided at the level of the client's understanding, that takes into consideration and respects their ethnic and cultural values and beliefs. It should include access to genetic and other counseling, further diagnostic options if needed or appropriate, appropriate therapeutic interventions, and/or preventative or prophylactic strategies. The environment for informed consent and the decision to participate should be free of coercion, and understanding should be evaluated. Before undertaking testing or screening, information on health, medical and life insurance coverage, both for the testing/screening and for follow-up care depending on the results, should be ascertained. For serious diseases such as Huntington disease, the client may be asked to bring a support person with him or her if they wish—this of course compromises privacy and confidentiality but may be desired by the client. Careful thought needs to be given as to who the person should be and if it is appropriate for the client. Long-term psychosocial counseling should be available for those undergoing presymptomatic testing. Clients should have the right to choose testing or screening without coercion into a clinical trial, although sometimes these circumstances may be protective. Sometimes the impetus to undergo testing is not from the client but is at the behest of an insurance company, other family member, adoption agency, potential mate, or employer. Testing should be the decision of the person being tested without repercussion. Information specific to predictive cancer testing is given in chapter 23. The following is information that should be provided by the health care provider to the client considering genetic testing:

- the reason that testing is appropriate for this person/family;
- what is being tested for;
- what estimation of risk and for surveillance can be done without genetic testing;
- what the procedure being considered entails, including description, cost, length of time, where it is to be done;
- what can and cannot be tested—if relevant, this should include the information that while some mutations will be looked for and detected, other rare ones might not be, and that negative results refer only to whatever was being tested or screened for and not to every genetic disorder; for example, if one is testing for CF, the most common mutations in that population group will be looked for but not every very rare mutation will be tested for;
- what would both positive and negative results mean, including that negative results do not necessarily translate to a zero risk, that a positive test may result in fear and anxiety, whereas negative results can also have emotional and relationship impact;
- he accuracy, validity, and reliability of the test, including the likelihood of false negative or false positive results and the suitability of this test for the information the client is seeking;

- the possibility that testing will not yield additional risk information;
- the length of time between the procedure and when the results are obtained;
- how the results will be communicated to the client;
- what will be analyzed;
- whether the actual test result will be revealed; for example, in Huntington disease, in some cases there may be some correlation between the number of CAG repeats and the predicted age-of-onset, but there is a gray area, so some centers do not disclose the actual number although the ACMG/ASHG (1998) have recommended such disclosure;
- what happens to the sample used for testing—who owns it, what uses are possible;
- a discussion of the possible risks of life and health insurance coverage and/or employment discrimination after testing results are done, although there may be benefits, such as if a person is free of a certain mutation, better insurance rates or coverage might result;
- the level of confidentiality of results and what this means (who can know or find out the results);
- risks of psychological distress and negative impact not only on the individual but also on the family, including stigmatization and altered self-image;
- risk of passing on the mutation in the disorder being tested for to children and the meaning of the risks;
- what disclosure might the client consider for other family members and who will he or she tell (if anyone) about the test results; and what obligation might the health provider feel to inform other family members;
- provision for referral for periodic surveillance, further testing, lifestyle changes, and/or treatment after testing if needed; and
- what these mean in the context of both positive and negative tests. As in other genetic testing, a negative test can have several meanings: that the individual is truly free of the disease, that the result is "false negative" due to laboratory error, that the case is sporadic, or there is the possession of alternate alleles than what could or was tested for.

PLANNING A GENETIC SCREENING PROGRAM

The major types of population-based genetic screening programs are those for (a) detecting genetic disease in newborns, (b) identifying carriers of recessive genes, (c) prenatal detection including maternal serum screening for various analytes (see chapter 12), and (d) predictive or presymptomatic screening in the workplace (see chapter 14).

The stimulus to begin a specific screening program may originate in a variety of ways, and pressure for screening services often arises out of enthusiasm instead of reason. Programs may be initiated because a test for a condition has been developed, and not by rational selection of a specific genetic disorder amenable to screening. Actual impetus may come from investigators or institutions interested in research or field testing, community groups at high risk for a specific disorder, legislators responding to constituent concerns, general public pressure generated by mass media information or citizen groups interested in a specific condition. Different groups, such as the ones just mentioned, may wish to actually provide the screening services alone or in conjunction with a local or state health department, hospital, school or community-based clinic, or these health care institutions may initiate screening. Important considerations in planning a genetic screening program are summarized in Table 11.1.

Because resources are not limitless, and not every condition is amenable to screening, certain criteria should be considered when deciding if, in fact, the disorder in question warrants the initiation of a new program or inclusion in a long-standing one. Genetic screening shares many principles and

TABLE 11.1   Considerations in Planning a Genetic Screening Program (order may vary)

Request for screening or recognition of problem

Assess the need

Justify the need

Determine feasibility and appropriateness

Decide on type of screening program

Designate target population, its health status, and its use of the health system

Establish goals and objectives based on sound ethical principles

Consider the cultural, ethnic, and religious beliefs and practices of the population

Identify and seek cooperation of both lay and professional community leaders

Plan program in conjunction with these leaders (include consumer representative)

Rank and prioritize goals

Identify alternative courses of action

Determine type and extent of program services to be provided

Identify program needs and resources—facilities, equipment personnel, and budget

Determine how program effectiveness will be measured and evaluated

Redefine objectives and goals in light of above

Establish policies and procedural guidelines

Assess awareness and knowledge of lay and professional communities at large

Plan and implement educational program by lay and professional workers

Recruit and train community volunteers

Plan publicity and media campaigns

Select screening site, technique or test, and services to be offered

If possible, run a small trial program, evaluate, and revise based on evaluation

Implement screening program

Evaluate and revise constantly, including cost/benefit ratio and cost-effectiveness

Note. The available budget may determine the components of the program and the extent of the services or vice versa. Provision for education, counseling, follow-up of those with positive results, diagnostic referral, recordkeeping, privacy, and treatment provisions are essential.

characteristics with mass screening for nongenetic disorders but some reflect the unique nature of genetic disorders. Genetic disorders are permanent, can be threatening to a person's self-esteem and identity, may have unintended consequences and implications for insurance and employment based on "pre-existing" conditions, and have implications not only for the person being tested but also for his/her relatives and descendants because screening is not only for the actual disease state but also for the carrier condition. Several basic major questions (described next) should be addressed before making a decision on whether or not a mass screening program should be initiated for a particular genetic condition.

Importance of the Disorder

Is the disorder or condition for which screening is being considered an important problem? "Important" can be interpreted to mean either that it is prevalent in the population or that it is a serious problem. Individually, each genetic disease is relatively rare. However, as a group, the burden is significant. By preventing mental retardation from occurring by neonatal screening for a disorder such as hypothyroidism, the cost to society of supportive or institutional care is eliminated, to say nothing of the elimination of financial and less tangible burdens to the family. Another way to evaluate the importance of a disorder is to examine its prevalence in a select high-risk population. An example of this would be considering the initiation of carrier testing for thalassemia in a community population of Greek ancestry, where the carrier rate would be substantially above that of the population as a whole. Such testing would consistently increase the cost effectiveness and maximize the resources available. Another consideration, especially for newborn screening, is whether importance is not only incidence, but also seriousness and potential prevention or modification of complications, short and long term morbidity, potential impact, and disability amelioration.

Availability of Screening Test

Is there a technique available that is suited for use in screening or detection as opposed to use in diagnosis? Such a test must meet certain criteria discussed later in this chapter. The test available may also determine the type of screening program to be offered. Testing should take place in an accredited, experienced laboratory to ensure quality of genetic tests. For some disorders, not every mutation known can be screened for due to logistical and cost considerations. There may also be variation in techniques used to screen for certain disorders—some may be more accurate than others.

Understanding and Potentially Altering the Natural History of the Disorder in Question

Can the disorder be favorably influenced with detection by screening as opposed to later diagnosis? For example, would there be a point in screening all Jewish infants in a community for Tay-Sachs disease when there is no known treatment at present? Or would the maximum benefit be derived from carrier testing and prenatal diagnosis in a high-risk population subgroup? What is the appropriate population to screen for the condition in question? If a disease state itself is screened for, is there some presymptomatic or latent period that is detectable by a screening test? Another consideration that follows is whether or not there is an effective, acceptable, recognized treatment available that improves survival or function. If the carrier state is screened for, what are the implications of being a carrier? It is not acceptable to screen populations, identify individuals with a disorder, and then have nothing to offer them in regard to treatment. For genetic disorders, genetic counseling and the offering of reproductive options or prenatal diagnosis is usually considered a legitimate screening goal. The collection of research data alone without some direct benefit to the client such as the above is usually not sufficient as the reason to establish screening. For newborn screening, in cases where little data are available for long-term outlook and impact, should this influence decisions about screening? In other words, should a disorder be included in the routine newborn screening programs if there is no clear evidence that early detection and/or treatment has significant impact upon the long-term outlook? Would it include the opportunity for supportive and anticipatory management, successful adapatation, education, offering genetic counseling and prenatal diagnosis, allowing reproductive and life planning, and prevention strategies to modify risk and severity of illness as well as complications. An example of the latter is the use of prophylactic treatment with penicillin and enrollment in comprehensive care to reduce the morbidity and mortality of children with sickle cell disease.

Appropriateness and Feasibility Including Facilities for Diagnosis and Treatment

Assuming that the previous considerations are met, what facilities are needed? What are available? What other resources are needed? Are there available resources for diagnostic referral for those patients with positive screening tests? What treatment facilities are available? Are laboratory facilities available and satisfactory? What else is needed? There needs to be a full program including education, counseling, testing recalls and confirmatory testing, further diagnostic procedures, referrals to specialists, and comprehensive treatment including a multidisciplinary approach. Is the agency considering screening the one that can best provide the service? Is it an appropriate one for the agency to expend resources on? Is the problem a major need for this population? Is there evidence of substantial benefit to the selected population? Is there evidence of acceptance on the part of the population? At a minimum, a screening program should include clear goals; appropriate education of the lay and professional segments of the target population; informed consent; policies based on ethical principles; provision for privacy and confidentiality; be voluntary without coercion; utilize a satisfactory, suitable screening technique; have laboratory facilities available; provide for diagnostic referral, follow-up, counseling, and recordkeeping; have enough personnel to implement the program; and include a means for evaluation. Questions have been raised as to whether or not screening programs, particularly for newborns, should be initiated for purposes of supportive and anticipatory management, life planning, and preventive strategies to modify risk and severity of illness as well as complications. Also in the case of newborns, the need for continued family-centered, community-coordinated treatment and care into adulthood is increasingly recognized.

Cost/Benefit and Cost/Effectiveness

A final consideration is that of program cost versus benefit. How can the cost of the screening program be justified when balanced against diagnosis after the disorder has manifested itself? For genetic disorders, the burden of disease is both tangible and intangible (see chapter 8). A few recent cost-effectiveness studies have been undertaken. They demonstrate that the cost-benefit ratio is favorable in neonatal screening for hypothyroidism. Others, like maple syrup urine disease (MSUD), may be cost effective when it is included with other disorders in newborn screening programs, but would be less cost-effective if a community-at-large was screened for carriers of MSUD given the low incidence and a relatively undefined population at risk. Also, using one specimen for multiple screening tests means that screening very early in life can miss some disorders such as PKU, whereas if it is done later, damage from others such as MSUD will already have occurred. Another issue is whether cost should include human suffering. Should, for example, newborn screening be done universally for all detectable metabolic conditions because no cost should be spared to detect even one affected newborn?

ELEMENTS IN ORGANIZATION OF THE PROGRAM

Once it has been determined that screening for a particular genetic disorder is appropriate, justified, and feasible, other planning should begin. These elements will vary, depending on the type of program. Some of these are discussed next.

Types of Screening

The choice of a type of screening program evolves from the previously discussed definition of genetic screening. Of these, the two most frequent purposes of screening are for either detection of the disease state itself or detection of the carrier state. The most common types of screening for actual genetic disease states is in newborns, usually to allow the earliest possible treatment and management to be instituted so that damage can be minimized. Programs for detection of carriers of deleterious autosomal or X-linked recessive disorders are most often conducted among young adults in specific population groups in an outpatient or community setting in order to provide genetic counseling, information on which reproductive choices can be made, and to offer prenatal diagnostic services. Screening for the carrier state is not always as feasible as detecting the actual disease state, even if it is desirable. A test may not be able to distinguish between the "normal" state and the carrier state but only between normal and diseased. Specific aspects of carrier screening are discussed later. Knowledge of elements of the genetic disorder such as its frequency in different population subgroups, available test capability, and choice of screening program type help to determine the population who should be screened in a specific community, whether it be on the basis of age, race, ethnic origin, or some other parameter. Some are geared to young adults in specific ethnic groups, as in premarital screening so that reproductive options can be clarified.

Target Population

Delineation of a target group at whom the screening program is directed also helps to make decisions about other program elements such as location, educational approach, time, format, types of counseling, facilities, equipment, and publicity. For example, if the screening is aimed at young adult couples, weekdays from 9 AM to 5 PM will not yield the largest number of participants. If young children or mothers are part of the target group, childcare facilities should be planned for, perhaps in conjunction with volunteer groups in the community. Any particular social, cultural, or religious practices affecting the population to be screened should be identified. For example, a Tay-Sachs screening program in an orthodox Jewish neighborhood held on a Saturday will show few, if any, attendees. These aspects are more important in screening populations other than newborns, as that setting (the hospital) usually is predetermined and the newborn is essentially a captive population, whereas for others screening is purely voluntary. The geographic area covered by screening will also delineate the target group. For a young population of high school education or less, educational information may be presented in a multimedia format or use a "soap opera" or "true confession" approach.

Site, Facilities, and Resources

An appropriate screening site must be selected. It should be easily accessible to the target population. It should have the space to include all the resources that are deemed necessary for the program such as an area and facilities (1) for intake and reception, (2) where education before screening can be carried out, (3) where needed personal data can be confidentially obtained, (4) for waiting before the actual screening test, (5) for child-care facilities if needed, (6) where the test procedure is done, (7) for administrative purposes, (8) for specimen collection and storage, (9) for maintenance of records, and (10) for genetic counseling. Requirements may vary if the actual processing of the specimen takes place on-site or somewhere else, and if diagnostic referral facilities, counseling, and follow-up services, or other program components are located on-site or elsewhere. The screening site will also be influenced by whether plans are for an ongoing program, a short-term program, or a one-shot type of screening. Screening programs have been held in such diverse locations as shopping malls, churches, schools, neighborhood health centers, barber and beauty shops, laundromats, street corners, hospitals, clinics, physicians' offices, and work settings. Selection depends on the aims of the program, the needs of the targeted population, and accessibility for that population. Selected steps in a community screening program are shown in Figure 11.1.

While screening in a temporary site such as a neighborhood facility may help to increase participation in the screening program, disadvantages also are possible. One important consideration is establishing some type of permanent location or base for the data collected during screening, such as the person's personal information and test results. After an initial mass screening program it may be most effective to incorporate screening of additional individuals into a permanent health-related institution such as a genetic counseling center. Records could then be maintained in one place, knowledgeable people could be available for later clarification about the disorder, and people needing further services could obtain them.

If personnel resources need supplementing, volunteers from the target population are sometimes used, but the clients' privacy and confidentiality

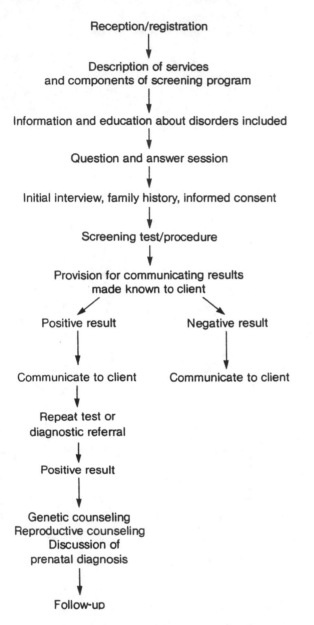

Reception/registration

↓

Description of services
and components of screening program

↓

Information and education about disorders included

↓

Question and answer session

↓

Initial interview, family history, informed consent

↓

Screening test/procedure

↓

Provision for communicating results
made known to client

↙   ↘

Positive result   Negative result

↓   ↓

Communicate to client   Communicate to client

↓

Repeat test or
diagnostic referral

↓

Positive result

↓

Genetic counseling
Reproductive counseling
Discussion of
prenatal diagnosis

↓

Follow-up

FIGURE 11.1   Selected steps in a community screening program at the site.

should be maintained. These issues should be addressed before recruitment, not afterwards.

Characteristics of a Suitable Screening Test

The qualities sought in selecting a test for use in a genetic screening program are listed in Table 11.2. Few tests fulfill all desired qualities equally well.

TABLE 11.2   Qualities of an Ideal Screening Test or Procedure

Rapid
Inexpensive
Simple
Sensitive
Specific } Few false-positives and false-negatives
Safe
Acceptable
Valid
Uses easily available specimens and material
Reproducible
Causes minimum of discomfort and inconvenience to
    client
Can be automated

Such qualities as absolute precision may be sacrificed for others such as low cost, since further confirmatory diagnostic workups need to be done anyway if positive results are found. The more quickly a test can be performed, the greater the benefit to both client and the provider. Waiting time will be decreased, minimizing the number of clients who may decide not to participate. In addition, a greater number of people can be served in a shorter time, adding to increased cost effectiveness as fewer provider personnel may be needed.

The test procedure and specimen should be subject to as little clerical processing, handling, and storage as possible in order to keep accuracy to a maximum. Simplicity in technique will also help to decrease error. Sensitivity and specificity are important in discussing screening tests, as are the related concepts of true positive, false positive, true negative, and false negative. Ideally, a screening test should be both highly sensitive and highly specific and have a low percentage of both false-positive and false-negative results. The sensitivity of a test measures the accuracy of the screening test in giving a positive result in all subjects actually having the disease being screened for. For a test to be 100% sensitive, it must correctly identify all people having the disorder in question. The specificity of a test is its accuracy in giving a negative result in all those who do not have the disease being screened for. For a test to be 100% specific, it must correctly discriminate all those who do not have the disorder in question. A test that is not sufficiently sensitive does not recognize all those who do have the disorder. A nonspecific test can falsely identify a healthy person as one who has the disorder. In the apparently healthy population group being screened, there are actually two subgroups of people—those who have the disorder and those who do not. There are also two possible results of the screening test used to discriminate between these two groups of people—normal (negative) and abnormal (positive). The term "true positive" is used to denote those people who had a positive (abnormal) test result and who also have the disorder. "False positive" is used for those who had a positive test result but do not have the disease. The term "true negative" is used to denote those individuals who had a negative (normal) test result and are truly free of the disorder. "False negative" refers to those individuals who have a negative test result but actually have the disorder in question. Tests giving low rates of both false positive and false negatives are most desirable. A high level of false positive results will lead to over-referral for further diagnosis and a high cost, whereas a high number of false negatives will lead to missing the individuals who are being sought, depriving them of treatment, and thus decreasing the effectiveness of screening.

As an example, if one were setting up a blood pressure screening program for the detection of hypertension, a decision would have to be made as to what would constitute an abnormal blood pressure reading. If a reading of 130/80 mm Hg were chosen, one would be relatively sure all those individuals with hypertension would be detected. However, one would also classify many individuals as hypertensive who were not (false positives). Thus, the detection program would be highly sensitive but nonspecific. If a reading of 160/100 mm Hg were chosen, one would be relatively sure all those who did not have hypertension were not classified as positive, but many of those who were hypertensive would be missed (false negatives). Thus, there would be a high level of specificity but low sensitivity.

Another term also associated with the previous discussion is that of "predictive value." Positive predictive value refers to the probability that the disorder screened for is present when the test is positive, while negative predictive value is the probability that disease is not present when the screening test is negative. The test or measure chosen for the screening

program being established should be a valid indicator of the disease—it should be a true measure of the disorder in question. It should not be subject to a wide variety of interpretation. There should be agreement on what the results mean. Establishing ranges of normal and abnormal for the measure being used should be done before beginning a screening program. An accredited, reputable, experienced laboratory with established quality-control standards should provide services. The Secretary's Advisory Committee on Genetic Testing (SACGT) (2000) for the Department of Health and Human Services recommended that any DNA or related test be formally evaluated to assess its analytic and clinical validity and suggested this be vested with the FDA. Despite all precautions, errors in results of tests can still occur. These are summarized in Table 11.3. Several of these errors can be minimized by proper handling of the specimen. Others are dependent on characteristics of the participant in screening, such as diet and medication ingested. Information regarding these should accompany the specimen submitted. A not uncommon source of error in newborn screening for metabolic errors occurs because the infant has not yet ingested enough formula or substrate to ascertain any abnormal processing. Another problem leading to false positive findings results when a test is done early in life and a particular infant has an immature enzyme system, which is not indicative of disease process but is only transient. An infant may need to be retested later if clinical evidence suggests the need, even if a screening test result was negative for the disorder in question. This is why further diagnostic investigation may be needed. Occasionally, missed detection results from failure to obtain a sample or failure to transport it to the lab. Regardless of the reason, nurses should anticipate that the parents will experience anxiety and apprehension when called for retesting. The qualities that most concern the client in a screening program are those of acceptability, convenience, comfort, and safety. Most clients participating in screening are volunteers who have been "recruited." They usually feel well. Therefore, although they may be convinced to submit a urine specimen or allow venous blood to be drawn, it is less likely that they would allow a skin biopsy to be done or to submit to proctoscopy. For a screening program to attract large numbers of individuals from the

TABLE 11.3   Factors Responsible for Inaccurate Screening Test Results

False negatives
    Unusual variant present
    Too early for defect present to be manifested
    Disorder is only detectable under certain conditions (i.e., stress)
    Inadequate nutritional intake
    Loss of specimen material

False positives
    Medications
    Special infant diets (i.e., soybean formulas)
    Hyperalimentation
    Transient metabolic aberration
    Production of a metabolite interfering with test
    Hypersensitivity of laboratory test used

Both
    Improper handling of specimen
    Improper storage of specimen
    Poor laboratory reliability
    Clerical error
    Delay in processing specimen
    Immature enzyme systems
    Improper laboratory procedures

group desired, specimens must be easily obtainable so that there is a minimum of inconvenience and discomfort.

PLANNING PROGRAM COMPONENTS AND SERVICES

The aims, objectives, and policies of the specific program should be clearly delineated. The most effective way is to involve community representatives and leaders from the population group in which screening is contemplated, local health professional representatives, and representatives from local foundations for that disorder, if any exist.

These individuals should be able to assess the readiness of the population to be screened in terms of their knowledge of the condition in question. The kind of education needed prior to the screening can then be planned. Thus education may be not only for the population being screened, but also for health professionals. For such professionals to participate by support, referral, and active involvement, they need to understand both the disorder and the aims, objectives, and components of the screening program. Policy guidelines should be established. If a carrier screening program is aimed

at young married couples, will a single person be allowed access? Will a couple in their fifties be allowed access? Equal access should be weighed against balancing harm and benefits, including test accuracy in different groups and cost-effectiveness. Such problems should be anticipated and discussed before program implementation.

The community advisory representatives will have knowledge of the sociocultural beliefs, practices, and language needs that may be unique or important to the population group and which can seriously affect the success of the program. For example, who are the decision-makers and authority-figures in this ethnic group? What are the cultural beliefs about genetic disease? How is gender valued? Are individuals empowered in regard to decision-making? How is the body viewed and treated? Will interpreters be needed? Knowledge of these practices should be used in preparing materials and determining methods for publicity, education, counseling, follow-up, and referral. They also may affect the screening test format to be used and the context in which it is explained.

Other decisions need to be made. What personal data will be collected from screening participants? What type and how long will records be kept? How will informed consent be obtained?

How will results be communicated to participants? How will confidentiality be safeguarded? To whom will results be released? What will happen to the sample? Have appropriate arrangements been made for diagnostic testing for those with positive test results? What type and degree of counseling is needed? How many and what type of professionals are needed in the screening program? How will the program be evaluated? Will those with positive results be entered into a registry?

GENETIC TESTING AND SCREENING FOR HETEROZYGOTE (CARRIER)

Each person is a carrier for five to seven recessive harmful genes for rare disorders. These are so rare that usually one's chosen mate does not carry the same ones. When this does occur, genetic disease can occur in the offspring. This is explained further in chapter 6. Both carrier testing and carrier screening are available. Carrier testing is more usually done in a specialized setting and involves individuals already known to be of high risk because of family history, whereas carrier screening usually involves those with no family history and takes place in other settings. The autosomal recessive (AR) disorders most commonly screened for are sickle cell anemia and Tay-Sachs disease. Cystic fibrosis (CF) screening is possible but at present there are more than 1,000 mutations of the *CFTR* gene that can result in CF, and so widespread population testing is somewhat difficult, particularly in some groups. Within families, genetic testing can be much more accurate, basically directed at the most common mutations, increasing the detection rate greatly. DNA testing for CF is 90–95% sensitive for those mutations common in Ashkenazi Jews, Bretons, French Canadians, and Native Americans; about 90% of the U. S. White population generally; about 75% accurate for African Americans; 57% accurate for Hispanic Americans; and only 30% accurate for Asian Americans. Thus the consensus statement issued by the National Institutes of Health (NIH) on genetic testing for CF in 1997 recommended offering testing for adults with a family history of CF, partners of a person with CF, couples planning pregnancy, and couples seeking prenatal testing. They estimate the cost of DNA testing for CF at between $50 and

$150. They did not recommend general population screening or newborn screening for CF in this report. The ACMG originally supported this, except that they believed that offering testing for couples who are planning pregnancy or already pregnant was premature until genetic counseling and educational supports were available and there was adequate experience with testing for mutations for CF in the ethnic and racial groups to be served (American College of Medical Genetics, 1998). In 2001, however, they issued a report about CF screening, encouraging preconception testing using either a sequential model in which one of the couple, usually the woman, is tested first, and if positive, then her partner, or doing both together. Among its recommendations was that CF population-based carrier screening be offered to Caucasians and made available to other ethnic and racial groups after education about the rarity of CF and the low detectability of the currently available test in their populations (most prevalent pan-ethnic mutations, about 25 including the most prevalent, ΔF508), will be included but this represents about 80% detection of all CF alleles) (Grody et al., 2001). Thus, there is some concern because about 20% of carriers can be missed, especially in non-White populations. They also specify including the R117H mutation which, along with the 5T and 7T variants, is associated with male infertility due to congenital bilateral absence of the vas deferens. The logistics of adding this to population screening programs because of the sheer numbers at potential risk (1 in 20 to 25 white Americans of Northern European ancestry are carriers) are enormous.

Some of the spectrum of *CFTR* found in black cystic fibrosis patients are in Feuillet-Fieux et al. (2004). It is important that screening or testing in patients and for carrier screening panels include *CFTR* mutation panels designed to serve the specific ethnic group that is being screened or diagnosed. The September/October 2004 issues of *Genetics in Medicine* devotes nearly the entire issue to cystic fibrosis screening and testing. ACOG also endorsed guidelines for preconception and prenatal carrier screening. Thus, if both members of a couple are carriers, amniocentesis may be done, although one of the mutations presents a risk only when the R117H and 5T variations are on the same allele, and R117H alone does not appear to present a risk for CF. A preliminary evaluation of the analytic validity of CF testing is very good and emphasizes the usefulness of confirmatory testing if a mutation is identified (Palomaki, Bradley, Richards, & Haddow, 2003). The American College of Obstetricians and Gynecologists (2004) has recommended as part of routine obstetric care offering preconceptional and prenatal carrier screening for individuals of French Canadian and Cajun descent and Ashkenazi Jews for Tay-Sachs disease, and for Ashkenazi Jews also the Canavan disease (an autosomal recessive disorder with developmental delay, seizures, blindness, and large head with death in early childhood usually due to deficiency of aspartoacylase), cystic fibrosis, and familial dysautonomia (see chapter 6). They further state that carrier screening is available for other genetic disorders with a relatively high frequency in those of Ashkenazi Jewish descent including mucolipidosis IV, Niemann-Pick disease type A, Fanconi anemia group C, Bloom syndrome and Gaucher disease but fall short of recommending offering these as a part of routine care, merely stating that persons may inquire about carrier testing and that materials be made available so they can make an informed decision. Obviously, genetic counseling could be of benefit to such couples. Widespread carrier population screening for PKU also will eventually be a reality.

For carrier screening where the person does not have the disease, the basic reasons for undertaking screening for detection of the heterozygous state is to provide genetic counseling, allow life and reproductive decision-making, and for prenatal diagnosis if desired later. The occurrence of genetic disease in the future children of someone who is a carrier for a specific recessively inherited disorder could be prevented in several ways. A future mate can be selected who is not a carrier for the same disorder. This can only be known if there is an accurate test for detection of the carrier state. If the person has selected, or wishes to select, a mate who is a carrier, then prevention can be achieved through exercising various reproductive options. The couple can choose to have natural children or not. If they choose to have natural children, prenatal diagnosis can often be done to detect disease in the fetus. If the fetus is affected, they can then elect to terminate the pregnancy or continue it. If they choose not to have natural children, then they could avoid contraception, practice birth control, or select sterilization for either or both individuals. If they wanted children, they could either adopt them or elect reproductive options such as gamete (sperm or egg) donation, in vitro fertilization, and/or embryo implantation. These choices are illustrated in Figure 11.2, and can be discussed with the individuals involved in the genetic counseling that accompanies the carrier detection program. Detection is not yet possible for carrier detection in many recessively inherited genetic disorders due to poor reliability of testing measures, lack of simple or acceptable techniques for screening, or expense resulting from lack of a defined population in which to screen. Carrier screening for Tay-Sachs, CF, β-thalassemia, and others have been carried out in high schools. There has been some concern regarding altered self-image, stigmatization, retention and understanding of information, understanding of impact, parental consent, the acting-out of adolescents in relation to rebellion from parents, and need for self-identity as reasons for making a testing decision without regard to all the consequences, and others. On the other hand, adolescents may be sexually active, and proper genetic counseling following carrier screening may be important in some high-risk groups. In a study (McConkie-Rosell, Spiridigliozzi, Iafolla, Tarleton, & Lachiewiez, 1997) of obligate carriers of the fragile X syndrome, the women interviewed stated that prior knowledge would have changed their reproductive plans, and they supported an aggressive approach for informing and testing their children. How intent translated into actual actions was not addressed.

In specific ethnic groups known to be at increased risk for specific autosomal recessive genetic diseases in which the carrier state can be readily detected, one way to proceed with preconceptional testing after appropriate education and informed consent is as follows: (1) First ascertain risk through family history including ancestry and genetic disorders in family; (2) then test the partner known to be a member of the ethnic group under consideration or with a positive family history; (3) if that partner is found to be a carrier, then the other partner should be tested. If that partner is not of the same ethnic descent, they could potentially have a rare mutation and carrier status might not be detected even if present so it is

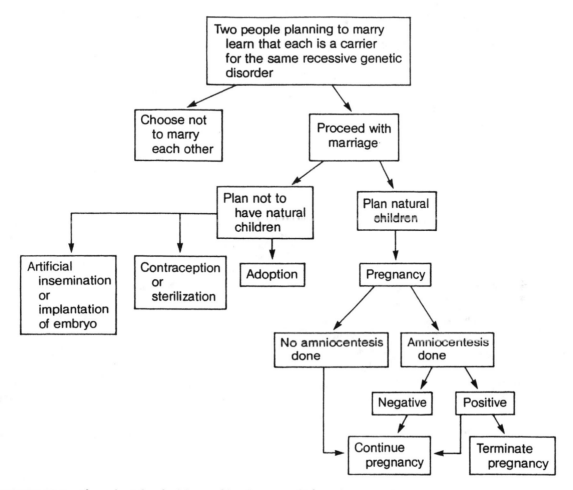

FIGURE 11.2   Flow chart for decision making in premarital carrier screening.

important that the couple understand this; (4) it is important to provide appropriate genetic counseling for the couple; (5) prenatal diagnostic options should be explored with the couple before pregnancy; and (6) preferably before testing the issue of disclosure to other relatives should be discussed because they may be carriers for the mutation in question. If a person is found to be a carrier, issues of disclosure to relatives who are potentially at risk are raised. American College of Obstetricians and Gynecologists (2004) states that "The provider does not need to contact these relatives because there is no provider-patient relationship with the relatives, and confidentiality must be maintained" (p. 428). As discussed elsewhere in this book, this is a controversial area, and other groups have published other opinions.

TAY-SACHS DISEASE: A PROTOTYPE

Tay-Sachs disease is considered to be the prototype for carrier screening. An infant born with this disease, in which GM_2 ganglioside accumulates in cells of the nervous system, appears normal until about 6 months of age. From then on, progressive mental and physical deterioration occurs, and death is inevitable, usually by 4 years of age. The basic defect is a lack of the enzyme hexosaminadase A (Hex A), which can result from a number of mutations in the *HEXA* gene. The following characteristics made this disorder very amenable to heterozygote screening programs: (1) there is a detectable reduction in Hex A activity in Tay-Sachs carriers (although now DNA testing is used); (2) a simple, inexpensive test is available for detection of carriers that meets the criteria specified earlier for screening tests; (3) prenatal diagnosis is available; (4) the mutant gene is concentrated in a specific population group—Jews of Eastern European (Ashkenazi) ancestry, particulary from one area of Poland and Lithuania. (5) the carrier rate in Ashkenazi Jews is approximately 1:27-30 individuals, thus defining a high-risk population group; (6) the natural course of the disease is inevitable and lethal, thus making it a severe burden; and (7) the lack of any treatment has made the option of terminating an affected pregnancy less controversial than it might have been otherwise. Success in Tay-Sachs carrier testing is evidenced by a 90% decrease in live born children with Tay-Sachs.

Jews who practice their religion according to the orthodox Jewish code do not generally subscribe to sterilization, abortion, or artificial insemination. Abortion can be permitted in specific cases with permission of Rabbinic authorities. Conservative and reform Judaism take more liberal views. All three groups maintain interest in premarital Tay-Sachs disease screening. In some traditional Jewish communities, the results of Tay-Sachs screening is considered as a factor when marital matchmaking is undertaken by professional matchmakers. A special program begun in Israel, and offered in other places as well, the Chevra Dor Yeshorim Program, was designed to avoid Tay-Sachs disease in Hasidic Jews, who oppose abortion and contraception. In essence, in this program, when a woman or man turns 18 or 20 years of age respectively, their blood is anonymously tested for Tay-Sachs, and the number recorded in a registry. When a couple is about to arrange a match, the matchmaker or a couple can query the registry. If both are carriers, they are told that another match will be arranged.

All of these considerations led many years ago to the initiation of large-scale Tay-Sachs disease screening in Jewish communities of Baltimore and Washington DC in 1972 by Kaback (1977) and his colleagues. Since then, a large number of Jewish communities have participated in Tay-Sachs disease screening, and research has been conducted on various aspects of the program. This program has served as a model for others. Some of the points discovered in this program are of interest and include: word of mouth and media were the most effective ways of drawing participants; when new members joined a synagogue, the rabbi provided information about Tay-Sachs screening availability; the highest ranking reasons for participation were desire to have children and perception of susceptibility. In their report of a genetic screening program for high school students in several Jewish high schools in Australia for both Tay-Sachs disease and cystic fibrosis heterozygotes, long-term follow up was also accomplished and revealed that 74% retained good knowledge, and 91% reported satisfaction with the program. Those who were found to be carriers had all told their extended family and 90% had also told close friends, but only 40% had informed their family physician. All carriers planned to inform their intended partners of their status and seek genetic counseling later. They did not report feelings of stigmatization (Barlow-Stewart et al., 2003). Grody (2003) described a carrier screening panel targeted for those of Ashkenazi Jewish origin including Tay-Sachs, cystic fibrosis, Gaucher disease, Canavan disease, familial dysautonomia, connexin-26 deafness, familial Mediterranean fever, Niemann-Pick disease, type A, Fanconi anemia, group C, and Bloom syndrome even though he points out that hemoglobinopathy carrier screening in the African-American population has never really been successful for societal reasons.

SCREENING FOR OTHER SELECTED GENETIC DISEASES

A number of selected genetic diseases have been proposed for inclusion in population screening programs of various types, including those with recessive inheritance and those with pharmacogenetic implications. Some have been suggested for inclusion in newborn screening as discussed below, and others for later screening. These include Factor V Leiden, prothrombin 2021A mutation, methylenetetrahydrofolate reductase variation, polymorphism of the angiotensin I-converting enzyme, hereditary hemochromatosis, the A1555G mutation in the mitochondrial genome associated with aminoglycoside ototoxicity, and others. Factor V is part of the coagulation cascade eventually forming clots. The Factor V Leiden mutation is present in about 2% to 15% of the general population and leads to a prevalent form of hereditary thrombophilia. It has a synergistic effect with both certain environmental factors such as contraceptive drugs, and other genes such as the prothrombin 2021A mutation. Factor V Leiden heterozygotes have a risk of about 10% for venous thrombosis while it may be up to 80% for homozygotes. It is considered as a risk factor for venous thromboembolism in pregnancy and needs to be assessed in the context of family history and past history of thrombosis. It can also result in pregnancy loss and placental abruption. It is still controversial as to whether to screen women for Factor V Leiden before prescribing oral contraceptives. Hereditary hemochromatosis has also been considered a candidate for widespread screening. This disorder is caused by mutations in *HFE*, especially C282Y. Mutations in this gene result in deposition of iron in organs, such as the pancreas, liver, and heart, causing disease. This is discussed in chapter 3. Despite the high population frequency, questions are raised about the natural history, effective intervention timing and type, and other issues such as penetrance and actual disease development. These issues raise some questions about the desirability of population screening for hemochromatosis especially if excellent education and counseling resources were not readily available.

NEWBORN SCREENING

Genetic knowledge from the Human Genome Project and the development of new technologies have led to a new era in newborn screening. Newborn screening is one of the great genetic public health success stories. Once phenylketonuria (PKU) was found to be associated with a type of mental retardation which could be prevented if a low phenylalanine diet was instituted soon after birth, a search began for a method to reliably detect PKU in newborns. Eventually, Robert Guthrie developed such a test using blood taken from the neonate by heel stick with a few drops placed on filter paper and dried. Testing was based on a bacterial growth inhibition assay using the dried blood spot. This test became the prototype for screening virtually the entire newborn population. If an abnormal screening test was identified, a low phenylalanine (phe) diet could be instituted, further diagnostic confirmation could be initiated, and effective treatment put in place for those whose diagnosis was confirmed. In the early 1960s, newborn screening for PKU, after some initial opposition to the concept of government-mandated testing, rapidly became part of state maternal-child health programs.

Other disorders were added to newborn screening tests over time, with inclusion varying by state as discussed later. A relatively constant group of conditions comprised the core conditions in newborn screening programs in the United States until recently. Newer technology such as tandem mass spectrometry (MS/MS) and the expansion of molecular and DNA-based techniques have identified additional mutations that fit accepted reasons for genetic screening and provided ways to detect them. Thus, the number of disorders that can be detected in the newborn has vastly increased.

The fact that some newborns will be screened for the full panel of available newborn screening tests and some will not, depending on the state in which they are born, has been called a major public health inequity. Advocacy by parents attracted popular press attention to this problem. Articles in the popular press and electronic media highlighted cases of adverse consequences of potentially detectable metabolic disease in newborns that were not detected because the state in which the parents resided did not include those conditions in their state screening programs. These articles also highlighted stories in which an infant was identified through newborn screening with a rare disorder and treated. One example that provoked activism by parents was that of a 6-month-old South Dakota infant who developed a rotavirus infection with diarrhea and vomiting. He took Pedialyte but had little else, but he was not dehydrated. He was found dead in his crib the next morning, and sudden infant death syndrome was thought to be the cause; however autopsy revealed fatty accumulation in the liver. These changes plus the history of reduced caloric intake led to further testing, which revealed that he had medium chain acyl-CoA dehydrogenase (MCAD) deficiency, described below. One of the reasons for including this disorder in routine newborn screening programs is that affected children can receive necessary preventive education and therapy and, in many cases, avert untoward incidents.

The major reason for newborn screening is to identify apparently healthy infants at-risk through universal newborn screening programs, provide early treatment for certain disorders as soon as possible and thereby prevent serious health consequences, especially severe mental retardation. Infants with abnormal initial testing results will usually have second screens and, depending on the results, further testing in order to confirm a diagnosis, but temporary treatment may be started in the interim if believed necessary. Many of the disorders detectable by newborn screening tests respond well to early treatment such as dietary restrictions. For others, treatment may be somewhat less successful. In recent years, a body of literature suggests that in some cases, despite early treatment, while severe retardation may be prevented, IQs are lower than those of siblings, and later neurological effects may be seen. The reasons for this may be varied and may involve extent and duration of dietary restriction, particular mutant genotype, adherence to therapy, and other parameters. Newborn screening must not only be concerned with screening and testing but with other components such as education; recalls and short-term follow up; diagnosis; referral to specialists; management; treatment; nursing, social and psychological services; assistance in other areas such as schools; genetic counseling; setting standards; quality assurance; and evaluation; ideally functioning as a coordinated system.

Newborn screening programs typically fall under a state's public health department but this is not universal. Typically, states screen for a set of metabolic disorders that have been mandated for years and that meet a set of criteria discussed below. States may also routinely screen newborns by blood specimen or other assessment for conditions of genetic or nongenetic causation such as congenital hearing loss, developmental hip dysplasia, human immunodeficiency virus (HIV) infection, congential toxoplasmosis, and others. There have been a variety of standards and guidelines developed regarding criteria for inclusion of a disorder within screening programs, some specific to universal state newborn screening. These are similar to those of screening programs in general and have been discussed previously under the section for planning a public health screening program.

States screen for a set of metabolic conditions that have been incorporated into regular legislation for universal mandated newborn population screening. From time to time, states may add disorders to pilot screening programs that may be universally applied, applied for specific selected populations deemed to be at greatest risk, included on a limited basis, or performed only by request. For example, California recently added the option of additional screening for 25 more disorders but still does not include biotinidase deficiency or CAH as routine. The Save Babies Through Screening advocacy group (http://www.savebabies.org/release1-07.02.htm) recommends screening newborns for 55 diseases, which would require considerable cost and personnel time as well as several procedures and might engender parental anxiety. Newborn screening typically includes diseases of metabolism such as PKU, hemoglobinopathies such as sickle cell disease, and endocrinopathies such as congenital hypothyroidism. Presently all states and the District of Columbia ($n = 51$) on a permanent basis routinely screen newborns for PKU, congenital hypothyroidism and galactosemia, and the majority also screen for sickle cell disease/hemoglobinopathies and congenital adrenal hyperplasia. Others typically include maple syrup urine disease, biotinidase deficiency, homocystinuria, cystic fibrosis, and medium-chain acyl-coA dehydrogase deficiency (MCAD) and two (the District of Columbia and Missouri) routinely screen for glucose-6-phosphate dehydrogenase (G6PD) deficiency. States also mandate newborn screening for other conditions such as congenital hearing loss which may be genetic or non-genetic, congenital toxoplasmosis, and, in the case of New York, human immunodeficiency virus infection. Other countries include conditions not currently mandated for inclusion in the United States' newborn screening programs and vice-versa.

Changes and proposed adjustments are now being made in screening programs due to new genetic knowledge which has made detection of a given disorder possible, new technology for detection and analysis, or the availability of new or better treatment options. These changes make new disorders fit the usual criteria for newborn screening, and provide reasons why ongoing assessment of which disorders to include must be an important component of the total program. The availability of tandem mass spectrometry (MS/MS) as an analytic technique allows about 30 different metabolic conditions to be screened for in the neonatal period using the same blood specimen. The technique does not, however, screen for every disorder presently included in screening programs, such as galactosemia, biotinidase deficiency, and others.

A mass spectrometer is a piece of equipment that separates and quantifies ions based on their mass/charge ratios that can use routinely obtained dried blood spot specimens. Data are transferred to a computer for analysis. Advantages include rapidity of analysis; greater accuracy than conventional methods, allowing screening for certain disorders to be more specific and sensitive; ability to detect disorders formerly difficult to detect; and the ability to screen for multiple diseases in a single run including amino acid, fatty acid oxidation, and organic acid disorders. Some concerns about the use of MS/MS have centered around cost issues, the need to provide alternate means of testing or instrumentation in case of breakdown, need for special personnel to be trained in this technology, and the issue of unknowns surrounding false positives and negatives because of lack of experience with detection of certain very rare disorders. Another issue is that some disorders can be detected by these means at 1 or 2 days after birth but others are not detectable until the newborn is 5 days old or older. This time is usually after hospital discharge, meaning that responsibility for additional specimen collection from a primary health provider or public health clinic is needed. Thus, primary care practitioners, including nurses, are responsible for ascertaining that newborns referred to their practices have been screened and results have been returned. Often nurses are instrumental in assuring that these initial and follow-up specimens are collected. Some of the disorders presently detectable through tandem mass spectrometry are listed in Table 11.4. The finding that, in Virginia, undiagnosed metabolic diseases were identified in 1% of unexpected deaths during a 5-year study period, and that 5% of all sudden infant deaths might be associated with metabolic diseases, suggests that the routine use of tandem mass spectrometry in newborn screening programs may have a positive impact (CDC, 2003). In some states, there is an option offered to parents to choose to test their newborn for additional disorders for an additional fee through the same channels that administer the mandated program and/or through other facilities, such as private or university laboratories. Options for many of these tests are available directly to the consumer through Internet offerings as well, and regulation of this kind of test offering has been proposed. Eventually DNA-based technology will be used routinely for newborn screening, replacing or augmenting current technology.

As briefly mentioned earlier, state regulation of newborn screening is highly variable . There is no national policy that determines which disorders should be screened for or establishes uniform components of newborn screening programs such as procedures for the communication of test results, especially in cases where initial specimens yield a "panic" result requiring immediate notification and action. States may vary in which tests they use to detect a given condition and in what results or parameters constitute an abnormal test result. One of the difficulties we had in reviewing data during the discussions of the PKU consensus panel was that different states may define an abnormal screening test result for PKU as greater than 4, 10, 12, or 15 mg/dL, or regulations may state "as determined by metabolic specialists." The end result is a great variety in newborn screening requirements. Thus, the newborn screening statutes and administrative regulations for each state may or may not:

- Specifically name the genetic or metabolic disorders that the newborn is to be tested for. Some screening statutes designate the disorders covered; others allow the state health department or an advisory commission to define and add additional ones. Some may be pilot programs, done in certain populations, or be by physician request.
- Specify the time after birth at which the sample must be taken. Some may specify only "before discharge," which may not be optimal for some disorders, particularly in a situation where the usual discharge time may be 24 to 48 hours after birth. Thus there should be specification for later screening, if needed, through primary health care providers.
- Provide for penalties to variously denoted health providers for not complying with the statutes. These, depending on the state, may include the physician, the hospital administration, the nurse, the midwife, or the person attending the newborn.
- Provide for penalties to the parents if testing is neglected.

TABLE 11.4   Selected Additional Disorders That Can be Screened for Using Tandem Mass Spectometry

Fatty Acid Oxidation Defects
    Carnitine palmitoyl transferase deficiency Type I (CPT-1)
    Carnitine palmitoyl transferase deficiency Type II (CPT-2)
    Carnitine/acylcarnitine translocase deficiency (CAT)
    Long-chain hydroxy acyl-CoA dehydrogenase deficiency (LCHAD)
    Multiple acyl-CoA dehydrogenase deficiency (GA-II)
    Short-chain acyl-CoA dehydrogenase deficiency (SCAD)
    Medium-chain acyl-CoA dehydrogenase deficiency (MCAD)
    Trifunctional protein deficiency
    Very-long-chain acyl-CoA dehydrogenase deficiency (VLCAD)
    Long-chain-acyl-CoA dehydrogenase deficiency (LCAD)
    2,4 Dienoyl-CoA reductase deficiency

Organic Acidemias
    Glutaric acidemia Type I (GA-1)
    Glutaric acidemia Type II (GA-2)
    3-Hydroxy-3-methylglutaryl-CoA lyase deficiency (HMG)
    Isobutyryl-CoA dehydrogenase deficiency
    Isovaleric acidemia (IVA)
    Malonic aciduria
    3-Methylcrotonyl-CoA carboxylase deficiency (3-MCC)
    Methylmalonic acidemia (MMA)
    Mitochondrial acetoacetyl-CoA thiolase deficiency (β-Ketothiolase deficiency)
    Propionic Acidemia (PA)
    2-Methylbutryl-CoA dehydrogenase deficiency

Urea Cycle Disorders
    Argininemia
    Argininosuccinate lyase deficiency (ASA)
    Citrullinemia
    Hyperammonemia, hyperornithinemia, homocitrullinuria (HHH)

Other Amino Acidemias
    5-oxoprolinuria
    Homocystinuria (CBS deficiency)
    Phenylketonuria
    Maple syrup urine disease
    Nonketotic hyperglycinemia
    Tyrosinemia type I
    Tyrosinemia type II

• Specify that specific informed consent be obtained from the parent or guardian. This varies as to what is specified for inclusion. Some hospitals hold classes for parents to explain the screening program, others verbally explain it, distribute written material, or cover it in a blanket way. Parents may not readily understand the language and concepts in these documents, and while medical literacy issues have received more attention and are addressed in many settings, understanding of newborn screening can still be limited. Many parents enter and leave the hospital without ever realizing that their infant has been screened unless there is an abnormal finding.

• Allow the newborn to be exempt from the test if the parent or guardian objects. The most common objection allowed is on religious grounds. In some states there must be a conflict with "the religious practices and principles of an established church ..." of which the parent is a member. Some states require that the objection be a written one, which is then submitted to the responsible institution.

• Establish an advisory council or commission on hereditary and metabolic disorders. The composition of the group may or may not be pre-scribed. It varies from all physicians to a mixture of health professionals to a combination of profes-sionals and consumers.

• Specify the length of time records of test results must be kept.

• Specify who is to be notified and of what type of results. States do not necessarily require that parents or physicians be notified if screening test results are negative.

• Maintain a registry of affected individuals. The intent is to use this to ensure adequate follow-up and treatment, but the establishment of such a registry is controversial for ethical reasons such as confidentiality and for issues such as insurability.

• Specify who is to pay for the screening tests performed. Some states assume the costs, whereas others allow hospitals and other institutons to charge parents for them. There is variation in what third party payers will contribute.

• Specify the procedure to be followed when an abnormal result is obtained.

• Specify who pays for diagnostic testing after an abnormal screening result.

• Supply treatment if a disorder is detected, or assume all or part of treatment-related costs.

• Establish laboratory standards with periodic review and evaluation as part of quality assurance protocols.

• Specify testing at one central or a few regional laboratories. This helps to avoid erroneous results by instituting a greater degree of quality control. A laboratory will then have experience in interpret-ing apparently positive results.

• Establish voluntary urine testing for research purposes. This is one way to perfect techniques so that they can be used later on a larger scale, if warranted.

• Mandate educational programs on genetic dis-orders for physicians, nurses, hospital staff, or the public. These may be either through continuing edu-cation or inclusion into basic professional curricula.

Professional societies including state nurses' associations may also advise the state agency responsible for newborn screening programs in regard to both technical issues and needed edu-cational programs. Nurses need to be aware of the newborn screening statutes and regulations governing the state in which they are practicing. If in practice in community health, pediatrics, obstet-rics, independent practice, or working as a nurse practitioner in joint practice, the nurse should be able to explain to a family the reasons for such screening, what it shows and does not show, whether or not the results will be communicated to them directly or at all if negative, and how. Impor-tant elements for inclusion in newborn screening programs are listed in Table 11.5. Nurses should also remember that if an infant has to be retested because of a positive initial screening result, parental anxiety will be severe, and every effort should be made to minimize such anxiety during this time.

TABLE 11.5 Important Elements in Newborn Screening Programs

• Inclusion of all neonates before hospital discharge according to state laws and guidelines
• Provision to include neonates not tested before discharge and those born outside the hospital as soon as possible
• Education of parents about screening at appropriate educational levels considering cultural beliefs—reasons, what is involved, how the communication of results is handled, etc.
• Informed parental consent within state laws
• Collection of appropriate specimen at proper time
• Reliable, accurate, standardized testing in centralized laboratory is ideal
• Provision for rescreening if tested too early; rescreening should be done at about 3 weeks of age for PKU
• Communication of positive screening results to local physician and parents quickly (by telephone with letter of con-firmation); ideally have counseling and psychosocial support available to help with anxiety engendered
• Follow-up all newborns with positive screening tests
• Ensure means of accurate diagnosis are available for all with confirmed positive screening tests
• Provision for genetic and other counseling that is culturally competent and educationally appropriate
• Provision for treatment and ongoing management of infant and family

In 2000, a report on newborn screening was issued by the Newborn American Academy of Pediatrics Newborn Screening Task Force at the request of the Maternal and Child Health Bureau, Health Resources and Services Administration (HRSA), Department of Health and Human Services. This report did not specify which tests should be included nationally although many had expected that it would. The designation of tests was left to the states, although efforts to try to establish a minimum core set of tests for the nation are underway through the Maternal and Child Health Bureau. Some of the decision-making of states has been based on the racial and ethnic population of those states and the most prevalent genetic disorders of those ethnic groups, since certain disorders are known to be very prevalent in certain ethnic groups and rare in others, with cost-effectiveness as a driving force. Some have suggested that some disorders do not need to be universally tested for but can be targeted by ethnic group, a practice that in our ethnically mixed society may be genetically as well as ethically unsound; however some states are at least piloting targeted newborn screening for certain disorders. While the recommendations in this report are too numerous to cover in their entirety, some of the other major emphases in this report (American Academy of Pediatrics, 2000) were that:

- Newborn screening is changing rapidly and public health departments may not be keeping up with changes in technology, genetic discoveries, and increased advocacy efforts; there was a need for federal and state public health agencies in partnership with health professionals and consumers to better define responsibilities;
- Public health agencies need to involve families, health professionals, and the public in the development, operation, and oversight of newborn screening information;
- Effective newborn screening systems require an adequate public health infrastructure and must be integrated within the health care delivery system, with children being linked to a medical home to assure appropriate care and treatment for medical, nonmedical, psychosocial, and educational needs of the child and family in the local community. This need

for comprehensive long-term care was also emphasized by the Consensus Panel on Phenylketonuria (PKU): Screening and Management;

- Public health agencies need to ensure adequate financial mechanisms;
- Cost-effectiveness may be defined in various ways;
- The cost of screening has not included the needed infrastructure in most studies; some studies have looked at cost only in regard to the screening test, but other elements including cost of finding and informing families and reporting results should be done;
- Model systems of care and support from infancy to adulthood for infants identified with disorders in newborn screening programs need to be designed and evaluated;
- National criteria need to be developed for adding disorders to state screening panels, but the report did not specify these or the disorders;
- Issues of state-to-state variance in uniformity about tests were identified, and as was educational information about the process to be sure that prospective parents are aware of the process;
- Parents have the right to be informed about screening and the right to refuse it; have the right to confidentiality and privacy protections for newborn screening results; and need to be informed about benefits as well as potential risks of tests and treatments, use of specimens in the future, storage policies, and how families will receive test results.

In response to this report, in 2000 the March of Dimes issued a statement which called for nationally mandated newborn testing for the following diseases: PKU, hypothyroidism, galactosemia, sickle cell disease, congenital adrenal hyperplasia, biotinidase deficiency, maple syrup urine disease, and homocystinuria. Since that time, they added MCAD and congenital hearing loss to this list.

The March of Dimes also called for the need for:

- abandoning currently available tests for new tests if the new test achieves a greater precision or a shorter turnaround time regardless of the cost differential;

- putting safeguards in place for timely reporting of test results;
- assuring uniform quality of newborn screening tests nationwide, including an overarching authority to ensure this; and
- ensuring that every newborn has the same core of screening tests by mandate, and that those be the best available even if the test is for a rare disease if that diagnosis can make a difference in the child's health (Howse & Katz, 2000).

Some states have opted to allow parents to choose to have supplemental screening tests at outside labs at a moderate extra cost, such as $25. Some of the companies and universities offering this service advertise on the Internet with full instructions for parents. One of the problems identified is not the cost of the $25 for testing, but the money needed to fund the infrastructure for recall and short term follow-up, diagnosis, treatment, management, quality assurance, and program evaluation for many more conditions than originally planned.

Disorders Included in Newborn Screening

Because newborn screening is in an ever-changing state, additions may be made to the disorders in current detection programs. Disorders may also be discontinued if the detection rate is low in a particular state. Genetic and metabolic disorders currently consistently and routinely screened for in the United States including the District of Columbia ($n = 51$) were discussed above. One congenital infection, toxoplasmosis (see chapter 13) is screened for as well. Because nurses are likely to need information about disorders routinely screened for in newborns in order to assess the newborn intelligently, to communicate with and educate parents of newborns and infants, and to explain the need for further testing if an abnormal result is found, a brief synopsis of these follows. The advent of mass newborn screening has shown that many of these disorders are more common than formerly believed. Infants dying from some inborn errors in the past were simply not diagnosed as having the

disorder. Many were thought to have died of overwhelming sepsis, so the true disease incidence was not recognized. Some symptoms that should lead the nurse to consider recommending or referring the infant for screening test batteries for inherited biochemical disorders are discussed in chapter 6. If the infant is diagnosed, siblings should be tested in case they have the disorder but have not manifested it, and they may benefit from treatment.

Another issue surrounding newborn screening is whether or not screening should be done for diseases that are not treatable, or for those with no known clinical repercussions such as histidinemia, formerly included in some state newborn screening programs but now believed to be benign. Some believe that screening for those with no known clinical significance may allow long-term follow-up of such individuals and reveal hitherto unrecognized subtle consequences. This must be balanced against expense and the anxiety engendered in the parents. Another issue is whether or not it is justifiable to screen for very rare disorders. Some believe that it yields a very low benefit/cost ratio, whereas others believe it is morally unjustifiable to do otherwise because of the potential to prevent adverse effects.

Phenylketonuria and Hyperphenylalaninemia

Phenylketonuria (PKU) was the first disorder to be included in mass newborn screening in the early 1960s. Years of experience with PKU screening revealed how little was really known about hyperphenylalaninemia heterogeneity when screening was begun, and pointed out the need for education of parents, informed consent for testing, and provision of genetic counseling services as integral parts of treatment programs. Worldwide, more than 10 million newborns are now screened for PKU each year.

The amino acid phenylalanine (phe) is essential for protein synthesis in humans. A complex reaction is involved in the hepatic conversion of phenylalanine to tyrosine (see Figure 11.3), and blockage causes elevations collectively refered to as hyperphenylalaninemias. These include transient hyperphenylalaninemia, persistent non-PKU hyperphenylalaninemia, classic PKU, and deficient tetrabiopterin biosynthesis that may result from impaired recycling of tetrahydropterin due to

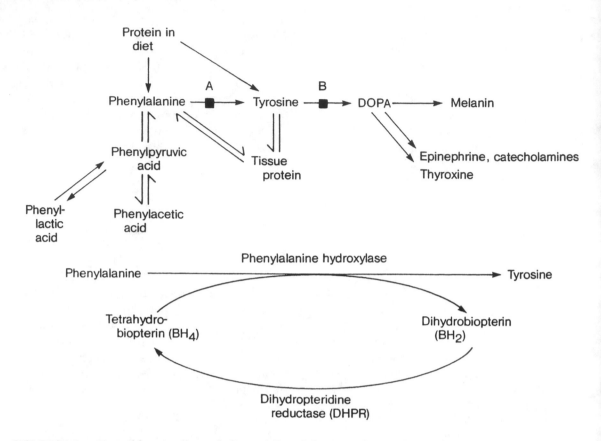

FIGURE 11.3   *(Top)* Abbreviated metabolism of phenylalanine and tyrosine. A = block in PKU (classical). B = block in albinism. *(Bottom)* Phenylalanine hydroxylating system (abbreviated). Note that some steps have been omitted for simplification.

dihydropteridine reductase deficiency. Hyperphenylalaninemia refers to phe levels above 2mg/dl (120µM), and may result from various mutations interfering with the conversion of phe to tyrosine including: (1) phenylalanine hydroxylase (PAH) deficiency resulting in classic PKU and a mild non-PKU hyperphenylalaninemia, (2) dihydropteridine reductase (DPHR) deficiency, (3) guanosine triphosphate cyclohydratase (GTP-CH), and (4) 6-pyruvoyltetrahydropterin synthetase (6-PTS) deficiency. The latter three involve impairment in tetrahydrobiopterin (BH₄) which is a coenzyme (cofactor) for PAH. Therefore, several defects in different steps in the metabolism of phenylalanine or its cofactor can result in elevated phe. The most common of these forms is classic PKU characterized by less than 1% of PAH activity. Deficiencies of >1% PAH activity result in milder hyperphenylalaninemia noted as non-PKU hyperphenylalan-

inemia caused by PAH deficiency. Those with mild persistent hyperphenylalaninemia (6 mg/dl or greater) may have a lower IQ if not treated, and so practitioners are being more aggressive in implementing diet therapy for these infants. Variants account for about 10% of all cases, and more than 400 mutations of the PAH gene are known to result in classic PKU. Hyperphenylalaninemia not resulting in classic PKU has different treatment approaches. It is important to rescreen infants who have positive early screening tests so that those with transient hyperphenylalaninemia are not placed on phenylalanine restricted diets that could be harmful to them.

It is now rare to see a child manifest the full spectrum of symptoms resulting from classic PKU because of screening programs and prompt treatment, but occasionally an affected infant is missed. Therefore, PKU should not be automatically ruled out in infants manifesting signs and symptoms associated with the disorder. Vomiting, eczema, and urine with a musty or mouselike odor are usually the only early symptoms. Delay in achieving developmental milestones may be noticed after 6 months of phenylalanine ingestion. Other symptoms that can occur are convulsions, increased muscle tone, agitated behavior, and delayed speech. A crossed-leg sitting position, tooth enamel hypoplasia, decalcification of the long bones, and a prominent maxilla are present. Pigment dilution occurs because of inhibition of tyrosinase by phenylalanine accumulation in the metabolic pathway leading to melanin synthesis (see Figure 11.3). Thus affected untreated patients commonly have fair hair and blue eyes; however, in darkly pigmented families, the affected patient will only be noticed to be less pigmented than other family members.

It is very important to institute a phe-restricted diet as soon as possible and before 1 month; continuous treatment throughout childhood, adolescence and probably lifelong, is now considered essential; diet restriction should be sufficient to keep plasma phe levels to normal ranges. Areas of controversy such as the length of time to restrict phenylalanine in the infant's diet, the rigidity of restriction, and how to approach maternal PKU is discussed in chapters 13 and 15.

It is estimated that only 5% of infants who have presumptive positive tests are eventually proven to have PKU. False-negative results also occur because of early screening, especially if the infant is feeding poorly. Nurses can note those infants in whom this is true, so that extra emphasis can be placed on another test being done at about 3 weeks of age. The amount of formula ingested in the last 24 hours, feeding difficulties if any, and type of feeding (bottle or breast) should be noted on the form that is sent with the specimen for testing. Between 5% and 10% of infants eventually found to have PKU had negative results from screening tests. Needless to say, any infant born into a family with a history of PKU needs more frequent than usual testing and monitoring. Another problem continuing to plague PKU screening has been the length of time taken in some cases to locate an infant with a positive screening test and conduct follow-up testing. This is problematic in instituting diet control to prevent retardation.

It has been suggested that all infants with persistent hyperphenylalaninemia and PKU be entered into a computerized registry for recontact in early adolescence in order to prevent the effects of maternal PKU on offspring. Questions of rights to privacy, confidentiality, and others must be balanced against the potential usefulness of such a registry.

Infants found to have hyperphenylalaninemia on newborn screening may eventually be placed after diagnosis into one of several categories. The major ones are: classic PKU, transient hyperphenylalaninemia without any further clinical significance, non-PKU hyperphenylalaninemia (phe levels are below 1,000 μM on a normal diet), and those with BH4 deficiency who need treatment for this.

The overall incidence of classic PKU in the general population in the United States is approximately 1 in 11,000 live births, whereas Irish and Scottish populations have an incidence as high as 1 in 5,000, and black, Japanese, and Ashkenazi Jewish populations show an incidence as low as 1 in 100,000. Inheritance is by the autosomal recessive mode of transmission. The human PAH gene has been identified and mapped. Carrier detection and prenatal diagnosis of classic PKU are possible. A complete discussion of PKU may be found in the National Institutes of Health Consensus Development Panel (2001).

Congenital Hypothyroidism

The inclusion of congenital hypothyroidism (CH) in neonatal screening programs represented a significant advance in the prevention of mental retardation. CH has an incidence of 1:3,600 to 1:5,000 live births, and thus is the most common preventable cause of mental retardation currently known. Congenital deficiency of thyroid hormone can result from a variety of transient and non-transient causes. Transient causes include prematurity and infants born to mothers taking antithyroid preparations. Nontransient causes include congenital deficiency of thyroid tissue, impaired activity of one of the enzymes involved in thyroid hormone biosynthesis, deficiency of thyroid stimulating hormone (TSH) secretion, tissue resistance or impaired response to TSH stimulation, deficiency of thyrotropin releasing hormone (TRH) itself, or impaired pituitary response to TRH. Familial hypothyroidism can result from either thyroidal or extrathyroidal dysfunction. Modes of transmission depend on the exact condition. For example, there can be autosomal dominant inheritance of mutations coding for transcription factors such as NKX2.1 as well as autosomal recessive inheritance of genes coding for thyroid peroxidase. Treatment is with thyroxine, sometimes with triiodothyronine. Current trends favor starting treatment as soon as possible, often with an initial higher dose.

Hypothyroidism may be one feature of another syndrome. Diagnosis of hypothyroidism by clinical symptoms is difficult. These infants, formerly called cretins, have a normal length and normal to increased weight at birth. They may be slow to feed, show placidity, not cry very often, and be constipated. Physical signs can include umbilical hernia, a protruding tongue, prolonged jaundice, and an increased fontanel size. Later, such signs as hoarse cry, dry skin, nasal congestion, choking during feedings, and coarse facies appear. By this time, irreversible mental retardation of some degree has already occurred.

States vary in whether they use thyroxine (T4) or TSH alone or in combination for initial screening. If T4 alone is used and is low, rescreening with both T4 and TSH is recommended. Infants under treatment for CH should be periodically reevaluated in case the disorder was transient. A review of the New England Regional Screening Program revealed that human error, including failures of collection and transmittal of blood specimens to the lab, was responsible for most of the 2% of undetected cases of neonatal hypothyroidism. Nurses should confirm that all newborns have had specimens collected and that they have been sent to the lab before discharge unless there is specific reason for not doing so.

Any infant with presumptive tests for hypothyroidism must undergo confirmatory diagnosis as quickly as possible. The American Academy of Pediatrics (1996) recommend returning results from a detection program no later than 3 1/2 weeks after birth, with therapy to be initiated by 1 month of age if it is needed. Nurses should understand how extremely critical time is in this disorder when getting an infant to diagnostic facilities or explaining the test results to parents. Formerly, between 1% and 2% of all admissions to institutions for the mentally retarded were from hypothyroidism; con-

genital hypothyroidism is a cause of mental retardation that can be virtually eliminated by newborn screening. Even though neonatal detection and treatment have virtually eliminated mental retardation from CH, long-term studies have indicated that IQs may be somewhat reduced, with subtle impairments occurring in language, visual spatial abilities, neuromotor skills, attention, memory, hearing, and auditory discrimination that may not be noted until adolescence. Assessment of cognitive abilities should be ongoing with appropriate actions. These impairments may be related to the cause or severity of the disorder present, adequacy and timing of treatment, as well as adherence to therapy. To promote adherence, nurses can use a variety of approaches. Infants with CH have also been found to have an excess of certain other congenital anomalies especially of the heart, eyes, and nervous system.

Galactosemia

Lactose (milk sugar) is a disaccharide composed of glucose and galactose. Defects in enzymes involved in the metabolism of galactose can result in galactosemia. The major types are classic galactosemia resulting from deficiency in galactose 1-phosphate uridyltransferase which has several variants (transferase deficiency), deficiency in uridine diphosphate galactose 4-epimerase (epimerase deficiency), and galactokinase deficiency. All are inherited in an AR manner. In the classic form, the infant usually appears normal at birth and before milk feeding begins. Once feeding begins, galactose and other metabolites accumulate in the blood and urine. Symptoms appear rapidly and include vomiting, diarrhea, jaundice, failure to thrive, hepatomegaly, cataract development, hypoglycemia, and eventually mental retardation. Death can occur before diagnosis. These infants are often susceptible to *E. coli* sepsis which may cause death. The disorder is sometimes mistaken for milk allergy or intolerance, and if the infant is withdrawn from milk for a period of time, diagnosis may be delayed until irreversible mental damage has occurred. The early elimination of galactose from the diet can prevent clinical symptoms. Diet is discussed in chapter 15. By late childhood, galactose ingestion may be tolerated without symptoms; however, current thinking does not support diet relaxation in older children. Lactose-restricted diets appear successful in preventing significant cataracts, severe infection, and severe liver disease. However, long-term studies reveal that a significant effect of galactosemia is central nervous system dysfunction manifested by delayed speech onset and language and learning disabilities, particularly involving spatial relationships and mathematics. Short attention spans and behavioral disorders have been noted as have ataxia and tremor. Recently, the majority of females with transferase deficient galactosemia have been found to have ovarian failure and hypogonadism and may exhibit amenorrhea. Premature menopause may be noted. Some galactosemic children show heights that are below the 3rd percentile, and Schweitzer, Shin, Jakobs and Brodehl (1993) found that about 83% of galactosemic children in their sample had IQs below 85; however, this was not found by Waggoner, Buist and Donnell (1990). In pregnancies at risk for galactosemia, some believe that the mother's galactose intake should be restricted prenatally, although there are little data on how restricted the diet should be or on how beneficial the restriction is. Infants treated between birth and 1 month of age appear to have the best outcomes, but late effects develop despite early treatment and good compliance with diet restrictions.

Epimerase deficiencies have been described in both a benign form and one that resemble transferase deficiency. The diet treatment involves the provision of small amounts of needed dietary galactose, and thus differs from transferase deficiency galactosemia.

The enzyme galactokinase is necessary for the first step in the metabolism of galactose to glucose. Its deficiency does not allow galactose to enter the cell and thus it accumulates, leading to galactokinase deficiency galactosemia. Clinical manifestations are milder than in the transferase type and consist mainly of cataract formation. The lifespan of affected children is essentially normal. The incidence is about 1 in 40,000–60,000 live births. Any infant or child with cataracts should be screened for galactosemia. Diet is as discussed previously.

Homocystinuria

Homocystinuria is a disorder of amino acid metabolism. It may result from impaired activity or deficiency of cystathionine β-synthetase (CBS) or methionine synthetase, and in each case can

result from genetic or nongenetic causes. The deficiency results in increased methionine, increased homocysteine, increased mixed disulfide, and decreased cysteine. CBS deficiency is most common. The overall incidence is about 1 in 150,000 to 200,000 live births, with considerable population variation. It is inherited in an AR manner. It is more frequent in Ireland, Great Britain, and Australia and relatively rare in Japan. There is both clinical variation and genetic heterogeneity. One form is responsive to pyridoxine (vitamin B₆) since cystathionine β-synthetase is a vitamin B₆ responsive enzyme. Thus some individuals are responsive to pharmacological doses of pyridoxine (vitamin B₆) and folic acid. Clinically, some patients may have all of the symptoms, whereas some show only a few. Those responsive to pyridoxine tend to be less severely clinically affected. The severity of the disease is usually constant within a family. Mental retardation that is mild or moderate is found in about half of the affected individuals. Skeletal abnormalities are common and may include scoliosis, kyphosis, and chest abnormalities such as pectus excavatum. Untreated patients tend to be tall with excessively long limbs and knobby knees, as in Marfan syndrome, a condition with which it is often confused. They have a flat-footed gait. Osteoporosis of the spine occurs, which causes back pain. Osteoporosis may be seen by age 20. Dislocation of the lens of the eye (ectopia lentis) is a classic finding that is not present at birth but usually develops by 6–10 years of age. Glaucoma and myopia are also frequent. Hair is fair, sparse, and breaks easily. If the individual with the pyridoxine responsive type is treated with it, the hair darkens. The skin tends to be thin except on the face where it is coarse. A malar flush is common. Spontaneous intravascular thromboses of both arteries and veins can occur in any area of the body, and 25% have an event by 15 to 20 years. These are the most severe disease manifestations and a major cause of early death. Seizures are one of the neurological manifestations present and may result from the thromboses. Early detection by newborn screening is aimed at prevention of these complications by supplying pyridoxine to the responsive patients, and by a low-methionine diet with cysteine supplementation in the others, beginning with a methionine-free formula in infancy. Betaine may be used as a dietary supplement if needed since it stimulates the remethylation of homocysteine, reducing its levels. This is a difficult diet to maintain because of the necessity of essentially eliminating meat, fish, eggs, and dairy products from the diet. Lentils and soybeans are relied on heavily for protein. Young women who are known to have homocystinuria should be counseled to avoid oral contraceptives when choosing birth control measures because of their tendency to develop thromboses. Heterozygotes are susceptible to premature occlusive vascular disease. Depending on the test used for newborn screening, those with the pyridoxine-responsive type may not be detected until later in infancy or childhood because the test used may be aimed at detecting hypermethioninemia. Homocystinuria should be considered in children or young adults with unexplained thromboses, acute psychoses, or dislocated lens. An illustration of the need to still consider inherited metabolic diseases in an older person even in the era of newborn screening is illustrated by the case of a 17-year-old who presented with auditory and visual hallucinations and paranoia who was found to have the pyridoxine-responsive form of homocystinuria. His symptoms normalized within several weeks of pyridoxine therapy. See Appendix B for support groups.

Maple Syrup Urine Disease

Maple syrup urine disease (MSUD) is also known as branched-chain ketoaciduria because the basic defect is in the second step (decarboxylation) of the metabolism of leucine, isoleucine, and valine, which are the amino acids having branched chains, and the corresponding ketoacids. Classification may be by clinical pheonotype such as classic, intermediate, intermittent, thiamine-responsive, and dihydrolipoyl dehydrogenase (E3) deficiency (extremely rare), or classified molecularly by affected gene loci as MSUD types Ia, Ib, II, and III. There are multiple allelic mutations known at each locus. Variants have different biochemical and clinical features with varying percents of decarboxylation activity. The incidence of MSUD in the general population overall is 1 in 100,000 live births. In Pennsylvania Old Order Mennonites the incidence may be as high as 1 in 176 live births.

In classic MSUD, enzyme levels may be 0% to 2% of normal. Infants appear normal until 3 to 7 days after birth when such early nonspecific symp-

toms as poor feeding, vomiting, lethargy, poor sucking, hypotonia, and a high-pitched frequent cry appear. These may not be seen in breast-feeding infants until the second week of life. The characteristic odor, described as burnt sugar or maple syrup, may be noticed in the urine, sweat, and ear cerumen of the affected infant as early as the 5th day of life. The buildup of leucine depresses blood glucose leading to hypoglycemic episodes and severe acidosis. Alternating periods of flaccidity and hypertonicity, the suppression of tendon reflexes, and loss of Moro's reflex occurs; convulsions, slow respiration with apneic periods, and coma appear. Death can occur as early as 10 to 14 days. If untreated, neurological problems, mental retardation, and physical delay may occur. The majority die in the first few months if untreated. By the time MSUD is identified in some screening programs, irreversible damage and death can occur. Classic MSUD is a newborn emergency because mental retardation occurs if dietary protein intake is not stopped within about 24 hours to prevent further accumulation of abnormal metabolites. At the same time, caloric intake must be maintained. The earlier treatment is begun, the better the potential outcome. Ideally, this should be before the 10th day of life, and it is believed that only a few infants with classic MSUD who receive treatment after 14 days of age achieve normal intellect. Permanent neurological damage and mental retardation can begin by 1 week of age and this is why treatment should be instituted while diagnostic confirmation is sought. When using the Guthrie screening method, often results were not reported as early as desirable but use of tandem mass spectrometry permits earlier identification and treatment. Nurses suspecting MSUD by virtue of the "nose" test or other observations should waste no time in seeking appropriate measures.

Once the diagnosis is established, maintenance on a diet that is nutritionally adequate and restricted in the branched chain amino acids (BCAA) is now considered necessary to some degree throughout life. Patients must be closely monitored because stresses such as infections, fever, illness, or surgery can cause metabolic changes leading to acute disease episodes. Thus, special management is needed in conjunction with elective surgery. Maintaining the diet can be difficult for the patient, family, and professionals because it is difficult to balance the amino acids needed for normal growth and development against the accumulation of toxic metabolites. Adjustments are needed frequently, and therefore close contact with the family should be maintained. Despite diet treatment, it has been reported that approximately one-third of affected persons achieved IQ scores greater than 90, with one-third between 70 and 90, and neurological impairment may also be seen.

In the intermediate form, no catastrophic illness is seen in infancy, but elevated BCAA, the characteristic odor, and neurologic impairment such as ataxia and retarded development are noted. Diagnosis is often made in late infancy or childhood, sometimes due to work-ups for the neurological symptoms or developmental delay. This form is rare. In the intermittent form, early development and intelligence are normal. Patients may show episodic attacks of unsteady gait, acute metabolic decompensation, and behavioral changes that are precipitated by infection or stress. Symptoms may appear anywhere from a few months to 2 years of age, or first be noticed in adulthood. The thiamine-responsive form is similar to intermediate MSUD. Thiamine is required as a cofactor in the decarboxylation step of the BCAA, and the thiamine-responsive form is responsive to large doses of thiamine (Vitamin B1) with diet restrictions. Variant forms require different diet adaptations. Infections or excessive protein intake may precipitate attacks. Details regarding optimum treatment are provided by Morton, Strauss, Robinson, Puffenberger, and Kelley (2002). Pregnancy in the MSUD woman may be stressful and precipitate decompensation during pregnancy or postpartum; thus careful monitoring and treatment, possibly including diet therapy is important. MSUD in an adult was featured in a mystery book by Patricia Cornwell titled, *Postmortem*. See Appendix B for support groups.

Hemoglobinopathies and Sickle Cell Disease

Included in this category are sickle cell anemia (HbSS), HbSC disease, thalassemia and sickle-thalassemia, and other hemoglobinopathies such as HbE, etc. (see chapter 6). In sickle cell anemia, the basic defect is caused by the substitution of the amino acid valine for glutamic acid in the sixth position of the beta chain of the hemoglobin molecule forming sickle cell hemoglobin (HbS) instead

of the normal adult hemoglobin (HbA). This changes the charge of the hemoglobin molecule, resulting in a different electrophoretic mobility that can be detected. When this occurs in only one of the two chains, the individual is said to have sickle cell trait. If the individual receives two of these recessive mutant genes from their parents, they are said to have sickle cell disease. Approximately 7% to 9% of Black Americans have sickle cell trait. Individuals of Mediterranean ancestry (e.g., Greek, Italian, Arabic) also have a higher frequency of sickle cell than other population groups. It is believed that these individuals are normally asymptomatic, but some may show exercise intolerance, especially at high altitudes. The chief reason to screen for sickle cell trait is to identify carriers so they can be counseled, and possibly to identify pregnant women who may be at higher risk for complications such as hematuria, urinary tract infections, and fetal distress at delivery. In sickle cell anemia itself, most of the symptoms arise from the vaso-occlusion resulting from red blood cell sickling. This sickling most often occurs in slow or reduced blood flow and in response to decreased oxygenation. Chronic hemolytic anemia, dactylitis (hand-foot syndrome resulting from bone necrosis and manifesting with soft tissue swelling), acute bacterial infection, especially pneumonia, and hepatosplenomegaly, occur around 6 months of age. Until this time infants have protection due to the presence of high levels of fetal hemoglobin.

In sickle cell anemia, periods of crisis occur that can be precipitated by stress. These are usually very painful, and result from sickling, stasis, and vascular occlusion. Many other manifestations occur, and the severity is variable. It is estimated that there is a death rate of 13% to 14% below 2 years of age, and as many as 50% used to die by age 20. Important therapeutic approaches such as hydroxyurea and comprehensive care in expert centers has markedly decreased mortality.

The rationale for the inclusion of sickle cell disease in these programs are as follows: (1) frequent uncomfortable diagnostic examinations are avoided later for a child with ambiguous symptoms resulting from sickle cell disease, (2) the expense of many diagnostic procedures are avoided for the family, (3) acute episodes can be recognized and treated promptly, (4) preventive health care can be stressed (i.e., prompt treatment of infections, prophylactic penicillin, good nutrition, and special immunizations such as for *Hemophilus influenzae* and meningococcal infections), and (5) genetic counseling can be extended to parents and siblings can also be screened. Sickle cell centers have the greatest experience and can usually offer support groups. A report from New York City on comprehensive care to families reported no deaths in infants followed from 8 to 20 months.

Tyrosinemia

Hypertyrosinemia may result from (1) transient tyrosinemia of the newborn, (2) tyrosinemia type 1 or hepatorenal tyrosinemia, (3) oculocutaneous tyrosinemia (type II, due to tyrosine aminotransferase deficiency), and (4) 4-hydroxyphenylpyruvate dioxygenase (pHPPD) deficiency, as well as nongenetic causes. Transient tyrosinemia in newborns improves spontaneously but can be accelerated by ascorbic acid intake and by restricting dietary protein temporarily. Many nurseries add Vitamin C to initial glucose feedings in order to minimize the incidence of false-positive screening tests due to the transient state. It is unclear whether this transient neonatal tyrosinemia is completely benign, because some investigators have reported its association with lethargy, poor feeding, reduced motor activity, and failure to thrive. It is common in the Arctic Inuit (12% of births).

The primary biochemical defect in tyrosinemia type I is deficiency of the enzyme fumarylacetoacetate hydrolase In the acute disorder, symptoms usually begin with failure to thrive, followed by lethargy, irritability, vomiting, edema, ascites, hypophosphatemia, hepatomegaly, cirrhosis, and renal tubular abnormalities such as aminoaciduria and phosphaturia. Hypoglycemia may occur. Blood and urine may both show increases in tyrosine and other amino acids, especially methionine. The urine may have an odor similar to boiled or rotten cabbage. Symptoms can begin in the 1st month of life, and if not treated, they can be fatal within the 1st year or so of life. Presentation may be with acute or chronic liver failure. The chronic form is usually manifested between 6 months of age and 3 years of age and symptoms may include renal tubule dysfunction, Vitamin D resistant rickets, peripheral neuropathy with painful neurologic crises and hypertonia that can result in rapidly

developing respiratory insufficiency; hypertension, hypertrophic cardiomyopathy, and hypoglycemia, as well as those symptoms previously mentioned. Death is caused by cirrhosis or hepatoma in childhood. Treatment usually consists of a diet that is low in tyrosine and phenylalanine (metabolized on an earlier path in the same metabolic pathway). Treatment, however, does not prevent eventual progression. Liver transplantation has now become the major treatment, and is implemented before age 2 years if possible. The mode of inheritance is AR. The overall incidence is 1 in 50,000 to 1 in 100,000, but is about 1 in 10,000 in Quebec province and 1 in 685 in the Chicoutini Lac St. Jean region of Quebec.

Biotinidase Deficiency

Biotinidase deficiency is also known as late-onset or juvenile multiple carboxylase deficiency. It results in the inability to recycle endogenous biotin and to release dietary protein-bound biotin resulting in the accumulation of lactate. Both profound (less than 10% of activity) and partial (10% to 30% activity) degrees of biotinidase deficiency are recognized. Biotinidase deficiency is an autosomal recessive disorder with an overall incidence worldwide of about 1 in 60,000 to 1 in 137,000. Symptoms may begin anywhere from 1 week to 2 years but typically begin at about 3 to 5 months; however, children presenting at 10 to 12 years of age have been reported. Clinical presentation may vary and can include myoclonic seizures, hypotonia, ketoacidosis, and organic aciduria as well as feeding difficulties, fungal infections, vomiting, diarrhea, and coma. Other signs/symptoms include alopecia, skin rash, ataxia, developmental delay, lethargy, vision problems, respiratory problems, and hearing loss. Metabolic ketoacidosis and organic acidemia may be seen with acute metabolic decompensation and coma in severe deficiency. Treatment consists of daily free biotin with usual dosages ranging from 5 to 20 mg per day. Known carrier mothers may be on biotin supplementation in pregnancy so that it may be taken up by the fetus.

Congenital Adrenal Hyperplasia

Congenital adrenal hyperplasia (CAH) includes a group of disorders all inherited in an AR manner, all of which have in common an enzyme defect in the steroidogenic path leading to decreases in cortisol production causing an increase in ACTH secretion and adrenal cortex hyperplasia. The most common form (about 90%) is 21-hydroxylase deficiency with an incidence of 1:10,000-18,000 live births that has early and late-onset forms; followed by 11β-hydroxylase deficiency that has early, late-onset, and mild forms; 17α-hydroxylase deficiency, and other very rare forms. CAH caused by 21-hydroxylase deficiency has both a simple virilizing form and a salt-losing form which may be considered together, as well as a nonclassic form which is typically mild, asymptomatic, or associated with postnatal androgen excess. The nonclassic form is more frequent in Ashkenazi Jews, and in this form one might see premature puberty in childhood as well as menstrual difficulties or infertility in adulthood. Hirsutism may be seen in women as well as oligomenorrhea and women. Hypersecretion of androgens results in masculinization of female fetuses and infants, manifesting itself in ambiguous external genitalia. In males, the first manifestation usually noticed is the premature appearance of pubic hair between 6 months and 2 years of age with advanced bone age. Treatment consists of cortisol replacement therapy and correction of ambiguous genitalia in female infants that is usually done at 6 to 12 weeks of age, a practice that has recently come under fire from some activists (see chapter 5). Some prefer to correct the vaginal opening in adolescence. In the late-onset form, androgen excess may not be noted in females until puberty or adulthood. In the salt-losing form, females are detected because of ambiguous genitalia, while males may be first detected later in infancy or early childhood because of symptoms such as poor feeding, diarrhea, weight loss, and vomiting which can resemble pyloric stenosis. If untreated, electrolyte imbalances result. Acute adrenal crisis occurs usually between the 4th and 15th day of life but can occur at 6 to 12 weeks which can result in cardiovascular collapse and death. Corticoids must be adjusted throughout life. In the mild form of 21-hydroxylase deficiency, females exhibit excess body and facial hair at puberty, and are usually treated with prednisone. CAH from 11β-hydroxylase deficiency is also manifested in females by ambigious genitalia seen at birth, or at puberty in the late-onset form. Hypertension is also noted. For couples at risk for 21-hydroxylase deficiency when pregnancy is

underway and before prenatal diagnosis, dexamethasone treatment in early pregnancy before genital differentiation has been used, although the safety of corticosteroids at this time is not established. If the fetus is normal, it may be discontinued. There has been interest in the correlation between genotype and phenotype. 21-hydroxylase deficiency results from mutations in the *CYP21* gene on chromosome 6p21.3 where there is also a pseudogene, *CYP21P*. Genotypes have been correlated with phenotypes in some cases allowing some prognostic predictions, however modifying genes such as those involved in tissue sensitivity to androgens and estrogens also play a role. For detailed information on treatment see Speiser and White (2003).

Medium-Chain Acyl-CoA Dehydrogenase Deficiency

Although medium-chain acyl-CoA dehydrogenase (MCAD) deficiency is rare, the first crisis, often misdiagnosed as sudden infant death syndrome (SIDS), is fatal in about 25% of cases. The crisis is manifested when an infant goes for a long time without eating, usually due to illness. The catabolic stress can result in hypoketotic hypoglycemia and hepatic encephalopathy and be mistaken for Reye syndrome. While symptoms may be seen in the neonatal period, episodes in the undiagnosed are most frequently seen between 3 months to 6 years of age and can result in neurological damage or death. Some affected individuals appear to be asymptomatic throughout their life, but long-term effects are not fully known. MCAD deficiency is a disorder of mitochondrial fatty acid oxidation affecting cellular energy and is especially common in those of northern European origin. A single mutation (A985G) accounts for more than 90% of the mutant alleles found in those who present clinically with MCAD deficiency. Maintaining carbohydrate intake and avoiding fasting can prevent episodes. Detection of MCAD became possible with the advent of MS/MS technology. Several states have added it to their mandated screening protocols, while others are piloting its inclusion. The March of Dimes added it as an addition to their recommended core of disorders to be included in a national newborn screening protocol. Some states have not instituted screening because of perceived concerns about the uncertainty of natural history, clinically effective treatment, and cost.

Cystic Fibrosis

Screening for cystic fibrosis (CF) in the newborn has been somewhat controversial, and is routinely performed in only a few states, although it is included in other pilot programs. CF is caused by mutations in the gene that encodes the cystic fibrosis transmembrane conductance regulator (CFTR) protein, one of a family of membrane proteins, and is considered a membrane transport disorder. The most common mutation is ΔF508 which accounts for about 70% of mutations in European Caucasian populations, but there are more than 1,000 mutations known. The result of mutation of the CFTR protein is dense mucous epithelial secretions in certain secretory cells. The incidence varies according to population, ranging from 1 in 1,800 in some Caucasian populations to 1 in 323,000 in some Japanese populations. An overall incidence in Caucasians is typically given at 1 in 2,500. Clinical features vary widely but typically involve gastrointestinal tract, respiratory tract, pancreas, liver, and reproductive tract. Modifier genes influence expression. The constellation of clinical features include chronic sinopulmonary diseases including colonization/persistent infection with certain microbial pathogens such as *Pseudomonas aeruginosa* and *Burkholderia cepacia,* chronic productive cough with persistent chest problems such as bronchiectasis, airway obstruction and nasal polyps; gastrointestinal and nutritional abnormalities that may include pancreatic insufficiency and recurrent pancreatitis, biliary cirrhosis, rectal prolapse or distal intestinal obstruction syndrome, chronic hepatic disease and nutritional problems including protein-calorie malnutrition, edema, failure to thrive, hypoproteinemia; salt-loss syndromes including chronic metabolic alkalosis; and male urogenital abnormalities resulting in obstructive azoospermia. Newborns may manifest meconium ileus. Growth reduction can be evident by 2 months of age. Particularly for pancreatic disease and sweat abnormalities there are genotype/phenotype correlations. These are less strong for the pulmonary manifestations. Two states (Colorado and Wisconsin) have been screening for CF in their newborn screening programs since the mid-1980s. In 1997, the National Institutes of Health issued a consensus development statement concluding that "Offering cystic fibrosis genetic testing to newborn infants is not recommended." The Centers for Disease Control and Prevention (1997) concluded that ". . . before recommending universal CF screening for newborns as a routine public health intervention, policymakers will need more compelling data about its effectiveness" (p. 21). That same year, a study was published finding nutritional benefits to children identified with CF as newborns and to whom adequate treatment was offered. However, flaws in methodology such as selection bias have been suggested, with the conclusion by others that there was no evidence of benefit. Since that time, the original study authors have reported additional subjects and responded to the methodological questions. They report both statistically and clinically significant findings, especially in regard to significantly better long-term growth in those patients detected through neonatal screening programs (Farrell et al., 2001). Recently, Koscik et al. (2004) have noted harmful effects on cognitive function in children with cystic fibrosis who had early malnutrition. Other studies indicate that pulmonary benefits could accrue from early diagnosis and treatment including less morbidity. A review of various ethical issues along with public health policy recommendations (Wilfond & Rothenberg, 2002) concludes that while early diagnosis offers benefits, that does not mean that routine newborn screening should be implemented. They also describe ways to maximize benefits and minimize harm by providing services such as a centralized communication system, genetic counseling services, and funding for CF centers for services such as nursing, dietary, social work, and so on. Because CF could be included in newborn screening programs using a two-tiered testing method of immunoreactive trypsinogen (IRT) followed by DNA testing for the most common mutation, ΔF508, and perhaps for other mutations, little additional cost would be added, and it is estimated that this method followed by diagnosis via sweat electrolyte testing would detect more than 97% of affected infants. Some researchers believe that now the burden of proof is on those who believe CF should not be included in screening programs to show why that is the case. In 2004, CDC published a statement recommending that "newborn screening for CF is justified" basing this on the basis of "moderate benefits and low risk of harm" (Centers for Disease Control and Prevention, 2004, p. 1). If gene therapy becomes available, the benefit of early identification would be obvious. CF is also discussed in chapter 6. A support group is the Cystic Fibrosis Foundation, http://www.cff.org.

Congenital Hearing Loss

Moderate to profound bilateral congenital hearing loss occurs in approximately 1 to 3 per 1,000 newborns in the United States, and is associated with delays in development of language, learning, and speech which can have lifelong consequences. Reliance on recognition by parents or health care providers or relying on family history has only identified, within the 1st year of life, a proportion of those affected. Thus, it was proposed that screening for hearing loss, including unilateral and milder loss, become part of universal newborn screening. A number of states have already included this in their programs, but some have not yet done so. A much awaited report from the U. S. Preventive Services Task Force on Newborn Hearing Screening (2001) concluded that "the evidence is insufficient to recommend for or against routine screening of newborns for hearing loss during the postpartum hospitalization" (p. 1995). Part of their rationale was based on the absence of prospective controlled studies to demonstrate "whether earlier treatment resulting from screening leads to clinically important improvement in speech or language skills at age three years or older . . ." (p. 1996), and stated that they could not determine whether potential benefits outweigh potential harm of false-positive tests. Other groups such as the American Academy of Pediatrics (Cunningham et al., 2003) have supported inclusion in newborn screening programs as well as throughout childhood. The Maternal and Child Health Bureau has financially supported states in implementing such programs, and more than 30 states have acted to incorporate such screening. Congenital deafness may arise from a variety of causes including in utero infection with cytomegalovirus and from a variety of genetic causes with varying modes of transmission. Eventually, methods of screening will include reliable DNA-based testing for common genetic forms of deafness such as connexin 26 and mitochondrial deafness that is syndromic or non-syndromic, and others since at least 50% of profound hearing loss is attributable to one or more gene mutations. For example, sensorineural hearing loss occurs in about 75% of children with profound biotinidase deficiency. It is important that all newborns with congenital hearing loss be evaluated for etiology and receive accurate genetic evaluation and counseling. This will not only benefit the family but may, depending on the etiology, indicate the involvement of other organs and systems requiring attention and treatment.

Other Fatty Acid Oxidation Defects, Organic Acidemias, Aminoacidemias and Other Metabolic Defects

With the advent of MS/MS technology, a large number of these disorders, shown in Table 11.6, can be detected using a single sample. In several states, one or more of these are being included in pilot programs within state newborn screening. In the New England Newborn Screening Program, there are 20 additional disorders for which testing is being piloted. Most of these disorders are individually rare but when looked at collectively are said to have an incidence of 1 in 4,000 to 1 in 5,000.

Other Disorders

A number of other genetic and nongenetic disorders have been suggested for potential inclusion in newborn screening programs. Examples include diabetes mellitus type 1, hyperlipidemia, familial hypercholesterolemia, neuroblastoma, fragile X and other chromosomal disorders, alpha-1- antitrypsin deficiency, Duchenne muscular dystrophy, hemochromatosis, BRCA1 and other gene mutations predisposing to cancer, Tay-Sachs disease, tuberous sclerosis, and Huntington disease. Arguments against inclusion of some of these have to do with one or more of the following: (1) the rarity of the disorder so that cost-effectiveness may be compromised; (2) the cost of the procedure, for example, in connection with chromosome analysis; (3) the lack of established ranges of normal; (4) lack of agreement as to what the variation or disorder means relative to any disease process or harmful event; (5) whether or not a disorder to which a genetic predisposition is identified will eventually become manifested, for example in BRCA1 mutations not all with the mutation eventually develop cancer; (6) disagreement on the need for early or any therapeutic intervention; (7) lack of treatment options available; (8) in the case of no available

TABLE 11.6   Potential Risks and Benefits Associated with Screening

	Type of screening		
	Carrier	Newborn	Predictive
Potential risks			
Uncovering misattributed parenthood	X	X	X
Stigmatization	X		X
Impaired self-concept	X		X
Increased insurance rates or loss of benefits	X		X
Loss of chosen marital partner	X		X
Social and cultural consequences	X		X
Interference with parent-child bonding		X	
Imposition of sick role	X	X	X
Anxiety associated with false-positive results	X	X	X
False feeling of security associated with false-negative results	X	X	X
Loss of the right *not* to know	X		X
Overprotection of child		X	X
Guilt feelings	X	X (parent)	X
Potential benefits			
Improved self-image if not a carrier or affected	X		X
Recover potential productive member of society		X	
Data collection for health planning	X	X	X
Allows for reproductive planning options	X	X	X
Institute plan for early detection of disease development			X
Initiation of early treatment		X	X
Alter disease process		X	X
Provide genetic counseling	X	X	X
Avoid costs associated with disease development		X	
Extend services to other relatives	X	X	X
If negative, avoidance of later unpleasant, expensive tests			X

treatment options, the possibility of psychological harm and discrimination; (9) for presymptomatic disorders such as Huntington disease, the possibility of psychological distress for a lifetime as well as discrimination as to education, jobs, and insurance; (10) if screening for one type of chromosome disorder such as fragile X is done, and another finding is identified, whether to reveal the incidental finding is an issue; (11) interference with the person's right not to know (in this case, the child might not want such information, but parents may already have obtained it); and (12) the inability to alter or affect the natural history of the disease. Not too long ago some screening of newborns was done for chromosomal abnormalities. Questions of cost, ethics, and ambiguity of the meaning of results forced their discontinuation. Hyperlipidemia and familial hypercholesterolemia had been suggested as diseases appropriate for inclusion in newborn screening programs. Here again there is a lack of agreement on the meaning of the test result

and what interventions (if any) would be appropriate to use. It is not clear whether or not a low-fat diet instituted early could retard the later development of coronary artery disease. In addition, the opportunity for early drug treatment such as with the statins might offer hope for improved outcomes. Part of the problem is the length of time involved in studying such cause and effect. In Britain and elsewhere, neonatal screening of male newborns is routine for Duchenne muscular dystrophy. Although no curative treatment is currently available, the family could receive genetic counseling thereby possibly preventing repeat cases in the family, and the family is spared anxiety during future diagnosis. However, they would have to live a longer time with the knowledge that their child is affected, and this could affect the entire family and familial relationships. Tuberous sclerosis is an autosomal dominant disorder characterized by white, leaf-shaped macules visible under a Wood's light, epilepsy, mental retardation, shagreen patches, and a typical rash on the nose and cheeks. It has been suggested for inclusion in newborn screening by using Wood's light to detect depigmented areas. Arguments against inclusion have included the argument that less than 100% of those affected show these "white nevi."

Conclusions

Newborn screening is not without problems. Changes in obstetric practice have shortened the hospital stay of both mother and infant. Thus, specimens are usually obtained just before the infant leaves the hospital. This can be as early as 24 hours after birth. Screening tests for some disorders may not be accurate this early. If they are not performed then, however, the compliance rate may be substantially lower. Infants transferred from one hospital to another might be missed. Many newborns will slip through the cracks in the health care system, not being detected until irreversible damage has occurred. Another criticism of mass newborn screening is the expense involved in screening low-risk infants for certain disorders. For example, it is relatively rare for a Black infant to have PKU. Should PKU testing thus be confined only to White infants in order to increase its cost effectiveness? Is the expense justified if disease in any child can be prevented or treated? On the other hand, if one blood or urine specimen can be used for disease screening for many disorders, this reduces the expense, but such multiplex testing may compromise accuracy in some cases. In addition, screening for many disorders at a time when accuracy may not be optimal for all may later lead to their erroneously not being considered as diagnostic possibilities. However, after diagnosis is made and treatment begins, vigilant monitoring is necessary to ensure not only optimal treatment, but also the exclusion of unnecessary treatment or misdiagnosis which also can be hazardous. There is a relatively high false-positive rate. Clayton reports that in New Jersey, for every newborn found to have PKU, 20 others are false-positives on their newborn screening. Effective newborn screening requires that there be a coordinated comprehensive multidisciplinary integrated system for delivery of care and that complex systems function effectively. This includes specimen collection, transport, tracking, laboratory analysis, data collection and analysis, locating and contacting families of infants with abnormal results on initial and subsequent screening for further evaluation and testing, and provision of follow-up services including diagnosis, treatment, and long-term management that includes education, psychological, nursing, and social services, genetic counseling, medical nutrition therapy, and medical foods. To date, parents have been minimally aware that their newborn has been screened for genetic disorders. It has been suggested that information about newborn screening be incorporated into standard prenatal care. As awareness of newborn screening opportunities and issues grows, public and professional voices will influence how newborn screening occurs in the U.S. in the future.

SCREENING GAMETE DONORS

A variety of assisted reproductive techniques have emerged including both gamete donation and embryo donation. Sperm donation for artificial insemination or in vitro fertilization is a genetic reproductive option when both parents are known carriers of a deleterious autosomal recessive gene or when the male is affected or at risk for carrying an autosomal dominant or X-linked mutant gene. Yet, there is still misunderstanding and inappropriate use of the procedure. A major issue lies in the screening of donors. A recent study showed inconsistencies between what screening actions should be taken, and those that are actually taken. There is a question of how far such screening should go. The couple should always understand that a normal infant cannot be guaranteed, although with the advent of various prenatal diagnostic techniques such as preimplantation genetic diagnosis, selection of embryos is possible but "normality" in all arenas can never be assured. For example, Gebhardt (2002) described a case of a man who had been a sperm donor for 18 children who was later found to have an adult-onset type of autosomal dominant neurologic disease. This type of situation is one reason to limit the number of inseminations per donor. Every effort should be taken to exclude those donors at greater risk than the general population. Some possible indications for exclusion include (1) presence of a single-gene disorder, chromosome abnormality, or serious multifactorial disorder in the donor or close blood relative; (2) Rh or ABO blood group that might cause incompatability between mother and fetus; (3) a donor who is 45 years of age or older; (4) exposure to drugs, radiation or chemical mutagens; (5) unexplained stillbirths, multiple miscarriages, or fetal deaths in their own children or close blood relative. Members of ethnic groups in which specific genetic disorders are more frequent should be tested for their carrier status. However, a non-hemophiliac male who has relatives with hemophilia could be a donor, as could the brother of a child with Tay-Sachs disease who is not a carrier. Such persons have been excluded by those with an inadequate knowledge of genetics. Couples considering artificial reproductive technologies may wish to discuss legal, ethical, and religious implications with a knowledgeable person and should be referred to an appropriate source. A particular issue is disclosure to the offspring that their conception was through gamete or embryo donation and what information to reveal. Guidelines have been developed that include information about counseling and information storage (Ethics Committee of the American Society for Reproductive Medicine, 2004).

Women who are donating eggs to a couple for genetic reasons would be subject to the same exclusionary criteria as sperm donors, with those 35 years and older being subject to exclusion because of the increased risk of chromosomal nondisjunction. In those couples using intracytoplasmic sperm injection as an assisted reproductive technique, there is an increased risk of birth defects as discussed in chapter 27. If the male partner is infertile, especially those with congenital bilateral absence of vas deferens, it has been suggested that they may have mutations in the CFTR gene, including unrecognized cystic fibrosis, or may have a chromosomal aberration. The combination of in vitro fertilization with the technique of preimplantation diagnosis is being used as described in chapter 27.

EARLY LEGISLATION AND GENETIC SCREENING

Not all legislative issues related to genetic screening can be discussed here. Information about potential genetic discrimination in relation to insurance and employment based on genetic testing and screening is summarized on the human genome project Web site. Information about screening in relation to PKU has been discussed previously. Early screening legislation in regard to sickle cell disease is discussed below because it points out how genetic information and misinformation may be used incorrectly even with good intent.

Sickle Cell Screening Legislation

The Civil Rights Movement and recognition given to sickle cell anemia as a Black health problem led to national attention. In 1971, President Nixon emphasized sickle cell anemia as a national health problem in a message to Congress. In July 1971, Massachusetts became the first state to mandate screening for sickle cell disease and trait, which was specified prior to school attendance. Other states followed suit. The purpose was to identify persons who were carriers for the sickle cell gene and allow for reproductive planning, thus decreasing high-risk pregnancies. Provisions of these acts were often both hastily written and passed without expert consultation. Thus many were defective both as to understanding of the disorder and as to adequate provision for counseling, education, and research. For example, one state mixed up homozygous disease status with carrier status. Another state erroneously provided for dietary control. Georgia entitled its bill "Education-Immunization for Sickle Cell Anemia Required for Admission to Public Schools," thus equating sickle cell anemia with a contagious disease, as did the District of Columbia. Other states associated it with syphilis in premarital blood testing, thus stigmatizing the carrier. Other states specified outdated or inaccurate testing methods.

New York State wrote its law to provide premarital screening to individuals "not of the Caucasian, Indian, or Oriental races," then stating that "no application for a marriage license shall be denied solely on the ground that such a test proves positive." Fears of eugenic restrictions were clearly aroused by this wording. Other problems arose as well. In states such as Georgia, preschool screening programs did not plan for what information about sickle cell could be offered entering school-age children.

They also did not plan for the uncovering of misattributed paternity in cases where a child was found to have sickle cell trait but neither putative parent was a carrier of the gene. The uncovering of individuals carrying the trait led to the implication that the trait itself was pathogenic. This led to unjustified job and insurance discrimination against such individuals. Another aspect of discrimination that was raised was why Whites of Mediterranean descent were not included in the laws being passed. Many Black leaders also questioned the loss of attention to more severe Black problems. In 1972 the National Sickle Cell Anemia Control Act was passed. This appropriated federal funds for voluntary sickle cell anemia screening and counselling and led to the establishment of ten comprehensive sickle cell centers. Many states repealed their early hastily written laws, and many rewrote them for incorporation into newborn screening programs. Damage to the credibility of genetic screening in general was a consequence of these poorly written laws.

PRESYMPTOMATIC AND PREDICTIVE TESTING

In presymptomatic or predictive screening or testing, the person is tested for the gene mutation (1) for the disease itself, for example in the case of Huntington disease (HD) or familial monogenic Alzheimer disease (discussed in chapter 21); or (2) for susceptibility to disease, such as in the case of *BRCA1* mutations and susceptibility to ovarian and breast cancer (discussed in chapter 23). In the case of predictive *screening*, a specific asymptomatic population or subpopulation would be screened for one of the two preceding situations, whereas for presymptomatic or predictive *testing*, the person being tested is deemed at higher risk usually because of family history or signs or symptoms. These terms usually apply to later onset disorders. In addition to the ones mentioned previously, other genetic conditions that fall into this category are hemochromatosis, familial hypercholesterolemia (both homozygous and heterozygous), neuroblastoma, adult polycystic kidney disease, and others. Such screening and testing has been controversial for several reasons. In some cases, there is not clarity about what possession of a given genetic variation or mutation means in terms of development of clinical manifestations or

disease. In other cases, there are fears related to the impact of discovering that one has a particular mutation that relate to the individual, family, community and society and may result in adverse (or beneficial) psychosocial effects, and effects on insurability, education, life choices, and jobs as well as potential discrimination. In this section, HD will be considered as an example while such testing related to the workplace, Alzheimer disease and cancer are considered in detail in chapters 14, 21, and 23, respectively.

HD is an autosomal dominant incurable neurodegenerative disorder most frequently manifesting itself in middle to late adulthood caused by expansion of CAG repeats in the HD gene. Its symptoms are discussed in chapter 6. Following many years of investigation, in 1986, presymptomatic testing for HD was first accomplished through DNA markers that were tightly linked to the HD gene. This method was limited to informative families, and accuracy was variable. In 1993, the HD gene was isolated, making direct presymptomatic diagnosis possible through ascertaining the number of the CAG repeat length. A large body of literature has emerged on predictive testing for HD. Since HD is not currently treatable, the benefits of testing relate to life and reproductive planning, and psychological parameters as discussed earlier. One of the revelations that emerged is that many fewer persons have sought testing for HD than were predicted to do so. In some cases, the original sets of guidelines for testing in Huntington disease were very prescriptive in terms of the entire procedure—the pretest, testing, result delivery, and post-test stages. While intentions are honorable, and designed in the best interests of the client, do such guidelines act to deny access to testing to some who would want to have it under more flexible conditions? Is this paternalistic? The most recent recommendations included not testing minors or children to be adopted. However, this is discussed further below.

A variety of studies have looked at why people decided to have testing or not. Some of the most frequent reasons for taking testing were for "wanting to know" and for planning and decision-making. Reasons for not choosing to be tested were because of the potential psychological burden of a positive test and fear of not being able to cope, because the risk to their children would increase, lack of treatment, potential loss of health and life insurance, no plan to have more children, cost of testing, not being able to "undo" the knowledge, and others. Some of those who were not found to have the gene experienced survival guilt, emotional numbness, and had difficulting in coping with the impact on the family. Many had lived for years struggling with the fear of development of HD and the adjustment that these emotional struggles were unnecessary was difficult. Others believed they were ostracized from those family members who had the HD gene, and were excluded. Partners of those who did not have HD were uniformly relieved. Some who have found that they have the HD gene mutation experienced hopelessness, depression, and suicide ideation. Others did not report long-term significant problems. Reported adverse effects have been fewer than anticipated. In a study looking at predictive testing and its impact on reproduction, it was found that 14% of those with the HD gene mutation had one or more subsequent pregnancies as compared with 28% of those without it. The majority of those with the HD gene mutation had prenatal testing (Evers-Kiebooms et al., 2002).

Many feel that HD testing should be available only to those who have reached the age of majority in whatever country they reside; others do not. Another issue has to do with whether or not to reveal the actual CAG length. This result is being increasingly asked for because the longer repeat length in the abnormal area may be related to the age of onset prediction. To not reveal it is paternalistic, and may not be consistent with right to know. However, the person may not understand this information and may compare their length to others. The ACMG/ASHG (1998) statement recommends disclosure. Some providers do not wish to disclose this because of potential bias to participation in research studies. Discrimination has occurred in those who have been shown to have the HD gene. In one case, it was reported that a person was denied entrance to medical school on the basis that the educational efforts would be "wasted." This points out the importance of guaranteeing confidential results and of legislating non-discrimination for genetic susceptibility or actual disease. Anonymous testing has been suggested for HD and other conditions similar to that done in HIV testing, and this has been done in a limited sort of way. Preserving anonymity, however, may limit support and counseling. In the situation where a pregnant woman requests prenatal diagnosis for her fetus for Huntington disease if the father is at risk, providing this information to her, depending on the outcome and her actions, may reveal the gene status of her partner resulting in violation of his right not to know. In a study by Roberts et al. (2003) of adult children with a parent with Alzheimer disease (AD), nearly 78% sought predictive or susceptibility testing. Among the reasons for doing so were for future research, to arrange personal affairs, and hoping for effective treatment development. The best predictor for seeking testing was their belief that other family members would need to be prepared for AD. In another study by Roberts et al. (2004), after family history was taken and risk assessment information was given persons most likely to seek predictive testing for AD had the following attributes: below 60 years of age, female gender and college education. Predictive testing for susceptibility gene mutations for certain disorders have a greater degree of uncertainty. Usually in these cases, such as with the apo E ε4 allele, the degree of risk for the development of late-onset AD is uncertain, and the results may offer few advantages in terms of knowledge to the person seeking information. For a position paper on genetic testing in late-onset adult disorders see McKinnon et al. (1997). Further points relating to presymptomatic and predictive testing are discussed in chapter 23 in relation to cancer and in chapter 21 in relation to Alzheimer disease, but they apply here as well.

GENETIC TESTING/SCREENING OF CHILDREN AND ADOLESCENTS

Should children or adolescents be tested for susceptibility to genetic disease, presence of the genes for late-onset diseases, and/or carrier status? The issue of genetic testing and screening of children and/or adolescents has been an area of great controversy. Some centers and groups have condemned such testing and refused to provide such services to children or adolescents even with parental consent, while others are more liberal. Newborn screening already tests infants for some disorders that do not have a direct therapeutic benefit. To be considered are personal issues such as medical, psychosocial, reproductive issues, and issues with a broader impact such as those affecting insurance, career, and future employment. A thoughtful report by the ASHG/ACMG (1995) discusses many related issues. In a study in Great Britain, pediatricians were more likely than geneticists to allow such testing at the request of parents or adoption agencies. There was great variation according to condition. In a study by Tibben (1992), parents were more favorable towards genetic testing than were health professionals. Michie, McDonald, Bobrow, McKeown, and Marteau (1996) reported on a family in which testing for familial adenomatous polyposis was done for the 2- and 4-year old sisters. Their hypothesis was that "complying with requests for predictive DNA testing . . . in parents wishing to reduce uncertainty about their children's future health is associated with good psychological outcomes regardless of the test results."

Reasons for considering testing in children commonly evolve from the diagnosis of a genetic disorder within a family, particularly one that has onset in late childhood, adolescence or adulthood rather than the necessity for diagnosis of a genetic disorder because of the presentation of symptoms or because of an immediate health implication. Some reasons for such testing include:

- the institution of preventive measures or therapy that can treat or ameliorate the severity or influence the natural history of the disease in question (a direct timely medical benefit or evidenced-based risk reduction program are the most compelling reasons for testing);
- sparing the child the unpleasantness and trauma of continued testing for disorders such as familial cancer when the child may not possess the gene in question;
- knowledge for the parent in terms of their own financial and reproductive planning given the future outlook for their present children;
- the elimination of the uncertainty of knowing whether or not they possess a gene for a serious disorder such as Huntington disease or adult polycystic kidney disease;
- the psychological benefit of a negative test; for a positive result, the chance for parents to

adjust to a diagnosis and plan ways to disclose and cope with the news at the appropriate time for their child; and
- the opportunity for life planning based on this information including choices related to education, career, lifestyle, and reproductive decisions. For example, a child at risk for retinitis pigmentosa could choose a career that did not require visual acuity or a child with familial hypertophic cardiomyopathy could receive early drug therapy for arrhythmia prevention.

Some reasons given for not performing such testing include:

- the child may not be able to understand the ramifications of testing, such as future insurability risks and possible effects on education and employability;
- the child may not be able to give informed consent or even assent, thus taking away the child's right to decide;
- the potential psychological consequences of learning that one has a genetic disorder or is a carrier, such as lowered self-esteem, changes in family dynamics and in parent-child bonding, loss of confidentiality of the child's condition since the parents will know the status;
- stimatization and labelling; and
- the potential negative psychological consequences of learning that one does not have a disorder and developing "survivor guilt" or feeling alienated from an affected sibling or family member.

Several legal principles may impact on the issue including the scope and limits of parental authority, the "mature minor rule," emancipated minor status, and recognition of the age of 7 years to assent to participate in human subject research. Competence to make decisions includes the ability to understand and communicate, reasoning and deliberation, the ability to develop and sustain moral values, and the child's developmental level. The Working Party of the Clinical Genetics Society (1994) believes that predictive genetic testing in children is appropriate when onset occurs in childhood or if there are medical interventions such as diet, medication, or surveillance for complications that can be offered; it does not believe it should be undertaken in a healthy child for an adult onset disorder if there are no useful medical interventions that can be offered. Clayton (1997) argues that parents should have latitude in deciding whether or not genetic testing is good for their child, and that other interests besides the child may be appropriately considered. In regard to genetic testing for cancer susceptibility (see chapter 23), the American Society of Clinical Oncology (2003) recommended that when cancer could develop during childhood and there are evidence-based risk reduction strategies, that the scope of parental authority includes deciding for the child participation or nonparticipation in such testing, and that if there is not an increased risk of childhood cancer that testing should be delayed until the person is of an age to make an informed decision. In a study of obligate fragile X carriers (McConkie-Rosell, Spiridigliozzi, Iafolla, Tarleton, & Lachiewiez, 1997), the women stated that the mean preferred age to test their children and to inform them about fragile X was 10 and 12 years, respectively. In studying siblings in an X-linked severe combined immunodeficiency, 89% would want their daughter tested before age 18 years, and 34% would test as a newborn; 51% would disclose the results before adolescence while 89% would do so before adulthood (Fanos, Davis, & Puck, 2001). In an interview study of children ages 10 to 17 years whose families had an increased risk of breast cancer or heart disease, initially children thought they would participate but as they considered further, they became more hesitant although they saw benefits of prevention, early detection, or treatment. The researchers concluded that the first reaction of children may not include an understanding of the benefits and risks and they encouraged further discussion and personalization (Bernhardt, Tambor, Fraser, Wissow, & Geller, 2003). It is also important to note that children may have limited options to refuse even if they wish to do so.

The provider needs to be able to discuss issues with families and help them to consider the risks and benefits in a non-adversarial, reasoned manner. As part of this the capacity of the child to understand and make decisions should be considered, and not based solely on age. Although parents are generally considered to act in the best interests of their children, many believe that the provider should be the advocate for the child's best interest, and that if the provider believes that it is not in the best interest of the child then the provider is not obligated to perform testing. Others believe that the decision does not rest with providers but is the choice of the family. Providers may not always have the necessary education to assist families with such decisions. In a study of pediatric residents, Rosen, Wallenstein, and McGovern (2002) found that there were no statistically significant differences in responses regarding ordering testing for children at risk for Huntington disease when analyzed by year of residency or by exposure to a genetics course. In the Huntington disease vignette, the percentage of pediatric residents believing it was appropriate to order a test at the request of the mother when the child is 10 years, with assent of the age-10 child prior to ordering, at age 17, and with assent prior at age 17 years was 39%, 24%, 52%, and 84%, respectively. When the son requested such testing at 10 years, 44% believed it was appropriate to order testing, while 89% felt it was appropriate at 17 years of age.

Decisions of both children and adolescents and their parents are also influenced by personal experiences with the illness being tested for. As Fanos (1997) points out, provision of genetic counseling and psychological support may be more important than the actual test decision. The joint statement by the American Society of Human Genetics Board and the American College of Medical Genetics Board of Directors (1995) states that "a request by a competent adolescent for the results of a genetic test should be given priority over parents' requests to conceal information" (p. 1234). The Task Force on Genetic Testing stated that "Genetic testing of children for adult onset diseases should not be undertaken unless direct medical benefit will accrue to the child and this benefit would be lost by waiting until the child has reached adulthood" (Holtzman & Watson, 1997, pg. 13). In general, there is support for testing children in childhood when they are symptomatic, when a genetic disorder generally appears in childhood, and presymptomatically when there is a benefit to preventive treatment. Testing children for the carrier status is even more complex. Commercial testing companies often do not ascertain the age of a person submitting a sample for testing through the mail.

ETHICAL, SOCIAL, AND LEGAL ISSUES

Genetic screening and testing entail certain risks as well as benefits. They are summarized in Table 11.6. Questions relating to the rights of the person being screened, such as the right to privacy, confidentiality of information, disclosure of findings, duty to warn, informed consent, refusal to participate, and the ownership of samples are also raised. Some have suggested that the option of anonymous genetic testing be available in much the same manner as anonymous HIV testing in order to minimize discrimination. This has not yet proved to be a widespread option, although some families and individuals have used false names or sought testing in another geographic locale in order to protect their privacy. Ethical principles in regard to genetic testing and screening include balancing various principles such as autonomy (the right of persons to decide), beneficience (the obligation to do good), justice, and nonmalificence (the obligation not to harm), and also include access. Hodge (2004) points out that there may be disadvantages to treating genetic information in a different sort of way and mentions that individual ethical rights have limits and "should not always trump the use of genetic tests or screening programs . . . for legitimate public health purposes (p. 66). Genetic screening/testing in the workplace setting may include testing related to the employment per se or merely be a convenient site for population screening but raises particular issues about confidentiality, the potential of coercion, privacy, autonomy, and dignity.

Right to Refuse to Participate

Although some newborn screening is compulsory, many states provide for exemption from screening of the newborn for genetic disorders if this is a violation of the parents' religious beliefs. This raises two interesting issues. The first is that often parents are not specifically asked to give informed consent for this type of screening, so that they never have the opportunity to refuse their child's participation. They may either never find out that testing has been done, or find out at the time of hospital discharge. The second point is whether or not the parents should have the right to deny the child the

privilege of discovering whether or not they may have disorders such as PKU and hypothyroidism, which are amenable to early treatment, thus preventing retardation. How does the principle of causing no harm apply? Whose rights are most important in this instance? What future influences will the legal rulings related to blood transfusions to save the lives of children whose parents object have on this type of genetic screening issue? Should parental refusal be honored or is it unjustifiable?

In other types of screening programs where participation is purely voluntary, exercising the right to refuse to participate in screening should not result in the denial of any other services. Subtle coercion should also be avoided. Care should be taken that promotional material is not unintentionally coercive, either by stigmatizing those who choose not to participate by playing on emotions such as for future children, or by subliminal means. For example, Clarke (2002) gives the example of the difficulty in distinguishing between popular consent or public coercion when screening is sponsored by the dominant social or religious institution, such as screening for β-thalassemia in Cyprus being sponsored by the Greek Orthodox church. Sometimes screening or testing can be coercive in that they are linked to research programs or protocols, and clients may be told that testing is dependent on enrollment in the protocol.

Informed Consent

The issue of informed consent is a major one. A full general treatment of this important issue is not possible here; however, some major points applicable to genetic testing and screening will be discussed. It is generally agreed that the physical risks resulting from testing and screening are minimal, usually limited to those resulting from having blood drawn. The major hazards are in the social, economic, and psychological domain, and these should be discussed. In addition, if the screening is voluntary, it is particularly necessary to apprise individuals of potential risks. The needed information should be described in terms understandable to the individual and should be included in the educational and promotional literature used in the program. The guidelines used nationally for the protection of human subjects are applicable to screening even though they were developed for experimental research consents, as it can be legitimately argued that many potential short- and long-term risks of screening are still not known. Thus the nature and purposes of the screening should be clearly spelled out. Some of the elements to be included were discussed at the beginning of this chapter.

Ownership and Future Use of Samples Taken for Testing/Screening

When blood or urine samples are used for either testing or screening, these are often stored away to use for additional testing. What happens to samples such as from newborns? Such a use and its implications may be unknown to the person from whom it has been taken. Thus consent is not usual or may be buried in a long complicated consent form. Could such samples be used for forensic or other legal identification reasons, and what does this mean in terms of the individual's right to privacy? Although these samples are generally considered to be a good source of material for research, it raises certain questions. What responsibilities are there if these samples are tested later and found to be positive for a different disorder, or if a future test or treatment becomes available? Is the researcher then responsible for locating that individual and communicating results? Who actually owns these samples? The question of asking for the individual's consent for use in later testing could be obtained along with instructions for whether or not the individual wants to be informed of the results, and this approach is being increasingly adopted. Individuals may also change their mind about the use of stored samples, and they should know the procedure for making their wishes known and acted upon. If identifying information is erased from the sample, both potential risks and benefits would be decreased but again many issues are raised. Knoppers and Laberge (1995) make the point that anonymous "samples are sources while participants in human research are persons." Epstein (1997) believes that researchers can use a sample that is anonymous because it does not violate rights, endanger the person, or expose him/her to personal risk. Here one weighs the value of respecting individuality with the potential to discover useful information. A controversy in the news media involved the obtaining and storage of

DNA samples from persons in armed services that were to be stored for 75 years. The reason given was for identification of combat casualties (see chapter 3). In 1995, two members of the U.S. Marine Corps asserted that this violated their rights but the military prevailed in a hearing. Statements on the storage and use of DNA samples have been formulated by various groups. In a proposed but not enacted bill that was referred to as the Domenici bill, (although a similar bill has been introduced in 1997) some of the points included the following thoughts:

1. The DNA molecule contains an individual's genetic information, and this information is written in a code that is being rapidly deciphered, sequenced, and understood.
2. Genetic information is uniquely private and personal information.
3. Genetic information has been misused resulting in harm to indiviuals.
4. The improper use and disclosure of genetic information can lead to significant harm to the individual, including stigmatization and discrimination.
5. The potential for misuse with respect to genetics is tremendous since genetics transcends medicine. It has the potential to penetrate many aspects of life including employment, insurance, forensics, finance, education, and even one's self-perception.
6. DNA samples and genetic information should not be collected, stored, analyzed, nor disclosed without the individual's authorization.
7. A genetic analysis of an individual's DNA provides information not only about an individual, but also about that individual's parents, siblings, and children, potentially infringing on individual and family privacy.
8. Because of its unique nature, DNA can be linked to a single identifiable individual, regardless of whether identifiers are limited to a DNA sample.
9. Existing legal protections for genetic information are inadequate to ensure genetic privacy.
10. Uniform rules for the collection, storage, and use of DNA samples, and genetic information obtained from such samples are

needed both to protect individual privacy and to permit legitimate genetic research. (S. 1898, U.D. Senate 1996, sec. 2)

Disclosure of Incidental or Unexpected Findings

It is wise for health professionals to thoroughly discuss and have a policy on what is to be done with unexpected findings before beginning testing or screening. Often a statement is included as part of informed consent as to what information will and will not be revealed. If a screening program has been undertaken for research purposes to determine the incidence of one disorder in the population, the discovery of another disorder may not need to be disclosed. A prescreening agreement may be worded in such a way that no responsibility will be incurred by the researcher. This problem is one that also accompanies prenatal diagnosis and is discussed in chapter 12. An example is the detection of newborns who have sickle cell trait rather than sickle cell anemia. The Institute of Medicine report (1994) raises the issue of whether parents should have this information because of possble stigmatization or whether this information would be of benefit to parents who may not realize that one or both is a carrier. Incidental findings could also impact upon stigmatization, insurance, and genetic discrimination issues.

Uncovering Misattributed Parenthood

One of the risks of screening is the discovery of misattributed parenthood, usually paternity. For example, if a screening program for sickle cell is undertaken in school screening and a child is discovered to have sickle cell trait, but neither putative parent has it, the chances are that one or both parents are not the natural parents of this child, barring a laboratory error. How is this situation to be handled? Does disclosure hold that such results must be shared? Can they be withheld? Can only the mother be informed of the result? The admonition to "do no harm" may be a guiding principle in making a decision. Again, incorporating a statement about policy into a pre-testing or screening consent can be valuable.

In cases of misattributed paternity, the choices of action depend on how strongly paternity impinges on risk. There are several choices that the counselor may have in AR disorders if the mother is unwilling to have misattributed paternity revealed and both partners have sought counseling. Some that have been used include counseling on the basis of a recurrence risk of 25% for having another child with the disorder, even though the woman's partner is not a carrier; counseling on the actual recurrence risk for the disorder for this couple, which is near zero if the partner is not a carrier, without giving complete information about patterns of transmission; suggesting that spontaneous mutation is the cause of the disorder, and giving the actual recurrence risk; and discussing options with the female partner separately. Problems, of course, also will result from the consequence of these choices, as they affect reproduction and childbearing of the couple. If the male partner subsequently finds a new mate, he may mistakenly believe he is a carrier if the counselor chooses the first option. In any case, conflicts are created between the ethics of the professional and the counselee's expectations. The President's Commission (1983) addresses these issues and recommends full disclosure accompanied by in-depth counseling, and failing that, accurate risk information even with incomplete understanding of the reasons by the counselees. However, each decision should be made on an individual basis. There is some fear that a precounseling or prescreening agreement may discourage some from seeking genetic services.

Confidentiality, Access to Information, and the Right to Privacy

Several types of problems can arise in this area. The first is to whom can the results of testing or screening be released? Ideally, only the person undergoing the screening should be given these results. In practice, testing or screening records may be kept and handled by a wide variety of nonprofessional personnel and volunteers. They may have access to other persons' identity for billing, insurance, and follow-up purposes. In small communities or neighborhoods, anonymity is not possible, and unintended stigmatization may result. In some screening programs, such as those for sickle cell, the actual sponsorship may be under the auspices of lay community groups. The obligations of such groups to maintain privileged communication is not legally clear. They also may not be cognizant of some of the ramifications of releasing information to unauthorized persons such as other family members, relatives, and even the patient's personal physician, without permission. Patients can consent to disclosure of the findings of screening. This may be specified. For example, the person may wish to have results sent to his or her physician or to certain relatives, which raises another issue. Should relatives who are at risk or whose offspring are at risk for developing genetic disease be informed of that risk even without the consent of the person being tested or screened? Does the health professional have a responsibility to these individuals as well that includes the duty to warn? This issue has been discussed previously in this document. It has also been found that clients have said they would notify relatives and then have selectively done this, so that some relatives have been informed and others have not received the information (Costalas et al., 2003). To some extent this may depend on their comfort level with those relatives and the closeness of the relationship. ASCO (2003) believes that the "health care provider's obligations (if any) to at-risk relatives are best fulfilled by communication of familial risk to the person undergoing testing, emphasizing the importance of sharing this information with family members so that they may also benefit" (p. 2403). They state that case law is not yet developed in regard to the "duty to warn," and that there are differences when the relatives are also patients of the health care provider. The American Society of Human Genetics (1998) lists conditions for disclosure of genetic information to family members at risk, and state that patients should be informed prior to testing that the results may have familial implications. Possible ways that it could come to pass would be for states to compel the reporting of positive screening results in the same way as they do for venereal or certain contagious disease, or for laws to be passed permitting the disclosure of significant information to relatives at risk. At present, this is not the case, and in fact the screener might be passing unwanted information on to relatives, thus interfering with their right not to know. In the case of HD, a grandparent might have had HD. The mother might have decided not to be tested and know her status. If her 18-year-old daughter is

tested and finds out she has the HD gene mutation, then the mother's status is revealed to the daughter and to the mother herself, interfering with her right not to know. Hopefully, education could prevent most involuntary disclosure issues from arising. The report of the President's Commission (1983) indicates that ethical obligations to prevent harm to relatives may override confidentiality if information is important in preserving the relatives' well-being. Offit and colleagues (2004) discuss 3 lawsuits against physicians that arose because they did not warn at-risk relatives about their risks for hereditary disease. All records should be kept in such a way that the individual is not immediately identifiable. Therefore, a code number instead of names should be used. Care must especially be taken when entering data in a central computer or data bank. Often these are accessible to individuals by means of telephone computer access. The same care should be taken when using registries for genetic disease. If patients are asked to give consent for such use, the extent must be spelt out in a way that the patient can understand.

Another type of a breach of confidentiality that can occur is by revealing statistical data that accidentally allow a person who has been tested to be identified. It is imperative to be sure that no individual can be identified in this way, even if it makes the research data presentation less detailed. Disclosure of information to unrelated third parties, such as insurance companies or employers, may have other consequences. These may include higher insurance rates, cancellation of insurance policies, or loss of job opportunities. Employers have long used various attributes in their selection process and now some include genetic information. New Jersey has enacted legislation prohibiting employment discrimination based on genetic information beyond testing. The President's Commission (1983) recommended that ". . . because of the potential for misuse as well as unintended social or economic injury, information from genetic testing should be given to people such as insurers or employers only with the explicit consent of the person screened." There should be specific rather than blanket consent forms for information so that the person being screened can ensure selective control. Screenees should be told when, what, and to whom information can be released before participating.

Genetic Disorders as Pre-existing Conditions

Frequently insurance companies cover people with the exception of pre-existing conditions. In a sense, all genetic disorders are pre-existing and permanent. This should be clarified before testing or screening is undertaken. If all possible conditions were tested for, however, probably no one would be left who did not have some pre-existing susceptibility to disease or a disease itself. Issues of discrimination in regard to insurance premiums or coverage are being discussed nationally. Some states have prohibited insurance companies from denying, limiting, or terminating coverage. National legislation is proposed. The Secretary's Advisory Committee on Genetic Testing (SACGT) for the Department of Health and Human Services (2000) recommended the support of legislation aimed at preventing genetic discrimination, and increased oversight of genetic testing though the FDA. Legislation designed to prohibit genetic discrimination in had reached the U.S. senate in 2004.

Interference With Parent–Child and Family Relationships

Identification of a child with a genetic variant that has not been shown to have any definite correlation with clinical disease, the carrier state, or an actual genetic disorder itself can change the relationship between the child and his or her parents. In the newborn, disruption of parent-infant bonding can occur. Overprotectiveness can occur at any age, leading to impaired psychological development. Parents can experience guilt at having given this disorder to the child, whether or not there is any basis in fact for these feelings. A sick role may be imposed on the child. These issues may be particularly prominent in population testing or screening for disorders for which there is no present treatment, such as Duchenne muscular dystrophy. The finding among siblings that one is a carrier and others are not can change their relationships with each other. Negative feelings for passing on a disease such as HD may be felt by those who have that testing and resentment may be directed at those who may have sought to hide the disorder. Those who are not found to carry the gene may be ostracized from some family affairs and be "left out" in various ways. Feelings of "survivor guilt" may be manifested by taking on the burden of caring for affected family members, such as in HD.

Stigmatization, Reduced Self-Worth and Damage to the Self-Concept

In the excitement of inducing participation in mass carrier screening or testing, it is easy to forget the risks that may occur. Impairment of self-image or self-worth is one such risk. Adolescents are particularly vulnerable because they are still searching and developing their self-identity. Views of their peers are extremely important in this development. Thus, for example, the effect of identifying all Jewish students in a high school population to volunteer for Tay-Sachs carrier testing can be extreme. First of all, they are identified as "different." Secondly, many of those who are then identified as carriers have been shown to have an impaired self-concept. Some researchers have attempted to justify this result by stating that many of the noncarriers had improved self-concepts. Because little long-term research has been done to date in this area, the long-term effects are not known. Nurses, with their understanding of growth and development, can assist in identifying these issues before screening begins. In a study of carrier testing for both Tay-Sachs disease and cystic fibrosis among Jewish high school students in Australia, follow-up 3 to 6 years later showed high levels of satisfaction, low concern and no reported stigma (Barlow et al., 2003). A few students thought they would need retesting at the time of reproduction indicating some misconceptions. Another question that arises is whether or not the identification of carrier status is really important to this age group. What are the anticipated uses to which it will be put? They can, however, begin to identify themselves in new and less favorable terms such as, "I am a Tay-Sachs carrier." In any school setting, it is difficult to prevent school officials from learning the results of the testing or screening. This should be considered in the planning phases of the program. Is it really the needs of the participants who are being met in the screening? Or is it the needs of the researchers? Once a person is identified as a carrier, regardless of age, there is no way to return to the pre-testing or screening state of ignorance.

In a rural Greek population, an intensive educational effort and screening program were instituted for carriers of thalassemia in an effort to reduce the incidence. Carriers were identified and the screeners left the village. When they returned several years later, they discovered that those individuals who were identified as carriers were virtually untouchable. Marriages could not be arranged for them, as was the custom. The social status of their families were impaired so that, in effect, all members were affected (Stamatoyannopoulos, 1974). It has been believed that education of an ethnic population as to the disorder will minimize stigmatization, but this might be a reflection of the culture of the health care provider, not of the population being tested. It also emphasizes the importance of understanding the culture of the group in which screening is to be done, before attempting to initiate a program. The participation of knowledgeable community individuals helps to minimize some of the negative aspects and to alert the providers to potential cultural problems. Although rationale for singling out ethnic groups for high-risk genetic screening centers on economic feasibility, the issue of discrimination can apply. Screening should be kept voluntary, and equal access for all to the screening should be allowed. Definition of groups on ethnic and racial lines may accrue both benefits and burdens for them. It was not long ago that arguments directed at improving the race through eugenics was popular in this country. The result of this thinking was the imposition of immigration restrictions, prohibitive marriage laws, sterilization acts, and the distraction from the real roots of labor and social problems. Between 1911 and 1930, about 30 states passed sterilization laws for a variety of conditions ranging from insanity to alcoholism to criminality. Thus many fears are founded in history. Although many states repealed those laws, some are still on the books, even though they are rarely if ever invoked. The rise of Nazi Germany contributed to the loss of respectability of many of the eugenic beliefs in the United States,

The misunderstanding of the health status of carriers, particularly in the case of sickle cell, has also led to unintended consequences. Loss of employment, loss of access to certain jobs, educational opportunities, and professions, discrimination for entry to the Air Force Academy, and increased insurance rates have been but a few. In addition some who are identified as carriers may not themselves understand the meaning of that status.

THE FUTURE

The potential for various types of genetic screening is expanding. These will include population and targeted genetic screening for actual diseases, for carrier state, for predictive screening, and for newborn screening as well as prenatal applications. Advances in scientific understanding and in the technology to translate the findings into practice will continue to grow. Many social, ethical, legal, and cultural factors impinge on genetic screening. They must be carefully considered before enthusiasm and good intentions lead unwittingly to harmful effects on individuals and groups. In regard to newborn screening, as there will be an increased ability to identify and treat an expanding list of disorders, there will be increased consumer advocacy to make broader universal detection available in a timely but responsible manner. As awareness of these issues grow, public policy decisions will increasingly influence genetic screening in the future. Nurses, among other health professionals, will need to be aware of the trends and issues surrounding screening, be informed so they can educate and interpret information correctly for their clients in a culturally sensitive and educationally appropriate manner, understand the emotional and psychological impact of results and the potential impact on such issues as insurability and future life planning, and understand the need for a coordinated comprehensive screening plan with appropriate follow-up of services.

BIBLIOGRAPHY

Ad Hoc Committee on Genetic Testing/Insurance Issues. (1995). Genetic testing and insurance. *American Journal of Human Genetics, 56,* 327–331.

American Academy of Pediatrics. Committee on Genetics. (1996). Newborn screening fact sheets. *Pediatrics, 98*(3 Part 1), 473–501.

American Academy of Pediatrics Newborn Screening Task Force. (2000). Serving the family from birth to the medical home. Newborn screening: A blueprint for the future. A call for a national agenda on state newborn screening programs. *Pediatrics, 106,* 389–427.

American College of Medical Genetics. (1998, Winter). Statement on genetic testing for cystic fibrosis. *American College of Medical Genetics College Newsletter, 10,* 9.

American College of Medical Genetics/American Society of Human Genetics. Huntington Disease Genetic Testing Working Group. (1998). ACMG/ASHG statement. Laboratory guidelines for Huntington disease genetic testing. *American Journal of Human Genetics, 62,* 1243–1247.

American College of Medical Genetics Board of Directors. (2004). ACMG statement on direct-to-consumer genetic testing. *Genetics in Medicine, 6,* 60.

American College of Medical Genetics, Storage of Genetics Materials Committee. (1995). Statement on storage and use of genetic materials. *American Journal of Human Genetics, 57,* 1499–1500.

American College of Obstetricians and Gynecologists (1996, February). Committee Opinion. *Genetic screening for hemoglobinopathies.* No. 168.

American College of Obstetricians and Gynecologists. (2004). Prenatal and preconceptional carrier screening for genetic diseases in individuals of Eastern European Jewish descent. Committee Opinion, No. 298. *Obstetrics & Gynecology, 104,* 425–428.

American Society of Clinical Oncology (2003). Policy statement update: Genetic testing for cancer susceptibility. *Journal of Clinical Oncolgy, 21,* 2397–2406.

American Society of Human Genetics. (1996). Statement on informed consent for genetic research. *American Journal of Human Genetics, 59,* 471–474.

American Society of Human Genetics Social Issues Subcommittee on Familial Disclosure. (1998). Professional disclosure of familial genetic information. *American Journal of Human Genetics, 62,* 474–483.

American Society of Human Genetics Board of Directors and the American College of Medical Genetics Board of Directors. (1995). Points to consider: Ethical, legal, and psychosocial impli-cations of genetic testing in children and adolescents. *American Journal of Human Genetics, 57,* 1233–1241.

American Society of Human Genetics and the American College of Medical Genetics. (2000). Statement: Genetic testing in adoption. *American Journal of Human Genetics, 66,* 761–767.

Andersen, L. K., Jensen, H. K., Juul, S., & Faergeman, O. (1997). Patients' attitudes toward detection of heterozygous familial hypercholesterolemia. *Archives of Internal Medicine, 157,* 553–560.

Anderson, P. J., Wood, S. J., Francis, D. E., Coleman, L., Warwick, L., Casanelia, S., et al. (2004). Neuropsychological functioning in children with early-treated phenylketonuria: Impact of white matter abnormalities. *Developmental Medicine and Child Neurology, 46,* 230–238.

Andrews, L., & Nelkin, D. (1998). Whose body is it anyway? Disputes over body tissue in a biotechnology age. *Lancet, 351,* 53–57.

Axworthy, D., Brock, D. J. H., Bobrow, M., & Marteau, T. M. for the UK Cystic Fibrosis Follow-up Study Group (1996). Psychological impact of population-based carrier testing for cystic fibrosis: 3-year follow-up. *Lancet, 347,* 1443–1446.

Bailey, D. B., Jr. (2004). Newborn screening for fragile X syndrome. *Mental Retardation and Developmental Disabilities Research Reviews, 10,* 3–10.

Barlow-Stewart, K., Burnett, L., Proos, A., Howell, V., Huq, F., Lazarus, R., et al. (2003). A genetic screening programme for Tay-Sachs disease and cystic fibrosis for Australian Jewish high school students. *Journal of Medical Genetics, 40,* e45–e57.

Beckwith, J. (1976). Social and political uses of genetics in the United States: Past and present. *Annals of the New York Academy of Science, 265,* 46–58.

Bernhardt, B. A., Tambor, E. S., Fraser, G., Wissow, L. S., & Geller, G. (2003). Parents' and children's attitudes toward the enrollment of minors in genetic susceptibility research: Implications for informed consent. *American Journal of Medical Genetics, 116A,* 315–323.

Blau, N. (2003). Tetrahydropbiopterin control in phenylketonuria. *Genetics in Medicine, 5,* 57–58.

Blau, N., & Erlandsen, H. (2004). The metabolic

and molecular bases of tetrahydrobiopterin-responsive phenylalanine hydroxylase deficiency. *Molecular and Genetic Metabolism, 82,* 101–111.

Bosch, A. M., Grootenhuis, M. A., Bakker, H. D., Heijmans, H. S., Wijburg, F. A., & Last, B. F. (2004). Living with classical galactosemia: Health-related quality of life consequences. *Pediatrics, 113,* e423–e428.

Bowles, L., & Cohen, H. (2003). Inherited thrombophilias and anticoagulation in pregnancy. *Best Practice & Research Clinical Obstetrics & Gynaecology, 17,* 471–489.

Bowman, J. E. (1978). Social, legal and economic issues in sickle cell programs. In J. J. Buckley (Ed.), *Genetics now: Ethical issues in genetic research.* Washington, DC: University Press of America.

Brandt-Raul, P. W., & Brandt-Raul, S. I. (2004). Genetic testing in the workplace: Ethical, legal, and social implications. *Annual Review of Public Health, 25,* 139–153.

Buchanan, G. S., Rodgers, G. M., & Branch, D. W. (2003). The inherited thrombophilias: Genetics, epidemiology, and laboratory evaluation. *Best Practice & Research Clinical Obstetrics & Gynaecology, 17,* 397–411.

Bundey, S. (1997). Few psychological consequences of presymptomatic testing for Huntington disease. *Lancet, 349,* 4.

Burgess, M. M., & Hayden, M. R. (1996). Patients' rights to laboratory data: Trinucleotide repeat length in Huntington disease. *American Journal of Medical Genetics, 62,* 6–9.

Camfield, C. S., Joseph, M., Hurley, T., Campbell, K., Sanderson, S., & Camfield, P. R. (2004). Optimal management of phenylketonuria: A centralized expert team is more successful than a decentralized model of care. *Journal of Pediatrics, 145,* 53–57.

Campbell, E. D., & Ross, L. F. (2004). Incorporating newborn screening into prenatal care. *American Journal of Obstetrics & Gynecology, 190,* 876–877.

Canadian Paediatric Society, Bioethics Committee. (2003). Guidelines for genetic testing of healthy children. *Paediatrics & Child Health, 8,* 42–45.

Canatan, D., Ratip, S., Kaptan, S., & Cosan, R. (2003). Psychosocial burden of β-thalassemia major in Antalya, south Turkey. *Social Science & Medicine, 56,* 815–819.

Cassio, A., Cacciari, E., Cicognani, A., Damiani, G., Missiroli, G., Corbelli, E., et al. (2003). Treatment for congenital hypothyroidism: Thyroxine alone or thyroxine plus triiodothyronine? *Pediatrics, 111(5 Pt. 1),* 1055–1060.

Cederbaum, S. (2002). Phenylketonuria: An update. *Current Opinion in Pediatrics, 14,* 702–706.

Centers for Disease Control and Prevention. (1997). Newborn screening for cystic fibrosis: A paradigm for public health genetics policy development. *Morbidity and Mortality Weekly Report, 46, (RR-16),* 1–24.

Centers for Disease Control and Prevention. (1998). Mortality among children with sickle cell disease identified by newborn screening during 1990–1994—California, Illinois, and New York. *Morbidity and Mortality Weekly Report, 47,* 169–172.

Centers for Disease Control and Prevention. (2003). Contribution of selected metabolic diseases to early childhood deaths—Virginia, 1996–2001. *Morbidity and Mortality Weekly Report, 52,* 677–679.

Centers for Disease Control and Prevention. (2004). Newborn screening for cystic fibrosis. *Morbidity and Mortality Weekly Report, 52(RR-13),* 1–36.

Clague, A., & Thomas, A. (2002). Neonatal biochemical screening for disease. *Clinica Chimica Acta, 315,* 99–110.

Clarke, A. (1994). The genetic testing of children. Working Part of the Clinical Genetics Society (UK). *Journal of Medical Genetics, 31,* 785–797.

Clarke, A. (2002). Ethical and social issues in clinical genetics. In D. L. Rimoin, J. M. Connor, R. E. Pyeritz, & B. R. Korf (Eds.), *Emery and Rimoin's principles and practice of medical genetics* (4th ed., pp. 897–928). New York: Churchill Livingstone.

Clarke, J. T. R. (2002). *A clinical guide to inherited metabolic diseases* (2nd ed.). Cambridge: Cambridge University Press.

Clayton, E. W. (1997). Genetic testing in children. *Journal of Medicine and Philosophy, 22,* 233–251.

Clayton, E. W. (2003). Ethical, legal and social implications of genomic medicine. *New England Journal of Medicine, 349,* 562–569.

Clayton, E. W., Hannig, V. L., Pfotenhauer, J. P., Parker, R. A., Campbell, P. W. III, & Phillips, J. A.

III. (1995). Teaching about cystic fibrosis carrier screening by using written and video information. *American Journal of Human Genetics, 57,* 171–181.

Comeau, A. M., Larson, C., & Eaton, R. B. (2004). Integration of new genetic diseases into statewide newborn screening: New England Experience. *American Journal of Medical Genetics, Part C (Seminars in Medical Genetics), 125C,* 35–41.

Committee for the Study of Inborn Errors of Metabolism. (1975). *Genetic screening.* Washington, DC: National Academy of Sciences.

Committee on Genetics. (2000). Molecular genetic testing in pediatric practice: A subject review. *Pediatrics, 106,* 1494–1497.

Costalas, J. W., Itzen, M., Malick, J., Babb, J. S., Bove, B., Godwin, A. K., et al. (2003). Communication of *BRCA1* and *BRCA2* results to at-risk relatives: A cancer risk assessment program's experience. *American Journal of Medical Genetics, Part C (Seminars in Medical Genetics), 119C,* 11–18.

Costello, P. M., Beasley, M. G., Tillotson, S. L., & Smith, I. (1994). Intelligence in mild atypical phenylketonuria. *European Journal of Pediatrics, 153,* 260–263.

Cunningham, G. (2002). The science and politics of screening newborns. *New England Journal of Medicine, 346,* 1084–1085.

Cunningham, M., Cox, E. O., the Committee on Practice and Ambulatory Medicine, and the Section on Otolaryngology and Bronchoesophagology. (2003). Hearing assessment in infants and children: Recommendations beyond neonatal screening. *Pediatrics, 111,* 436–439.

Deodato, F., Boenzi, S., Rizzo, C., Abeni, D., Caviglia, S., Picca, S., et al. (2004). Inborn errors of metabolism: An update on epidemiology and on neonatal-onset hyperammonemia. *Acta Paediatrica Supplement, 93*(445), 18–21.

Dillard, J. P., Carson, C. L., Bernard, C. J., Laxova, A., & Farrell, P. M. (2004). An analysis of communication following newborn screening for cystic fibrosis. *Health Communication, 16,* 197–205.

Dugan, R. B., Wiesner, G. L., Juengst, E. T., O'Riordan, M. A., Matthews, A. L., & Robin, N. H. (2003). Duty to warn at-risk relatives for genetic disease: Genetic counselors' clinical experiences.

American Journal of Medical Genetics, Part C (Seminars in Medical Genetics), 119C, 27–34.

Epstein, C. J. (1997). 1996 AHSG presidential address. Toward the 21st century. *American Journal of Human Genetics, 60,* 1–9.

Epstein, C. J. (2004). Genetic testing: Hope or hype? *Genetics in Medicine, 6,* 165–172.

Evers-Kiebooms, G., Nys, K., Harper, P., Zoetewiej, M., Durr, A., Jacopini, G., et al. (2002). Predictive DNA-testing for Huntington's disease and reproductive decision making: A European collaborative study. *European Journal of Human Genetics, 10,* 167–176.

Falk, M. J., Dugan, R. B., O'Riordan, M. A., & Matthews, A. L. (2003). Medical gneticists' duty to warn at-risk relatives for genetic disease. *American Journal of Medical Genetics, 120A,* 374–380.

Fanos, J. H. (1997). Developmental tasks of childhood and adolescence: Implications for genetic testing. *American Journal of Medical Genetics, 71,* 22–28.

Fanos, J. H., Davis, J., & Puck, J. M. (2001). Sib understanding of genetics and attitudes toward carrier testing for X-linked severe combined immunodeficiency. *American Journal of Medical Genetics, 98,* 46–56.

Farrell, P. M. (2004). Cystic fibrosis newborn screening: Shifting the key question from "Should we screen?" to "How should we screen?" *Pediatrics, 113,* 1811–1812.

Farrell, P. M., Kosorok, M. R., Rock, M. J., La Yova, A., Zeng, L., & Lai, H. C. (2001). Early diagnosis of cystic fibrosis through neonatal screening prevents severe malnutrition and improves long-term growth. *Pediatrics, 107,* 1–13.

Fisher, N. L. (Ed.). (1996). *Cultural and ethnic diversity. A guide for genetics professionals.* Baltimore: Johns Hopkins University Press.

Fryer, A. (1995). Genetic testing of children. *Archives of Disease of Childhood, 72,* 97–99.

Gason, A. A., Aitken, M., Delatycki, M. B., Sheffield, E., Metcalfe, S. A. (2004). Multimedia messages in genetics: Design, development, and evaluation of a computer-based instructional resource for secondary school students in a Tay Sachs disease carrier screening program. *Genetics in Medicine, 6,* 226–231.

Gebhardt, D. O. (2002). Sperm donor suffers years later from inherited disease. *Journal of Medical Ethics, 28,* 213–214.

Gotto, A. M., Jr. (2004). Targeting high-risk young patients for statin therapy. *Journal of the American Medical Association, 292,* 377–378.

Green, J. M., Hewison, J., Bekker, H. L., Bryant, L. D., & Cuckle, H. S. (2004). Psychosocial aspects of genetic screening of pregnant women and newborns: A systematic review. *Health Technology Assessment, 8,* 1–124.

Grodin, M. A. (1994). *Children as research subjects.* New York: Oxford University Press.

Grody, W. W. (2003). Molecular genetic risk screening. *Annual Review of Medicine, 54,* 473–490.

Grody, W. W., Cutting, G. R., Klinger, K. W., Richards, C. S., Watson, M. S., & Desnick, R. J. (2001). Laboratory standards and guidelines for population-based cystic fibrosis carrier screening. *Genetics in Medicine, 3,* 149–154.

Grody, W. W., Griffin, J. H., Taylor, A. K., Korf, B. R., & Heit, J. A. (2001). American College of Medical Genetics consensus statement on factor V Leiden mutation testing. *Genetics in Medicine, 3,* 139–148.

Gruters, A., Biebermann, H., & Krude, H. (2003). Neonatal thyroid disorders. *Hormone Research, 59*(Suppl. 1), 24–29.

Gruters, A., Jenner, A., & Krude, H. (2002). Long-term consequences of congenital hypothyroidism in the era of screening programmes. *Best Practices in Research Clinical Endocrinology and Metabolism, 16,* 369–382.

Guidelines for the molecular genetics predictive test in Huntington's disease. *Neurology, 44,* 1533–1536.

Hankey, G. J. (1997). How will society handle people with presymptomatic genetic disease? *Medical Journal of Australia, 166,* 55.

Harper, P. S., Gevers, S., de Wert, G., Creighton, S., Bombard, Y., & Hayden, M. R. (2004). Genetic testing and Huntington's disease: Issues of employment. *Lancet Neurology, 3,* 249–252.

Henthorn, J. S., Almeida, A. M., & Davies, S. C. (2004). Neonatal screening for sickle cell disorders. *British Journal of Haematology, 124,* 259–263.

Hilliges, C., Awiszus, D., & Wendel, U. (1993). Intellectual performance of children with maple syrup urine disease. *European Journal of Pediatrics, 119,* 46–50.

Hirtz, D. G., & Fitzsimmons, L. G. (2002). Regulatory and ethical issues in the conduct of clinical research involving children. *Current Opinion in Pediatrics, 14,* 669–675.

Hodge, J. G., Jr. (2004). Ethical issues concerning genetic testing and screening in public health. *American Journal of Medical Genetics, Part C, Seminars in Medical Genetics, 125C,* 66–70.

Hoffmann, D. E., & Wulfsberg, E. A. (1995). Testing children for genetic predispositions: Is it in their best interest? *Journal of Law, Medicine & Ethics, 23,* 331–344.

Holtzman, N. A. (1998). Bringing genetic tests into the clinic. *Hospital Practice, 33*(1), 107–128.

Holtzman, N. A., & Watson, M. S. (1997, September). *Promoting safe and effective genetic testing in the United States. Final Report of the Task Force on Genetic Testing.* National Human Genome Research Institute, NIH.

Howse, J. L., & Katz, M. (2000). The importance of newborn screening. *Pediatrics, 106,* 595.

Hunter, M. K., Mandel, S. H., Sesser, D. E., Miyabira, R. S., Rien, L., Skeels, M. R., et al. (1998). Follow-up of newborns with low thyroxine and nonelevated thyroid-stimulating hormone-screening concentrations: Results of the 20-year experience in the Northwest Regional Newborn Screening Program. *Journal of Pediatrics, 132,* 70–74.

Institute of Medicine. (1994). *Assessing genetic risks. Implications for health and social policy.* Washington, DC: National Academy Press.

Joint LWPES/ESPE CAH Working Group. (2002). Consensus statement on 21-hydroxylase deficiency from the Lawson Wilkins Pediatric Endocrine Society and the European Society for Paediatric Endocrinology. *Journal of Clinical Endocrinology & Metabolism, 87,* 4048–4053.

Kaback, M. (Ed.). (1977). *Tay Sachs disease: Screening and prevention.* New York: Alan R Liss.

Kaufman, S. (1998). Genetic disorders involving recycling and formation of tetrahydrobiopterin. *Advances in Pharmacology, 42,* 41–52.

Kenna, M. A. (2003). Neonatal hearing screening. *Pediatric Clinics of North America, 50,* 301–313.

Kent, A. (2003). Consent and confidentiality in genetics: Whose information is it anyway? *Journal of Medical Ethics, 29,* 16–18.

Khoury, M. J., McCabe, L. L., & McCabe, E. R. B. (2003). Genomic medicine: Population screening in the age of genomic medicine. *New England Journal of Medicine, 348,* 50–58.

Knoppers, B. M., & Laberge, C. M. (1995). Research and stored tissues. Persons as sources, samples as persons? *Journal of the American Medical Association, 274,* 1806–1807.

Koscik, R. L., Farrell, P. M., Kosorok, M. R., Zaremba, K. M., Laxova, A., Lai, H. C., et al. (2004). Cognitive function of children with cystic fibrosis: Deleterious effect of early malnutrition. *Pediatrics, 113,* 1549–1558.

Kruse, B., Riepe, F. G., Krone, N., Bosinski, H. A., Kloehn, S., Partsch, C. J., et al. (2004). Congenital adrenal hyperplasia—how to improve the transition from adolescence to adult life. *Experiments in Clinical Endocrinology and Diabetes, 112,* 343–355.

Kvittingen, E. A. (1995). Tyrosinaemia—treatment and outcome. *Journal of Inherited Metabolic Diseases, 18,* 375–379.

Laird, L., Dezateux, C., & Anionwu, E. N. (1996). Neonatal screening for sickle cell disorders: What about the carrier infants? *British Medical Journal, 313,* 407–411.

Lam, W. K., Cleary, M. A., Wraith, J. E., & Walter, J. H. (1996). Histidinaemia: A benign metabolic disorder. *Archives of Disease of Childhood, 74,* 343–346.

Lashley, F. R. (2002a). Ethically speaking. *Chart, 99*(1), 10.

Lashley, F. R. (2002b). Newborn screening: New opportunities and new challenges. *Newborn and Infant Nursing Reviews, 2,* 228–242.

Lashley, F. R. & Durham, J. D. (Eds.). (2002). *Emerging infectious diseases: Trends and issues.* New York: Springer Publishing.

Lee, P. J., Lilburn, M., Wendel, U., & Schadewaldt, P. (2003). A woman with untreated galactosaemia. *Lancet, 362,* 446.

Leonard, J. V., & Morris, A. A. M. (2002). Urea cycle disorders. *Seminars in Neonatology, 7,* 27–35.

Leung, W-C. (2000). Results of genetic testing: When confidentiality conflicts with a duty to warn relatives. *British Medical Journal, 321,* 1464–1465.

Levy, H. L. (2003). Lessons from the past—looking to the future. Newborn screening. *Pediatric Annals, 32,* 505–508.

Levy, H. L. & Waisbren, S. E. (1994). PKU in adolescents: Rationale and psychosocial factors in diet continuation. *Acta Paediatrica, Suppl. 407,* 92–97.

Li, Y., Scott, C. R., Chamoles, N. A., Ghavami, A., Pinto, B. M., Turecek, F., et al. (2004). Direct multiplex assay of lysosomal enzymes in dried blood spots for newborn screening. *Clinical Chemistry, 3.*

Lucassen, A., & Parker, M. (2001). Revealing false paternity: Some ethical considerations. *Lancet, 357,* 1033–1035.

Mandl, K. D., Feit, S., Larson, C., & Kohane, I. S. (2002). Newborn screening program practices in the United States: Notification, research, and consent. *Pediatrics, 109,* 269–273.

Mansfield, E. (2003). Genetic testing and personalized medicine: An FDA view. *Preclinica, 1,* 155–158.

Mariman, E. C. M. (2000). Act to resolve conflict. *British Medical Journal, 321,* 1465.

Matalon, R., Koch, R., Michals-Matalon, K., Moseley, K., Surendram, S., Tyring, S., Erlandsen, H., et al. (2004). Biopterin responsive phenylalanine hydroxylase deficiency. *Genetics in Medicine, 6,* 27–32.

McCabe, L., & McCabe, E. R. B. (2004). Direct-to-consumer genetic tesing: Access and marketing. *Genetics in Medicine, 6,* 58–59.

McConkie-Rosell, A., & Spiridigliozzi, G. A. (2004). "Family matters": A conceptual framework for genetic testing in children. *Journal of Genetic Counseling, 13,* 9–29.

McConkie-Rosell, A., Spiridigliozzi, G. A., Iafolla, T., Tarleton, J., & Lachiewiez, A. M. (1997). Carrier testing in the fragile X syndrome: Attitudes and opinions of obligate carriers. *American Journal of Medical Genetics, 68,* 62–69.

McKinnon, W. C., Baty, B. J., Bennett, R. L., Magee, M., Neufeld-Kaiser, W. A., Peters, K. F., et al. (1997). Predisposition genetic testing for late-onset disorders in adults. A position paper of the National Society of Genetic Counselors. *Journal of the American Medical Association, 278,* 1217–1220.

Mehlman, M. J., Kodish, E. D., Whitehouse, P., Zinn, A. B., Sollitto, S., Berger, J., et al. (1996). The need for anonymous genetic counseling and testing. *American Journal of Human Genetics, 58,* 393–397.

Merz, B. (1987). Matchmaking scheme solves Tay-Sachs problem. *Journal of the American Medical Association, 258,* 2636–2639.

Michie, S., McDonald, V., Bobrow, M., McKeown, C., & Marteau, T. (1996). Parents' responses to predictive genetic testing in their children: Report of a single case study. *Journal of Medical Genetics, 11,* 313–318.

Morton, D. H., Strauss, K. A., Robinson, D. L., Puffenberger, E. G., & Kelley, R. I. (2002). Diagnosis and treatment of maple syrup disease: A study of 36 patients. *Pediatrics, 109,* 999–1008.

National Institutes of Health. (1997, April 14–16). Genetic testing for cystic fibrosis. *NIH Consensus Statement No. 106, 15*(4), 1–37.

National Institutes of Health, Consensus Development Panel. (2001). National Institutes of Health Consensus Development Conference Statement: Phenylketonuria (PKU): Screening and management, October 16–18, 2000. *Pediatrics, 106,* 972–982.

National Institutes of Health, Workshop on population screening for the cystic fibrosis gene (1990). *New England Journal of Medicine, 323,* 70–71.

Nelson, R. M., Botkjin, J. R., Kodish, E. D., Levetown, M., Truman, J. T., Wilfond, B. S., et al. (2001). Ethical issues with genetic testing in pediatrics. *Pediatrics, 107,* 1451–1455.

Newborn Screening Task Force. (2000). Serving the family from birth to the medical home: Newborn screening: A blueprint for the future. *Pediatrics, 106,* 389–422.

Nisselle, A. E., Delatycki, M. B., Collins, V., Metcalfe, S., Aitken, M. A., du Sart D., et al. (2004). Implementation of HaemScreen, a workplace-based genetic screening program for hemochromatosis. *Clinical Genetics, 65,* 358–367.

Northam, E. A. (2004). Neuropsychological and psychosocial correlates of endocrine and metabolic disorders—a review. *Journal of Pediatric Endocrinology and Metabolism, 17,* 5–15.

Offit, K., Groeger, E., Turner, S., Wadsworth, E. A., & Weriser, M. A. (2004). The "duty to warn" a patient's family members about hereditary disease risks. *Journal of the American Medical Association, 292,* 1469–1473.

Olivieri, A., Stazi, M. A., Mastroiacovo, P., Fazzini, C., Medda E., Spagnolo, A., et al. (2002). A population-based study on the frequency of additional congenital malformations in infants with congenital hypothyroidism: Data from the Italian Registry for Congenital Hypothyroidism (1991–1998). *Journal of Clinical Endocrinology & Metabolism, 87,* 557–562.

Palomaki, G. E., Bradley, L. A., Richards, C. S., & Haddow, J. E. (2003). Analytic validity of cystic fibrosis testing: A preliminary estimate. *Genetics in Medicine, 5,* 15–20.

Pandor, A., Eastham, J., Beverley, C., Chilcott, J., & Paisley, S. (2004). Clinical effectiveness and cost-effectiveness of neonatal screening for inborn errors of metabolism using tandem mass spectrometry: A systematic review. *Health Technology Assessment, 8,* 1–121.

Parsons, E. P., Clarke, A. J., Hood, K., Lycett, E., & Bradley, D. M. (2002). Newborn screening for Duchenne muscular dystrophy: A psychosocial study. *Archives of Diseases of Childhood, Fetal Neonatal Edition, 86,* F91–F95.

Pey, A. L., Desviat, L. R., Gámez, A., Ugarte, M., & Pérez, B. (2003). Phenylketonuria: Genotype-phenotype correlations based on expression analysis of structural and functional mutations in *PAH. Human Mutation, 21,* 370–378.

Pinto, G., Tardy, V., Trivin, C., Thalassinos, C., Lortat-Jacob, S., Nihoul-Fékété, C., et al. (2003). Follow-up of 68 children with congenital adrenal hyperplasia due to 21-hydroxylase deficiency: Relevance of genotype for management. *Journal of Clinical Endocrinology & Metabolism, 88,* 2624–2633.

Potter, N. T., Spector, E. B., & Prior, T. W. (2004). Technical standards and guidelines for Huntington disease testing. *Genetics in Medicine, 6,* 61–65.

President's Commission for the Study of Ethical Problems in Medicine and Biomedical and Behavioral Research. (1983). *Screening and counseling for genetic conditions.* Washington, DC: GPO.

Quaid, K. A., & Morris, M. (1993). Reluctance to undergo predictive testing: The case of Huntington disease. *American Journal of Medical Genetics, 45,* 41–45.

Refsum, H., Fredriksen, A., Meyer, K., Ueland, P. M., & Kase, B. F. (2004). Birth prevalence of homocystinuria. *Journal of Pediatrics, 144,* 830–832.

Reilly, P. R., Boshar, M. F., & Holtzman, S. H. (1997). Ethical issues in genetic research: Disclosure and informed consent. *Nature Genetics, 15,* 16–20.

Rhead, W. J., & Irons, M. (2004). The call from the newborn screening laboratory: Frustration in the afternoon. *Pediatric Clinics of North America, 52,* 803–818.

Rimoin, D. L., Connor, J. M., Pyeritz, R. E., & Korf, B. R. (Eds.). (2002). *Emery and Rimoin's principles and practice of medical genetics* (4th ed.). New York: Churchill Livingstone.

Roberts, C. G. P., & Ladenson, P. W. (2004). Hypothyroidism. *Lancet, 363,* 793–803.

Roberts, J. S., Barber, M., Brown, T. M., Cupples, L. A., Farrer, L. A., LaRusse, S. A., et al. (2004). Who seeks genetic susceptibility testing for Alzheimer's disease? Findings from a multisite randomized clinical trial. *Genetics in Medicine, 6,* 197–203.

Roberts, J. S., LaRusse, S. A., Katzen, H., Whitehouse, P. J., Barber, M., Post, S. G., et al. (2003). Reasons for seeking genetic susceptibility testing among first-degree relatives of people with Alzheimer disease. *Alzheimer Disease and Associated Disorders, 17,* 86–92.

Roe, C. R. (2002). Inherited disorders of mitochondrial fatty acid oxidation: A new responsibility for the neonatologist. *Seminars in Neonatology, 7,* 37–47.

Rohr, F. J., Lobbregt, D., & Levy, H. L. (1998). Tyrosine supplementation in the treatment of maternal phenylketonuria. *American Journal of Clinical Nutrition, 67,* 473–476.

Rosen, A., Wallenstein, S., & McGovern, M. M. (2002). Attitudes of pediatric residents toward ethical issues associated with genetic testing in children. *Pediatrics, 110,* 360–363.

Ross, L. F. (2002). Predictive genetic testing for conditions that present in childhood. *Kennedy Institute Ethics Journal, 12,* 225–244.

Rothenberg, K., Fuller, B., Rothstein, M., Duster, T., Kahn, M. J. E., Cunningham, R., et al. (1997). Genetic information and the workplace: Legislative approaches and policy challenges. *Science, 275,* 1755–1757.

Rouse, B., & Azen, C. (2004). Effect of high maternal blood phenylalanine on offspring congenital anomalies and developmental outcome at ages 4 ad 6 years: The importance of strict dietary control preconception and throughout pregnancy. *Journal of Pediatrics, 144,* 235–239.

Rovet, J. F. (2005). Children with congenital hypothyroidism and their siblings: Do they really differ? *Pediatrics, 115,* e52–57.

Rovet, J., & Daneman, D. (2003). Congenital hypothyroidism: A review of current diagnostic and treatment practices in relation to neuropsychologic outcome. *Paediatric Drugs, 5,* 141–149.

Rovet, J. F. (2004). In search of the optimal therapy for congenital hypothyroidism. *Journal of Pediatrics, 144,* 698–700.

Sankar, P. (2003). Genetic privacy. *Annual Review of Medicine, 54,* 393–407.

Saudubray, J. M., Nassogne, M. C., de Lonlay, P., & Touati, G. (2002). Clinical approach to inherited metabolic disorders in neonates: An overview. *Seminars in Neonatology, 7,* 3–15.

Schweitzer, S., Shin, Y., Jakobs, C., & Brodehl, J. (1993). Long-term outcome in 134 patients with galactosaemia. *European Journal of Pediatrics, 152,* 36–43.

Scriver, C. R., Beaudet, A. L., Sly, W. S., & Valle, D. (Eds.). (2001). *The metabolic and molecular bases of inherited disease* (8th ed.). New York: McGraw Hill.

Seckl, J. R., & Miller, W. I. (1997). How safe is long-term prenatal glucocorticoid treatment? *Journal of the American Medical Association, 277,* 1077–1079

Secretary's Advisory Committee on Genetic Testing. (2000). Enhancing the oversight of genetic tests: Recommendations of the SACGT. Online at http://www4. od. nih. gov/oba/sacgt. htm.

Simoneau-Roy, J., Marti, S., Deal, C., Huot, C., Robaey, P., & Van Vliet, G. (2004). Cognition and behavior at school entry in children with congenital hypothyroidism treated early with high-dosc levothyroxine. *Journal of Pediatrics, 144,* 747–752.

Speiser, P. W., & White, P. C. (2003). Congenital adrenal hyperplasia. *New England Journal of Medicine, 349,* 776–788.

Stamatoyannopoulos, G. (1974). Problems of screening and counseling in the hemoglobinopathies. In A. G. Motulsky, & W. Lenz (Eds.), *Birth Defects.* Amsterdam: Excerpta Medica.

Statement of the American Society of Human Genetics on cystic fibrosis carrier screening. (1992). *American Journal of Human Genetics, 51,* 1443–1444.

Steinfeld, R., Kohlschutter, A., Ullrich, K., & Lukacs, Z. (2004). Efficiency of long-term tetrahydrobiopterin monotherapy in phenylketonuria. *Jouranl of Inherited and Metabolic Diseases, 27,* 449–453.

Strange, C., Dickson, R., Carter, C., Carpenter, M. J., Holladay, B., Lundquist, R., et al. (2004). Genetic testing for alpha$_1$-antitrypsin deficiency. *Genetics in Medicine, 6,* 204–210.

Sugarman, E., Rohlfs, E. M., Silverman, L. M., & Allitto, B. A. (2004). *CFTR* mutation distribution among U.S. Hispanic and African American individuals: Evaluation in cystic fibrosis patient and carrier screening populations. *Genetics in Medicine, 6,* 392–399.

Susceptibility testing for children. (2003). *Health Progress, 84*(3), 11–12.

Sutton, V. R. (2002). Tay-Sachs disease screening and counseling families at risk for metabolic disease. *Obstetrics and Gynecology Clinics of North America, 29,* 287–296.

Tassicker, R., Savulescu, J., Skene, L., Marshall, P., Fitzgerald, L., & Delatycki, M. B. (2003). Prenatal diagnosis requests for Huntington's disease when the father is at risk and does not want to know his genetic status: Clinical, legal, and ethical viewpoints. *British Medical Journal, 326,* 331–333.

Taylor, S. D. (2004). Predictive genetic test decisions for Huntington's disease: Context appraisal and new moral imperatives. *Social Science & Medicine, 59,* 137–149.

Tibben, A. (1993). On psychological effects of presymptomatic DNA-testing for Huntington's disease. PhD thesis. Netherlands, Rotterdam University. Cited in Michie, S., McDonald, V., Bobrow, M., McKeown, C., & Marteau, T. (1996). Parents' responses to predictive genetic testing in their children: Report of a single case study. *Journal of Medical Genetics, 11,* 313–318.

Tibben, A., Vegter-van der Vlis, M., Skraastad, M. I., Frets, P. G., van der Kamp, J. J. P., Niermeijer, M. F., et al. (1992). DNA-testing for Huntington's disease in the Netherlands: A retrospective study on psychosocial effects. *American Journal of Medical Genetics, 44,* 94–99.

Twomey, J. G. (2002). Genetic testing of children: Confluence or collision between praents and professionals? *AACN Clinical Isues, 13,* 557–566.

Tyler, A., & Morris, M. (1990). National symposium on problems of presymptomatic testing for Huntington's disease, Cardiff. *Journal of Medical Ethics, 16,* 41–42.

U.S. Senate. (1996). A bill to protect the genetic privacy of individuals, and for other purposes. 104th Congress, 2d sess, SR 1898.

U.S. Preventive Services Task Force. (2001). Newborn hearing screening: Recommendations and rationale. *American Family Physician, 4,* 1995–1999.

Vastag, B. (2003). Cystic fibrosis gene testing a challenge. *Journal of the American Medical Association, 289,* 2923–2924.

Wagener, J. S., Sontag, M. K., & Accurso, F. J. (2003). Newborn screening for cystic fibrosis. *Current Opinion in Pediatrics, 15,* 309–315.

Waggoner, D. D., Buist, N. R. M., & Donnell, G. N. (1990). Long-term prognosis in galactosaemia: Results of a survey of 350 cases. *Journal of Inherited Metabolic Diseases, 13,* 802–818.

Walter, J. H., & White, F. J. (2004). Blood phenylalanine control in adolescents with phenylketonuria. *International Journal of Adolescent Medicine and Health, 16,* 41–45.

Wang, C., Gonzalez, R., & Merajver, S. D. (2004). Assessment of genetic testing and related counseling services: Current research and future directions. *Social Science & Medicine, 58,* 1427–1442.

Warren, N. S., Carter, T. P., Humbert, J. R., & Rowley, P. T. (1982). Newborn screening for hemoglobinopathies in New York State: Experience of physicians and parents of affected children. *Journal of Pediatrics, 100,* 373–377.

Waters, P. J. (2003). How *PAH* gene mutations cause hyper-phenylalaninemia and why mechanism matters: Insights from in vitro expression. *Human Mutation, 21,* 357–360.

Watson, M. S., Cutting, G. R., Desnick, R. J., Driscoll, S. A., Klinger, K., Mennuti, M., et al. (2004). Cystic fibrosis population carrier screening: 2004 revision of American College of Medical Genetics mutation panel. *Genetics in Medicine, 6,* 387–391.

Weber, P., Scholl, S., & Baumgartner, E. R. (2004). Outcome in patients with profound biotinidase deficiency: Relevance of newborn screening. *Developmental Medicine and Child Neurology, 46,* 481–484.

Wertz, D. C., Fanos, J. H., & Reilly, P. R. (1994). Genetic testing for children and adolescents: Who decides? *Journal of the American Medical Association, 272,* 875–881.

Wilcox, W. R., & Cederbaum, S. D. (2002). Amino acid metabolism. In D. L. Rimoin, J. M. Connor, R. E. Pyeritz, & B. R. Korf (Eds.), *Emery and*

Rimoin's principles and practice of medical genetics (4th ed., pp. 2405–2440). New York: Churchill Livingstone.

Wilcken, B., Wiley, V., Hammond, J., & Carpenter, K. (2003). Screening newborns for inborn errors of metabolism by tandem mass spectrometry. *New England Journal of Medicine, 348,* 2304–2312.

Wilfond, B., & Rothenberg, L. S. (2002). Ethical issues in cystic fibrosis newborn screening: From data to public health policy. *Current Opinion in Pulmonary Medicine, 8,* 529–534.

Williams, J. K., & Schutte, D. L. (1997). Benefits and burdens of genetic carrier identification. *Western Journal of Nursing Research, 19,* 71–81.

Witt, D. R., Schaefer, C., Hallam, P., Wi, S., Blumberg, B., Fishbach, A., et al. (1996). Cystic fibrosis heterozygote screening in 5,161 pregnant women. *American Journal of Human Genetics, 58,* 823–835.

Wolf, B., Spencer, R., & Gleason, T. (2002). Hearing loss is a common feature of symptomatic children with profound biotinidase deficiency. *Journal of Pediatrics, 140,* 242–246.

Zeesman, S., Clow, C. L., Cartier, L., & Scriver, C. R. (1984). A private view of heterozygosity: Eight year follow up study of carriers of the Tay-Sachs gene detected by high-school screening in Montreal. *American Journal of Medical Genetics, 18,* 769–778.

12

Prenatal Detection and Diagnosis

Prenatal detection and diagnosis are integral components of "routine" prenatal care due to:

- availability of relatively safe techniques and tests that are cost-effective for hundreds of genetic conditions;
- rapid communication of new techniques by the mass media that have closed the time gap between research and practice;
- increased emphasis on quality of life;
- effectiveness of family planning techniques, allowing couples to have the number of children they desire;
- smaller family size, so that the "quality" of each child assumes a relatively greater value;
- an increased number of women in the workforce, and seeking higher education, so that conception is postponed until many are in a high-risk group because of age;
- liberalization of abortion laws so that abortion became a legal, acceptable, obtainable reproductive alternative to an affected infant, allowing viable choices after prenatal diagnosis; and
- increased availability of antenatal fetal treatment, more sophisticated antepartum and intrapartum management, and neonatal intensive management.

Methods of prenatal detection and diagnosis are both invasive and noninvasive and include the following techniques:

- amniocentesis (diagnosis),
- chorionic villus sampling (diagnosis),
- ultrasonography (detection and diagnosis),
- embryofetoscopy (diagnosis),
- fetal blood and tissue sampling (diagnosis),

- maternal serum screening (detection), and
- techniques that are still largely investigational such as preimplantation diagnosis (diagnosis) and the analysis of fetal cells and cell-free fetal DNA in maternal circulation (diagnosis).

Maternal serum screening is a detection-and-screening technique applied to the pregnant population. Criteria for screening tests as described in chapter 11 apply to this discussion. Ideally, preconception counseling can precede pregnancy and therefore prenatal diagnosis, so that potential preventive steps such as rubella titer determination and vaccination before conception can be taken if necessary, folic acid, other vitamin supplementation, and other preventive measures can be accomplished to reduce some risks. Techniques such as radiography, amniography, and fetography are rarely used today. Each of the prenatal genetic detection and diagnostic techniques is discussed below.

IDENTIFYING CANDIDATES FOR PRENATAL DIAGNOSIS

Current obstetrical practice in the U.S. usually includes the second trimester prenatal screening/detection techniques of maternal serum analyte screening for alpha fetoprotein and for other markers considered part of the popularly called "multiple marker" screen, such as human chorionic gonadotropin and unconjugated estriol with or without additional markers such as inhibin-A. Ultrasonography may be used for routine screening in both the first and second trimester as discussed below as well as for diagnosis at more sophisticated levels.

Practicing nurses should be able to recognize which individuals may be candidates for prenatal diagnosis beyond the standard screening and should include this information with the rest of the care being provided. This assessment includes both maternal and paternal information. It may be appropriate to identify candidates for prenatal diagnosis before the individual is pregnant, and include that information in preconceptional counseling when it occurs. This assessment may be accomplished by interview, questionnaire, and history (see chapter 9). Amniocentesis and chorionic villus sampling (CVS) are the most common invasive diagnostic methods presently used. Indications for prenatal diagnosis are listed in Table 12.1. These indications identify those individuals who will be at increased risk, and thus form the basis for assessing which pregnant women are likely candidates for prenatal diagnosis. The most common reason for recommending prenatal diagnosis is advanced maternal age (usually defined as age 35 years and older), a reflection of a trend for many women to have children later in their lives, after they have embarked on a career. However, Meyers, Adam, Dungan and Pranger (1997) as well as Goetzl and D'Alton (2001) believe that prenatal diagnosis for chromosomal problems should be offered for maternal age of 31 years if there is a twin gestation. The former have found that the risk of at least one aneuploid twin at age 31 years is 1/190 for White and 1/187 for Black American women. Most of the reasons for such increased risk have been discussed in earlier chapters, but a few merit special discussion.

Individuals who belong to an ethnic group with an identified high frequency of a specific detectable inherited disorder should be asked whether they have had their carrier status determined. If they have not, a first approach (depending on the stage of the pregnancy) may be to ascertain the carrier status of the father because, for some disorders, pregnancy makes accurate maternal determinations inaccurate. If he is a carrier, or if the pregnancy is already advanced to a time period when carrier determination could not be carried out before the optimal time for amniocentesis was past, then amniocentesis may be appropriate and should be discussed. An example of how to proceed for prenatal carrier testing in a specific ethnic group, those of Eastern European Jewish descent, is given in the document

by the American College of Obstetricians and Gynecologists (2004), and is discussed in more detail in chapter 11. Those pregnancies at risk for an X-linked recessively inherited disorder for which no specific assay or molecular diagnosis is available are especially problematical, but this is less common with advances in tests and techniques. The usual procedure has been to determine the fetal sex. One option for this in addition to the more common techniques is preimplantation genetic diagnosis, discussed below. If the fetus is a male, and the mother is a known carrier, there is a 50% risk for it to be affected. If a decision is made to terminate such a pregnancy, then the risk of aborting a normal male fetus is 50%. Obviously, such a situation calls for support for parental decisions from all professional staff involved with the patient, and also for the provision of supportive counseling that may need to be ongoing. It is not the place of anyone involved with the clients to express their own views, especially if they differ from those of the clients. An extreme degree of parental anxiety, regardless of actual risk, is considered by many to be an acceptable psychological indication for prenatal diagnosis. Such an indication demands more intensive counseling and explanation of what can be determined before the procedure is undertaken. Both young and advanced paternal age can increase the risk of chromosome aberrations and other birth defects in the fetus. It is also known to increase the risk of some dominant gene mutations (as discussed in chapter 4) that are potentially detectable by ultrasound. It has been suggested that prenatal diagnosis for genetic reasons should be offered to all women, even if at low risk, rather than limit testing to those at increased risk (Caughey et al., 2004). This brings up issues of access and disparities in health care based on ability to pay.

It is the role of the professional practitioner and a standard of care to thoroughly inform those clients who may be at increased risk of the availability of prenatal diagnosis, and to inform all pregnant women of the option of maternal serum alpha-fetoprotein screening, either alone or as part of a multiple marker test, discussed below, as well as for level I ultrasound. Many require that an informed consent be signed whether the procedure is desired or not desired. If such diagnosis or

TABLE 12.1   Some Current Genetic Indications for Prenatal Diagnosis

Indication	Possible standard prenatal diagnostic technique(s)
Pregnancy at Risk for Chromosome Aberration	
Maternal age of 35 years and above	Amniocentesis, CVS
Previous child with chromosome abnormality or instability disorder	Amniocentesis, CVS
Chromosomal abnormality in parent (mosaicism, translocation carrier, other aneuploidy)	Amniocentesis, CVS
Previous stillbirth or perinatal death (cause unknown)	Amniocentesis, CVS
History of infertility in either parent	Amniocentesis, CVS
Habitual abortion history	Amniocentesis, CVS
Previous child with malformations (no chromosomes analyzed)	Amniocentesis, CVS, Ultrasound
Intracytoplasmic sperm injection	Amniocentesis, CVS
Abnormal serum levels of multiple markers	Amniocentesis, CVS, Ultrasound
Pregnancy at Risk for NTD	
High maternal serum level of AFP	Amniocentesis, Ultrasound
Previous child with NTD	Amniocentesis, Ultrasound
NTD in either parent or close relative	Amniocentesis, Ultrasound
Pregnancy at Risk for X-Linked Inherited Disorders	
Mother a known carrier	Amniocentesis, CVS
Close maternal male relative affected	Amniocentesis, CVS
Pregnancy at Risk for Detectable Inherited Biochemical Disorder	
Parents known carriers or affected	Amniocentesis, CVS
Previous child born with known detectable biochemical disorder	Amniocentesis, CVS
Close family member with known inherited biochemical disorder	Amniocentesis, CVS
Other	
High degree of parental anxiety	Amniocentesis, CVS, Ultrasound
Significant exposure to radiation, infection, chemicals, or drugs	Amniocentesis, Ultrasound, CVS
Diabetes mellitus in mother	Ultrasound, Amniocentesis
Previous child with structural abnormality	Ultrasound, Amniocentesis, CVS
Family history of structural abnormality	Ultrasound, Amniocentesis, CVS

NTD = neural tube defects, AFP = alpha-fetoprotein, CVS = chronic villus sampling, Ultrasound refers to targeted or extended ultrasound.

expertise is not available in the area, it is the professional's responsibility to refer the client to a center that does provide the needed expertise or service, and assist in making arrangements for the service.

CLIENT INFORMATION BEFORE PRENATAL DIAGNOSIS

Before clients can make a decision of whether or not to have prenatal diagnosis, they should understand basic information. Even what obstetrical practitioners may consider "routine screening" (such as an initial ultrasound or maternal serum screening) for their population may not seem so to the clients. The nurse should be able to explain, clarify, and interpret the information at a level that

the client can understand, that is culturally sensitive and appropriate, free from any coercion, and to evaluate that understanding. This should be accomplished as early as possible in the pregnancy, so that the client can think about the options and discuss then again. Written reinforcement that the client can take with her is an excellent way to supplement information. Information provided should include the following:

- the reason prenatal diagnosis is considered appropriate for this woman or couple;
- what will be analyzed (e.g., chromosome and alpha-fetoprotein analysis are usually routinely done regardless of the primary reason for seeking amniocentesis, thus unexpected results could occur);

- what information will be obtained (e.g., the couple should know that a search for chromosome abnormalities is broader than only for Down syndrome even if the latter is the reason that the couple is interested in prenatal diagnosis);
- the risk of having an affected child in this pregnancy before prenatal diagnosis;
- what the procedure being considered entails, including description, cost, length of time, where it is to be done, and aftercare;
- what the risks of the procedure are—the magnitude and the kind;
- what can and cannot be detected—this should include the information that while some disorders can be virtually excluded (e.g., chromosome disorders if an amniocentesis is being done), a completely normal infant cannot be assured, both because of a slight risk of error and because no procedure can detect every possible defect;
- the length of time between the procedure and when the results are obtained;
- how the results will be communicated to them;
- that prenatal diagnosis can be done even if the couple does not wish to consider abortion as a viable alternative; if the results are negative, it may relieve anxiety, and if they are positive, the couple may either change their minds, seek fetal therapy, plan for the delivery of the infant in an expert care center, and/or have time to think about alternative plans for care of the infant;
- in those now relatively uncommon cases where an X-linked recessively inherited disorder is in question and cannot be assayed for specifically, they should understand that a specific test will not be done; the fetal sex will be determined and that decision-making will proceed on that basis;
- unintended possible psychological consequences if a problem is detected. In one instance, Angier (1996) describes her feelings of dismay when she was told that her fetus had a clubfoot on ultrasound (which turned out not to be the case). She poignantly describes the disclosure and the aftermath; and
- potential unintended consequences such as pressure from insurance companies not to carry an affected child to term, or termination or diminution of benefits or coverage for the pregnancy, for the child, and aftercare.

An integral part of the nurse's goal for the client at this time should be the establishment and building of a supportive relationship for counseling during the rest of the pregnancy, and especially after prenatal diagnosis, if this is the option that has been chosen, as well as for pregnancy termination if that option has been selected, and after delivery.

AMNIOCENTESIS

Amniocentesis preceded by ultrasound is still the most extensively used method of prenatal diagnosis. Amniocentesis was proposed in the 1880s but not performed until 1919, when it was used to relieve pressure on the fetus. In the 1950s it was done to determine fetal sex and for the diagnosis of Rh isoimmunization. The 1960s saw the first use of cultured amniotic fluid cells for chromosome analysis and the detection of enzyme deficiencies.

Rapid advances in the field make a list of specific disorders that are diagnosable obsolete before this goes to press. In order to provide up-to-date information for the concerned parents-to-be who are at risk for a known specific disorder, referral should be made either to a geneticist who keeps abreast of the current developments in that particular disorder and knows the location of major research centers, or directly to a major center. At the present time, all chromosome disorders are potentially diagnosable, but as some may arise sporadically in women who are younger than 35 years of age and who are not at risk for another disorder, not all will be detected prenatally unless all pregnant women were to have fetal chromosome analysis. Sicherman, Bombard, and Rapport (1995) have suggested that an age-specific threshold should be abandoned, or if policy makers wish to have a cost-effective age level, then 23 years of age and older would be more appropriate in balancing the cost of the procedure versus the cost of the birth of an affected child. The risk of chromosome abnormalities at different maternal ages is discussed in chapter 5. The determination of amniotic alpha-fetoprotein (AFP) levels and other parameters for neural tube defects (NTDs) is usually routine at the time of amniocentesis. Maternal serum may have already been tested for AFP and other markers. Many inherited biochemical disorders can be diagnosed either by specific biochemical assays, by DNA assays. The latter are used to detect hemoglobinopathies (e.g., sickle cell disease and the thalassemias). Thus, prenatal testing may be at the level of the mutant gene (DNA), chromosome, gene product (i.e., enzyme), or phenotype (morphology). Some disorders can arise from more than one mutation in the same gene that produces the same phenotype, and therefore, to perform accurate analysis the practitioner may need to know the specific mutation segregating in a given family.

Amniocentesis refers to the withdrawal of a sample of amniotic fluid from the amniotic sac. It is usually done at the 15th to 18th week of gestation, when the uterus has reached the pelvic brim, the amniotic fluid volume is adequate (150–250 ml), and enough fetal cells are present to be able to carry out analysis (see Figure 12.1). Fetal cells in the amniotic fluid come from the skin and mucous membranes of the respiratory, digestive, genital, and urinary tracts as well as the umbilical cord and amnion. This also allows for the analysis to be completed in time for the parents to exercise the option of termination of the pregnancy if they so choose. The actual procedure is usually done on an outpatient basis, paying careful attention to asepsis. A local anesthetic may be used. Ultrasound guidance with continuous needle visualization is done. A 20 to 22 gauge spinal needle is used to enter the amniotic sac through the abdomen and withdraw 20 ml to 30 ml of amniotic fluid. Often the first few ml obtained are discarded because of potential maternal cell contamination. The necessary amount and quality of fluid is successfully obtained about 95% of the time. Analysis of the sample depends on the initial indication for the amniocentesis, but presently, most centers routinely do chromosome and AFP analysis regardless of the initial indication. Most practitioners recommend a dose of Rh immunoglobulin to all unsensitized Rh negative women to prevent Rh isoimmunization. Many centers use ultrasound after the amniocentesis to assess fetal wellbeing. In cases of multiple gestation, amniocentesis is still possible, but it is more complex. The availability of appropriate DNA analytic techniques now makes

the detection of certain fetal gene mutations possible through the use of amniocentesis instead of other more risky prenatal techniques such as fetal blood sampling.

With increased frequency of use, amniocentesis has become a safer procedure than it initially was. Comparisons of fetal loss in women having amniocentesis with controls may be difficult depending on the time period during which fetal loss was attributed to amniocentesis, because this varies from study to study. An accepted risk figure for fetal loss due to amniocentesis that is above the figure for losses in the same period of pregnancy has been given as 0.25% to 0.5%. An increased incidence of fetal loss and of other complications was associated with an increased number of needle insertions to obtain a sample, uncertain placentation or anterior placentation, and the use of needles with gauges of 19 or larger. The idea that the decrease in amniotic fluid and pressure following amniocentesis might cause harmful developmental effects in the fetus has been explored, with no reporting of short-term adverse effects. No long-term cognitive studies showing negative effects have yet been reported.

Overall complications from amniocentesis are relatively infrequent. There have been questions raised as to whether infants of mothers having amniocentesis are more likely to develop respiratory problems and emphysema that may be caused by chronic leakage of amniotic fluid, interfering with normal lung development, and this continues to be a concern, although it is estimated to occur in a very small percentage. Maternal complications can include vaginal bleeding, amniotic fluid leakage, infection, Rh sensitization, precipitation of labor, and perforation of the bladder or placenta. Fetal risks include spontaneous abortion, needle puncture injuries, and injury because of withdrawal of amniotic fluid such as amniotic band syndrome. It is not uncommon for the woman to have cramping, vaginal spotting, and amniotic fluid leakage as transient aftereffects. Simpson and Elias (2003) state that following amniocentesis serious maternal complications and fetal injuries are remote (p. 349).

Proper handling of the sample is important. Today, the failure rate of amniotic cell culture is only 1% to 2%, but it will necessitate repeat amniocentesis. Amniocyte culture failures have been associated with single-use plastic syringes, so

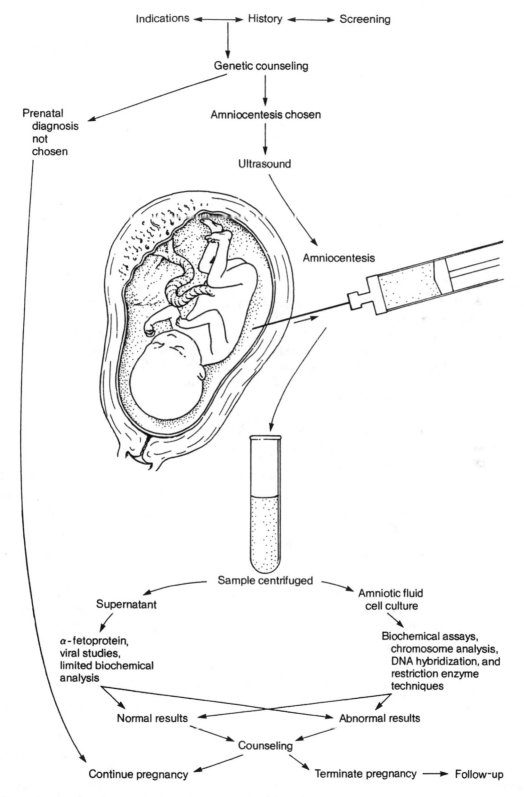

FIGURE 12.1   Amniocentesis: Options and disposition of sample.

these should not be used. The accuracy of the results is about 99.4%. Inaccurate results can occur because of culture contamination by mycoplasma or fungi, contamination of the culture by maternal cells or blood, loss of enzyme activity because of handling or transportation, inaccurate results due to an inexperienced laboratory or a rare disease variant, and laboratory mix-ups or clerical errors. One precaution against maternal cell contamination is to discard the first 2 to 3 ml of amniotic fluid obtained. If the sample is contaminated by blood, AFP values will be falsely elevated. These figures are for experienced centers, and standardization and quality control are critical issues.

After amniocentesis is done, the waiting period between the procedure and obtaining the results can be 2 to 3 weeks, although rapid chromosome culture techniques can be used to provide results in about a week or earlier. This may be a time of anxiety and apprehension for the couple, particularly if they have undertaken amniocentesis because of a previous birth with a genetic disorder. Indeed, amniocentesis has been referred to as a "crisis situation" in terms of the psychosocial stresses and anxiety imposed on the normal stresses surrounding a pregnancy. The still important study by Fletcher (1979) found that unresolved past problems, unconscious feelings of guilt, and failure and stresses within the family were exacerbated during this period, especially in families who had experienced the birth of a child with a genetic disorder. In Tymstra's study (1991), some mothers felt that a "conditional relationship" was imposed between the mother and fetus. Rapp (1997) reported that other families did not have anxiety or depression. Awareness of these aspects, the establishment of a good relationship with the family, and a clear, mutual understanding of the information prenatal diagnosis provides, as discussed earlier, will be helpful during this period.

If abnormal findings result from the prenatal diagnosis, the couple has a limited time period in which to make a decision in regard to the continuation or termination of the pregnancy, if they have not already done so. They may need discussion and specialized counseling that may include conferences with experts in treating the disorder, and with parents of children with the disorder, in addition to other supports. Giving the results to the family must be done sensitively and skillfully,

and both members of the couple should be told in person by the practitioner in a private setting when there is time to discuss issues and options. Issues regarding this discussion are discussed in chapter 8. Liberalized abortion laws have made amniocentesis a meaningful procedure in terms of removing the "Russian roulette" atmosphere of attempting pregnancy when in a high-risk group. For many couples who have had a child with an inherited genetic disorder, and who have a high risk for another child with the same disorder, the availability of prenatal diagnosis offers them the chance to have an unaffected child. Without it, from 50% to 90% of couples who have a 25% to 50% risk of an affected child would not have attempted another pregnancy. In one study of Hispanic and African American pregnant women, acceptance of amniocentesis was lower than in Caucasian populations, and was lowest for Hispanic women. They reported a decline in amniocentesis acceptance from 1995 to 2001 (Baker et al., 2004). Any influence of religious factors was not reported. In a pluralistic society, it is important for the nurse and other professional practitioners to support the right of the individual clients to make a decision that is compatible with their personal philosophy and lifestyle and to provide support for that decision. The World Health Organization (WHO) (1996) states that decisions following prenatal diagnosis should be made by the *couple* and that the responsibility of the health care worker is to provide the information in a manner that can be understood. Some of the difficulties surrounding these aspects are discussed later in this chapter.

Although abortion for genetic indications after prenatal diagnosis is regarded by many who disapprove of abortion in general as legitimate, there can be a great deal of stress that accompanies that decision-making. While prenatal diagnosis is more routine currently, both maternal and paternal feelings of depression after hearing that the fetus is affected may occur. Family disruption can also occur after the birth of an affected child. Thus, the nurse should be aware that ongoing counseling and contact is necessary after pregnancy termination and should make every effort to ensure access to such counseling for both partners. Studies of stress associated with amniocentesis indicate stress is greatest when waiting for results, and if the results are abnormal, when making a decision.

Feelings may be similar to those experienced while waiting for the results of diagnosis following abnormal screening tests discussed later. If the pregnancy is terminated, then stress is great after the procedure, as well as just before it. Plans for nursing intervention should include support during these periods.

Early Amniocentesis

Early amniocentesis (EA) is another form of prenatal diagnosis. Very early amniocentesis was defined by Evans, Johnson, and Holzgreve (1994) as at or less than 11 weeks gestation, and early amniocentesis as 12 to under 14 weeks gestation, while others define EA as under 15 weeks gestation. Problems include difficulty in obtaining adequate amniotic fluid. In Canada, a randomized trial compared EA and mid-trimester amniocentesis and found an increased risk for talipes equinovarus and fetal loss in the EA group, especially before 13 weeks gestation. ("Randomised trial to assess . . ., 1998). Sundberg et al. (1997) found a significant increase in talipes equinovarus in patients in an EA group as opposed to a CVS group as did Philip et al. (2004), who also found a greater increase in unintended pregnancy loss. Wilson et al. (1997) found no significant difference in pregnancy loss or neonatal outcome between EA and usual amniocentesis in a study of 695 women, whereas Eiben et al. (1997) found no statistical difference between EA (3,277 cases) and standard amniocentesis (1,808 cases) in regard to spontaneous abortion; however, they did note hip and foot dislocations occurring in a small percentage of fetuses. Congenital foot deformities were also found in a study by Nikkilä, Valentin, Thelin, and Jorgensen, (2002). Other concerns are the possibility of increased culture failure and the questions about validity of AFP and acetylcholinesterase measures before 13 weeks' gestation. ACOG (2001) and Simpson and Elias (2003) conclude that CVS is safer than EA and that amniocentesis is safer than either of the others.

CHORIONIC VILLI SAMPLING

Earlier methods of prenatal diagnosis are inherently desirable. Chorionic villus sampling (CVS) is typically done at 10 to 12 weeks gestation, but has

been performed earlier. Usually, CVS is done by the transcervical or transabdominal route. For the transcervical procedure, under concurrent ultrasound guidance, a catheter (1.5 mm) with an internal obturator is inserted through the vagina and cervix, and is guided to the chorion of the placenta. The obdurator is withdrawn, a syringe with nutrient medium is attached and gentle negative pressure is applied as the catheter is pulled back so that 10 to 20 mg of the chorionic villi is obtained. For the transabdominal procedure, again under ultrasound guidance, a 20 gauge spinal needle with obdurator is inserted through the chorion, the obturator is withdrawn, and a syringe with medium is attached and gentle pressure is applied as the needle is moved back through the chorion. Early detection allows wider scope for in utero treatment or, if chosen, safer early pregnancy termination. Cytogenetic, enzymatic, and DNA studies can all be performed on chorionic villi, and the amount of material obtained makes this method preferable for DNA analysis. A disadvantage of CVS is that neither AFP testing nor any other assay needing amniotic fluid can be done on CVS specimens. Thus, women who have CVS should be referred for maternal serum alpha-fetoprotein (MSAFP) screening at 15 to 20 weeks. Another disadvantage is the higher rate of cytogenetic ambiguous results than are seen in amniocentesis samples. These are caused by maternal cell contamination or culture-related mosaicism. The rate ranges from 1.1% to 2.0% and is sometimes known as confined placental mosaicism (CPM) or chromosomal anomalies confined to the placenta (CACP) and not present in the fetus. CPM has been associated with adverse fetal outcomes including intrauterine growth restriction and an increased rate of fetal loss. False negative mosaicism has also been detected with an error rate of about 0.1%. In the previous instances, amniocentesis should be offered to the mother to clarify results. Few effects immediately follow CVS except for vaginal bleedings which occurs more frequently after the transcervical procedure. However, the major serious fetal sequelae from CVS are for transverse limb deficiencies or reduction defects. Possible mechanisms for limb reduction defects might be through vascular disruption and uteroplacental insufficiency leading to fetal hypoperfusion, by limb entrapment, or by pressor substance release. After studying the results from cohort studies in the United States, various European countries, and Australia, the United States Multistate Case-Control Study and European registry results, it has been concluded that there is a small but real risk of transverse limb deficiency that overall is 0.03% to 0.14%. These rates, as well as severity of the defect, were said to be higher if CVS was performed before 10 weeks gestation (0.20%) than after 10 weeks (0.07%). The risk for spontaneous fetal loss from CVS is approximately 1.64% to 2.5%. Fetal loss has been reported as higher before 13 weeks. As with most of the other prenatal diagnostic procedure, CVS should be done in the context of an experienced center, practitioner, and program for best results. Usually chromosome results from direct preparations are available as early as 24 to 36 hours, with cultures available for confirmation in about 1 to 2 weeks. Discussion of issues after CVS are similar to those discussed under amniocentesis.

ULTRASONOGRAPHY

Ultrasonography alone is the major method for detecting fetal malformations. Ultrasound consists of vibrations that are inaudible to the human ear. This high-frequency sound produces a mechanical pressure wave, causing vibration consisting of the contraction and expansion of the body tissues and fluids through which it passes. The waves are transmitted into the body through a transducer and echoes at boundaries between adjacent tissues are reflected. These are converted into electrical signals and are amplified and processed so that they can be visually displayed on an oscilloscope and videotaped or photographed. Fluid-filled or surrounded structures are visualized especially well. The use of oil or gel on the abdominal wall is necessary to diminish the loss of waves. Ultrasound can be used in different ways or modes. In pregnancy, the frequencies used usually avoid known tissue effects from ultrasound that in some instances are the basis for its use, such as heat and tissue destruction. Ultrasound is noninvasive and non-ionizing. Patient preparation is minimal; a full bladder is often useful for aiding visualization.

Screening ultrasound in early pregnancy, at 10 to 13 weeks, is usually done to accurately date the pregnancy by measures such as crown-rump, but because of better resolution than previously, part of the scan includes examining the fetal anatomy and measuring fetal nuchal translucency (abnormal thickness at the posterior aspect of the neck of a fetus less than 13 weeks, after which it is called nuchal thickening, nuchal fold, or cystic hygroma). Nuchal translucency is used to assess risk for certain chromosome abnormalities such as Down syndrome and trisomies 13 and 18. In the first trimester, this parameter in experienced hands has been estimated to detect about 80% of Down syndrome with a 5% false-positive rate (McLennan, 2003). The absence of the fetal nasal bone may also be assessed since it is associated with Down syndrome. Alone, a nonvisualized nasal bone during the second trimester of pregnancy was said to identify 40% to 45% of Down syndrome pregnancies. This parameter increases the detection rate, lowering the need for invasive diagnostic testing.

The prenatal uses of ultrasound may be either primary or adjunct. The placenta and internal and external fetal structures can be visualized. Ultrasound is used in conjunction with: (a) amniocentesis, chorionic villus sampling, fetoscopy, and fetal blood and tissue sampling as a guide to increase safety and diagnostic accuracy; and (b) abnormal AFP and/or multiple serum analyte test levels to rule out false-positives and false-negatives due to inaccurate gestational age assessment, fetal death, multiple pregnancy, or to define the abnormality present. Alone ultrasound can be used to:

- detect certain fetal abnormalities in pregnancies identified as high risk; this now can include such features as increased nuchal translucency or cystic hygroma, abnormal fetal bone length, or absent fetal nasal bone, and certain other indicators that might be associated with fetuses with trisomy 21 and other aneuploidies;
- monitor fetal growth and allow fetal measurements such as crown-rump length and biparietal fetal head diameter to be made;
- determine the number of fetuses;
- determine fetal presentation;
- assess gestational age;
- ascertain fetal hypoxemia;
- ascertain if the fetal environment is normal, including amniotic fluid volume, assessment of the umbilical cord, blood flow, and

evaluation of the placenta for anomalies or maturity;

- detect ectopic pregnancy;
- assess structural and functional integrity;
- evaluate immediate fetal risk for optimum management and treatment;
- assess fetal viability; and
- detect hydatidiform mole.

Guidelines for obstetric ultrasound examination have been published by the American Institute of Ultrasound in Medicine (1996), and include minimum guidelines for routine examination. In addition, the extended or detailed examination and targeted imaging for fetal anomalies (TIFFA) are terms used for examination to detect fetal anomalies. Those who should be referred for targeted, detailed ultrasonography are:

- those with previous child or family history of detectable structural malformation or anomaly (including congenital heart defects),
- those who are at known high risk for other detectable fetal anomalies such as:
  - ◆ maternal condition predisposing to fetal anomaly,
  - ◆ drug/alcohol exposure in pregnancy,
  - ◆ maternal infection in pregnancy,
- abnormal pregnancy progression,
- abnormal maternal serum AFP or abnormal multiple serum analyte screening results,
- abnormal AFP results on amniocentesis,
- intrauterine growth retardation, and/or
- suspicious findings on routine ultrasound.

The availability of high-resolution ultrasound machines incorporating both curvilinear and multifocal transducers allow for obtaining good views of the fetus and making a diagnostic interpretation in the hands of the skilled ultrasonographer. These can be translated into clinical outcomes. For example, if esophageal atresia is diagnosed, the esophageal pouch can be aspirated at birth and oral feedings avoided until repair is accomplished, thus preventing aspiration and pneumonia and decreasing morbidity. Moving structures such as the beating fetal heart (using Doppler), the placenta, and fetal movement can be observed, and four chamber views of the heart allow for referral for fetal echocardiography and other procedures, if needed.

Sonographic screening effectiveness for detection of cardiac lesions varies with the type of defect. Advances in ultrasound imaging in three (3D) and four dimensions (real-time 3D imaging) are beginning to be used in prenatal diagnosis.

Basic ultrasound is a screening procedure that is done on pregnant women who have no clinical indication (low risk) for ultrasound. Increasingly in the U.S., ultrasound may be first offered during the first trimester at about 10–13 weeks followed by an option of more detailed ultrasound screening early in the second trimester for women who have no known risk factor. Some structural abnormalities may be identified during the first trimester as discussed below. It is estimated that about 70% of all pregnant women in the United States have ultrasound evaluation. However, although routine ultrasound is used in many countries such as Great Britain, it has not yet been recommended for routine use in the United States. The major reason for this are cost-benefit issues. Significant effects overall on infant outcome are not demonstrated in some trials. The routine antenatal diagnostic imaging with ultrasound (RADIUS) trial enrolled more than 15,000 women, and essentially found no difference in adverse perinatal outcome between the screened or the control group although there were significant differences in the detection of fetal anomalies before 24 weeks gestation (Crane et al., 1994). The Eurofetus study reported by Grandjean, Larroque, and Levi (1999) reported the detection of a large proportion of fetal anomalies. However, there is variation in the degree of sensitivity and specificity of detection of anomalies such as cleft lip and palate. In the case of Down syndrome and other aneuploidies, more accurate data results from combining the use of certain maternal serum markers (described below) with ultrasound measurements to reduce false-positives. A major consideration in the use of ultrasound, particularly in targeted situations, is the experience of the ultrasonographer and the quality of the equipment. While cost-benefit ratios of routine ultrasound have been questioned in the past, these have been reconsidered. Data from short-term human studies of embryo exposure indicate the relative harmlessness of the procedure, but not its absolute safety. Nurses should be sure that ultrasound is used only when really needed for the minimum time of exposure and at the least intensity that will yield necessary data. The popularity of using ultrasound images as prenatal keepsake portraits with names such as "fetal fotos" or as videos has prompted a statement from the FDA that this is regarded as an unapproved use of a medical device. Nurses should also be aware that early fetal sex determination by screening ultrasound may not be accurate. The author knows of one family who were told after this method that they would have a boy. They decorated a room for a boy, gave away the clothes from their little girl, prepared their daughter for her new brother even by name, and were surprised when a girl was delivered!

FETAL BLOOD AND TISSUE SAMPLING

Presently these methods of prenatal diagnosis carry a greater risk of fetal loss than do the others discussed. However, these methods may be chosen when there is not another way to ascertain the desired information about the particular genetic disorder in the fetus.

Fetal Blood Sampling

Fetal blood sampling (FBS) is known by several other names depending on the sampling site used to collect the specimen including funipuncture, funicentesis, cordocentesis and percutaneous umbilical blood sampling (PUBS). FBS is used prenatally for the following indications:

- diagnosis of genetic disorders, particularly those that need fetal DNA samples, that cannot be diagnosed by other prenatal diagnostic methods; these may include hemoglobinopathies (although DNA analysis of amniotic fluid cells or chorionic villi cells have largely replaced FBS), certain immunologic deficiencies and disorders, and certain coagulation disorders;
- rapid chromosome analysis (often within 24 hours) particularly if ambiguous results, mosaicism, or culture failure resulted from amniocentesis or CVS;
- diagnosis of fetal red cell and platelet alloimmunization;
- diagnosis of fetal infections such as toxoplas-

mosis, cytomegalovirus, rubella, and others, often allowing treatment to be given (usually done after 22 weeks);
- evaluation of nonimmune hydrops fetalis;
- to perform certain fetal blood chemistry tests such as acid-base status; and
- evaluation of twin-to-twin transfusion syndrome.

FBS is usually done as an outpatient procedure with maternal sedation and local anesthesia as needed. Sometimes fetal paralysis with a neuromuscular blocker is done to prevent fetal movement and injury. Today, ultrasound guidance instead of fetoscopy (in utero visualization of the fetus and placenta by means of an endoscope about 1.7 to 2.2 mm in diameter) is the norm before FBS. FBS is most commonly accomplished at 17–18 weeks or later but has been done as early as 12 weeks. Using strict aseptic tecnique, a 20 or 22 gauge spinal needle is inserted transabdominally with continuous ultrasound guidance and visualization of the needle tip. Fetal blood may be obtained from the umbilical cord or the fetus. The most common sites are the cord root and the intrahepatic vein. Up to 3–4 ml may be safely obtained. After the sample is obtained, it is necessary to verify by a variety of laboratory techniques that it is not maternally contaminated. FBS is not used as a technique of first choice for most disorders because of the higher risks accompanying it. Fetal loss rates from the North American PUBS registry have ranged from 2% to 9.4%. Goetzl and D'Alton (2001) estimate an overall risk of about 1% to 2% over background. This may be higher in early gestation and more compromised fetuses. Various studies support the finding that pregnancy loss related to FBS is increased when the fetus is abnormal over loss when the fetus is normal. The chief complications are chorioamnionitis or other maternal or fetal infection, Rhesus sensitization (which should be prevented by the administration of Rh immune globulin following the procedure), premature rupture of membranes and premature labor, fetal hemorrhage, severe bradycardia, and others. Fetal complications increase with longer procedure times and the number of attempts to obtain a sample. It is important that FBS be done by expert personnel in specialized centers.

Fetal Tissue Sampling/Biopsy

The major fetal tissues sampled in prenatal diagnosis are skin, muscle and liver. Fetal skin sampling may be obtained by the percutaneous insertion of biopsy forceps with the use of continuous ultrasound guidance as well as by fetoscopy. More commonly, a biopsy forceps can be inserted through an angiocath that has been placed in the amniotic cavity. Indications are skin diseases (a) that are not diagnosable by DNA analysis of a sample obtained through amniocentesis or CVS (most are now diagnosable in this manner) or (b) in which the DNA analysis is uninformative in the specific family seeking the information. Postnatal scarring is a complication, and the site of the skin biopsy must be carefully selected. Preferable sites are the buttocks, back, thorax, or scalp. The face, neck, and genitalia should be avoided. Fetal liver and muscle biopsy may be used to diagnose inborn biochemical disorders with detectable manifestations in these tissues that are not amenable to DNA analysis through samples from amniocentesis or CVS or in cases in which the DNA analysis is not informative; however, but usually this is not the case and this procedure is rarely used. Examples of disorders detected by fetal liver biopsy are ornithine transcarbamylase deficiency and glycogen storage disease type Ia. Fetal muscle biopsy has been used to detect Duchenne muscular dystrophy, but other methods usually suffice. Simpson and Elias (2003) report, in a small sample, a 17% fetal loss rate.

MATERNAL SERUM ANALYTE SCREENING

The use of maternal serum screening for alphafetoprotein (MSAFP) and for other markers for detection of certain defects, particularly open neural tube defects (NTDs) and certain chromosome disorders, depending upon the markers used, has become commonplace in pregnancy. In 1985, ACOG recommended offering MSAFP screening to every pregnant woman, and it rapidly became a standard of care. It is important to stress, however, that this is a screening test and not a diagnostic test. Therefore, the finding of any abnormal results requires prompt diagnostic investigation. About 90% of infants with NTDs are born to mothers with no prior history or known high risk; therefore they would not be pre-determined to be at high risk and would not be referred for amniocentesis or targeted ultrasound. The severe burden of NTDs made this screening highly desirable. Success in the fortification of food with folic acid as well as folic acid supplementation both preconceptionally and in early pregnancy has diminished the number of women found to have high MSAFP values on testing, emphasizing a successful public health prevention approach. Low levels of MSAFP are now used in the detection of Down syndrome and other chromosome abnormalities, usually in conjunction with other markers. In maternal serum, typically these tests are called the multiple marker tests or screen and include determination of AFP, human chorionic gonadotropin (hCG), either total or free β, and unconjugated estriol (μE_3). These are used in screening maternal serum for fetal aneuploidy, currently usually with at least one other indicator depending on trimester, such as pregnancy-associated plasma protein-A (PAPP-A), inhibin-A, often in conjunction with ultrasound-determined fetal nuchal translucency measurements, and sometimes determination of the presence or absence of the nasal bone. In this section, AFP, acetylcholinesterase, detection and diagnosis of NTDs, MSAFP and multiple marker screening will be discussed.

Alpha-Fetoprotein, Acetylcholinesterase, and Neural Tube Defects

AFP is a glycoprotein, similar to albumin, that is first synthesized in the fetal yolk sac and later in the fetal liver. It can be detected in the amniotic fluid or in the maternal serum. Its initial use was as an oncofetal antigen tumor marker, especially for hepatomas; but in the early 1970s, elevated AFP levels in amniotic fluid were associated with open NTDs. Later, low AFP levels were associated with certain chromosomal abnormalities discussed below. The source of AFP in amniotic fluid and maternal blood originates from the fetal cerebrospinal fluid, gastric fluid, meconium, bile, and urine. The outcome of AFP's variety of origins in the fetus means that elevation of AFP occurs not only with open NTDs, but also with other fetal anomalies, making AFP a nonspecific test. For example, in gastrointestinal anomalies such as esophageal atresia, normal clearance of AFP through fetal swallowing cannot occur. In renal disorders, such as congenital nephrosis, excess fetal serum AFP is excreted and thus is elevated in the amniotic fluid. AFP is used as a specific test when both parents are known carriers of congenital nephrosis, especially of the type frequent in persons of Finnish extraction. In renal agenesis, AFP is very low or absent. In closed NTDs, the layer of skin or tissue present prevents AFP from leaking out through the fetal cerebrospinal fluid, and so AFP levels are not elevated. Thus, AFP cannot be used to detect the approximate 20% of spina bifidas and 94% of encephaloceles that are closed, while 90-100% of anencephaly is detected. The major genetic conditions identified by elevated MSAFP levels during pregnancy are:

- open neural tube defects—spina bifida, anencephaly (more than 90% are open), and encephalocele (only about 6% are open);
- ventral wall defects—omphalocele (midline defect with herniation of abdominal organs into a membrane covered sac), and gastroschisis (extrusion of abdominal organs anteriorly with no covering membrane);
- congenital nephrosis (Finnish type);
- cystic hygroma (sometimes in association with Turner syndrome);
- other fetal defects such as Turner syndrome, teratomas, hydrocele, certain congenital skin conditions, and esophageal and duodenal atresia.

AFP in maternal blood rises during pregnancy until the 30th gestational week and then falls. The optimal time for MSAFP is between 16 and 18 weeks' gestation but it can be done between 15 and 22 weeks. The concentration of amniotic fluid AFP (AFAFP) is highest at the end of the first trimester. AFP levels are reported in multiples of the median (MoM). The normal median is population-based and is established from the unaffected pregnancies tested in that laboratory, and thus is influenced by the characteristics of the population served by that laboratory. Some degree of overlap occurs in AFP levels between normal pregnancies and pregnancies with NTDs (see Figure 12.2). If the cutoff level is set low enough to include almost all NTD pregnancies, then a large proportion of non-NTD pregnancies will be included, giving a high proportion

of false-positive results. If the cutoff level is set so high that few unaffected pregnancies would be included, then a large proportion of NTD pregnancies will be missed, giving a high proportion of false-negative results. The usual cutoff is 2.0 to 2.5 MoM. These must be interpreted in relation to other factors. For example the identical MSAFP raw value that is 2.5 MoM at 15 weeks' gestation will be only 1.2 MoM at 19 weeks. Women who weigh less may have higher AFP than the norm because of smaller blood volumes and less dilution. Black women with unaffected pregnancies have MSAFP distributions that are 10% to 15% higher than Asian or White women. Women with type 1 diabetes mellitus may have lower MSAFP levels than nondiabetic women, although they may be at higher risk for NTDs, and many believe that maternal screening is inappropriate for such women, preferring to offer amniocentesis instead. Obese women may show lower levels of AFP, and Asian woman have levels that may be 6% lower than White women. Various formulas and tables have been developed to determine the probability of a given woman with particular findings and characteristics for having a fetus with an NTD that are also population-adjusted for the population frequency of NTDs, and combination with the results from testing other analytes increases diagnostic accuracy.

While the chief reasons for elevated AFP levels other than diseases being screened for are error in calculation of gestational age, low maternal weight, and membership in the Black race, there can be other reasons for high MSAFP levels. Some of these relate to pregnancy outcome, whereas others are population-related or biological in nature necessitating interpretation when the MSAFP results are being evaluated. These include:

- multiple pregnancy,
- prior amniocentesis or fetoscopy,
- fetal death,
- severe Rh incompatibility,
- threatened abortion,
- placental distress,
- levels in past pregnancies, and
- bloody contamination.

When MSAFP levels are elevated, the reason is sought. Typically, an ultrasound examination is

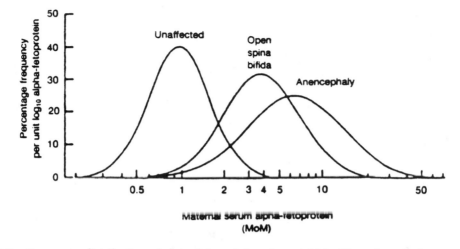

FIGURE 12.2   Frequency distribution of alpha-fetoprotein values at 16 to 18 weeks gestation.
From the United Kingdom Collaborative Study on Alpha-Fetoprotein in Relation to Neural Tube Defects (1977). Reproduced with permission from Elsevier (*The Lancet*, 1977, Vol. 1, p. 1323).

performed that includes confirming gestational age and fetal viability, and ruling out multiple gestation if possible. If the gestational age used for the MSAFP interpretation was wrong, then a recalculation is done. If gestational age is correct, then targeted ultrasound is done to look for the malformations known to result in high MSAFP levels. Some clinicians will repeat the MSAFP while others believe that targeted ultrasound and/or amniocentesis is warranted immediately for analysis of both AFP and acetylcholinesterase (AChE). Another identified consequence of elevated MSAFP levels in women during the second trimester is an increased risk of sudden infant death syndrome (SIDS) in their infant, but the reason for this is not yet known (Smith et al., 2004).

AChE is derived mostly from the tissues of the fetal nervous system, and increased levels of AChE in the amniotic fluid have been associated with NTDs. AChE determination has been used in conjunction with AFP and has successfully reclassified about 90% of non-NTD pregnancies with elevated AFP, reducing the cost of more expensive/extensive procedures. Those cases of increased AFP and normal AChE may represent abnormalities other than NTDs, some of which may be surgically correctable.

The finding that those women with high serum AFP, but normal values on amniocentesis, are still at increased risk for an adverse pregnancy outcome

of different types reflects a need to closely monitor those pregnancies. These outcomes include premature rupture of the membranes, fetal demise, abruptio placentae, preterm labor, pregnancy-associated hypertension, and infants that are small for gestational date. Waiting for serum analyte screening results engenders anxiety. Parents should be informed promptly of both normal and abnormal results. They should not be told to assume normality if they do not hear from the clinic or center. Those having abnormal results require sensitive and appropriate counseling and referral for appropriate prenatal diagnosis.

Maternal Serum Screening for Chromosome Abnormalities

In the mid 1980s, the association of low MSAFP levels and certain fetal chromosomal abnormalities, particularly Down syndrome, was made. The advantages of this screening test were immediately recognized. Although prenatal diagnosis has long been a standard of care for women 35 years and older, women younger than 35 years now deliver 75% to 80% of all infants born with Down syndrome. These younger women would not ordinarily be candidates for prenatal diagnosis. Thus the potential for one blood specimen to serve as a multiple screening method was very exciting. Decreased MSAFP levels can also result from fetal demise, increased maternal weight, hydatidiform mole, older gestational age, and congenital very low AFP levels (about 1 in 100,000).

While maternal serum screening was usually done in the second trimester, because of AFP levels the ideal would be detection of Down syndrome and other chromosome disorders in the first trimester. Expected detection levels for some analytes have now been determined for first trimester screening, and increasingly prenatal care is incorporating serum screening for chromosomal abnormalities with ultrasound in the first trimester.

MoM levels adjusted according to the above factors are used to detect Down syndrome and autosomal trisomies such as trisomy 13 and 18. The median MSAFP value for a woman whose fetus has Down syndrome is about 0.74 MoM of normal pregnancies. Cutoff levels for screening may range from 0.4 to 0.8 MoM to determine those at increased risk who need further diagnosis such as amniocentesis, and may be combined with other serum markers, maternal age calculations, as well as factors influencing MSAFP, as discussed previously. Other markers available include human chorionic gonadotropin, maternal serum estriol, pregnancy-associated plasma protein A (PAPP-A), and inhibin A. Human chorionic gonadotropin (hCG) levels of about 2.5 MoM were found to be associated with fetal Down syndrome but are normal in NTDs, and are now part of the screening panel, being very sensitive for trisomy 21 detection. Total hCG and/or free beta hCG levels may be used. hCG is produced by the trophoblast after uterine wall implantation and increases rapidly during the first two months of gestation, then decreasing steadily until 20 weeks, followed by a plateau. Maternal serum unconjugated estriol (μE_3) is a steroid hormone produced by the placenta from precursors originating in the fetal liver and adrenal glands. It has been found to be lower in women with fetuses with Down syndrome (0.79 MoM). Maternal serum PAPP-A measured in the second trimester appears to be significantly lower in fetal trisomies 21, 18, and 13 when compared to controls. Combinations of these markers may be used together with maternal age adjustments in the second trimester to screen for women who are then identified as being at a higher risk to bear a child with Down syndrome or other chromosomal trisomy. When nuchal translucency is found during

the early pregnancy ultrasound scan, it can serve as an additional marker. Using a first semester screening protocol of maternal age at or above 35 years, nuchal translucency, PAPP-A, and free β-hCG, the detection rate for Down syndrome was estimated at 86% with a false-positive rate of 4.25%; and for second trimester, maternal age plus MSAFP, unconjugated estriol, hCG, and INH-A, the detection rate was estimated at 82% with a false-positive rate of 6.9% (Benn, 2003). Another screening marker for Down syndrome is the proform of eosinophil major basic protein (proMBP), which has been suggested as a substitute for INH-A but is still being evaluated. McLennan (2003) in Australia reports that using first trimester nuchal translucency with first trimester serum screening of free β-hCG and PAPP-A resulted in detection of about 90% for trisomy 21 with a false positive rate of 5%. Cuckle (2001) estimated that the detection rate for Down syndrome at 10 to 11 weeks gestation using MSAFP, β-hCG, μE_3, PAPP-A, nuchal translucency, and absent nasal bone as indicators is 97.5%. However, some centers report lower detection rates of about 75%. ACOG has recommended multiple marker screening as standard care for women under 35 years of age. The American College of Medical Genetics recommended that multiple marker (MM) screening should replace MSAFP screening for women under 35 years of age, believing that women above that age should have CVS or amniocentesis. This is because MM fails to detect Down syndrome in those 35 years and 40 years old at 30% and 10%, respectively, as well as about 30% of those with trisomy 18 and about 50% of those with other chromosome abnormalities. All results need to be adjusted for ethnic group differences when interpreted. False positive results may recur in subsequent pregnancies, and Wald, Huttly, and Rudnicka (2004) have suggested an approach for adjusting the markers to counterbalance this problem. The American College of Obstetricians and Gynecologists (2004a) has supported first-trimester screening for Down syndrome and for trisomy 18 using nuchal translucency, free β-hCG, and PAPP-A if: (1) appropriate ultrasound quality monitoring programs are in place, (2) sufficient information and resources are available to provide comprehensive counseling regarding the options and limitations, and (3) the test is positive that there is access to appropriate diagnostic testing. They further recommend the use of combined first and second trimester screening as useful and support integrated tests.

Clinicians should be sure that clients receive clear, non-biased information about the meaning of the results of the MM screen, and that those with abnormal levels are promptly referred for ultrasonography and amniocentesis. Table 12.2 summarizes serum screening results for NTDs and chromosomal abnormalities.

FETAL CELLS AND FETAL CELL-FREE DNA CIRCULATING IN MATERNAL BLOOD

The analysis of maternal blood in early pregnancy for fetal cells and/or fetal cell-free circulating DNA holds the exciting potential for eventually allowing biochemical, DNA, and chromosome analysis of the fetus with a simple low-risk procedure (venipuncture), allowing for further diagnosis, early therapy, and early selective pregnancy termination, if desired. It is known that from at least the 2nd month of pregnancy on, fetal cells such as trophoblasts, nucleated erythrocytes, and leukocytes, enter the maternal circulation but in very small numbers ranging from 1 in 10^5 to 1 in 10^9. Thus, in order to perform analyses, fetal cells must be sorted and isolated from maternal ones, and enhanced through polymerase chain reaction (PCR) or another method for induction of rapid and accurate division of fetal cells. Newer techniques such as FISH (see chapter 5) for chromosome analysis can then be used. Enrichment of fetal DNA may aid analysis. Prenatal diagnosis of the fetal RhD blood type, fetal sex, and some chromosomal

abnormalities have been accomplished by this method. Limitations exist in addition to those mentioned above and include difficult technical considerations. It is expected that individual fetal cell isolation can be accomplished. This technique could potentially be combined with use of DNA technology and microchip arrays to screen for hundreds of mutations from one maternal blood sample. Fetal cell-free DNA analysis circulating in maternal serum has been used to determine fetal sex between 10 to 13 weeks of gestation, and Costa, Benachi, and Gautier (2002) report 100% accuracy in one series. Following fetal sex determination in this way, in the case of X-linked disorders, further techniques can be pursued only for male fetuses, thus preventing unnecessary risks if the fetus is a female. Ultrasonography may also be used to verify fetal sex determination. More recently, the demonstration of fetal RNA in maternal plasma opens possibilities for use as markers for prenatal gene expression profiling and other uses. Fetal epigenetic markers hold promise for use in the future.

PREIMPLANTATION DIAGNOSIS

Successful preimplantation genetic diagnosis was reported in 1990. In this technique, genetic analysis is usually carried out on embryos at the 4- to 8-cell stage (2 to 3 days), and unaffected embryos are transferred back into the uterus. Often this is done in conjunction with standard assisted reproductive techniques such as in vitro fertilization (IVF). Usually, multiple embryos are produced by this method, and the unaffected embryo(s) would then be transferred to the uterus. The present uses are mainly for determining fetal sex, detecting some

TABLE 12.2   Association of Selected Maternal Serum Analytes and Selected Fetal Abnormalities

Analyte	Abnormality		
	NTDs	Trisomy 21	Trisomy 18
Maternal serum AFP**	↑	↓	↓
hCG	Normal	↑	↓
uE3	Normal	↓	↓
PAPP-A	NA	↓*	↓
Inhibin A**	NA	↑	NA

* = 1st trimester
** = 2nd trimester

chromosome abnormalities, and some limited detection of inherited biochemical disorders such as cystic fibrosis, myotonic dystrophy, and thalassemia. Couples using this method currently are those already identified as at risk for a specific genetic disorder, especially X-linked ones, for which there is no specific DNA analysis; those who have had fertility and reproductive problems; and those with objections to pregnancy termination. Another potential use is to identify affected fetuses to permit gene therapy before embryonic organogenesis. Most centers recommend CVS or amniocentesis to confirm the results after a normal embryo is transferred to the uterus and pregnancy ensues. Little data are available on the risk of fetal anomalies resulting from preimplantation diagnostic manipulation. However, some reports indicate there is a relatively high incidence of postzygotic chromosomal abnormalities arising early. Concern has been expressed over the ethical implications of this testing, especially for "social" sex selection, and the possible dangers of eugenic manipulation. Assisted reproductive technologies and the use of preimplantation genetic diagnosis are further discussed in chapter 27.

OTHER TECHNIQUES

The development of a thin-gauge embryofetoscopic technique (TGEF) for endoscopy in the first trimester, with advances in optical systems, may revitalize prenatal diagnosis by direct visualization when that is needed. The transabdominal approach is most common, as transvaginal approaches are associated with higher fetal losses. This method may also be used for access to the embryo for blood and tissue sampling and for fetal therapy. Reece (2001) estimates procedure-related losses of 2.0% to 2.5%. Radiography may be useful for the diagnosis of certain skeletal defects but is not commonly used. Another technique that might become useful is the analysis of fetal cells obtained by transcervical retrieval by lavage, cytobrush, and mucous aspiration; however the problems of maternal cell contamination and confined placental mosaicism need to be overcome. Fetal MRI is being developed by some investigators as a supplemental technique for confirmation of inconclusive ultrasound findings and for the evaluation of certain neurologic conditions as well as some abdominal and genitourinary abnormalities.

ETHICAL, SOCIAL, AND LEGAL ISSUES ASSOCIATED WITH PRENATAL DIAGNOSIS

Some of the issues surrounding prenatal diagnosis really relate to the option of pregnancy termination after the results are available, because a second trimester abortion is viewed by some as both an ethical and a medical problem. One may, on the other hand, view prenatal diagnosis as protective of life because it allows many couples with a high genetic risk to undertake pregnancies that they would not have dared to risk otherwise; or if the pregnancy is unplanned, it allows them to carry to term an unaffected fetus that might otherwise have been aborted. The option of selective abortion allows meaningful reproductive alternatives to be presented to a couple at risk for a fetus with a known defect. The entire question of abortion is a very complex one, fraught with emotion, which cannot be addressed here adequately, but will only be looked at in a limited way as it relates to prenatal diagnosis. A professional nurse may have to recognize and separate his or her personal beliefs from those of the clients in order to provide quality care. It is important that clients get accurate, clear, unbiased, comprehensible information, and then are assisted in carrying out whatever decision they make.

Many of the same issues that were explored in chapters 10 and 11 are also applicable to prenatal detection and diagnosis. These include the right of the person to refuse to participate or to have a prenatal diagnostic procedure, issues of autonomy and choice, disclosure, confidentiality, access to information, the right to privacy, ownership of the samples taken, and ambiguous finding (see chapter 11). Others, discussed next, include aspects of autonomy and choice, sex selection and "trivial" reasons for prenatal diagnosis, and the related issue of enhancement, individual versus societal rights, obligations of the health care provider, and testing for diseases with uncertain outcomes or manifestations in adulthood. Other issues not unique to genetic related situations include access of clients to prenatal diagnosis and how socioeconomic factors might influence the availability of prenatal diagnosis especially for women who may not be defined as at high risk, thus creating conditions of health disparity.

Patients seeking to determine fetal sex as the primary reason for prenatal diagnosis fall into two categories—those at risk for an X-linked inherited disorder for which no specific assay is available, and those who wish to exercise sex selection. In the first situation, there is little problem if the fetus is a female. If the fetus is a male, and the mother is a carrier, then the chance for him to be affected is 50%. If pregnancy termination is selected without further testing, 50% of the time a normal fetus will be aborted. This is a very difficult situation for the family. Genetic counseling before prenatal diagnosis will clarify some of the issues. Parents may be less inclined to seek abortion if the condition is a treatable one. If it is one that is ultimately fatal (e.g., Duchenne muscular dystrophy), then the couple may find it totally unacceptable for them to give birth to this child. Molecular diagnosis is now offering new testing options for these conditions. Additionally the use of preimplantation genetic diagnosis offers additional choices.

The second group poses a different type of problem. Generally, prenatal diagnosis for social sex selection, and the implied pregnancy termination if the 'wrong" sex is being carried, is considered a trivial reason for procedures which, although generally safe, do carry a small risk of fetal loss and injury above that which would normally be expected. In one survey of geneticists, Wertz et al. (1997) found that about one third would perform amniocentesis for social sex selection or non-disease-related reasons. Arguments against performing prenatal diagnosis for sex selection are the following:

1. When a center is already over-burdened with clients and is experiencing delay in processing and communicating results to high-risk clients, then most would agree that prenatal diagnosis purely for sex choice should be a low-priority reason for use of a scarce resource. Scarce resource could also include misallocation of limited personnel.
2. The idea of selective abortion because of sex choice is morally offensive to many.

3. Although the risk of error and ill effects is low, it still is above that present normally in pregnancy, and sex choice is not a disease.
4. In our culture there still seems to be a general sex preference for males, especially for the first-born, so that allowing sex selection might have long-term societal effects.

Arguments for performing diagnosis are the following:

1. The 1973 Supreme Court decision does not require a woman to state reasons for abortion, but stated that a woman has the right to control reproduction and associated risks (but does this include prenatal diagnosis?).
2. If the sex of the child is so important to a couple that a woman undertakes prenatal diagnosis for sex choice, a child born who was of the undesired sex might be seriously disadvantaged in life with that couple.
3. A policy against sex selection could endanger the rights of the majority of women.

Fletcher (1979) in a still relevant statement stated that it is inconsistent to have a law that allows abortion with absolute rights of women to decide, and yet not provide amniocentesis for information about fetal sex for fear that abortions for minor reasons will result. Yet it appears clear that the practitioners cannot be forced into providing prenatal diagnosis for those reasons but that they do have an obligation to refer the couple to a center where this can be done. Some further believe that couples desiring prenatal diagnosis in order to exercise social sex selection should assume the costs themselves, and if they do so they should be allowed to "purchase" this service. Inconsistencies in policy at various centers have led some women to construct false histories for genetic risk in order to obtain prenatal diagnosis for sex selection. The President's Commission for the Study of Ethical Problems in Medicine and Biomedical and Behavioral Research (1983) concluded that individual physicians are free to follow their consciences on the use of amniocentesis for sex selection but that public policy should discourage but not prohibit such use. The Committee on Assessing Genetic Risks (Andrews et al., 1994) recommends not using prenatal diagnosis for sex selection. Prenatal diagnosis for sex selection has been called "home-made eugenics" by Kevles and Hood (1992). In the past, some centers did not routinely release information on the sex of the fetus until after the 24th week of pregnancy, unless such information was specifically requested. In China, the situation might be different. Female children are not valued, and Beardsley (1997) notes that millions "vanish." Therefore prenatal sex selection might offer some advantages. Pennings (2002) raises the question of whether sex selection really differs from other acceptable specifications such as health, and raises the question of the validity of the technique for family balancing.

Another situation is that in which the pregnancy is at risk for a relatively minor defect, such as cleft lip and palate. One must ask whether or not the practitioner can judge what is a minor defect to the couple concerned. Coping with necessary surgery and rehabilitation may be beyond the capacity of that particular couple's resources—financial, emotional, and physical. It may produce additional stresses on the rest of the family or on the marital relationship, of which the practitioner cannot be aware. A positive action that can be taken is to provide immediate (because the time element is so critical), expert counseling for the couple in order to try to elicit the true concerns and problems, and help them to arrive at a decision that is realistic for the couple, not the practitioner. A broader question is: Who decides normality? Should abortion be condoned or condemned for a defect such as an extra digit on the extremities? WHO (1996) has stated that it found no evidence of general abuse of prenatal diagnosis for minor or frivolous reasons.

Unexpected or ambiguous findings can result from prenatal diagnosis and can present dilemmas. The practitioner may or may not feel obligated to completely disclose such findings, if there was an agreement before testing that limited what would be disclosed. For example, if a woman at risk for Down syndrome in the fetus was found to be carrying a fetus with a small chromosome inversion about which little is known, the practitioner may only wish to tell her that the fetus does not have Down syndrome, and not mention the inversion. However, this paternalistic approach is probably not legally nor morally viable. Current knowledge and trends favor openness and honesty in informing the parents of such situations, combined with expert supportive counseling. The limitations of current knowledge should be made clear. Issues relating to the sex chromosome variations are discussed in chapter 5. Ambiguous findings may also arise after ultrasound screening that identifies what is called fetal "soft" markers, such as choroid plexus cysts in the fetal brain or mild renal dilatation, which not too long ago was believed to be associated with Down syndrome but is now known to be present in 1% to 2% of normal fetuses. Baillie, Smith, Hewison, and Mason (2000) conducted interviews with women who had fetal soft markers identified during second trimester ultrasound screening and who were referred for further evaluations. They found that they were in a state of crisis, ambivalence, and alienation, and a majority "put their pregnancy on hold." In one case, the mother, while awaiting further diagnostic testing, closed the door to the nursery. Weinans et al. (2000) found that 13% of the women in their study with abnormal serum screening results continued anxiety throughout pregnancy even though further diagnostic tests were normal.

Cases have been heard in the courts regarding the birth of a child with a genetic disorder for which the parents were carriers at a high risk or the mother was at risk, prenatal diagnosis was available, but the parents were not informed of their risk or the option of prenatal diagnosis by their physician. Although all physicians are obviously not qualified to perform prenatal diagnosis, court decisions point to the necessity of providing the necessary information and referring the clients to a center that has the needed services. Even today, health care workers may not have up-to-date information. The author had an inquiry from a couple who were known carriers for Tay-Sachs disease. The woman was 7 months pregnant, and her obstetrician had not mentioned the availability of prenatal diagnosis. A magazine article had sparked her inquiry. Fortunately, the eventual outcome was that the infant did not develop Tay-Sachs disease. But, her confidence in her obstetrician was undermined, and she sought a new physician for the delivery of her infant. Based on the implications of the case, *Darling v. Charleston Memorial Hospital,* it appears that not only physicians but other health practitioners have the professional obligation to remain aware of current developments, to recognize inadequate care, and to provide referral.

In the early days of amniocentesis, many centers would not perform the procedure without the prior agreement of the couple to pregnancy termination if the fetus was affected. The reasoning behind this had to do with the use of scarce resources and that many believed that there was no point to doing an amniocentesis and undergoing the risk if outcome was not affected. Today, such prior agreement would be thought of as coercive, and if it exists, nurses may need to inform the parents that they have the right to change their minds about any decision reached before the procedure is done and results are obtained, and after that as well. Knowing about an affected fetus allows the parents to prepare and plan for employment and living arrangements, placement, treatment, use of their resources, telling their families, obtaining specialized perinatal care, optimizing delivery and aftercare. Thus, it can enhance autonomy. Because 95% of amniocenteses have resulted in the detection of a normal fetus, the procedure may be very reassuring to couples at risk. In addition, some parents who before the procedure though that they would not consider pregnancy termination, may in fact change their minds if they discover that they are carrying a fetus with a poor prognosis or inevitable death. In some cultures, it may be preferable to "accept what is given" and have a child with a birth defect rather than no child.

Other issues regarding prenatal diagnosis have more recently been discussed. For example, suppose a test for a behavior such as homosexuality were to be available. Would a couple be able to select testing and what would be the ethical issues involved if they were to select pregnancy termination? An interesting dramatization of this dilemma is *Twilight of the Golds,* a television movie and play. What are the issues for diseases that emerge in adulthood? What are the issues, concerns, and rights of parents to select pregnancy termination or life for a fetus for a disease such as Huntington disease or some types of Alzheimer disease that will most likely not be symptomatic until that fetus is an adult? What about the risk for inherited, or susceptibility to, cancer? What is the meaning of the finding of a gene mutation such as *BRCA1* in the fetus? What will guide decisions when cancer development is not certain? These issues may not only involve disease states but issues of living such as life insurance, health benefit coverage, stigmati-

zation, and other issues. An issue that has occurred in preimplantation genetic diagnosis is that of late onset genetic disorders such as Huntington disease in which parents wish to ensure that their offspring is disease free but do not wish to know their own carrier status, and ask that a disease-free embryo be selected. Another application has been using preimplantation genetic diagnosis for selection of an embryo based n HLA type to serve as a stem cell donor for a sibling in need of such treatment. Other issues also include the possibility of the finding of a future cure for a late onset disease that is not now available. In the future, will selection of embryos after preimplantation genetic diagnosis be only for disease, or will preferred traits eventually be sought, for example taller stature or pleasing facial features if those could be determined, and should this be allowed?

A somewhat related situation is that in which prenatal diagnosis reveals that the mother is carrying a fetus with a disorder that will be extremely costly to society to treat and to educate, and which she decides to carry to term. How will society regard such families in the future? Will society continue to assume financial responsibility? Should the values of the individual or of society prevail? If a woman has the right to choose to terminate a pregnancy, shouldn't she also have the right to choose not to terminate it? Can society morally deny services to a disabled child because of his or her parents' decision? All of these are complex fundamental issues that have to do with the rights of the individual and the good of society, freedom and equality, and the quality of and right to life. Certainly, simplistic, rigid methods cannot be used to solve them, but a thoughtful, individualized approach should be taken. Professionals can help to emphasize the importance of the preservation of choice and to safeguard these choices in their practice.

BIBLIOGRAPHY

ACMG Position Statement on Multiple Marker Screen in Women 35 and older. (1994, January). *American College of Medical Genetics College Newsletter, 2.*
ACMG Statement on multiple marker screening in pregnant women. (1996). *American College of Medical Genetics College Newsletter, 4.*

American College of Medical Genetics. (2002). *Standards and guidelines for clinical laboratories* (3rd ed.).

American College of Obstetricians and Gynecologists. (1996, September). Educational Bulletin. Maternal serum screening, *228*, 1–9.

ACOG Technical Bulletin Number 187, December 1993. (1994). Ultrasonography in pregnancy. *International Journal of Gynecology and Obstetrics, 44*, 173–183.

American College of Obstetricians and Gynecologists. (1995, October). Committee Opinion. Chorionic villus sampling. *160*, 1-3.

American College of Obstetricians and Gynecologists. (2001, May). Prenatal diagnosis of fetal chromosomal abnormalities. *ACOG Practice Bulletin, No. 27*, 1–12.

American College of Obstetricians and Gynecologists. (2004a). First-trimester screening for fetal aneuploidy. ACOG Committee Opinion No. 296. *Obstetrics & Gynecology, 104*, 215–217.

American College of Obstetricians and Gynecologists. (2004b). Nonmedical use of obstetric ultrasonography. ACOG Committee Opinion No. 297. *Obstetrics & Gynecology, 104*, 423–424.

American College of Obstetricians and Gynecologists. (2004c). Prenatal and preconceptional carrier screening for genetic diseases in individuals of Eastern European Jewish descent. Committee Opinion, No. 298. *Obstetrics & Gynecology, 104*, 425–428.

American Institute of Ultrasound in Medicine. (1996). Guidelines for performance of the antepartum obstetrical ultrasound examination. *Journal of Ultrasound in Medicine, 15*, 185–187.

Andrews, L. B., Fullarton, J. E., Holtzman, N. A., & Motulsky, A. G. (1994). *Assessing genetic risks: Implications for health and social policy.* Washington, DC: National Academies Press.

Angier, N. (1996, November 26). Ultrasound and fury: One mother's ordeal. *New York Times*, online edition, http://www.nytimes.com/yr/mo/day/news/national/sonogram-sci.html.

Annas, G. J. (1981). Righting the wrong of wrongful life. *Hastings Center Report, 11*(2), 8–9.

Baillie, C., Smith, J., Hewison, J., & Mason, G. (2000). Ultrasound screening for fetal abnormality: Women's reactions to false positive results. *British Journal of Health Psychology, 5*, 377–394.

Baker, D., Teklehaimanot, S., Hassan, R., & Guze, C. (2004). A look at a Hispanic and African American population in an urban prenatal diagnostic center: Referral reasons, amniocentesis acceptance, and abnormalities detected. *Genetics in Medicine, 6*, 211–218.

Beardsley, T. (1997). China syndrome. *Scientific American, 276*(3), 33–34.

Benn, P. A. (2002a). Advances in prenatal screening for Down syndrome: I. General principles and second trimester testing. *Clinica Chimica Acta, 323*, 1–16

Benn, P. A. (2002b). Advances in prenatal screening for Down syndrome: II. First trimester testing, integrated testing, and future directions. *Clinica Chimica Acta, 324*, 1–11.

Benn, P. A., Egan, J. F. X., Fang, M., & Smith-Bindman, R. (2004). Changes in the utilization of prenatal diagnosis. *Obstetrics & Gynecology, 103*, 1255-1260.

Benn, P. A., Fang, M., Egan, J. F. X., Horne, D., & Collins, R. (2003), Incorporation of inhibin-A in second-trimester screening for Down syndrome. *Obstetrics & Gynecology, 101*, 451–454.

Bianchi, D. W. (1995). Prenatal diagnosis by analysis of fetal cells in maternal blood. *Journal of Pediatrics, 127*, 847–856.

Brun, J-L., Mangione, R., Gangbo, F., Guyon, F., Taine, L., Roux, D., et al. (2003). Feasibility, accuracy and safety of chorionic villus sampling: A report of 10,741 cases. *Prenatal Diagnosis, 23*, 295–301.

Bunduki, V., Ruano, R., Miguelez, J., Yoshizaki, C. T., Kahhale, S., & Zugaib, M. (2003). Fetal nasal bone length: Reference range and clinical application in ultrasound screening for trisomy 21. *Ultrasound in Obstetrics & Gynecology, 21*, 156–160.

Cameron, C., & Williamson, R. (2003). Is there an ethical difference between preimplantation genetic diagnosis and abortion? *Journal of Medical Ethics, 29*, 90–92.

Caughey, A. B., Washington, E., Gildengorin, V., & Kuppermann, M. (2004). Assessment of demand for prenatal diagnostic testing using willingness to pay. *Obstetrics & Gynecology, 103*, 539–545.

Centers for Disease Control and Prevention. (1995). Chorionic villus sampling and amniocentesis: Recommendations for prenatal counseling. *Morbidity and Mortality Weekly Report,* 44(No. RR-9), 1–11.

Chan, A. K., Chiu, R. W., & Lo, Y. M. (2003). Cell-free nucleic acids in plasma, serum and urine: A new tool in molecular diagnosis. *Annals of Clinical Biochemistry, 40*(Pt. 2), 122–130.

Chasen, S. T., & Skupski, D. W. (2003). Ethical dimensions of nuchal translucency screening. *Clinics in Perinatology, 30,* 95–102.

Chiu, R. W. K., & Lo, Y. M. D. (2004). Recent developments in fetal DNA in maternal plasma. *Annals of the New York Academy of Sciences, 1022,* 100–104.

Coakley, F. V., Glenn, O. A., Qayyum, A., Barkovich, A. J., Goldstein, R., & Filly, F. A. (2004). Fetal MRI: A developing technique for the developing patient. *American Journal of Radiology, 182,* 243–252.

Costa, J-M., Benachi, A., & Gautier, E. (2002). New strategy for prenatal diagnosis of X-linked disorders. *New England Journal of Medicine, 346,* 1502.

Crane, J. P., LeFevre, M. L., Winborn, R. C., Evans, J. K., Ewigman, B. G., Bain, R., et al. (1994). A randomized trial of prenatal ultrasonographic screening: Impact on the detection, management, and outcome of anomalous fetuses. The RADIUS Study Group. *American Journal of Obstetrics and Gynecology, 171,* 392–399.

Cuckle, H. (2001). Time for total shift to first-trimester screening for Down's syndrome. *Lancet, 358,* 1658–1659.

Cunniff, C., and the Committee on Genetics. (2004). Prenatal screening and diagnosis for pediatricians. *Pediatrics, 114,* 889–894.

Dhallan, R., Au, W-C., Mattagajasingh, S., Emche, S., Bayliss, P., et al. (2004). Methods to increase the percentage of free fetal DNA recovered from the maternal circulation. *Journal of the American Medical Association, 291,* 1114–1119.

Eiben, B., Hammans, W., Hansen, S., Traecki, W., Osthelder, B., Stelzer, A., et al. (1997). On the complication risk of early amniocentesis versus standard amniocentesis. *Fetal Diagnosis and Therapy, 12,* 140–144.

Evans, M. I., Johnson, M. P., & Holzgreve, W. (1994). Early amniocentesis: What exactly does it mean? *Journal of Reproductive Medicine, 39,* 77–78.

Evans, M. I., Llurba, E., Landsberger, E. J., O'Brien,

J. E., & Harrison, H. H. (2004). Impact of folic acid fortification in the United States: Markedly diminished high maternal serum alpha-feto-protein values. *Obstetrics & Gynecology, 103,* 474–479.

Failure to inform of AFP test: Birth defects—$4.3 million damages. Case in point: Basten by and through Basten v. U.S., 848 F. Supp. 2d 962 (AL 1994). *Regan Report on Nursing Law, 35*(2), 2.

Fletcher, J. C. (1979). Ethics and amniocentesis for fetal sex identification. *New England Journal of Medicine, 301,* 550–553.

Getz, L., & Kirkengen, A. L. (2003). Ultrasound screening in pregnancy: Advancing technology, soft markers for fetal chromosomal aberrations, and unacknowledged ethical dilemmas. *Social Science & Medicine, 56,* 2045–2057.

Goetzl, L., & D'Alton, M. (2001). Prenatal diagnosis. In F. W. Ling, & P. Duff (Eds.), *Obstetrics and gynecology: Principles for practice* (pp. 69–89). New York: McGraw-Hill.

Grandjean, H., Larroque, D., & Levi, S. (1999). The performance of routine ultrasonic screening of pregnancies in the Eurofetus Study. *American Journal of Obstetrics and Gynecology, 181,* 446–454.

Hampton, T. (2004). Markers in prenatal ultrasound debated. *Journal of the American Medical Association, 291,* 170–171.

Harris, R. A., Washington, E., Nease, R. F., Jr., & Kupperman, M. (2004). Cost utility of prenatal diagnosis and the risk-based threshold. *Lancet, 363,* 276–282.

Kevles, D. J., & Hood, L. (Eds). (1992). *Code of Codes.* Cambridge, MA: Harvard University Press.

Kumar, S., & O'Brien, A. (2004). Recent developments in fetal medicine. *British Medical Journal, 328,* 1002–1006.

Learman, L. A., Kuppermann, M., Gates, E., Nease, R. F., Jr., Gildengorin, V., & Washington, A. E. (2003). Social and familial context of prenatal genetic testing decisions: Are there racial/ethnic differences? *American Journal of Medical Genetics, Part C (Seminars in Medical Genetics), 119C,* 19–26.

Lee, W., DeVore, G. R., Comstock, C. H., Kalache, K. D., McNie, B., Chaiworapongsa, T., et al. (2003). Nasal bone evaluation in fetuses with Down syndrome during the second and third trimesters of pregnancy. *Journal of Ultrasound in Medicine, 22,* 55–60.

Lees, W. (2001).U ltrasound imaging in three and four dimensions. *Seminars in Ultrasound, 22,* 85–105.

Lo, U. M. D., & Poon, L. L. M. (2003). The ins and outs of fetal DNA in maternal plasma. *Lancet, 361,* 193–194.

Lo, Y. M. D., Tein, M. S. C., Lau, T. K., Haines, C. J., Leung, T. N., Poon, P. M. K., et al. (1998). Quantitative analysis of fetal DNA in maternal plasma and serum: Implications for noninvasive prenatal diagnosis. *American Journal of Human Genetics, 62,* 768–775.

Ludomirsky, A. Data presented at Sixth International Conference on Cordocentesis, Philadelphia, PA, October 21, 1991. Cited in R. L. Berkowitz, & L. Lynch (1994). *Fetal blood sampling* (pp. 359–369). In R. K. Creasy, & R. Resnick (Eds.), *Maternal-fetal medicine: Principles and practice.* Philadelphia: W.B. Saunders.

McIntosh, G. C., Olshan, A. F., & Baird, P. A. (1995). Paternal age and the risk of birth defects in the offspring. *Epidemiology, 6,* 282–288.

McLennan, A. (2003). Advances in prenatal screening. *Australian Family Physician, 32,* 107–112.

Meyers, C., Adam, R., Dungan, J., & Prenger, V. (1997). Aneuploidy in twin gestations: When is maternal age advanced? *Obstetrics & Gynecology, 89,* 248–251.

Mezei, G., papp, C., Tóth-Pál, E., Beke, A., & Papp, Z. (2004). Factors influencing parental decision making in prenatal diagnosis of sex chromosome aneuploidy. *Obstetrics & Gynecology, 104,* 94–101.

Muller, F., Dreux, S., Sault, C., Galland, A., Puissant, H., Couplet, G., et al. (2003). Very low alpha-fetoprotein in Down syndrome maternal serum screening. *Prenatal Diagnosis, 23,* 584–587.

Nelson, L. J. (2003). Preimplantation diagnosis. *Clinics in Perinatology, 30,* 67–80.

Ng, F. K. O., Tsui, N. B. Y., Lau, T. K., Leung, T. N., Chiu, R. W. K., Panesar, N. S., et al. (2003). mRNA of placental origin is readily detectable in maternal plasma. *Proceeding of the National Academy of Sciences, USA 100,* 4748–4753.

Nicolaides, K. H., Heath V., & Cicero S. (2002). Increased fetal nuchal translucency at 11–14 weeks. *Prenatal Diagnosis, 22,* 308–315.

Nikkilä, A., Valentin, L., Thelin, A., & Jorgensen, C. (2002). Early amniocentesis and congenital foot deformities. *Fetal Diagnosis and Therapy, 17,* 129–132.

Pennings, G. (2002). Personal desires of pathients and social obligations of geneticists: Applying preimplantation genetic diagnosis for non-medical sex selection. *Prenatal Diagnosis, 22,* 1123–1129.

Penso, C. A., Sandstrom, M. M., Garber, M-F., Ladoulis, M., Stryker, J. M., & Benacerraf, B. B. (1990). Early amniocentesis: Report of 407 cases with neonatal follow-up. *Obstetrics & Gynecology, 76,* 1032–1036.

Petrau, S., & Mugford, M. (2004). Should prenatal diagnostic testing be offered to all pregnant women on economic grounds? *Lancet, 363,* 258–259.

Philip, J., Silver, R. K., Wilson, R. D., Thom, E. A., Zachary, J. M., Mohide, P., et al. (2004). Late first-trimester invasive prenatal diagnosis: Results of an international randomized trial. *Obstetrics & Gynecology, 103,* 1164–1173.

President's Commission for the Study of Ethical Problems in Medicine and Biomedical and Behavioral Research. (1983). *Screening and counseling for genetic conditions.* Washington, DC: Government Printing Office.

Puñales-Morejon, D. (1997). Genetic counseling and prenatal diagnosis: A multicultural perspective. *Journal of the American Medical Womens Association, 52,* 30–32.

Rados, C. (2004). FDA cautions against ultrasound 'keepsake' images. *FDA Consumer Magazine, 38,* 12–16.

Randomized trial to assess safety and fetal outcome of early and midtrimester amniocentesis. (1998). The Canadian Early and Mid-trimester Amniocentesis Trial (CEMAT) Group. *Lancet, 351,* 242–247.

Rapp, R. (1997). Communicating about chromosomes: Patients, providers, and cultural assumptions. *Journal of the American Medical Women's Association, 52,* 28–32.

Reece, E. A. (2001). Looking beyond conception using first-trimester embryofetoscopy. In M. Evans, L. Platt, & F. De La Cruz (Eds.), *Fetal therapy* (pp. 21–26). New York: Parthenon Publishing Group.

Robertson, J. A. (2003). Extending preimplantation genetic diagnosis: The ethical debate: Ethical issues in new uses of preimplantation genetic diagnosis. *Human Reproduction, 18,* 465–471.

Rode, L., Wojdemann, K. R., Shalmi, A. C., Larsen, S. O., Sundberg, K., Nørgaard-Pedersen, B., et al. (2003). Combined first-and second-trimester screening for Down syndrome: An evaluation of proMBP as a marker. *Prenatal Diagnosis, 23,* 593–598.

Senyei, A. E., & Wassman, E. R. (1993). Fetal cells in the maternal circulation. *Obstetrics and Gynecology Clinics of North America, 20,* 583–598.

Sermon, K., Van Steirteghem, A., & Liebaers, I. (2004). Preimplantation genetic diagnosis. *Lancet, 363,* 1633–1641.

Sicherman, N., Bombard, A. T., & Rappoport, P. (1995). Current maternal age recommendations for prenatal diagnosis: A reappraisal using the expected utility theory. *Fetal Diagnosis and Therapy, 10,* 157–166.

Simpson, J. L., & Bischoff, F. (2004). Cell-free fetal DNA in maternal blood. *Journal of the American Medical Association, 291,* 1135–1137.

Simpson, J. L., & Elias, S. (2003). *Genetics in obstetrics and gynecology* (3rd ed.). Philadelphia: W.B. Saunders.

Smith, G. C. S., Wood, A. M., Pell, J. P., White, I. R., Crossley, J. A., & Dobbie, R. (2004). Second-trimester maternal serum levels of alpha-feto-protein and the subsequent risk of sudden infant death syndrome. *New England Journal of Medicine, 351,* 978–986.

Spencer, K., Bindra, R., Cacho, A. M., & Nicolaides, K. H. (2004). The impact of correcting for smoking status when screening for chromosomal anomalies using maternal serum biochemistry and fetal nuchal translucency thickness in the first trimester of pregnancy. *Prenatal Diagnosis, 24,* 169–173.

Strong, C. (2003). Fetal anomalies: Ethical and legal considerations in screening, detection, and management. *Clinics in Perinatology, 30,* 113–126.

Sundberg, K., Bang, J., Smidt-Jensen, S., Brocks, B., Lundsteen, C., Parner, J., et al. (1997). Randomized study of risk of fetal loss related to early amniocentesis versus chorionic vilus sampling. *Lancet, 350,* 697–703.

Thornhill, A. R., Dedie-Smulders, C. E., Geraedts, J. P., Harper, J. C., Harton, G. L., Lavery, S. A., et al. (2005). ESHRE PGD Consortium "Best practice guidelines for clinical preimplantation genetic diagnosis (PGD) and preimplantation genetic screening (PGS)." *Human Reproduction, 20,* 35–48.

Tymstra, T. (1991). Prenatal diagnosis, prenatal screening, and the rise of the tentative pregnancy. *International Journal of Technological Assessment in Health Care, 7,* 509–516.

Verlinsky, Y., Rechitsky, S., Sharapova, T., Morris, R., Taranissi, M., et al. (2004). Preimplantation HLA testing. *Journal of the American Medical Association, 291,* 2079–2085.

Wald, N. J., Huttly, W. J., & Hackshaw, A. K. (2003). Antenatal screening for Down's syndrome with the quadruple test. *Lancet, 361,* 835–836.

Wald, N. J., Huttley, W. J., & Rudnicka, A. R. (2004). Prenatal screening for Down syndrome: The problem of recurrent false-positives. *Prenatal Diagnosis, 24,* 389–392.

Wald, N. J., Rodeck, C., Hackshaw, A. K., Walters, J., Chitty, L., & Mackinson, A. M. (2003). First and second trimester antenatal screening for Down's syndrome: The results of the Serum, Urine and Ultrasound Screening Study (SURUSS). *Health Technology Assessment, 7*(11), 1–88.

Weinans, M. J. N., Juijssoon, A. M. G., Tymstra, T., Gerrits, M. C. F., Beekhuis, J. R., & Mantingh, A. (2000). How women deal with the results of serum screening for Down syndrome in the second trimester of pregnancy. *Prenatal Diagnosis, 20,* 705–708.

Wetz, D. C. (1997). Is there a "women's ethic" in genetics: A 37-nation survey of providers. *Journal of the American Medical Women's Association, 52,* 33–38.

Wilson, R. D., Johnson, J., Windrim, R., Dansereau, J., Singer, J., Winsor, E. J. T., et al. (1997). The early amniocentesis study: A randomized classical trial of early amniocentesis and mid-trimester amniocentesis. *Fetal Diagnosis and Therapy, 12,* 97–101.

World Health Organization. (1996). WHO Technical Report Series, 865. *Control of hereditary diseases.* Geneva, Switzerland: World Health Organization.

13

The Vulnerable Fetus

The concept of the fetus as totally protected by a placental barrier was cracked by the association of specific birth defects with rubella infection, and shattered by the thalidomide disaster of the early 1960s. It is now known that the fetus is vulnerable to many influences, some of which may emerge many years postnatally. The practitioner treating a pregnant woman has two patients—the mother and the fetus.

The term "teratogen" is often used to describe those agents acting during pregnancy that cause structural or functional damage to the unborn child, in contrast to "mutagen," which damages genetic material. Low-risk teratogens are defined as "agents that produce congenital defects in less than 10 infants among 1,000 maternal exposures" (Shepard, 2002, p. 275). Terms such as embryotoxic, fetotoxic, or developmental toxicity may also be used. The term "fetus" as used in this chapter also includes the embryo. In a given exposure during pregnancy, a teratogen can have any of the following consequences:

- no apparent effect,
- prenatal or perinatal fetal death,
- congenital anomalies,
- altered fetal growth (e.g., growth retardation),
- postnatal functional and behavioral deficits and aberrations, and
- carcinogenesis.

Complex and multifaceted maternal and fetal factors influence the consequences to the fetus of drugs, radiation, and chemical and infectious agents. These include the following:

- Agents often act differently in different species, and on individuals within the species

(e.g., differences in genetic constitution, variability in metabolic pathways, etc.). This applies to both the mother and fetus.
- The age of the fetus at the time of exposure: generally when exposed to agents affecting the period from fertilization to implantation the result is either death or regeneration; during the period of organogenesis the result is usually gross structural alterations; and after organogenesis in the fetal period the result is usually related to alterations in cell size and number, although the central nervous system and external genitalia remain vulnerable through most of pregnancy (see Figure 13.1).
- The agent's access to, and disposition within, the fetus.
- The chemical, biologic, and physical properties of the agent (for microorganisms—type, virulence, and number) have varying effects.
- Interactions with other agents and factors (e.g., environmental, nutritional, other drugs, etc.) can have negative consequences.
- Level and duration of dosage or exposure influence the agent's effect.
- Maternal biochemical pathways and mechanisms for handling drugs and chemicals are altered by pregnancy.
- The degree of interference with maternal systems and the extent of modulation that occurs determine the effect on the fetus.
- The genetic constitution of both mother and fetus; dizygotic twins have been born with one having anomalies typical of a drug effect, whereas the other was normal.

Drugs and chemicals can cause fetotoxic effects not only by direct fetal interaction, but also through interference with maternal systems (circulatory,

The Vulnerable Fetus   311

endocrine, excretory, appetite regulating, etc.). Some of the problems involved in determining whether or not a specific substance is injurious to the fetus include:

- Different effects may be seen depending on the time of gestation at which the fetus is exposed, and the exact date of pregnancy is not always known;
- The number of pregnant women getting a certain drug or disease at the same time of gestation are few and a slight increase in an anomaly may not be statistically significant; even then differences in their environment, the reason for giving the drug, ethnic differences, and so on make associations and generalizations difficult;
- The difficulty in detecting minor anomalies or delayed deficits;
- One fetotoxic agent can have several different effects; drugs rarely produce only one type of defect;
- Many fetotoxic agents can show the same effect;

- Long-term problems cannot be detected easily (e.g., the administration of diethylstilbestrol [DES] in pregnant women and the appearance of clear cell adenocarcinoma of the vagina in their daughters);
- In humans, all of the interacting and modulating factors, such as genotype of both mother and fetus, environmental chemicals, nutrition, and so forth, may differ and cannot be controlled;
- Bias in recall; mothers who give birth to infants with defects are more likely to recall adverse events such as illness, medications, and so on in their pregnancies than women who have normal infants;
- Effects may be subtle (e.g., behavioral alteration);
- Agents do not need to harm the mother in order to damage the fetus;
- Difficulties in extrapolating data from animal studies; and
- More than one drug may interact as may the drug and the disease process.

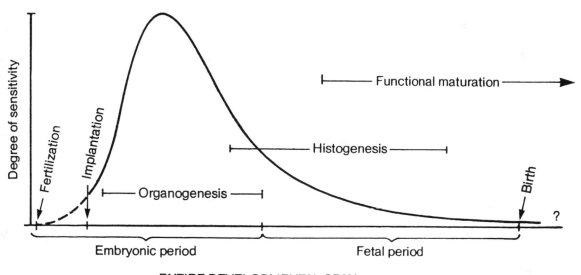

ENTIRE DEVELOPMENTAL SPAN

FIGURE 13.1   Periods of fetal growth and development and susceptibility to deviation. The highest sensitivity, at least to structural deviation, occurs during the period of organogenesis, from about days 18 to 20 until about days 55 to 60. The absolute peak of sensitivity may be reached before day 30 postconception. As organogenesis is completed susceptibility to anatomical defects diminishes greatly, but probably minor structural deviation is possible until histogenesis is completed late in the fetal period. Deviations during the fetal period are more likely to involve growth or functional aspects because these are the predominant developmental features at this time. (Wilson JG: Environment and Birth Defects. New York, Academic Press, 1974).

This chapter considers the effect of drugs, alcohol, cigarette smoking, infectious agents, ionizing radiation, and unfavorable maternal environment on the fetus. Environmental effects are considered in chapter 14.

DRUGS AND CHEMICAL AGENTS IN PREGNANCY

In spite of the bitter lesson of thalidomide, pregnant women still continue to take a substantial number and variety of self- or physician-prescribed drugs. In an early study, Forfar and Nelson (1973) found that all of the women in their study took prescribed drugs, including iron, and 64.4% took nonprescription drugs; Doering and Stewart (1978) found that all patients took at least two different drugs, and 93.4% took five or more; Bonassi, Magnani, Calvi, Repetto, and Publisi (1994) reported that in their Italian sample, only 17.3% of pregnant women did not take any drug, and the mean number of drugs taken was 2.17; a large collaborative study of 14,778 women found that 14% took no drugs and the mean was 2.9; Rubin, Ferencz, and Loffredo (1993) found that 68% of women used at least one drug; in the study by Dow-Clarke, MacCalder, and Hessel (1994), 43% used non-prescribed medications in pregnancy, although more than 92% knew these should be avoided; and Hill (1973) found that 65% of the women took self-prescribed drugs, while at some time in their pregnancy all women took between 3 to 29 drugs, with a mean of 10.3. Splinter, Sagraves, Nightengale and Rayburn (1997) reported that the mean number of medications women in their study took during the first, second, and third trimesters excluding vitamins and minerals was 1.57, 2.01, and 2.85, respectively. These women reported that they decreased their use of tobacco, alcohol, caffeine, and illicit drugs during this pregnancy. Henry and Crowther (2000) reported that pregnant women took between 2.3 and 2.6 nonprescription medications during pregnancy. In looking at the use of illicit substances in pregnancy during a period from 1996–1998, Ebrahim & Gfroerer (2003) found that 2.8% of pregnant women reported such use as did 6.4% of women of childbearing age who were not pregnant. Andrade and colleagues (2004) examined prescription drug use in pregnancy in regard to the FDA categories described later in this chapter. They found that over 47% of women in their study were prescribed drugs from categories C, D, or X. Nordeng and Havnen (2005) found that 36% of the 400 women studied reported use of herbal drugs during pregnancy.

Most drugs taken by the pregnant woman are transported to the fetus. Although most attention to the harmful effects of drugs on the fetus has been devoted to those mediated by the mother, attention has been given to male-mediated drug effects occurring around the time of conception. It is postulated that these might occur by damaging the sperm itself, by the presence of a drug or its metabolites in seminal fluid, or by altering paternal metabolic systems. Those believed to possibly affect the fetus in this manner are anticonvulsants, methadone, lead, alcohol, sex hormones, various chemicals (see chapter 14), morphine, smoking, and caffeine.

Most data on paternal effects come from animal studies that have shown decreased birth weight, increased infant mortality, and behavioral alterations due to methadone. These data are only speculative, but practitioners should advise males to restrict their use of drugs, particularly recreational ones, around the time of planned conception.

Several questions must be asked before recommending a drug for a pregnant woman.

1. Is pharmacologic intervention necessary for this condition?
2. Are other effective alternative therapies available?
3. Is the risk increased if no treatment is given?
4. Is this specific drug the agent of choice for both the condition and the pregnancy?
5. Does the risk of the disorder or its consequences outweigh the risk of the drug?
6. Does the value of the drug to the mother for treatment of the disorder weigh favorably against any possible detrimental effects to the fetus?

These questions are not always easy to answer. To begin with, the statement that a drug "has not been shown to be a human teratogen" does not mean that it is safe, as it may never have been adequately tested in the pregnant human female. Establishing drug safety is difficult because of the previously discussed problems and factors influencing fetal effects. In addition, drug testing for safety when doing animal and laboratory studies may not use a species that is sensitive to the effects of the drug. Thalidomide had appeared harmless in the species in which it was tested. Some testing is now carried out on primates, but their expense and long generation time mean that small number of animals are used, and so a small increase in malformations or a subtle effect will not be detected. Drugs tested in humans before mass marketing may be in specific population groups from which generalizations should not be made, or have few or no pregnant women in the sample because of ethical concerns for safety. If the effect is one in which the increased incidence of defects is small and nonspecific, then the number of subjects in preliminary tests before marketing may not be sufficient to demonstrate the effect. Cost and time are also limiting factors on the extent of testing that is carried out because there are pressures to get new drugs on the market quickly.

After distribution, the association of a drug with detrimental fetal effects can be made by case reports, surveillance, and epidemiologic studies. The teratogenicity of thalidomide was discovered because of the sudden increased incidence of a previously rare type of limb defect (phocomelia) that coincided with the widespread use of thalidomide in pregnant women in the early 1960s. The numerous case reports appearing at the same time in the literature led to the establishment of the association and its withdrawal from the market at that time. Thalidomide is available again, this time in the treatment of leprosy, various dermatological and autoimmune conditions, and is being studied for other uses. Surveillance for associated birth defects is planned. Retrospective studies can be done after the birth of a malformed child when a woman is asked to recall details of her illnesses and medications used during her pregnancy, but is subject to recall bias. Epidemiologic surveillance and reporting of congenital anomalies, especially the frequency of certain "sentinel" defects, is carried out by the Centers for Disease Control and Prevention (CDC) at several sites across the United States to detect any changes in patterns or incidence that might reflect an environmental influence. Amalgamated criteria for human teratogenesis are given by Shepard (2002).

Prescription drugs are labeled as to their pregnancy category. The FDA has established five categories as follows:

A. Controlled studies show no risk. Adequate, well-controlled studies in pregnant women have failed to demonstrate risk to the fetus.
B. No evidence of risk in humans. Either animal findings show risk, but human findings do not, or, if no adequate human studies have been done, animal findings are negative.
C. Risk cannot be ruled out. Human studies are lacking, and animal studies are either positive for fetal risk, or lacking as well. However, potential benefits may justify the potential risk.
D. Positive evidence of risk. Investigational or post-marketing data show risk to the fetus. Nevertheless, potential benefits may outweigh the potential risk.
X. Contraindicated in pregnancy. Studies in animals or humans, or investigational or post-marketing reports have shown fetal risk which clearly outweighs any possible benefit to the patient.

Even those drugs listed in Category A should not be used unless "clearly needed." About two-thirds of drugs listed in the *Physician's Desk Reference* are in Category C. There has been a great deal of criticism of the present system since many drugs have not been tested in pregnant women.

In order for nurses to stay up-to-date on recent advances in recognizing drugs with adverse effects in pregnancy, the periodic teratogen updates that appear in the journal *Birth Defects Research*, the *Morbidity and Mortality Weekly Report (MMWR)*, and the *FDA Drug Bulletin* can be used. On-line information such as Development and Reproductive Toxicology (DART) and Environmental Teratology Information Center (ETIC) are part of TOXNET (available through the National Library of Medicine) and the REPRORISK system. The organization of Teratology Information Services located throughout the U.S. and Canada can be accessed through their organization (http://www.otispregnancy.org), as well as MotherRisk (http://www.motherisk.org), and The Clinical Teratology Web at TERIS, and may be helpful. Certain fetotoxic drugs are discussed next, and others are presented in Table 13.1. Absence from the table

TABLE 13.1   Selected Drugs Known or Suspected to be Harmful or Teratogenic to the Fetus

Drug	Reported effects
Alcohol	See text
Antibiotics	
Aminoglycosides	Amikacin, gentamycin, kanamycin, tobramycin (see streptomycin)
Chloramphenicol	Effects in neonate from administration in second and third trimester include gray baby syndrome, hypothermia, failure to feed, collapse, and death
Streptomycin	Ototoxic to fetal ear, eighth cranial nerve damage, other aminoglycosides may also cause this
Tetracycline	Yellow/brown discoloration of tooth enamel, enamel hypoplasia, inhibits bone growth
Anticancer drugs	
Alkylating agents	Chlorambucil has been associated with renal agenesis
	Busulfan has been associated with growth retardation, cleft palate, microphthalmia, and increased incidence of multiple malformations; all apparently cause a risk of increased spontaneous abortion
Aminopterin	Cranial dystosis, hydrocephalus, hypertelorism, micrognathia, limb and hand defects, multiple congenital malformations
Antimetabolites	Cyclophosphamide has been associated with increased incidence of multiple malformations, especially skeletal defects, cleft palate
Methotrexate	Increased incidence of miscellaneous congenital malformations, especially of the central nervous system and limbs
Anticoagulants	
Warfarin (Coumadin)	Fetal warfarin syndrome, facial abnormalities, nasal hypoplasia, respiratory difficulties, hypoplastic nails, microcephaly, hemorrhage, ophthalmic abnormalities, bone stippling, developmental retardation
Anticonvulsants	Also see text
Phenytoin	Fetal hydantoin syndrome, growth retardation, mental deficiency, dysmorphic feature, short nasal bridge, mild hypertelorism, cleft lip and palate, cardiac defects, transplacental carcinogenesis (neuroblastoma)
Trimethadione (Tridione)	Apparent syndrome of developmental delay, V-shaped eyebrows, and paramethadione low-set ears, high or cleft palate, irregular teeth, cardiac defects, (Paradione) growth retardation, speech difficulties, increased risk of spontaneous abortion
Valproic acid	Spina bifida
Antimalarial	
Chloroquine	Slight risk of chorioretinitis, may cause ototoxicity
Quinine	Deafness, limb anomalies, visceral defects, visual problems, other multiple congenital anomalies
Antithyroid	
Iodides and thiouracils	Depression of fetal thyroid hypothyroidism, goiter
Carbimazole	Scalp defects, dysmorphic facial features, other possible anomalies
Hormones	
Adrenocorticoids	Intrauterine growth retardation, neonates may show adrenal suppression and possible increased susceptibility to infection; there are conflicting reports of increased incidence of cleft lip and palate
Androgens	Masculinization of female fetus
Clomiphene	Questionable increase in incidence of NTDs
Diethylstibestrol	Development of vaginal adenocarcinoma, usually in adolescence or young adulthood, reproductive tract structural alterations, in exposed males, testicular abnormalities, sperm and semen abnormalities have been reported.
Oral contraceptives	Association of increased incidence of cardiac and limb defects, (progestogen/estrogen) VACTERL syndrome; conflicting research reports, may not be teratogenic
Psychotropics	
Chlordiazepoxide (Librium)	Possible overall increased incidence of congenital malformations
Diazepam (Valium)	Hypotonia, hypothermia, withdrawal symptoms at birth(?), increase in incidence of cleft lip and palate

TABLE 13.1 *(Continued)*

Drug	Reported effects
Haloperidol tifluoperazine, prochlorperazine	Suspected of causing slight increase in incidence of limb defects in exposed fetuses; weigh against need for mother
Lithium	Increase in stillbirths, neonatal deaths; edema, hypothyroidism, goiter, hypotonia, cardiovascular anomalies such as Ebstein's anomaly; use another drug during pregnancy if possible
Meprobamate	Possible increase in cardiac defects or major malformations
Others	
Aminoglutethamide (Cytadren)	Pseudohermaphroditism, increased incidence of fetal deaths, increased incidence of malformations
Angiotensin-converting-enzyme inhibitors	Hypoplasia of skull, some skeletal anomalies, oligohydramnios, IUGR, patent ductus ateriosus (degree of risk uncertain)
Metronidazole (Flagyl)	Midline facial defects, cleft lip and palate (?), chromosome aberrations with long-term use (?); carcinogenic and mutagenic in nonhuman systems, debated in humans
Misoprostol (a prostaglandin E₁)	Moebius sequence
Nonsteroidal inflammatory drugs Indomethacin (others may also have these effects)	Premature closure of ductus arteriosus, oligohydramnios
Penicillamine	Connective tissue defects (e.g., cutis laxa)
Retinoids	(see text)
Salicylates	The use of aspirin has been associated with "postmaturity syndrome" and with a slight possible increase of hemorrhage, especially in premature infants, and possibly some anomalies (debated)
Sulfonylureas	Chlorpropamide and tolbutamide may be associated with increased congenital anomalies and increased fetal mortality (debated)
Thalidomide	Phocomelia and other limb defects, eye and ear malformations and abnormalities

Note: All exposed fetuses will not show these effects. Absence from this table does not imply safety. Heavy metals and anesthetic gases and hyperthermia are discussed in chapter 14. See text for discussion.

does not imply safety. Some adverse fetal effects are not teratogenic. Women may also be taking herbal or botanical products and may not think of them as drugs per se. The effects of these products on the fetus, alone or in combination, are largely unknown. It is not possible to present an all-inclusive list here, and reports on the safety (or non-safety) of drugs in pregnancy often conflict. Nevertheless, these drugs are best avoided where another less harmful, efficacious one can be substituted. Selected drugs are discussed in more detail next.

Diethylstilbestrol

Diethylstilbestrol (DES) is a synthetic estrogen that was introduced in the 1940s and used extensively in pregnant women in the 1950s and 1960s to treat habitual abortion, bleeding, premature delivery, and toxemia. Many women (as many as 7% of all pregnant) took DES before the hazards to the fetus were identified. In 1971, the association between an epidemic in young women of clear cell adenocarcinoma of the vagina and cervix (CCA) and the use of DES during pregnancy in their mothers was made. The magnitude of the DES exposure problem is not completely known, because many women did not know the precise medication they took or only knew the trade name and did not recognize that they had been exposed despite wide publicity in the lay press. It is estimated that there may have been about 4,000,000 male (DES sons) and female (DES daughters) exposed offspring. The association between DES use by the mother and CCA in their daughters years later has been well documented. Less widely recognized consequences in women include nonneoplastic alterations of the reproductive system, especially in the vagina, uterus (often T-shaped), or cervix which may be seen in 25% to 35% of exposed women; and an increased incidence of spontaneous abortion, ectopic pregnancies, and prematurity. Despite the increased prevalence of adverse pregnancy outcomes, long-term studies show that more than 80% of those who became pregnant had at least one liveborn infant. In exposed males (DES sons), sperm and semen abnormalities; testicular abnormalities, including benign cysts in the epididymis; and small and undescended testes have been reported as more prevalent than in controls. There is a possible increased risk of testicular and prostate cancer thus pointing up the need for these men to practice screening recommendations for these conditions. Some investigators report altered social behavior but others disagree. DES daughters should not be given estrogen and should be advised to have continuing care. DES sons should see a urologist and be taught the technique and importance of self-examination of the testes. In recent years the children of DES sons and daughters (DES grandchildren) have been followed. Many have been born prematurely. An increased risk of hypospadias in sons of DES daughters has been noted by Klip et al. (2002). The National DES action groups or the National Cancer Institute can supply information and referrals. DES is a proven teratogen.

Antiepileptic Drugs

The use of antiepileptic drugs (AEDs) for maternal seizures such as epilepsy during pregnancy needs to be carefully considered, balancing the risk of malformations with the risk to the fetus of uncontrolled seizures. The increased risk of congenital malformations in the pregnancy outcomes of epileptic vs. non-epileptic women might be due to direct drug effects, indirect effects through interference with metabolic processes such as folate metabolism, maternal or fetal genetic variances in drug or folate metabolism, effects on the embryonic heart, and/or other unknown factors. A very detailed review is in Barrett and Richens (2003). Phenobarbital and phenytoin (Dilantin) are given together about three quarters of the time, so that individual effects of the two have been hard to separate. Phenytoin and other hydantoins are associated with a risk of orofacial clefts, especially cleft lip and palate, and with congenital heart disease

that is 5 to 10 times and 2 to 3 times that of the general population, respectively. In general, the risk of major congenital malformations in women taking anti-epileptic drugs is approximately 4% to 9% vs. 2% to 3% for the general population (Morrow & Craig, 2003) as well as increased risk for minor defects and cognitive and developmental delay. In addition, a fetal hydantoin syndrome consisting of any or all of the following has been reported: growth retardation; mental retardation; dysmorphic facial features such as short nasal bridge, bowed upper lip, and mild ocular hypertelorism; and hypoplastic fingers and nails. These consequences must be weighed against the ill effects of prolonged uncontrolled seizures. Risks have been variously estimated and appear to be about 10% for the full, and up to an additional 30% for a part of the syndrome. The problem of seizure control should be discussed by the female with epilepsy before conception with her health care practitioner, so that they can agree on an appropriate course of action. There is some evidence that certain fetuses may be more vulnerable to damage from hydantoin because of the slow activity of the enzyme epoxide hydrolase. If possible, it seems best to use monotherapy or a single agent at the lowest possible effective dose that might be divided, particularly in the first trimester, taking into consideration the stage of pregnancy most affected by the particular agent, coupled with monitoring of blood levels and untoward effects. Nurses should be aware that Vitamin K deficiency is sometimes seen in infants about 48 to 72 hours after birth whose mothers took phenytoin with hemorrhage occurring. Such infants should be observed for this complication. This may be ameliorated by the administration of Vitamin K during labor. The anticonvulsant trimethadione is associated with a very high rate of spontaneous abortion or with fetal malformations such as cardiovascular defects, craniofacial anomalies, and others, and effects such as mental deficiency and speech disorders. Valproic acid (Depakote, Depakene) has been specifically associated with a risk of spina bifida in 1% to 2%, hypospadias, radial aplasia (rare), and possibly an autism-like disorder. Carbamazepine (Tegretol) has been associated with neural tube defects, and possibly other defects (such as eye malformations) as well. A fetal valproate syndrome has been described that may include orofacial clefts, cardiovascular defects, and craniofacial abnormalities such as trigonocephaly, midface hypoplasia, high forehead, small mouth with thin upper lip, and low nasal bridge. Other features may include overlapping toes, poor lower limb musculature, clumsy gait, learning and behavioral abnormalites, delayed development including speech, and hypoglycemia after birth. In carbamazepine exposure, effects can also include minor facial dysmorphy such as short nose, broad nasal bridge, and small chin; and nail hypoplasia with some reported learning difficulties. Another anticonvulsant, ethosuximide (Zarontin), is not presently known to be teratogenic. It should be noted that often various antiepileptic drugs are used in combinations and there may be inter-drug effects generated.

Management of the pregnancy should include folic acid supplementation before and during pregnancy for prevention. Prenatal diagnosis, including maternal alpha fetoprotein determination and ultrasound, should be considered for women so exposed to detect fetal effects to the extent possible. Nulman, Scolnik, Chitayat, Farkas, & Koren (1997) believe that malar hypoplasia, epicanthus, micrognathia, and other facial findings are associated with offspring of women with untreated epilepsy.

Anticancer Drugs

In general these drugs are both teratogenic and mutagenic. They can cause spontaneous abortion, fetal death, congenital anomalies, and systemic toxicity in the fetus (e.g., hematopoietic depression) particularly in the first trimester. The severe effects of these drugs must be weighed against the risk that delay in treatment may jeopardize the health and life of the mother. If possible, therapy should be delayed until the second trimester and combination therapy should be avoided, with the least toxic agent used. Antimetabolites such as methotrexate and aminopterin (no longer in general use) have a reported fetal malformation incidence of more than 50% when given in the first trimester. As with radiation exposure, the importance of the pregnancy to the parents and the willingness to take a substantial risk should be considered when discussing possible termination of the pregnancy. For some drugs in this category, data are difficult to obtain because of the multimodal

agent therapy and small numbers treated. Both males and females taking anticancer drugs should avoid pregnancy or procreation for at least one year after therapy is discontinued. Males may wish to take advantage of sperm banking before beginning therapy, and women may wish to consider harvesting and saving ova for later use via assisted-reproductive techniques.

Oral Contraceptives and Other Hormonal Agents

Oral contraceptives are usually only given inadvertently during pregnancy. The grouping together of hormonal pregnancy tests, oral contraceptives, and hormonal therapy when searching for adverse fetal effects has "muddied the waters" and made it difficult to clarify individual effects. The association of limb defects and congenital heart disease with the administration of oral contraceptives has been suggested but not subsequently proven. It has also been suggested that oral contraceptives are not teratogenic (Koren, Pastuszak, & Ito, 1998). The administration of androgens and progestational agents has resulted in masculinization of the external genitalia of the female fetus, whereas feminization of the male fetus has been reported with estrogen administration as it has with ingestion of soy products in pregnancy. These effects do not occur in all exposed fetuses.

Other Drugs

From time to time, concern arises about the potential teratogenicity of certain drugs or agents, and so some brief comments that are additions to Table 13.1 are stated here. There is some disagreement as to the extent of fetal danger from aspirin intake during pregnancy, especially in the last trimester. However, nurses should remember that this is rarely an essential drug, and generally acetaminophen, which appears to carry little risk, can be recommended instead. Among the antibiotics, because of the effects of tetracycline on bones and teeth and of the high level of toxicity of chloramphenicol, another less fetotoxic antibiotic such as amoxicillin or the cephalosporins can usually be substituted. Streptomycin, amikacin, gentamicin, kanamycin, and tobramycin may be ototoxic and damage the eighth cranial nerve. Tuberculosis (TB) in pregnancy is increasing worldwide. The present regimen of choice for TB treatment in pregnancy is isoniazid, rifampin, and ethambutol for 9 months. Ethionamide has been associated with central nervous system abnormalities in one series and streptomycin is ototoxic. For TB, capreomycin, aminoglycosides, ciprofloxacin, ofloxacin, cycloserine, and clofazimine should be avoided during pregnancy. Pyrazinamide is probably safe. Pyridoxine supplementation when taking isoniazid is recommended.

Caffeine has been associated in some studies with an increased level of spontaneous abortion and prematurity or major malformations, but other studies have not supported this. The effects of caffeine are difficult to separate from smoking, and studies have examined caffeine from various sources, such as coffee, colas, and tea which may contain other substances. In addition, there are genetic differences in the way caffeine is metabolized. Women should probably be advised to limit caffeine intake and be given information on caffeine-containing foods, over-the-counter drugs, and beverages. Caffeine may be associated with low birth weight and intrauterine growth retardation (IUGR), particularly if more than 300 mg per day is used. Vitamin A derivatives such as isotretinoin (Accutane) used for acne treatment, and etretinate (Tegison) used for psoriasis have shown teratogenic effects. Isotretinoin used orally has been linked to increases in spontaneous abortion, central nervous system malformations such as hydrocephalus, heart anomalies, ear anomalies, renal and optic nerve effects and other defects. Etretinate may be associated with excess central nervous system malformations. Pregnancy should be avoided within 6 months of use. Isotretinoin may be used by teenage girls who accidentally become pregnant; thus those taking it should receive information about how to avoid pregnancy. At issue is the fact that teenage girls at risk for unplanned pregnancies may share their prescription drugs with each other. Fluconazole, used in fungal infections, is a teratogen giving rise to characteristic craniofacial anomalies such as exorbitism, synostosis, and a "pear-shaped" nose.

Concern has also been raised about the use of antidepressant drugs in pregnancy. Fluoxetine (Prozac) is the most widely prescribed. While an increase in three or more minor anomalies decreased

birth weight and perinatal complications was found in children of women who took it in the first trimester, these data were confounded because of nonrandomness and the fact that many of the women were also taking other psychotropic medications. Lithium and the monoamine oxidase inhibitors should be avoided in pregnancy. Trazodone and Nefazodone use does not appear to be contraindicated in pregnancy. Nulman, Rovet, et al. (1997) did not find effects on global IQ, language development, or behavior in preschool children who had been exposed to fluoxetine or tricyclic antidepressant drugs.

Nursing Points

- Be proactive. Do pre-conception counseling which should include assessment of current alcohol and drug use, environmental exposures and smoking and provide education.
- Females of reproductive age seen in various settings should be taught that medical and social drug exposure of certain types can affect the fetus, especially in the 1st month or trimester when she may not realize she is pregnant. This should include the dangers of medication sharing.
- Encourage the client to tell her pharmacist, physician, nurse, and other health practitioners involved in her care that she is pregnant.
- Identify those most likely to be users of medications and drugs (including alcohol, caffeine, and cigarettes) and inform those who are considering pregnancy or who are already pregnant of the hazards.
- Teach women that over-the-counter products, including extra vitamins, herbals, or iron, are considered drugs and should not be taken without discussion with her health care provider.
- Integrate the previous information into school health programs.
- Educate men that taking certain drugs just prior to conception may affect the sperm and be injurious to the fetus; advise waiting 90 days after the last dose before conceiving.
- Educate women as to the dangers of self-medication in pregnancy.
- Provide teaching related to nondrug management of common conditions, such as relaxation techniques for tension instead of medication.

- Involve the client in decision-making if drug therapy is being considered, as an informed partner in her own care.
- Instruct her to keep an accurate list of all medications ingested during pregnancy with the date, dose, length of time taken, and the reason for it.
- Maintain a record of all prescription or recommended drugs with the same information; this should be in a handy form for easy reference as part of the patient profile.
- If drug therapy is necessary, the lowest effective therapeutic dose of the least toxic agent should be used.
- The risks and benefits should always be considered, and doses should be individualized.
- Question any drug that appears contraindicated in pregnancy because the practitioner prescribing it may not know that the patient is pregnant.

ALCOHOL IN PREGNANCY

The harmful effects of alcohol in pregnancy were noted long ago. Aristotle observed that drunken women often had feebleminded children and the Old Testament (Judges 13:7) states: "Behold, thou shalt conceive, and bear a son; and now drink no wine or strong drink. . . ." From time to time other references have been made, but Lemoine in France in 1968 and Ulleland in the United States in 1972 were the first to make the association between maternal alcohol consumption in pregnancy and abnormalities in their infants. In 1973 the name "fetal alcohol syndrome" (FAS) was applied to a distinct pattern of anomalies by Jones, Smith, Ulleland, and Streissguth. In late 1980 the Surgeon General advised pregnant women not to drink alcoholic beverages and to be aware of alcohol content in other foods. A warning addressed to pregnant women is on alcohol containers, and in stores selling alcohol that contains language such as, "According to the Surgeon General, women should not drink alcoholic beverages during pregnancy because of the risk of birth defects. . . ." Many commercials, some using popular music artists, continue that message. A National Task Force on Fetal Alcohol Syndrome and Fetal Alcohol Effect (Bertrand et al., 2004) has developed an agenda that ranges from uniform clinical case and surveillance case definitions for FAS and ARND to development and dissemination of various educational and curricular material. The Public Affairs Committee of the Teratology Society has also issued a recent statement addressing FAS, particularly in regard to improved recognition, risk factors for and prevention of FAS. Some believe that the definition of FAS is too narrow and believe that the term should be changed to include fetal alcohol effects (FAE) and be called Fetal Alcohol Spectrum Disorder. One issue has been that most of the signs used in diagnosis of FAS are "soft" although researchers at the University of Washington have attempted to more succinctly define features such as the smooth philtrum, palpebral fissures and thin vermillion upper lip border by use of a numerical guide (Astley & Clarren, 1999). CDC has launched a massive initiative aimed at educating health professionals, teachers, and the public about fetal alcohol syndrome.

Influences on Effects of Alcohol in Pregnancy

Factors such as genetic susceptibility, genetically determined differences in the metabolism of alcohol, time of fetal exposure, maternal nutritional status, gene-gene interactions, multidrug-interactions, and the dose of alcohol all play a role in the extent of fetal consequences. Consequences include decreased birth rate, growth retardation, increase in spontaneous abortion rates, and stillbirths, as well as congenital anomalies and functional deficits. FAS may represent the extreme upper end of the spectrum of effects that occur as a result of maternal consumption of alcohol in pregnancy, whereas lowered birth weight and minimal functional deficits represent the lower end.

Alcohol freely crosses the placenta and reaches the fetus. Alcohol elimination in the fetus is slower than the adult rate. At present, it is not known whether it is the alcohol itself that causes the fetal effects or whether they are caused by some intermediate metabolite of the alcohol, such as acetaldehyde. The effects of alcohol on the male have not been fully determined, but it is known that spermatogenesis is adversely affected. The effects of maternal alcohol abuse in pregnancy are difficult to separate from the use of other drugs, cigarette smoking, and malnutrition.

Fetal Alcohol Syndrome and Alcohol-Related Effects

To standardize usage, the Committee to Study Fetal Alcohol Syndrome (FAS) of the Institute of Medicine in its 1996 report (Stratton et al., 1996) recommended new diagnostic criteria for FAS and alcohol-related effects (ARE). Three categories define FAS and two potentially co-occurring categories define ARE—alcohol-related birth defects (ARBD) and alcohol-related neurodevelopmental disorder (ARND). The diagnostic criteria for these are in Tables 13.2 and 13.3. Other terms that have been used include prenatal exposure to alcohol (PEA) and fetal alcohol spectrum disorder (FASD). FASD is becoming a preferred term. Besides its teratogenic and fetotoxic effects, in utero exposure to alcohol may enhance the chance for neoplasia, especially neuroblastoma, in later life. Thus alcohol consumption can affect reproduction and offspring in the following phases: (1) before conception—lowered fertility; (2) prenatal—risk of spontaneous abortion and prematurity; (3) perinatal and birth—stillbirth, low birth weight, growth retardation, FAS, alcohol-related effects, ARBD, and other anomalies; (4) newborn and infant—hyperactivity, fretfulness, failure to thrive, poor sucking and feeding, sleep disturbances, and behavioral and learning deficits which may be part of FAS or ARND; (5) childhood—hearing loss, vision impairment, ARND, behavioral and learning deficits, hyperactivity, sleep disturbances and others; (6) adolescence—behavioral and learning deficits, maladaptive behaviors, and ARND.

Long-term studies of adolescents and adults with FAS by Streissguth (1993) and Streissguth and O'Malley (2000) found deficits in socialization, communication skills, attention deficits, and hyperactivity; also about half were mentally retarded. The facies were not as distinct, but microcephaly and shortness persisted.

Incidence and Risk

The incidence of FAS is estimated at 0.6 to 2.2 per 1000 live births overall. Alcohol-related effects may be more frequently seen. These may be low estimates because diagnosis may not be made until later in life when functional deficits are more noticeable. FAS is many times higher among those

of low socioeconomic status (SES) and is higher in some ethnic populations, but these data may be confounded because of SES. Various researchers have examined the outcomes from women who used alcohol in pregnancy. The results of studies vary because of different definitions of mild, moderate, and severe alcohol use; different alcohol content in different alcoholic beverages; and because of varying patterns of alcohol consumption, ranging from a constant daily amount to periodic binges to a combination of both. Nevertheless, it is estimated that the risk for any major or minor congenital anomaly in an alcohol-abusing pregnancy ranges from 38% to 71%, with an overall adverse pregnancy outcome average of 50%. Data as to the magnitude of risk for the pregnant woman who ingests a minimal amount of alcohol either consistently or sporadically are less clear-cut. Some researchers suggest that alcohol does not need to be totally avoided during pregnancy and that it may be more realistic for women to restrict their intake to one standard measure (1 oz equivalent of absolute alcohol) per day. Researchers fear that unnecessary guilt may arise in mothers of children with birth defects who drank mildly during pregnancy. However, others disagree and presently, no minimum safe level for alcohol consumption in pregnancy has been established. Alcohol is metabolized by various enzymes such as alcohol dehydrogenase and members of the cytochrome P450 group that are known to have considerable genetic variation. Thus fetal susceptibility to the effects of alcohol may be influenced by the genetic makeup of the pregnant woman who drinks in pregnancy in terms of the metabolism and handling of alcohol as described under pharmacogenomic variation in chapter 18. Pregnant women should avoid drinking alcohol and be aware of the alcohol content in food and drugs.

Prevention

Nearly 19% of women drink alcohol while pregnant. In one study (Naimi, Lipscomb, Brewer, & Gilbert, 2003), preconceptual binge drinking was associated with unintended pregnancy. Effects of alcohol consumption in pregnancy are potentially preventable. Prevention can be at various levels—universal (for all persons in a particular community or society), selective (targeted to those at

TABLE 13.2   Diagnostic Criteria for Fetal Alcohol Syndrome

1. FAS with confirmed maternal alcohol exposure

   A. Confirmed maternal alcohol exposure
   B. Evidence of a characteristic pattern of facial anomalies that includes features such as short palpebral fissures and abnormalities in the premaxillary zone (e.g., flat upper lip, flattened philtrum, and flat midface)
   C. Evidence of growth retardation, as in at least one of the following:
      • low birth weight for gestational age
      • decelerating weight over time not due to nutrition
      • disproportional low weight to height
   D. Evidence of CNS neurodevelopmental abnormalities, as in at least one of the following:
      • decreased cranial size at birth
      • structural brain abnormalities (e.g., microcephaly, partial or complete agensis of the corpus callosum, cerebellar hypoplasia)
      • neurological hard or soft signs (as age appropriate), such as impaired fine motor skills, neurosensory hearing loss, poor tandem gait, poor eye-hand coordination

2. FAS without confirmed maternal alcohol exposure

   B, C, and D as previously stated.

3. Partial FAS with confirmed maternal alcohol exposure

   A. Confirmed maternal alcohol exposure
   B. Evidence of some components of the pattern of characteristic facial anomalies
   Either C, D, or E
   C. Evidence of growth retardation, as in at least one of the following:
      • low birth weight for gestational age
      • decelerating weight over time not due to nutrition
      • disproportional low weight to height
   D. Evidence of CNS neurodevelopmental abnormalities, as in
      • decreased cranial size at birth
      • structural brain abnormalities (e.g., microcephaly, partial or complete agenesis of the corpus callosum, cerebellar hypoplasia)
      • neurological hard or soft signs (as age appropriate), such as imparied fine motor skills, neurosensory hearing loss, poor tandem gait, poor eye-hand coordination
   E. Evidence of a complex pattern of behavior or cognitive abnormalities that are inconsistent with developmental level and cannot be explained by familial background or environment alone, such as: learning difficulties; deficits in school performance; poor impulse control; problems in social perception; deficits in higher level receptive and expressive language; poor capacity for abstraction or metacognition; specific deficits in mathematical skills; or problems in memory, attention, or judgment.

From: *Fetal Alcohol Syndrome, Diagnosis, Epidemiology, Prevention, and Treatment* (pp. 76–77), by K. Stratton, C. Howe, & F. Battaglia, 1996. Committee to Study Alcohol Syndrome, Institute of Medicine, Washington, DC: National Academy Press. Reprinted with permission.

higher risk because of a factor such as age group), and indicated (targeted to high-risk individuals). The nurse should be part of or initiate preventative efforts with different emphases, as appropriate, that include the following:

1. Increasing public awareness of the effects of alcohol in pregnancy so that it becomes part of the general health knowledge of a population. This can be done by media campaigns (e.g., radio talk shows, television); distribution of literature in such areas as laundromats, liquor stores, beauty salons, and marriage license bureaus; inclusion of such information in school health programs; informational signs on public transportation; displays at health fairs; local businesses that complement information disseminated by local health departments, clinics, and hospitals. One drawback to these methods is that often the very people these are aimed at are not reached by these methods. In general, the aims are to recommend abstinence as a way of assuring safety and to create a climate in which nondrinking in pregnancy is the accepted behavioral norm. Aiming the media campaign at a wide audience creates awareness in friends and relatives of the pregnant woman so that support for

TABLE 13.3 Diagnostic Criteria for Alcohol-Related Effects

Clinical conditions in which there is a history of maternal alcohol exposure and where clinical or animal research has linked maternal alcohol ingestion to an observed outcome.

There are two categories that may co-occur. If both diagnoses are present, then both diagnoses should be rendered:

1. Alcohol-related birth defects (ARBD)

List of congenital anomalies, including malformations and dysplasias

Cardiac	Atrial septal defects	Aberrant great vessels
	Ventricular septal defects	Tetralogy of Fallot
Skeletal	Hypoplastic nails	Clinodactyly
	Shortened fifth digits	Pectus excavatum and carinatum
	Radioulnar synostosis	Klippel-Feil syndrome
	Flexion contractures	Hemivertebrae
	Camptodactyly	Scoliosis
Renal	Aplastic, dysplastic, hypoplastic kidneys	Ureteral duplications
	Horseshoe kidneys	Hydronephrosis
Ocular	Strabismus	Refractive problems secondary to small globes
	Retinal vascular anomalies	
Auditory	Conductive hearing loss	Neurosensory hearing loss
Other	Virtually every malformation has been described in some patient with FAS. The etiologic specificity of most of these anomalies to alcohol teratogenesis remains uncertain.	

2. Alcohol-related neurodevelopmental disorder (ARND)

Presence of:

A. Evidence of CNS neurodevelopmental abnormalities, as in any one of the following:
   - decreased cranial size at birth
   - structural brain abnormalities (e.g., microcephaly, partial or complete agenesis of the corpus callosum, cerebellar hypoplasia)
   - neurological hard or soft signs (as age appropriate), such as impaired fine motor skills, neurosensory hearing loss, poor tandem gait, poor eye-hand coordination

   and/or:

B. Evidence of a complex pattern of behavioral or cognitive abnormalities that are inconsistent with developmental level and cannot be explained by familial background or environment alone, such as learning difficulties; deficits in school performance; poor impulse control; problems in social perception; deficits in higher level receptive and expressive language; poor capacity for abstraction or metacognition; specific deficits in mathematical skills; or problems in memory, attention, or judgment

From: *Fetal Alcohol Syndrome, Diagnosis, Epidemiology, Prevention, and Treatment* (pp. 76–77), by K. Stratton, C. Howe, & F. Battaglia, 1996. Committee to Study Alcohol Syndrome, Institute of Medicine. Washington, DC: National Academy Press. Reprinted with permission.

nondrinking will be available. Such information should be routinely given at family planning clinics as well so that effects can be realized when pregnancy is being contemplated, not after several weeks or months have gone by.

2. Targeting prevention and information for specific groups.

3. Increasing awareness and knowledge of the health practitioner by integration into the curricula in schools of nursing, medicine, public health, health education, and social work; through professional seminars and continuing education programs; and by inclusion in professional journals. Professionals who have been out of school for a while may not realize the extent of the alcohol problem in women or its effects in pregnancy.

4. Making knowledge about the effects of alcohol on the fetus an integral part of prenatal and preconcptual care.

5. Making the same knowledge an integral part of alcohol treatment programs for women of reproductive age.

6. Training professionals to identify women at risk.

7. Establishing support groups and agencies for services to pregnant women at risk.

8. Advocating for access to services such as detoxification for women using alcohol.

Secondary prevention can be targeted to early detection of infants and children with alcohol-related effects. Some clinicians believe that any infant whose birth weight is below 3,000 gms should be evaluated for alcohol-related effects. Alertness to the possibility of FAS or other effects should continue past birth. In infancy, childhood, and adolescence, intervention in terms of medical and health services, special education, and counseling and parenting classes for parents can lead to improvements in functioning.

Identifying Pregnancies at Risk

Although there is a relationship between the dose of alcohol consumed, the time of pregnancy, and the severity of defects in the fetus, studies in animals and humans have determined that benefits are accrued if maternal consumption of alcohol ceases, even if this occurs after the first trimester. Thus it is important to identify those individuals who are still using alcohol by the first prenatal visit if not at a contraceptive or general gynecologic visit. In general, women want to have healthy babies, and this provides motivation even in the severe alcoholic. It has also been found that there is a decrease in the desire for alcohol during pregnancy. Both of these factors may help to further support efforts by the concerned nurse geared at eliminating alcohol use in pregnancy. All assessment and teaching should be culturally sensitive, specific, and appropriate. Several tools are available to use for identifying the person who is using alcohol to excess. They include the Michigan Alcohol Screening Test (MAST), the Severity of Alcohol Dependence Questionnaire, the CAGE test, T-ACE test, and the TWEAK test. A properly conducted interview is important. Problems with such an interview may arise because the patient may feel guilty, threatened, or stigmatized and may practice various defense mechanisms such as denial. In turn, the nurse may be uncomfortable in asking questions about alcohol abuse, feel inadequate in handling the patient's responses, or be unsure about facilities available in the community for help. Most patients do not respond truthfully to a question such as, "How much do you drink?" or "You don't drink, do you?" Sokol, Martier, and Ager (1989) suggest that an initial question when taking the family history is a good place to begin. One can ask, "Has anybody in your family ever had a drinking problem?" When investigating the patient's own health habits, one asks, "Do you ever drink any wine, beer, or mixed drinks?" If a positive answer or indication results, then in order to prevent resistance, these researchers suggest focusing on past behavior; for example, asking "When did you first start drinking?" "How often did you drink at that time?" All questions should be asked in a nonjudgmental way. The use of the past tense in these questions may not prove too threatening to the patient and pave the way to ask questions about current behavior, such as, "How much can you hold now?" or "How many drinks does it take to make you high?" In order to elicit the information of how much the patient is drinking now, one may ask, "How much are you drinking now?" and to suggest a range of amounts such as "Two six-packs a day?" to the woman who drinks beer. It is important, in this instance, to suggest a relatively high amount, so that the woman feels that it is all right to tell the nurse how much she really drinks and that it is not out of line with the nurse's expectations. The responses of the majority of women will indicate early in the interview that they do not abuse alcohol, and so all of these questions may not be necessary. For those who appear to abuse alcohol, the exact circumstances, amounts, and patterns can be elicited. Positive responses in this area, as in any other part of an interview, should provoke fuller assessment. Those who appear to be abusing alcohol should be referred specifically to a treatment center in the area (if possible one that specializes in women or pregnant women), recommending a specific contact person or program. The nurse should ease the process by making the contact, because it is necessary that therapy be instituted as early as possible in the pregnancy to minimize damage. If nurses cannot locate treatment resources in their community, help may be sought from Alcoholics Anonymous; the National Institute on Alcohol Abuse and Alcoholism, National Institutes of Health; CDC, National Center on Birth Defects and Developmental Disabilities; and the National Clearinghouse for Alcohol Information. Women who abuse alcohol may fear that their infant will be taken from them and therefore hide their use. Even if a woman does not accept referral and treatment, contact should be maintained and both the practitioner and the patient should keep an open mind. Using the harm reduction model, the suggestion can be made that the woman limit her drinking if she cannot quit. Ascertainment of the problem and the outcome should be documented in the client's record. It is the opinion of some practitioners and legal experts that the alcoholic mother should be offered a therapeutic abortion.

Nursing Points

Other nursing points include the following:

- Awareness of alcohol-related effects and FAS when assessing newborns and infants. In children who have some features of of ARBD or ARND, the nurse should ask him/herself the question, "What is the probability that this problem is secondary to alcohol exposure in utero?"
- A woman with chronic alcohol consumption is likely to be at increased risk in the perinatal period for abruptio placenta, precipitous delivery, tetanic contractions, or infection, and the nurse should anticipate these problems.
- The infant of an alcohol-abusing mother may be at risk for altered glucose metabolism, withdrawal symptoms, or show FAS at birth. Therefore, the nurse should be alert for respiratory problems, seizures, and tremors. The need for resuscitation is not uncommon.
- If FAS or alcohol-related effects are detected in newborns, other defects should be looked for carefully.
- Nurses working with women of reproductive age should familiarize themselves with common signs and symptoms of alcoholism—neglect, family disruption, partners who abuse alcohol, agitation, tremors, and laboratory signs (e.g., macrocytic anemia or liver function abnormalities).
- The growth-retarded infant resulting from FAS or alcohol-related effects can be masked by the appearance of an apparent cause such as placental insufficiency; therefore all small-for-date infants should be closely followed for several years.
- Nurses should be aware that the infant with alcohol-related effects may have poor sucking; therefore failure to thrive may be compounded by the difficulty the mother finds in feeding the infant.
- Support and help should begin in the immediate postpartum period and be reassessed and reinforced on return to the clinic or health practitioner.
- In the postpartum period, mothers with alcohol problems may be unable to form adequate bonding with their infant; therefore the nurse should look for these problems and promote bonding. There may be a prolonged recovery period, and alcohol abuse in the hospital should be watched for. Home follow-up should be arranged before the mother leaves the hospital.
- Education in parenting with demonstrations may be useful at various stages.
- Nurses do not necessarily need to become alcohol experts, but they do need to know where to obtain information and where to refer clients for help.
- Affected children and families should be referred to early intervention programs, counseling, family therapy, and for appropriate language, speech, and learning services.
- Ongoing contact with a family who had alcohol problems during pregnancy is necessary; children who later manifest fretful behavior, hyperactivity, and abnormal sleep may be more prone to child abuse in an already unstable situation.
- School nurses may need to continue follow-up of the children, as some have learning deficits that become manifest in the school years. These children often superficially appear to have a large vocabulary and thus may not be detected early.
- Practitioners should take care not to cause women who drink to relieve tension or

depression to switch to drugs as an alternative, as these may be more harmful than the alcohol.

- Women identified as alcohol abusers should be encouraged to discontinue or decrease their intake before conception.
- The rest of the family should be included when the nurse makes assessments and referrals.

COCAINE AND USE OF OTHER SOCIAL AND STREET SUBSTANCES

The use of cocaine and crack cocaine has become epidemic and it is estimated that 1% of the U.S. population has tried cocaine. Frank et al. (1988) reported that 10% to 45% of women patients at urban teaching hospitals used cocaine during pregnancy. Zuckerman et al. (1989) estimated that of women delivering at a hospital in Boston, 31% used marijuana and 18% used cocaine during the pregnancy, and national data estimate that in women 15 to 44 years of age, 8.9% used marijuana or cocaine. In the 1999 report from the National Household Survey on Drug Abuse, the rate of use for each of the following among pregnant women was: 3.4% for illicit drugs, 17.6% for tobacco, and 13.8% for alcohol (see Lester et al., 2002). Parallels have been noted between increases in maternal drug use and increases in the number of low-birth-weight infants born and in infant mortality. Many women who use cocaine also use other street drugs and/or alcohol, and may also suffer from poor nutrition, stress, infections and other confounding conditions, making effects on the fetus difficult to isolate to one agent. Multiple drug use may also be synergistic. Street-drug use is probably more dangerous to the homeless woman without prenatal care than to the middle-class woman. Volpe (1992) in a review of effects of cocaine indicated that the incidence of congenital malformation in infants whose mothers used cocaine was 10% as compared with 2% in controls. Cocaine use in pregnancy has been reported as resulting in IUGR, low birth weight, increased fetal loss, prematurity, abruptio placentae, urogenital and other congenital malformations, cerebral infarctions, and neurological and behavioral effects such as irritability, poor sleep, poor state regulation, small head circumference at birth, poor visual and auditory tracking, tremors,

and poor feeding. The latter effects appear to be long term, and in a study by Tronick, Frank, Cabral, Mirochnick, and Zuckerman (1996), when controlling for a variety of variables, after 3 weeks, infants heavily exposed to cocaine continued to show excitability and poorer state regulation than others. Mayes, Granger, Bornstein, and Zuckerman (1992) found only minimal neurobehavioral deficits after prenatal cocaine exposure, and Chasnoff, Griffith, Freier, and Murray (1992) did not find differences on the Bayley scales between exposed and control infants. Frank, Augustyn, Knight, et al. (2001) reviewed a variety of studies regarding crack and cocaine exposure in utero and found that many of the effects previously reported may result from multisubstance use. Another review by Vidaeff and Mastrobattista (2003) found that teratogenicity had not been established by large-scale studies except possibly for urogenital malformations. However, cognitive and attentional process deficits, some of which are subtle, have been shown in longer term studies into childhood. Language delays and behavioral problems, even while controlling for other variables, persisted in studies reported by Delaney-Black et al. (2000a, 2000b). Both cocaine and opiate fetal exposure were shown by Lester et al. (2003) to adversely affect neural transmission. However, the image of the "crack" baby is an image said not to be based on fact. When offspring of heroin-dependent parents were compared to controls in one study, they demonstrated more hyperactivity, inattention, and behavior problems (Ornoy, 2003).

Marijuana also has been investigated as a teratogen. Recent studies are somewhat inconclusive; however, fetal oxygenation and growth are affected in the same way that cigarette smoking affects oxygenation. Growth retardation appears to be a sequela. There have been reports of some cognitive and verbal abnormalities among children prenatally exposed to heavy marijuana use, and older children may exhibit hyperactivity and learning problems. Attentional behavior and executive function have been reported to be affected. For all studies of illicit drug use in pregnancy, there is confounding by multiple drug use, infection such as syphilis, use of alcohol and cigarettes, and environmental influences such as violence exposure, abuse, and poor nutrition that can influence study short-term and long-term results. The nurse should try to identify the woman using drugs, and assist in enrolling her in a treatment plan (see Alcohol section earlier in this chapter). Women using drugs such as cocaine are likely to have late or no prenatal care.

CIGARETTE SMOKING

Between 16% and 30% of pregnant women continue to smoke. Maternal cigarette smoking in pregnancy is related to detrimental effects. These include an increased spontaneous abortion rate, an increased perinatal mortality rate, an increased incidence of maternal complications such as placenta abruptio and placenta previa, decreased birth weight and size in later childhood, an increased incidence of preterm delivery, and lower Apgar scores at 1 min and 5 min after birth. The latter is a source of particular concern because low Apgar scores have been associated in other studies with developmental and neurologic disabilities in later life. The finding of lower mental functioning and lower scholastic ability among the offspring of mothers who smoked in pregnancy may be related to oxygen deprivation and exposure to the products of cigarette smoke. Reduced birth weight, length, and head circumference have been associated with maternal smoking of 10 or more cigarettes a day, and Karatza, Varvarigou, and Beratis (2003) found that at age 2 years, weight tended to return to normal but the children of smokers tended to have length retardation below the fifth percentile. Head circumference remained reduced, particularly in those whose mothers smoked 20 or more cigarettes per day.

Talipes equinovarus or idiopathic clubfoot appears to be associated with maternal cigarette smoking and a dose-response relationship appears likely. Maternal smoking during pregnancy appears to increase the risk for orofacial clefts. This association was strong enough that the Bulletin of the World Health Association stated that it could be used in antismoking campaigns (Little, Cardy, & Munger, 2004). One factor in this association appears to be polymorphic variation in genes encoding fetal acetyl-N-trasferase 1 (NAT1), an enzyme involved in the biotransformation of certain tobacco compounds that leads to genetic susceptibility to the effects of tobacco smoke

(Lammer et al., 2004). It can be difficult to sort out the effects of smoking from confounding variables such as caffeine, alcohol, and drug use. Cigarette smoking is associated with high fetal lead in the blood. Nurses should regard as an important part of any prenatal program education about the effects of smoking in pregnancy, and an active prenatal smoking cessation program. Cessation may be easier for women at this time because early nausea and vomiting may make smoking distasteful. This may be a protective mechanism. Nurses should also consider smoking cessation important for themselves before considering or during pregnancy (or any other time). Bishop, Witt, and Sloane (1997) list cigarette smoke as a possible teratogen.

IONIZING RADIATION

A frequent reason for seeking genetic counseling is because of radiation exposure during pregnancy. The question of the consequences of the effects of low-dose radiation to the fetus is presently still somewhat unsettled. There is probably no threshold level that can be considered absolutely safe for radiation exposure. Factors, in addition to those considered for all agents during pregnancy, are the type of radiation emitted, its affinity for certain tissues, and the actual dose absorbed by the fetus. The most sensitive stage for spontaneous abortion due to radiation is just before or after the time of the first menstrual period after becoming pregnant, when neither pregnancy nor the loss may be realized. However, radiation may be detrimental to the fetus in any stage of pregnancy and include outcomes such as fetal death, malformation, tissue effects, or cancer, especially leukemia. In the past, pelvimetry was used in pregnancy to detect fetopelvic disproportion but it is no longer useful in making decisions to perform cesarean sections.

The major hazard associated with in utero radiation exposure is an increased risk of childhood cancer for the fetus, especially, but not limited to the third trimester. Estimates vary, but the chance for leukemia to develop after in utero exposure of 1-2 centiGray (cGy) (1 cGy = 1 rad) is increased by a factor of 1.5 to 3 over the natural incidence. Doll and Wakeford (1997) estimated the excess risk for childhood cancer after irradiation of 10 mGy or more is approximately 6% per Gy. Larger doses of radiation (i.e., 50 cGy) have been known to result in microcephaly, mental retardation, microphthalmia, genital and skeletal malformations, retinal changes, and cataracts. A major concern is that low-level radiation exposure may kill developing brain cells that are not replaced. Chromosome breakage, gaps, and rearrangements such as duplications or partial trisomies in peripheral leukocytes have been noted in workers chronically exposed to low-dose radiation, and aneuploidy leading to Down and Turner syndromes has been associated with radiation exposure. It is also known that some genotypes are more susceptible to damage by ionizing radiation than others. The use of therapeutic radioisotopes is known to cause fetal thyroid destruction.

Experts vary on what action to take when a pregnant woman is inadvertently exposed to X-rays in the first trimester. Increases in childhood cancer aside, some believe that if the dose is less than 1 cGy, the mother can be told that there are no documented reports of any deleterious effects. For doses of below 5 to 10 cGy, many support telling the mother that it is unknown what the ill effects may be, but that the exposure is not believed to be teratogenic, while others believe total reassurance is appropriate. A chest X-ray is about .008 cGy and a barium enema about 1 cGy exposure. Paternal exposure to radiation before conception has been described to result in an increased incidence of leukemia and non-Hodgkins lymphoma in their offspring. It is obviously preferable to prevent inadvertent or unnecessary radiation exposure of the pregnant woman, and sometimes ultrasound can be an alternative to diagnostic X-rays. Some measures that nurses should be aware of to do this are as follows:

- In women of reproductive age, limit radiation exposure to that which is clearly indicated, necessary, and for which information or treatment cannot be obtained any other way.
- Women of reproductive age who receive radiation to the lower abdomen or pelvis should be advised to use contraception and delay conception for several months after exposure.
- All clients should be encouraged to ask exactly why an X-ray film is being ordered and how necessary it is.

- Clients should keep records of the X-ray films that they have had, so unnecessary duplication does not occur.
- Women should be encouraged to let a health professional know if there is a possibility of pregnancy before receiving radiation.
- Health professionals should always ask female patients in a nonjudgmental way if there is a possibility of pregnancy before the woman receives any radiation. It is particularly important to be nonjudgmental and appropriate in manner when asking this of an adolescent.
- Be aware that pregnancy can mimic some gastrointestinal and genitourinary disorders.
- Pregnant nurses and other female employees should not work with patients receiving radioisotopes.
- The minimum number of radiographs in the smallest field, with the lowest duration and intensity of exposure should always be used.
- Before X-ray or radioisotope therapy is given to a female patient, determine the date of the last menstrual period, determine if pregnancy is possible, and if it is, communicate this information to the physician ordering the therapy and ask that necessity and risk be discussed with the woman with the possibility of delay being considered.
- A pregnancy test may be done if there is considerable doubt.
- The gonads should always be effectively shielded; clients should be encouraged to request this as shielding is still not always used.
- If possible, delay the procedure until onset of next menstruation or within the 10 days following the 1st day of the last menstrual period, unless data are important because of immediate illness of the woman.

INFECTIOUS AGENTS AND INTRAUTERINE INFECTIONS

The first recognized association between an infectious disease in the mother and congenital abnormalities in the newborn was made for syphilis in 1850. A definitive cause-and-effect relationship between a virus and specific congenital malformations was first established by Gregg after a rubella epidemic in Australia in 1941 led to a significant excess of congenital cataracts and heart disease in infants whose mothers had contracted rubella in the first trimester. Fetal consequences of maternal infection may include (a) embryonic/fetal death— if in the first few weeks, the embryo may resorb; otherwise, spontaneous abortion or stillbirth will occur; (b) premature or term delivery of a normal infant or one with IUGR/low birth weight, congenital infection, congenital anomalies, and/or persistent postnatal infection. Congenitally infected infants may show clinical or subclinical infection with or without immediate or long-term consequences. Fetal death may be caused by direct fetal invasion by the microorganism or by severe maternal damage (e.g., fever, toxins). Some problems that nurses should be aware of in identifying the stage of fetal development or relating abnormalities to maternal infection include doubt as to the date of the last menstrual period; infection may have been subclinical or very mild; lack of maternal awareness of the importance of the infectious disease and failure to note the dates her illness encompassed; and lack of objective evidence of infection (e.g., laboratory tests because of expense, limited availability, nonrecognition of illness, or difficult techniques). The degree of damage to the fetus is not related to the severity of the maternal infection.

Many infections with severe fetal consequences can occur in mothers with few or no signs of illness. The most important intrauterine infections in the United States traditionally were syphilis, toxoplasmosis, rubella, cytomegalovirus, and herpes simplex, known by the acronym "STORCH." Since others such as human immunodeficiency virus (HIV) infection have become important, the acronym is not used as widely. Infection with some organisms is so rare in pregnancy that its effects are almost impossible to distinguish from chance events. Some cases of cerebral palsy are linked to infectious diseases such as herpes simplex virus and cytomegalovirus. Table 13.4 lists some agents and their fetal effects after maternal infection.

Most congenital anomalies due to microorganisms are caused by viruses. This may be because other microorganisms can release toxins and cause fetal death rather than a milder tissue effect leading to malformation. The American College of Obstetricians and Gynecologists (1993) estimated the

incidence of viral and parasitic infectious complications in pregnancy at 5–15% of all pregnancies, with consequent congenital structural damage occurring in 1–2% of all exposed fetuses. Sorting out sequelae from viruses causing "the flu" and the common cold are hard to distinguish since different viruses may cause these diseases, and fever may occur concomitantly. One of the chief roles for nursing lies in prevention of infection in pregnancy. Pregnant women are at risk by virtue of living in the community and by increased exposure to young children, who often have infectious diseases. The most important diseases resulting in congenital anomalies in the fetus are individually discussed next.

Rubella

An epidemic of rubella resulted in the birth of more than 20,000 infants with congenital rubella syndrome in the United States in 1964. The development of a vaccine in 1966, concerted vaccination efforts, recognition of the effects of maternal infection, and increased social acceptance of therapeutic abortion resulted in a marked decrease in cases of congenital rubella syndrome. Cases of rubella result when there are low levels of vaccinated persons in the community, and outbreaks may occur among religious communities refusing vaccination. There are an estimated 10% to 15% of women of childbearing age who lack rubella antibody and are therefore at risk for developing rubella during pregnancy, and more young males remain susceptible, posing a potential source of infection. However, in 2000–2001, only 11 infants with congenital rubella were born in the United States, emphasizing the effectiveness of vaccination. Cases are higher in Hispanic communities than in others, and this may indicate a target group for prevention. Since 50% of individuals with rubella may not develop a rash, and because the disease can be mild in adults, about one-third of pregnant women who contract rubella either do not recognize or do not report their illness.

The risk of fetal infection is about 90% in the first two months of pregnancy and about 50% in the third, declining thereafter. The risk of fetal eye and cardiac malformations is greatest when infection occurs in the first 8 weeks of pregnancy, whereas the risk of deafness is greatest between 5

TABLE 13.4   Harmful Effects of Selected Infectious Agents During Pregnancy

Agent/disease	Effects		
	Increased reproductive loss	Congenital malformations	Prematurity or growth retardation
Viral			
Coxsackie B	+	?	0
Cytomegalovirus	+	+	+
Chicken pox (Varicella-zoster)	0	+	+
Herpes simplex 1 and 2	+	+	+
Mumps	+	?	0
Parvovirus B19	+	?	+
Polio	+	0	+
Rubella	+	+	+
Rubeola (measles)	+	?	+
Venezuelan equine encephalitis	+	+	0
Bacterial			
Syphilis *(Treponema pallidum)*	+	+	?
Tuberculosis	+	0?	+
Listeriosis *(Listeria monocytogenes)*	+	0	+?
Group B streptococcus infection	+	0	?
Chlamydia trachomatis	+	0	+
Neisseria gonorrhoeae	0	0	+
Q fever	+	0	0
Parasitic			
Malaria *(Plasmodium spp)*	+	0	+
Toxoplasmosis *(T. gondii)*	+	+	+
Chagas' disease *(Trypanosoma cruzi)*	+	0	?
Fungal			
Valley fever *(Coccidioides immitis)*	+	0	+

+ = established, 0 = no present evidence, ? = possible, not established.

and 15 weeks of pregnancy. Data are insufficient for the consequences of infection acquired after the 4th to 5th month, but delayed development and hearing deficits have been described when infection occurred as late as the 31st week of pregnancy. Congenital rubella has been described in fetuses whose mothers had the disease weeks before conception. The persistence of the virus in maternal tissues probably accounts for this finding.

The frequency of specific clinical features of the rubella syndrome vary. Approximately one third of defects are missed in the neonatal period and become noticeable later in childhood. The classic features described in early literature, such as cardiac malformations (especially patent ductus arteriosus and pulmonary stenosis), eye abnormalities (especially cataracts, retinopathy, microphthalmia, and glaucoma), and permanent hearing loss (bilateral and unilateral) are still seen. To them, the following features of the expanded syndrome can now be added: growth retardation, one manifestation of which is low birth weight for gestation; microcephaly; bone lesions and radiologic changes in long bones often described as "celery stalk"; thrombocytopenia, petechiae, and purpura, which give the newborn a "blueberry muffin" appearance; jaundice; hepatosplenomegaly; pneumonitis; and encephalitis. Among the abnormalities often not detected in infancy are genitourinary anomalies, adrenal insufficiency, behavioral manifestations of minimal brain dysfunction, mental retardation, autism, various thyroid disorders including hypothyroidism, and growth hormone deficiency. Hearing loss caused by Organ of Corti damage may not be evident until later childhood after secondary learning and speech disabilities have accrued. These findings plus progressive panencephalitis seen in the second decade, and diabetes mellitus, which develops in 10% to 20% of affected infants, may be caused by the persistence of virus in tissues. Between one third and two thirds of affected infants lose their antibody to rubella and are therefore again susceptible to the virus. The comparatively recent recognition of the delayed long-term sequelae makes it difficult to estimate the percentage of newborns who actually have disease effects. Approximately 30% of infants with congenital rubella syndrome die in the first 4 months. Because the risk of fetal damage is substantial, therapeutic termination of pregnancy should be discussed with any pregnant woman known to have contracted rubella during pregnancy, one with known exposure, or one to whom rubella vaccine was inadvertently administered during pregnancy.

Nursing Points

- Because there is no treatment for congenital rubella, all efforts must be directed at prevention. Women who are considering pregnancy should have serologic evaluation to determine whether or not rubella antibody is present.
- Susceptible women of childbearing age should only be vaccinated in the documented absence of pregnancy; instructions should include the necessity to use contraception and avoid pregnancy for at least 3 menstrual cycles after vaccination.
- Such vaccination should be followed by serologic determination that appropriate antibody response has occurred.
- Vaccination as a routine part of childhood immunization programs should be supported and encouraged.
- Identified pregnant women who are susceptible to rubella should be vaccinated immediately postpartum and post-abortion.
- Rubella titers and vaccination if indicated should be done for all female staff on obstetrics and newborn units or clinics, in day care centers, schools, prisons, and facilities for the mentally retarded.
- Seek confirmation of suspected exposure to rubella (e.g., examination of contact).
- Because infected infants shed virus through the nasopharynx and urine, they should be kept away from women in their childbearing years, isolated in the hospital, and be kept apart from susceptible women in clinics and offices.

Cytomegalovirus

Cytomegalovirus (CMV) belongs to the same family as the herpes virus. Approximately 0.2% to 2.9% with an average of 1% of liveborn infants have congenital CMV, but this varies considerably in different populations. It is said to be the current most frequent cause of intrauterine infection in the United States, estimated to occur in about 44,000 U.S. infants per year. Intrauterine infection usually occurs because of primary maternal infection, but it can also result from reactivation of latent infection. Primary CMV infection in pregnancy occurs in about 1% to 2% of pregnant women. The rate of transmission to the fetus after primary maternal infection in pregnancy can vary but is about 40% to 50%; however, these rates are far lower for those with recurrent infection. Those at highest risk for primary CMV in pregnancy are young primiparas of the lower socioeconomic groups.

Classic cytomegalic inclusion disease is seen in only about 10% of infected newborns, and can include the following: microcephaly, hepatosplenomegaly, jaundice, petechial rash, cerebral calcifications, motor disabilities, chorioretinitis, microphthalmia, hydrocephalus, and hernia. A small percent have milder disease. Primary teeth may show characteristic enamel defects such as discoloration, opacity, and rapid wearing. However, the majority of infants are asymptomatic at birth, and many later show long-term sequelae such as sensorineural hearing loss, minimal brain dysfunction, mental retardation, dental defects, motor defects, or poor school performance. Chorioretinitis may not be detected at birth but seen later. Necrotizing enterocolitis and fetal death have also been associated with recurrent CMV infection. The magnitude of long-term insidious effects, such as mild intellectual impairment, has only begun to be appreciated. Early detection helps children to achieve their maximum potential through early remedial efforts.

Nursing Points

- Because even the asymptomatic group of infected newborns sheds virus through urine and saliva for up to 3 years after birth, thus disseminating infection, they should be kept from direct contact with pregnant women, including the staff, when in the hospital, home, office, or clinic.

- Infants with suspected or proven disease should be closely followed up for detection of delayed effects (including perceptual and intellectual deficits, dental defects), and for appropriate medical, educational, and family support.
- Serologic testing should be done on the first prenatal visit in order to detect seroconverters, especially in high-risk groups.
- CMV should be suspected in women with mononucleosis-type symptoms, and diagnosis should be pursued.
- Documented maternal infection, especially in the first trimester, is a reason to discuss pregnancy termination with the client. Tests such as ultrasound to assess the fetus or amniocentesis to confirm infection and viral load may be useful.
- Antibody determinations should be done in female employees. Those without antibodies who are planning pregnancy should not be assigned to obstetric or newborn units or seek employment in day care centers, schools, or facilities for the mentally retarded.
- If a blood transfusion is needed for a pregnant woman, use citrated blood that is more than 3 days old, if possible, because CMV can be transmitted in fresh whole blood.
- Emphasis should be placed on good hand washing for women throughout pregnancy, and especially after contact with potential infective sources.
- Care in handling blood and urine specimens is essential.
- Enforcement of good hand-washing techniques in hospitals, day care centers, and clinics is essential. Hospital personnel appear at increased risk for CMV, and full infection control measures may be warranted with known infected cases.

Herpes Simplex Virus

Both herpes simplex virus-1 (HSV-1) and HSV-2 can cause perinatal infection. HSV-1 asymptomatically infects most individuals before 5 years of age in the oral area, becomes latent and may reactivate at any time, but particularly under stress, fever, or malnutrition, to form a "cold sore." It can also produce genital infection in infants. HSV-2 is important as a sexually transmitted disease, it primarily affects genital areas, and is found in about one in five persons over 12 years of age in the United States. The most important effects are in the neonate due to infection when passing through the birth canal, and some authors recommend cesarean section. ACOG recommends antiviral therapy during pregnancy. The rates of spontaneous abortion and premature births are higher in women with genital herpes infection than comparable uninfected women. HSV has been recovered from abortuses. Primary HSV infection is associated with a 50% risk of neonatal infection, while in recurrent HSV, intrapartum transmission is about 5% to 8%. The association of congenital malformations with HSV infection in the first trimester includes microcephaly, cerebral atrophy, intracranial calcification, and chorioretinitis. Herpes simplex virus infections, especially type 2, can also be vertically transmitted to the fetus causing neonatal herpes simplex virus sepsis syndrome and encephalitis. Since HSV reaches the central nervous system of the fetus, like rubella and CMV, it may be that long-term effects have not yet been identified. Nurses should be sure that infants born to infected mothers are isolated, and that isolation technique is used when handling such infants. Nurses can identify some women at greatest risk by ascertaining a history of a sexual partner with genital herpes, or by a past history of another sexually transmitted disease. Virus can be shed from external genitalia and the cervix, so good hand washing is important.

Syphilis

Syphilis is caused by the spirochete *Treponema pallidum*. It is still a significant sexually transmitted disease in this country, with about 6,000 new cases of primary and secondary syphilis and 441 cases of congenital syphilis reported in 2001. A new surveillance case definition was implemented by the CDC in 1996, and infants with reactive tests or whose mother had untreated or inadequately treated syphilis are classified as not infected, confirmed case, or probable case. The major route of infection is through sexual contact, but it can also be transmitted through contaminated injection equipment, especially among drug users, or through direct nonsexual contact with infectious lesions. It is now known that the infected pregnant woman can transmit syphilis to the fetus at any stage of her pregnancy and in any stage of the disease. Transmission occurs in 70% to 100% of cases, and if the fetus is not treated, 25% die in utero.

Congenital syphilis can be manifested as "early" (before 2 years of age) or "late" (after 2 years of age), but overlap occurs. In early syphilis the most common symptoms are rhinitis or "snuffles," hepatosplenomegaly, generalized lymph node enlargement, jaundice, rash, and bone involvement including osteomyelitis. Often attention is first sought for affected infants because of rhinitis, persistent diaper rash, or failure to thrive. If not diagnosed or not treated completely, the manifestations of late congenital syphilis may be seen, including teeth changes (Hutchinson's teeth, Moon's or mulberry molars), eye lesions (keratitis, photophobia, uveitis, corneal scarring), deafness, bone changes (saddle nose, hard palate perforations, saber shins, impaired maxillary growth), neurologic involvement (paresis, convulsive disorders), and mental retardation.

Nurses should be aware that all pregnant women should be tested for syphilis at their first prenatal visit because of the success in minimizing fetal damage when treated with penicillin. Antepartum syphilis screening is required in 46 states and the district of Columbia, and 34 states mandate one early prenatal test, whereas the other 12 states included additional testing in the third trimester (Hollier, Hill, Sheffield, & Wendel, 2003). Usually a nonspecific test such as the Venereal Disease Research Laboratory (VDRL) or rapid plasma reagin (RPR) can be used at the point of patient contact, but the test can give false-positive results in hepatitis, mononucleosis, malignancies, tuberculosis, autoimmune disease, narcotics abuse, and pregnancy. Thus if a pregnant woman has a positive result, the underlying cause should be determined so that treatment can be instituted if necessary, and a more sensitive, specific test for syphilis should be done. These include tests that detect antibodies to components of T. pallidum such as the T. pallidum hemagglutination (TPHA) test, the fluorescent treponemal antibody-absorption test (FTA-abs), and the enzyme-linked immunosorbent assay (ELISA). Those women at the greatest risk for

developing syphilis should be retested later in pregnancy. Some factors identified as associated with increased risk are: women who are unmarried, very young mothers, drug use in the woman or her partner, sexual promiscuity, contact with known syphilitics or those with STDs, history of past STDs including HIV, tattooed women, members of disadvantaged urban minority groups, or those who have unexplained lesions or rashes. Syphilis is disproportionately prevalent in the southeastern United States. A high index of suspicion is needed to consider syphilis in pregnant woman. Factors associated with risk at the time of delivery are premature delivery with no explanation, unexplained large placenta, hydrops fetalis, unexplained stillbirth, or no prenatal care. Further investigation and a blood test should be carried out in order to minimize severe fetal effects. The CDC recommends blood tests for pregnant women at both 20 and 28 weeks.

Toxoplasmosis

Toxoplasmosis is caused by the protozoan *Toxoplasma gondii.* Adults may acquire the organism from the ingestion of raw or undercooked meat, or by contamination of soil, litter, and food by the feces of infected cats. Acquired infection is usually found in children or young adults, and can be detected by serum antibody screening. Overall 20% to 30% of women of reproductive age in the United States have such serum antibodies, but this varies with geographic location, socioeconomic level, and cultural practices. The following rates of transmission to the fetus are estimated: if the mother acquires toxoplasmosis in the first trimester, 15%; second trimester, 25%; and third trimester, 50% to 65%, with an overall risk of about 40%. Accurate transmission rates are difficult to determine because 70% of newborns later found to have congenital toxoplasmosis are asymptomatic at birth. The risk for severe manifestations is highest in the first trimester.

Congenital toxoplasmosis is almost always caused by acute primary infection in pregnancy (estimated at 0.2–1.0%), which can be asymptomatic or consist of any of the following: mild fever, enlarged lymph glands, headache, or muscles aches—all of which may be easily dismissed or unappreciated. Thus only those who became infected during pregnancy would be at risk for fetal complications or stillbirths. Antenatal testing would usually have to be done twice to determine this, once to detect negative individuals and a second time to see if seroconversion occurred. Drugs used in treatment are considered toxic with possible teratogenic effects, therefore, therapeutic abortion is an option that should be discussed with patients who clearly have had seroconversion.

Congenital toxoplasmosis shows varying manifestations that may include chorioretinitis, cerebral calcification, hydrocephalus, microcephaly, convulsions, anemia, seizures, hepatosplenomegaly, anemia, rash, and mental retardation. Late manifesting sequelae include intellectual impairment, developmental delay, hearing loss, nystagmus, strabismus, and late-developing chorioretinitis resulting in blindness. Screening has been proposed for women before or during pregnancy, and also for newborns, but current tests do not meet criteria for universal screening (see chapter 11). Prenatal diagnosis of fetal toxoplasmosis can be accomplished by organism detection in fetal blood samples or in amniotic fluid. Detailed, specialized ultrasound examination can detect abnormal morphologic signs such as bilateral, symmetrical ventricular dilatation. Treatment has been attempted during pregnancy, and there is indication that it may be of benefit to the fetus without harm. The current recommendation is for spiramycin therapy as soon as possible. After fetal infection is confirmed then a combination of pyrimethamine, sulfadiazine, and folinic acid can be given alternately with spiramycin. Eventually, it is hoped that treatment could be accomplished by intraamniotic drug infusion.

Other points that nurses should include in health teaching are to advise pregnant women to do the following:

- Eat only well-cooked meat (heated to 66°C) or freeze all meat if they have to cook it less than well done.
- Avoid close contact with cats.
- If the woman already has a cat in her home, someone else should change the cat's litter daily and dispose of feces in a sanitary manner. It should be fed only cooked, dry, or canned food; it should be kept away from wild rodents.
- Practice good hand washing before eating or

handling food and after gardening, handling uncooked meat, or touching pets.
- Do not eat raw eggs.
- Wash all raw fruits and vegetables carefully.
- Control flies, roaches, and so on, and limit their access to food.
- Use special precautions if their work involves animals in a lab or as a veterinarian.
- Cover children's sandboxes.

Maternal Genital and Urinary Tract Infections

The impact of some of these infections has only relatively recently been appreciated. In 1982, Martin and coworkers did a prospective study of women infected with *Chlamydia trachomatis* in pregnancy and found a 10-fold increased risk of perinatal death and a significantly higher prematurity rate when matched with uninfected controls. Untreated gonorrhea in pregnancy may be associated with premature birth, low birth weight, premature rupture of the membranes, and postnatal infection. Genital mycoplasmas such as *Ureaplasma urealyticum* have been implicated in habitual abortion, prematurity, and low birth weight as well as fetal pneumonia. The evidence is less compelling for *Mycoplasma hominis*. Bacterial vaginosis may result in preterm labor and premature rupture of the membranes. Prevention may be accomplished before infection by recommending that women have their sexual partners use condoms, especially in groups determined to be at highest risk. Urinary tract infections have been shown to be associated with stillbirths, low birth weight, and with both poor motor ability and lower intelligence quotient values in early childhood. The nature of the association is unknown.

Other Infections

A few other infections should be mentioned. Maternal varicella zoster (chicken pox) infections are relatively rare. Outcomes from first trimester infections include prematurity and low birth weight, and in the literature, congenital varicella syndrome has been identified in 0% to 9% of infected fetuses depending on the study. This consists of abnormal limbs (hypoplasia, abnormal digits, and equinovarus), skin scarring, eye abnormalities (chorioretinitis, Horner's syndrome, microphthalmia, cataract), and brain abnormalities including mental retardation. Counseling is important, and Pastuszak et al. (1994) believe that the absolute risk is about 2% while Henderson and Weiner (1995) estimate a risk of 0.5–2.0% for embryopathy after infection in the first 20 weeks of pregnancy; however, Harger et al. (2002) in a prospective study found a frequency of only 0.4%. Herpes zoster may occur in the first year of life but this may be modified by the administration of zoster immune globulin. The availability of live attenuated varicella vaccine should mean that congenital varicella syndrome will become even rarer, but vaccination is not recommended during pregnancy and immediate pregnancy should be avoided after vaccination. The human parvovirus B12 is the cause of erythema infectiosum (fifth disease). In the fetus it may cause excessive fetal loss or nonimmune fetal hydrops, for which the risk is about 15% if maternal infection occurs in the first 20 weeks of pregnancy.While group B streptococcal disease has not been associated with fetal malformation in mothers infected during pregnancy, it has been associated with increased stillbirths, premature delivery, and postnatal infection and thus affects fetal outcome. HIV infection is transmitted to the fetus during pregnancy if the mother is infected, and HIV has been detected in abortuses as early as 8 weeks. The early reports of cases of HIV-associated embryopathy have not been confirmed. Transmission is influenced by various factors including the maternal viral load, resistance, response to infection, and the CD4 count. Various medication regimes involving highly active antiretroviral therapies are now used during pregnancy and the intrapartum period, with treatment of the infant after birth. For a review of regimens and potential adverse effects of medication see Minkoff (2003). Maternal-fetal HIV transmission has been reduced to about 1% to 2% in developed countries. Cesarean sections have also been proposed to reduce transmission.

Maternal influenza infection has been linked to stillbirth, miscarriage and premature birth, and certain investigators link maternal viral infections to autism but this is unproven. Viral hepatitis infections are not known to cause congenital malformations, and vertical transmission may occur in relation to other factors such as maternal viral load and stage of infection. The hepatitis A, B, C, and E viruses may be transmitted to the fetus, possibly resulting in fetal infection but is not a common occurrence. Maternal hepatitis B infection can result in low birth weight infants and premature birth. Hepatitis C vertical infection rates ranges from 5% to up to 15%. Hepatitis E can also be associated with preterm labor and higher rates of perinatal mortality. The recent concern about bioterrorism and the deliberate release of anthrax in the U.S. has led to concern about smallpox vaccination and anthrax in pregnancy. Although there is little information regarding anthrax in pregnancy, especially early in pregnancy, management guidelines for exposed persons have been issued by ACOG. Preterm delivery appears to be one outcome. Smallpox vaccine administered during pregnancy can result in fetal vaccinia, fetal or neonatal death, and premature birth and low birth weight—thus the vaccine should not be administered to pregnant women, persons in close contact with pregnant women, or those who might become pregnant within 4 weeks after vaccination. Smallpox itself is particularly lethal in pregnancy. Other recommendations regarding immunization in pregnancy are suggested by the CDC national immunization program (http://www.cdc.gov/nip). As new or newly recognized infectious diseases emerge, there is a need to address the effects of the causative microbial agent on pregnancy outcomes. For example, little information is available on monkeypox, a zoonotic disease caused by an orthopoxvirus. In one case, a woman infected at 24 weeks gestation delivered an infant with a monkeypox-like rash who subsequently died at 6 weeks of age. In regard to those pregnant women infected by severe acute respiratory syndrome (SARS) associated coronavirus, their own clinical course appeared more severe. There infants did not show congenital malformations but two of the five in one study had growth retardation, and two of five had severe gastrointestinal complications including necrotizing enterocolitis. These mothers had received therapy with antiviral agents including ribavirin, a potential teratogenic agent (Shek et al., 2003). In regard to West Nile virus infection caused by a flavivirus, CDC has issued interim guidelines and is collecting data on the effects of maternal infection in pregnancy. It is noted that in one case a pregnant woman with encephalitis due to West Nile virus had an infant with congenital infection, chorioretinitis and cerebral tissue destruction (Centers for Disease Control and Prevention, 2004). *Coccidioides immitis*, the fungus responsible for coccidioidomycosis (San Joaquin fever, Valley fever) is associated with infection in endemic areas such as the Southwest, Mexico, and many Latin American countries. In endemic areas, primary infections occur in 0.1% to 0.5% of pregnant women. *C. immitis* is associated with a 50% mortality for the fetus due to premature delivery and deaths of pregnant women rather than direct fetal effects. Nonimmune pregnant individuals should minimize spore inhalation by avoiding dust in endemic areas even if only traveling through them. *Listeria monocytogenes* in pregnancy is a foodborne illness which can cause fetal death or congenital infection and growth retardation.

MATERNAL ENVIRONMENT

The maternal environment and metabolism affect the developing fetus in many ways. Effects derive from interaction of maternal and fetal genotypes, as well as their interaction with internal and external environmental effects. The influence of maternal nutrition and risks of pregnancy and childbirth to adult women with genetic disorders such as Marfan syndrome are beyond the scope of this book. Major genetically-determined alterations, such as diabetes mellitus and maternal PKU, are discussed below.

Diabetes Mellitus

Pregnant women may have diabetes before pregnancy (pregestational diabetes mellitus) or have gestational diabetes mellitus (GDM). GDM is defined as glucose intolerance with onset or first recognition during pregnancy. After delivery, in most cases of GDM, glucose regulation will become normal. GDM is believed to affect from 1% to 14% of all pregnancies, depending on the population (Engelgau, 1995), and in examining data from the U.S. Nurses' Health Study, 4.9% reported GDM in pregnancy (Solomon et al., 1997). Evidence of adverse effects among women who have milder hyperglycemia in pregnancy is less clear than that among women who have been diagnosed with diabetes mellitus before pregnancy,

and groups are split on the advisability for screening for GDM. Potential risks may be macrosomia, stillbirth, metabolic and respiratory complications in the infant, and hypertension and need for cesarean section in the mother, but GDM is generally considered non-teratogenic, perhaps because it usually appears after organogenesis. The U.S. Preventive Services Task Force (2003) in not recommending for or against routine screening for GDM stated that evidence was insufficient that screening for GDM substantially reduced important adverse health outcomes for mothers or infants and stated that evidence is not available to determine if the benefits outweigh the harm. The American Diabetes Association (2004) recommends screening all women who are not at low risk for GDM. The American Diabetes Association (2004) approaches the risk recommendation a little differently, and states that certain factors place women at low risk for GDM, and that pregnant women who fulfill all of these criteria do not need to be screened for GDM. These low-risk factors includes women who are below 25 years of age, are of normal body weight, have no first-degree relative with diabetes, have no history of abnormal glucose metabolism, have no history of poor obstetric outcome, and are not members of an ethnic/racial group with a high prevalence of diabetes mellitus such as Hispanic American, Native American, Asian American, African American or Pacific Islander (p. S9–S10). These criteria result in about 90% of pregnant women being screened for GDM. ACOG (2001) recommends screening for GDM in all pregnant women in some manner while noting the American Diabetes Association criteria.

The picture is different for women with diabetes mellitus who become pregnant. The incidence of major congenital anomalies in the offspring of diabetic women is three to four times that of controls. Maternal metabolic influences appear to be the primary determining factor. Direct genetic effects are unlikely, because anomalies and defects are not elevated in the offspring of diabetic men whose wives were not diabetic, but these effects may play a future role. Although all major anomalies are increased, those of the cardiovascular system (especially a hypertrophic type of cardiomyopathy), kidneys, and skeletal system are most prominent with caudal dysplasia or sacral agenesis present in 1%. Infants frequently have macrosomia—they are large for their gestational age but are physiologically immature, have increased total body fat, and enlarged viscera. Nurses should anticipate that the infant of a diabetic mother frequently exhibits lethargy, hypotonia, polycythemia (hematocrits >65%) leading to other complications, a poor sucking reflex, and metabolic imbalances such as hypocalcemia (present in up to 50%), hypomagnesemia (present in up to 38%), hyperbilirubinemia, and hypoglycemia, and they should plan accordingly. Careful observation is necessary because the neuromuscular system is often very excitable. Respiratory distress syndrome, formally known as hyaline membrane disease, is five to six times that found in normal newborns. Long-term effects include obesity (by 8 years of age, 50% of the weight of offspring were over the 90th percentile), cognitive impairment, and developmental delays. All these effects are more frequent with suboptimal control. Perinatal and maternal mortality is higher in diabetic women. Increase in glycosolated hemoglobin is seen in poorly controlled diabetics and correlates with increased hyperglycemia. There is some evidence that defective insulin secretory response may be seen in adults exposed to an in utero diabetic environment that is independent of genetic factors. Diabetic women wanting children should probably be helped to plan them at a younger age before diabetic-related pathology worsens. Prenatal diagnosis that includes ultrasound, amniocentesis, and AFP level determination should be used to monitor the pregnant woman. Before conception an addition of folic acid in recommended doses to help to prevent neural tube defects is recommended. The time of delivery may be geared to the determination of fetal lung maturity.

Nursing Implications

It is currently believed that poor diabetic control (hyperglycemia) and ketoacidosis are responsible for the above findings. In order to minimize these effects, it is necessary to rigorously control metabolic balance and blood sugar from preconception through delivery, carefully monitor other potential risks such as hypertension, follow thyroid function closely, and use folic acid supplements daily. Success is best if an expert in the management of diabetic pregnancy is consulted. Because this control may be more stringent than that needed for everyday management of the nonpregnant diabetic, the mother's full cooperation and understanding is vital. Too strict control can result in hypoglycemia. Basic education as to the benefits of such control beginning prior to planned conception should be integrated in teaching programs for diabetics of reproductive age, since it is estimated that about two-thirds of women with diabetes mellitus have unplanned pregnancies. Recommendations are detailed in American Diabetes Association (2004). Nurses should also be aware of some risk factors associated with potential gestational diabetes, such as family history of diabetes, marked obesity, glycosuria, glucose intolerance, membership in an ethnic group at increased risk for diabetes mellitus as discussed previously, or a personal history of GDM. The nurse should ensure that those pregnant women who should be screened for GDM receive such services. It is estimated that 20% to 30% of women who develop gestational diabetes become overt diabetics within 5 years, so such women should be followed with this in mind. It may be useful to start a group of pregnant diabetics for support, sharing of concerns, and teaching, if there is a large enough population in the area. Referral can be made to the American Diabetes Association.

Maternal Phenylketonuria and Hyperphenylalaninemia

The successful early dietary treatment of children with PKU or hyperphenylalaninemia (PHP) has prevented early, severe mental retardation and resulted in nonretarded adult women with PKU or PHP who then had their own children. In the late 1950s and early 1960s, it became apparent that a substantial number of non-PKU, non-hyperphenylalaninemic (non-PHP) offspring of these women were retarded. Fetal damage appears because of the prenatal exposure to the high concentration of either phenylalanine or its metabolites in the mother. Such women also have an increased frequency of spontaneous abortion. The major untoward fetal effects include various degrees of poor cognitive outcomes including mental retardation, microcephaly, congenital heart disease, esophageal atresia, neurologic problems (convulsions and spasticity), and growth retardation.

Longer-term increases in behavioral difficulties have been described. Although diet restrictions are now thought to be necessary throughout life, even relatively recently diet therapy for PKU typically ceased in childhood and so many women were on a normal diet (see chapters 11 and 15). Among untreated women, the degree of fetal complications appears positively related to the maternal blood level of phenylalanine, and positively to inadequate protein intake in pregnancy as well. The maintenance of a low phenylalanine (phe) diet throughout pregnancy is believed to prevent or minimize the fetal effects. Maternal weight and nutrient intake need to be monitored. Diet recommendations are those that maintain blood phenylalanine concentrations of 2–6 mg/dL. Too low levels can impair fetal growth. Reports of the success of these efforts have been both positive and negative and adherence may be one factor. It is believed that such therapy should begin before conception and be in effect at conception for optimal benefit. Indeed, the current trend is to maintain phe-restricted diets throughout adulthood, as discussed in chapter 11. Thus females with PKU or PHP should be followed over a long period and information about maternal PKU should be included in their health teaching. Recalling women at 12 years of age for information about maternal PKU and reproductive counseling may be effective. To do this, all PKU persons would need to be entered into a registry at diagnosis, presenting logistical and ethical problems. Adolescents with PKU or PHP may need to accept a greater level of responsibility if they choose to become sexually active.

Some women with PKU or PHP may not be aware of the potential danger to the fetus, or believe erroneously that treatment can begin successfully, early in pregnancy. Others may not inform their health care practitioner that they have had PKU or PHP, either out of ignorance or because they do not wish to return to the stringent and unpleasant diet they remember from childhood. For these reasons, it may be beneficial to screen all women of childbearing years for PKU or PHP, but this may not be practical or successful. The nurse should see that data regarding the outcome of maternal PKU or PHP are discussed with women known to be at risk, so that the women may explore the options available. The nurse should then assist her in obtaining optimum

dietary counseling with monitoring from a nutritionist experienced with maternal PKU and also help her to obtain products and recipes. Tyrosine supplementation may be useful during pregnancy. It is recommended that serum levels of phe be monitored twice a week, and that fetal development be monitored with ultrasound. The restricted phe diet can be costly, and help may be needed from such programs as Women, Infants, and Children. Support through morning sickness will also be necessary.

Other Maternal Metabolic and Genetic Disorders

Improved detection and treatment in infancy and childhood has led to women with other biochemical disorders reaching adulthood and becoming pregnant. This is also true of women with disorders such as congenital heart disease, which can affect the fetus in an indirect biochemical sense, for example through anoxia. This number is expected to increase in the coming years. Because of their rarity, there are not too much data available, but some indications have emerged. Women with hyperhomocysteinemia have a higher frequency of pre-eclampsia, placenta abruptio, and a higher number of fetal losses than expected, and women with myotonic dystrophy have increased rates of spontaneous abortions, stillbirths, and perinatal deaths, and polyhydramnios in such women may be correlated with an affected fetus. Women with acute intermittent porphyria have exacerbations of disease in pregnancy and increased rates of prematurity and spontaneous abortion. Other problems experienced in pregnancy may not be directly connected to the biochemical milieu, but will not be discussed here. For example, women with Marfan syndrome may experience stress on the already compromised cardiovascular system, and women with Ehlers Danlos syndrome may have a higher incidence of hernias and delivery complications. Women with sickle cell anemia may deliver infants who are small for gestational age, and they need to be watched for complications; those with spina bifida can be at risk for premature labor. Prepregnancy maternal obesity has been associated with a variety of birth defects such as neural tube defects, omphalocele, congenital heart defects, and multiple anomalies.

Emotions and Stress

The vulnerability of fetus to stressful maternal life events and/or anxiety occurring during organogenesis has been suggested. A full review is beyond the scope of this chapter. Carmichael and Shaw (2000) reported that experiencing at least one stressful event in the periconceptual period was associated with an increased prevalence odds ratio of having an infant with conotruncal heart defects, neural tube defects, and cleft lip with or without cleft palate. Hansen, Lou, and Olsen (2000) found that the frequency of cranial-neural-crest malformations was higher in the infants in their study who are exposed to severe life events during pregnancy. Catalano and Hartig (2001) found anxiety to be associated with low birth weight in their study. There has been a link described between maternal anxiety and reduced fetal cerebral circulation.

Hyperthermia

Hyperthermia has been shown to be teratogenic in animals. Major sources of hyperthermia for pregnant women include fever, baths, saunas, hot tubs, and electric blankets. Data on fevers are confounded by effects of the microorganism such as a virus. For example, possible teratogenic effects of influenza and the common cold may be related to the accompanying fever. Milunsky et al. (1996) have reported that heat exposure in early pregnancy from hot tubs, saunas, and fever, but not from electric blankets, poses an increased risk for neural tube defects; others have not confirmed this.

Noise

The American Academy of Pediatrics (1997) issued a statement on noise which stated that exposure to noise during pregnancy can damage the fetus. They review studies indicating that exposure to excessive noise during pregnancy may result in prematurity, intrauterine growth retardation, and high-frequency hearing loss in the newborn. Nurses should help pregnant women reduce such risks, which may result from occupational or environmental exposure including such things as "boom boxes" and airport noise.

BIBLIOGRAPHY

American Academy of Pediatrics. Committee on Environmental Health. (1997). Noise: A hazard for the fetus and newborn. *Pediatrics, 100,* 724–727.

American College of Obstetricians and Gynecologists. (2002). ACOG Committee Opinion 268. Management of asymptomatic pregnant or lactating women exposed to anthrax. *Obstetrics & Gynecology, 99,* 366–368.

American College of Obstetricians and Gynecologists. (2003). ACOG Practice Bulletin. No. 44. Neural tube defects. *Obstetrics & Gynecology, 102,* 203–213.

American College of Obstetricians and Gynecologists. (1994). ACOG Technical Bulletin No. 195. Substance abuse in pregnancy. *International Journal of Gynecology & Obstetrics, 47,* 73–80.

American College of Obstetricians and Gynecologists. (1993, February). ACOG Technical Bulletin Number 177. Perinatal viral and parasitic infections. *International Journal of Gynecology & Obstetrics, 42,* 300–307.

American Diabetes Association. (2004). Diagnosis and classification of diabetes mellitus. *Diabetes Care, 27*(Suppl. 1), S5–S10.

American Diabetes Association. (2004). Gestational diabetes mellitus. *Diabetes Care, 27*(Suppl. 1), S88–S90.

American Diabetes Association. (2004). Preconception care of women with diabetes. *Diabetes Care, 27*(Suppl. 1), S76–S78.

Andrade, S. E., Gurwitz, J. H., Davis, R. L., Chan, K. A., Finkelstein, J. A., Fortman, K., et al. (2004). Prescription drug use in pregnancy. *American Journal of Obstetrics and Gynecology, 191,* 398–407.

Anselmo, J., Cao, D., Karison, T., Weiss, R. E., & Refetoff, S. (2004). Fetal loss associated with excessive thyroid hormone exposure. *Journal of the American Medical Association, 292,* 691–695.

Astley, S. J., & Clarren, S. K. (1999). *Diagnostic guide for fetal alcohol syndrome and related conditions: The 4-digit diagnostic code* (2nd ed.). Seattle, WA: University Publication Services.

Atreya, C. D., Mohan, K. V. K., & Kulkarni, S. (2004). Rubella virus and birth defects: Molecular insights into the viral teratogenesis at the cellular level. *Birth Defects Research, (Part A), 70,* 431–37.

Balducci, J., Rodis, J. F., Rosengren, S., Vintzileos, A. M., Spivey, G., & Vosseller, C. (1992). Pregnancy outcome following first-trimester varicella infection. *Obstetrics & Gynecology, 79,* 5–6.

Bale, J. F., Jr. (2002). Congenital infections. *Neurological Clinics, 20,* 1039–1060.

Barrett, C., & Richens, A. (2003). Epilepsy and pregnancy: Report of an Epilepsy Research Foundation Workshop. *Epilepsy Research, 52,* 147–187.

Bauer, C. R., Shankaran, S., Bada, H. S., Lester, B., Wright, L. L., Krause-Steinrauf, H., et al. (2002). The Maternal Lifestyle Study: Drug exposure during pregnancy and short-term outcomes. *American Journal of Obstetrics and Gynecology, 186,* 487–495.

Bertrand, J., Floyd, F. L., Weber, M. K., O'Connor, M., Riley, P., Johnson, D. A., et al. (2004). *Fetal alcohol syndrome: Guidelines for referral and diagnosis.* Atlanta, GA: Centers for Disease Control and Prevention.

Bishop, J. B., Witt, K. L., & Sloane, R. A. (1997). Genetic toxicities of human teratogens. *Mutation Research, 396,* 9–43.

Black, R. A., & Hill, D. A. (2003). Over-the-counter medications in pregnancy. *American Family Physician, 67,* 2517–2524.

Blazer, S., Moreh-Waterman, Y., Iller-Lotan, R., Tamir, A., & Hochberg, Z. (2003). Maternal hypothyroidism may affect fetal growth and neonatal thyroid function. *Obstetrics & Gynecology, 102,* 232–241.

Bonassi, S., Magnani, M., Calvi, A., Repetto, E., & Publisi, P. (1994). Factors related to drug consumption during pregnancy. *Acta Obstetricia Gynecologica Et Scandinavica, 73,* 535–540.

Bouhours-Nouet, N., May-Panloup, P., Coutant, R., de Casson, F. B., Descamps, P., Douay, O., et al. (2005). Maternal smoking is associated with mitochondrial DNA depletion and respiratory chain complex III deficiency in placenta. *American Journal of Physiology, Endocrinology & Metabolism, 288,* E171–E177.

Brent, R. L., Tanski, S., & Weitzman, M. (2004). Pediatric perspective on the unique vulnerability and resilience of the embryo and child to environmental toxicants: The importance of rigorous research concerning age and agent. *Pediatrics, 113,* 935–944.

Brody, S. C., Harris, R., & Lohr, K. (2003). Screening for gestational diabetes: A summary of the evidence for the U.S. Preventive Services Task Force. *Obstetrics & Gynecology, 101,* 380–392.

Cardonick, E., & Iacobucci, A. (2004). Use of chemotherapy during human pregnancy. *Lancet Oncology, 5,* 283–291.

Carmichael, S. L., & Shaw, G. M. (2000). Maternal life event stress and congenital anomalies. *Epidemiology, 11,* 30–35.

Catalano, R., & Hartig, T. (2001). Communal bereavement and the incidence of very low birthweight in Sweden. *Journal of Health and Social Behaviour, 42,* 333–341.

Centers for Disease Control and Prevention. (1994). Rubella and congenital rubella syndrome—United States, January 1, 1991–May 7, 1994. *Morbidity and Mortality Weekly Report, 43*(21), 397–401.

Centers for Disease Control and Prevention. (2002). National task force on fetal alcohol syndrome and fetal alcohol effect. *Morbidity and Mortality Weekly Report, 51*(RR14), 9–12.

Centers for Disease Control and Prevention. (2003). Treatment of tuberculosis. American Thoracic Society, CDC, and Infectious Diseases Society of America. *Morbidity and Mortality Weekly Report, 52*(No. RR-11), 1–88.

Centers for Disease Control and Prevention. (2003). Women with smallpox vaccine exposure during pregnancy reported to the National Smallpox Vaccine in Pregnancy Registry—United States, 2003. *Morbidity and Mortality Weekly Report, 52,* 386–388.

Centers for Disease Control and Prevention. (2004). Interim guidelines for the evaluation of infants born to mothers infected with West Nile virus during pregnancy. *Morbidity and Mortality Weekly Report, 53,* 154–157.

Chambers, C. D., Johnson, K. A., Dick, L. M., Felix, R. J., & Jones, K. L. (1996). Birth outcomes in pregnant women taking fluoxetine. *New England Journal of Medicine, 335,* 1010–1015.

Chasnoff, I. J. (2002). *Drug use in pregnancy: Mother and child.* Kluwer Academic Publishing.

Chasnoff, I. J., Griffith, D. R., Freier, C., & Murray, J. (1992). Cocaine/polydrug use in pregnancy: Two-year follow-up. *Pediatrics, 89,* 284–289.

Clarren, S. K., & Smith, D. W. (1978). The fetal alcohol syndrome. *New England Journal of Medicine, 298,* 1063–1067

Cohen, F. L. (1986). Paternal contributions to birth defects. *Nursing Clinics of North America, 21,* 51–66.

Collinet, P., Subtil, D., Houfflin-Debarge, V., Kacet, N., Dewilde, A., & Puech, F. (2004). Routine CMV screening during pregnancy. *International Journal of Obstetrics & Gynecology, 114,* 3–11.

Correa, A., Botto, L., Liu, Y., Mulinare, J., & Erickson, J. D. (2003). Do multivitamin supplements attenuate the risk for diabetes-associated birth defects? *Pediatrics, 111,* 1146–1151.

Daniel, K. L., Honein, M. A., & Moore, C. A. (2003). Sharing prescription medication among teenage girls: Potential danger to unplanned/undiagnosed pregnancies. *Pediatrics, 111,* 1167–1170.

Day, N. L., & Richardson, G. A. (2004). An analysis of the effects of prenatal alcohol exposure on growth: A teratologic model. *American Journal of Medical Genetics, Part C (Seminars in Medical Genetics), 127C,* 28–34.

Delaney-Black, V., Covington, C., Templin, T., Kershaw, T., Nordstrom-Klee, B., Ager, J., et al. (2000a). Expressive language development of children exposed to cocaine prenatally: Literature review and report of a prospective cohort study. *Journal of Communication Disorders, 33,* 463–480.

Delaney-Black, V., Covington, C, Templin, T., Ager, J., Nordstrom-Klee, B., Martier, S., et al. (2000b). Teacher-assessed behavior of children prenatally exposed to cocaine. *Pediatrics, 106,* 782–791.

Doering, P. L., & Stewart, R. B. (1978). The extent and character of a drug consumption during pregnancy. *Journal of American Medical Association, 239,* 843–846.

Doll, R., & Wakeford, R. (1997). Risk of childhood cancer from fetal irradiation. *British Journal of Radiology, 70,* 130–139.

Dow-Clarke, R. A., MacCalder, L., & Hessel, P. A. (1994). Health behaviours of pregnant women in Fort McMurray, Alberta. *Canadian Journal of Public Health, 85,* 33–336.

Ebrahim, S. H., & Gfroerer, J. (2003). Pregnancy-related substance use in the United States during 1996–1998. *Obstetrics & Gynecology, 101,* 374–379.

Einarson, A., Bonari, L., Voyer-Lavigne, S., Addis, A., Matsui, D., Johnson, Y., et al. (2003). A multicentre prospective controlled study to determine the safety of trazodone and nefazodone use during pregnancy. *Canadian Journal of Psychiatry, 48,* 106–110.

Engelgau, M. M. (1995). Screening for NIDDM in nonpregnant adults. *Diabetes Care, 18,* 1606–1618.

Enright, A. M., & Prober, C. G. (2004). Herpesviridae infections in newborns: Varicella zoster virus, herpes simplex virus, and cytomegalovirus. *Pediatric Clinics of North America, 51,* 889–908.

Expert Committee on the Diagnosis and Classification of Diabetes Mellitus. (2003). Report of the Expert Committee on the Diagnosis and Classification of Diabetes Mellitus. *Diabetes Care, 26*(Suppl. 1), S4–S21.

Eyler, F. D., Behnke, M., Conlon, M., Woods, N. S., & Wobie, K. (1998). Birth outcome from a prospective, matched study of prenatal crack/cocaine use: I. Interactive and dose effects on health and growth. *Pediatrics, 101,* 229–237.

Feigin, R. D. (Ed.). (2003). *Pediatric infectious diseases.* Elsevier Science.

Forfar, J. O., & Nelson, M. M. (1973). Epidemiology of drugs taken by pregnant women: Drugs that may affect the fetus adversely. *Clinical Pharmocology & Therapuetics, 14*(Pt. 2), 632–642.

Foulds, N., Walpole, I., Elmslie, F., & Mansour, S. (2005). Carbimazole embryopathy: An emerging phenotype. *American Journal of Medical Genetics, 132A,* 130–135.

Fraga, C. G., Motchnik, P. A., Wyrobek, A. ., Rempel, D. M., & Ames, B. N. (1996). Smoking and low antioxidant levels increase oxidative damage to sperm DNA. *Mutation Research, 351,* 199–203.

Frank, D. A., Zuckerman, B. S., Amaro, H., Aboagye, K., Bauchner, H., Cabral, H., et al. (1988). Cocaine use during pregnancy: Prevalence and correlates. *Pediatrics, 82,* 888–895.

Friedman, J. M., & Hanson, J. W. (2002). Human teratology. In D. L. Rimoin, J. M. Connor, R. E. Pyeritz, & B. R. Korf (Eds.), *Emery and Rimoin's principles and practice of medical genetics* (4th ed., pp. 1011–1045). New York: Churchill Livingstone.

Friedman, J. M., & Polifka, J. E. (2000). *Teratogenic effects of drugs: A resource for clinicians (TERIS)* (2nd ed.). Baltimore: Johns Hopkins University Press.

Gaytant, M. A., Rours, G. I., Steegers, E. A.,

Galama, J. M., & Semmekrot, B. A. (2003). Congenital cytomegalovirus infection after recurrent infection: Case reports and review of the literature. *European Journal of Pediatrics, 162,* 248–253.

Getz, L., & Kirkengen, A. L. (2003). Ultrasound screening in pregnancy: Advancing technology, soft markers for fetal chromosomal aberrations, and unacknowledged ethical dilemmas. *Social Science & Medicine, 56,* 2045–2057.

Gibbs, R. S. (2002). The origins of stillbirth: Infectious diseases. *Seminars in Perinatology, 26,* 75–78.

Gilbert, G. L. (2002). Infections in pregnant women. *Medical Journal of Australia, 176,* 229–236.

Hague, W. M. (2003). Homocysteine and pregnancy. *Best Practice & Research Clinical Obstetrics & Gynaecology, 17,* 459–469.

Hansen, D., Lou, H. C., & Olsen, J. (2000). Serious life events and congenital malformations: A national study with complete follow-up. *Lancet, 356,* 875–880.

Harger, J. H., Ernest, J. M., Thurnau, G. R., Moawad, A., Thom, E., Landon, M. B., et al. (2002). Frequency of congenital varicella syndrome in a prospective cohort of 347 pregnant women. *Obstetrics & Gynecology, 100,* 260–265.

Havens, P. L., & Waters, D. (2004). Management of the infant born to a mother with HIV infection. *Pediatric Clinics of North America, 51,* 909–937.

Henderson, J. L., & Weiner, C. P. (1995). Congenital infection. *Current Opinion in Obstetrics and Gynecology, 7,* 130–134.

Henry, A., & Crowther, C. (2000). Patterns of medication use during and prior to pregnancy: The MAP study. *Australia and New Zealand Journal of Obstetrics and Gynecology, 40,* 165–172.

Hepper, P. G., Dornan, J. C., & Little, J. F. (2005). Maternal alcohol consumption during pregnancy may delay the development of spontaneous fetal startle behaviour. *Physiology of Behavior, 83,* 711–714.

Hill, D., & Dubey, J. P. (2002). Toxoplasma gondii: Transmission, diagnosis and prevention. *Clinics in Microbiology and Infection, 8,* 634–640.

Hill, R. M. (1973). Drugs ingested by pregnant women. *Clinical Pharmcology and Therapeutics, 14*(Pt. 2), 654–659.

Holier, L. M., Hill, J., Sheffield, J. S., & Wendel, G. D., Jr. (2003). State laws regarding prenatal syphilis screening in the United States. *American Journal of Obstetrics and Gynecology, 189,* 1178–1183.

Holmes, L. B., Coull, B. A., Dorfman, J., & Rosenberger, P. B. (2005). The correlation of deficits in IQ with midface and digit hypoplasia in children exposed in utero to anticonvulsant drugs. *Journal of Pediatrics, 146,* 118–122.

Hoyme, H. E., May, P. A., Kalberg, W. O., Kodituwakku, P., Gossage, J. P., Trujillo, P. M., et al. (2005). A practical clinical approach to diagnosis of fetal alcohol spectrum disorders: Clarification of the 1996 Institute of Medicine criteria. *Pediatrics, 115,* 39–47.

Jacobsson, B., Pernevi, P., Chidekel, L., & Platz-Christensen, J. J. (2002). Bacterial vaginosis in early pregnancy may predispose for preterm birth and postpartum endometritis. *Acta Obstetricia et Gynecologica Scandinavica, 81,* 1006–1010.

Joffe, J. (1979). Influence of drug exposure of the father on perinatal outcome. *Clinical Perinatology, 6*(1), 21–36.

Joffe, J. M., & Soyka, L. F. (1982). Paternal drug exposure. Effects on reproduction and progeny. *Seminars in Perinatology, 6,* 116–124.

Jones, J., Lopez, A., & Wilson, M. (2003). Congenital toxoplasmosis. *American Family Physician, 67,* 2131–2138.

Jones, K. L., Smith, D. E., Ulleland, C. N., & Streissguth, A. P. (1973). Patterns of malformation in offspring of chronic alcoholic mothers. *Lancet, 1,* 1267–1271.

Kadanali, A., Tasyaran, M. A., & Kadanali, S. (2003). Anthrax during pregnancy: Case reports and review. *Clinical Infectious Diseases, 36,* 1343–1346.

Källén, K. (1997a). Maternal smoking and orofacial clefts. *Cleft Palate Craniofacial Journal, 34,* 11–16.

Källén, K. (1997b). Maternal smoking during pregnancy and limb reduction malformations in Sweden. *American Journal of Public Health, 87,* 29–32.

Karatza, A., Varvarigou, A., & Beratis, N. G. (2003). Growth up to 2 years in relationship to maternal smoking during pregnancy. *Clinical Pediatrics, 42,* 533–541.

Klip, H., Verloop, J., van Gool, J. D., Koster, M. E., Burger, C. W., van Leeuwen, F. E., et al. (2002). Hypospadias in sons of women exposed to diethylstilbestrol inutero: A cohort study. *Lancet, 359,* 1102–1107.

Koren, G., Pastuszak, A., & Ito, S. (1998). Drugs in pregnancy. *New England Journal of Medicine, 338,* 1128–1137.

Lammer, E. J., Shaw, G. M., Iovannisci, D. M., Van Waes, J., & Finnell, R. H. (2004). Maternal smoking and the risk of orofacial clefts: Susceptibility with *NAT1* and *NAT2* polymorphisms. *Epidemiology, 15,* 150–156.

Lester, B. M., LaGasse, L., Seifer, R., Tronick, E. Z., Bauer, C. R., Shankaran, S., et al. (2003). The maternal lifestyle study (MLS): Effects of prenatal cocaine and/or opiate exposure on auditory brain response at one month. *Journal of Pediatrics, 142,* 279–285.

Levy, H. L., Guldberg, P., Güttler, F., Handley, W. B., Matalon, R., Rouse, B. M., et al. (2001). Congenital heart disease in maternal phenylketonuria: Report from the maternal PKU collaborative study. *Pediatric Research, 49,* 636–642.

Little, J., Cardy, A., & Munger, R. G. (2004). Tobacco smoking and oral clefts: A meta-analysis. *Bulletin of the World Health Organization, 82,* 213–218.

Martin, D. H., Koutsky, L., Eschenbach, D. A., Daling, J. R., Alexander, E. R., Benedetti, J. K., et al. (1982). Prematurity and perinatal mortality in pregnancies complicated by maternal *Chlamydia trachomatis* infections, *Journal of the American Medical Association, 247,* 1585–1588.

Mayes, L. C., Granger, R. H., Bornstein, M. H., & Zuckerman, B. (1992). The problem of prenatal cocaine exposure: A rush to judgment. *Journal of the American Medical Association, 267,* 406–408.

Menegola, E., Broccia, M. L., Di Renzo, F., & Giavini, E. (2003). Pathogenic pathways in fluconazole-induced branchial arch malformations. *Birth Defects Research (Part A), 67,* 116–124.

Messinger, D. S., Bauer, C. R., Das, A., Seifer, R., Lester, B. M., Lagasse, L. L., et al. (2004). The maternal lifestyle study: Cognitive, motor, and behavioral outcomes of cocaine-exposed and opiate-exposed infants through three years of age. *Pediatrics, 113,* 1677–1685.

Michals-Matalon, K., Platt, L. D., Acosta, P. P., Azen, C., & Walla, C. A. (2002). Nutrient intake and congenital heart defects in maternal phenylketonuria. *American Journal of Obstetrics and Gynecology, 187,* 441–444.

Milunsky, A., Ulcickas, M., Rothman, K. J., Willett, W., Jick, S. S., & Jick, H. (1996). Maternal heat exposure and neural tube defects. *Journal of the American Medical Association, 268,* 882–885.

Minkoff, H. (2003). Human immunodeficiency virus infection in pregnancy. *Obstetrics & Gynecology, 101,* 797–810.

Montoya, J. G., & Liesenfeld, O. (2004). Toxoplasmosis. *Lancet, 363,* 1965–1976.

Morgan, W. F. (2003). Non-targeted and delayed effects of exposure to ionizing radiation: I. Radiation-induced genomic instability and bystander effects *in vitro. Radiation Research, 159,* 567–580.

Morgan, W. F. (2003). Non-targeted and delayed effects of exposure to ionizing radiation: II. Radiation-induced genomic instability and bystander effects *in vivo,* clastogenic factors and transgenerational effects. *Radiation Research, 159,* 581–596.

Morrow, J. I., & Craig, J. J. (2003). Anti-epileptic drugs in pregnancy: Current safety and other issues. *Expert Opinion in Pharmacotherapy, 4,* 445–456.

Mylonakis, E., Paliou, M, Hohmann, E. L., Calderwood, S. B., & Wing, E. J. (2002). Listeriosis during pregnancy: A case series and review of 222 cases. *Medicine, 81,* 260–269.

Ng, T. W., Rae, A., Wright, H., Gurry, D., & Wray, J. (2003). Maternal phenylketonuria in Western Australia: Pregnancy outcomes and developmental outcomes in offspring. *Journal of Paediatrics and Child Health, 39,* 358–363.

Naimi, T. S., Lipscomb, L. E., Brewer, R. D., & Gilbert, B. C. (2003). Binge drinking in the preconception period and the risk of unintended pregnancy: Implications for women and their children. *Pediatrics, 111,* 1136–1141.

Nordeng, H., & Havnen, G. C. (2005). Impact of socio-demographic factors, knowledge and attitude on the use of herbal drugs in pregnancy. *Acta Obstetrica et Gynecological Scandinavica, 84,* 26–33.

Nulman, I., Rovet, J., Stewart, D. E., Wolpin, J., Gardner, H. A., Theis, J. G. W., et al. (1997). Neurodevelopment of children exposed in utero to antidepressant drugs. *New England Journal of Medicine, 336,* 258–262.

Nulman, I., Scolnik, D., Chitayat, D., Farkas, L. D., & Koren, G. (1997). Findings in children exposed in utero to phenytoin and carba-mazepine monotheapy: Independent effects of epilepsy and medications. *American Journal of Medical Genetics, 68,* 18–24.

Ornoy, A. (2003). The impact of intrauterine exposure versus postnatal environment in neu-rodevelopmental toxicity: Long-term neurobe-havioral studies in children at risk for develop-mental disorders. *Toxicology Letters, 140–141,* 171–181.

Pastuszak, A. L., Levy, M., Schick, B., Zuber, C., Feldkamp, M., Gladstone, J., et al. (1994). Out-come after maternal varicella infection in the first 20 weeks of pregnancy. *New England Jour-nal of Medicine, 330,* 901–905.

Physicians' Desk Reference (58th ed.). (2004). Montvale, NJ: Medical Economics.

Pinelli, J. M., Symington, A. J., Cunningham, K. A., & Paes, B. A. (2002). Case report and review of the perinatal implications of maternal lithium use. *American Journal of Obstetrics and Gynecol-ogy, 187,* 245–249.

Polifka, J. E., & Friedman, J. M. (2002). Medical genetics: 1. Clinical teratology in the age of genomics. *Canadian Medical Association Jour-nal, 167,* 265–273.

Prasad, K. N., Cole, W. C., & Hasse, G. M. (2004). Health risks of low dose ionizing radiation in humans: A review. *Experimental Biology and Medicine, 229,* 378–382.

Project CHOICES Intervention Research Group. (2003). Reducing the risk of alcohol-exposed pregnancies: A study of a motivational interven-tion in community settings. *Pediatrics, 111,* 1131–1135.

Rappaport, V. J., Velazquez, M., & Williams, K. (2004). Hemoglobinopathies in pregnancy. *Obstetrics and Gynecology Clinics of North America, 31,* 287–317.

Revello, M. G., & Gerna, G. (2002). Diagnosis and management of human cytomegalovirus infec-tion in the mother, fetus, and newborn infant. *Clinical MIcrobiology Reviews, 15,* 680–715.

Rouse, B., & Azen, C. (2004). Effect of high mater-nal blood phenylalanine on offspring congenital anomalies and developmental outcome at ages 4 and 6 years: The importance of strict dietary control preconception and throughout preg-nancy. *Journal of Pediatrics, 144,* 235–239.

Rubin, J. D., Ferencz, C., & Loffredo, C. (1993). Use of prescription and non-prescription drugs in pregnancy. *Journal of Clinical Epidemiology, 46,* 581–589.

Schaefer, C. (Ed.). (2001). *Drugs during pregnancy and lactation.* Amsterdam: Elsevier.

Schrager, S., & Potter, B. E. (2004). Diethylstilbe-strol exposure. *American Family Physician, 69,* 2395–2402.

Scialli, A. R., Buelke-Sam, J. L., Chambers, C. D., Friedman, J. M., Kimmel, C. A., Polifka, J. E., et al. (2004). Communicating risks during preg-nancy: A workshop in the use of data from ani-mal developmental toxicity studies in preg-nancy labels for drugs. *Birth Defects Research, (Part A), 70,* 7–12.

Shea, K. M., & Little, R. E. (1997). Is there an asso-ciation between preconception paternal X-ray exposure and birth outcome? The ALSPAC Study Team. Avon Longitudinal Study of Preg-nancy and Childhood. *American Journal of Epi-demiology, 145,* 546–551.

Shek, C. C., Ng, P. C., Fung, G. P., Cheng, F. W., Chan, P. K., Peiris, M. J., et al. (2003). Infants born to mothers with severe acute respiratory syndrome. *Pediatrics, 112,* e254–e256.

Shepard, T. H. (2002). Annual commentary on human teratogens. *Teratology, 66,* 275–277.

Shepard, T. H., Brent, R. L., Friedman, J. M., Jones, K. L., Miller, Moore, C. A., et al. (2002). Update on new developments in the study of human teratogens. *Teratology, 65,* 153–161.

Singer, L. T., Minnes, S., Short, E., Arendt, R., Farkas, K., Lewis, B., et al. (2004). Cognitive outcomes of preschool children with prenatal cocaine exposure. *Journal of the American Med-ical Association, 291,* 2448–2456.

Skelly, A. C., Holt, V. L., Mosca, V. S., & Alderman, B. W. (2002). Talipes equinovarus and maternal smoking: A population-based case-control study in Washington state. *Teratology, 66,* 91–100.

Smeenk, R. J. (1997). Immunological aspects of con-genital atrioventricular block. *Pacing and Clinical Electrophysiology, 20*(8 Pt. 2), 2093–2097.

Sobngwi, E., Boudou, P., Mauvais-Jarvis, F., Leblanc, H., Velho, H., Vexlau, P., et al. (2003). Effect of a diabetic environment in utero on predisposition to type 2 diabetes. *Lancet, 361,* 1861–1865.

Sokol, R. J., Martier, S. S., & Ager, J. W. (1989). The

T-ACE questions: Practical prenatal detection of risk-drinking. *American Journal of Obstetrics and Gynecology, 160,* 863–868.

Solomon, C. G., Willett, W. C., Carey, V. J., Rich-Edwards, J., Hunter, D. J., Colditz, G. A., et al. (1997). A prospective study of pregravid determinants of gestational diabetes mellitus. *Journal of the American medical Association, 278,* 1078–1083.

Splinter, M. Y., Sagraves, R., Nightengale, B., & Rayburn, W. F. (1997). Prenatal use of medications by women giving birth at a university hospital. *Southern Medical Journal, 90,* 498–502.

Stegmann, B. J., & Carey, J. C. (2002). TORCH infections. Toxoplasmosis, other (syphilis, varicella-zoster, parvovirus B19), rubella, cytomegalovirus (CMV), and herpes infections. *Current Women's Health Report, 2,* 253–258.

Stoler, J. M., & Holmes, L. B. (2004). Recognition of facial features of fetal alcohol syndrome in the newborn. *American Journal of Medical Genetics, Part C (Seminars in Medical Genetics), 127C,* 21–27.

Stratton, K., Howe, C., & Battaglia (Eds.). (1996). *Fetal alcohol syndrome: Diagnosis, epidemiology, prevention, and treatment.* Washington, DC: National Academy Press.

Streissguth, A. P. (1993). Fetal alcohol syndrome in older patients. *Alcohol & Alcoholism, Suppl. 2,* 209–212.

Streissguth, A. P., Landesman-Dwyer, S., Martin, J. C., & Smith, D. W. (1980). Teratogenic effects of alcohol in humans and laboratory animals. *Science, 209,* 353–361.

Streissguth, A. P., & O'Malley, K. (2000). Neuropsychiatric implications and long-term consequences of fetal alcohol spectrum disorders. *Seminars in Clinical Neuropsychiatry, 5,* 177–190.

Surgeon General's Advisory on Alcohol and Pregnancy. (1981). *FDA Drug Bulletin, 11*(2), 9–10.

Tronick, E. Z., Frank, D. A., Cabral, H., Mirochnick, M., & Zuckerman, B. (1996). Late dose-response effects of prenatal cocaine exposure on newborn neurobehavioral performance. *Pediatrics, 98,* 76–83.

Ulleland, C. N. (1972). The offspring of alcoholic mothers. *Annals of the New York Academy of Science, 197,* 167–171.

U.S. Preventive Services Task Force. (2003). Screening for gestational diabetes mellitus: Recommendations and rationale. *Obstetrics & Gynecology, 101,* 393–395.

Vidaeff, A. C., & Mastrobattista, J. M. (2003). In utero cocaine exposure: A thorny mix of science and mythology. *American Journal of Perinatology, 20,* 165–172.

Volpe, J. J. (1992). Effects of cocaine use on the fetus. *New England Journal of Medicine, 327,* 399–407.

Watkins, M. L., Rasmussen, S. A., Honein, M. A., Botto, L. D., & Moore, C. A. (2003). Maternal obesity and risk for birth defects. *Pediatrics, 111,* 1152–1158.

Weiner, C. P., & Buhimschi, C. (Eds.). (2004). *Drugs for pregnant and lactating women.* Philadelphia: Churchill Livingstone.

Wendel, G. D. Jr., Sheffield, J. S., Hollier, L. M., Hill, J. B., Ramsey, P. S., & Sanchez, P. J. (2002). Treatment of syphilis in pregnancy and prevention of congenital syphilis. *Clinical Infectious Diseases, 35*(Suppl 2), S200–S209.

Wilson, J. G. (1977). Embryotoxicity of drugs in man. In J. G. Wilson, & F. C. Fraser (Eds.), *Handbook of Teratology, Vol 1.* New York: Plenum Press.

Wilson, J. G. (1973). *Environment and Birth Defects.* New York: Academic Press.

Yudin, M. H., Steele, D. M., Sgro, M. D., Read, S. E., Kopplin, P., & Gough, K. A. (2005). Severe acute respiratory syndrome in pregnancy. *Obstetrics & Gynecology, 105,* 124–127.

Zuckerman, B., Frank, D. A., Hingson, R., Amaro, H., Levenson, S., Kayne, H., et al. (1989). Effects of maternal marijuana and cocaine on fetal growth. *New England Journal of Medicine, 320,* 762–781.

14

Reproductive and Genetic Effects of Environmental Chemicals and Agents

EXTENT OF THE PROBLEM

Potentially hazardous chemicals are present in our environment both deliberately, such as in food additives, agricultural chemicals, industrial compounds, and fuel, and inadvertently through contamination, pollution, and accidents. The effects of environmental agents on genetic material is an increasing source of public concern as well as a public health problem. Hazardous chemicals may cause: damage to the developing fetus directly (teratogenesis, see chapter 13), cancer, or mutation by direct damage of genetic material in the germ cells, resulting in hazards to future generations. There is a myriad of different chemicals in worldwide use, with new ones added each year. They are distributed widely, and are present in natural and synthetic forms, alone and in combination, and are used for commerce, agriculture, industry, and military purposes. Once in the environment, they may enter the food chains and attain even greater concentration. A minimum safe dose or level or safe time exposure has not been established for most of these. Relatively few have been investigated with respect to their mutagenic, carcinogenic, or teratogenic effects. Most carcinogens (80%–90%) are also mutagens, but mutagens are not necessarily carcinogens. The study of genotoxic chemicals presently is analogous to the study of radiation effects a few decades ago. The term toxicogenomics, defined as the study of genes and their products important in adaptive responses to toxic exposures, is a relatively new one. Exposures to certain environmental agents can result in genetic consequences to the exposed individuals them-

selves, their immediate offspring, or future generations because of structural or functional disruption of the genetic material or apparatus in either germ or somatic cells. It is difficult to connect cause and effect between a specific agent and most birth defects, genetic disorders, and neoplasms, as discussed in this chapter. Those agents with delayed, indirect, or subtle effects are hardest to identify.

Damage to genetic material may have different outcomes depending on the agent, exposure, and the person's genetic constitution. Each person has their own constellation of metabolizing enzymes and receptors, and so handles chemicals in a unique manner. Damage to the germ cells may result in a dominant or recessive single-gene mutation, a chromosomal mutation involving a gain, loss, or rearrangement of parts of chromosomes, or genomic mutation affecting chromosome number (gain or loss) but not structure. Agents can also cause changes in DNA functioning such as imprinting (see chapter 4). A dominant gene mutation may result in visible anomalies in the offspring or infertility in the individual if the damage is so great that normal offspring cannot be produced. Production of abnormal germ cells may also result in repetitive spontaneous abortions or fetal death when reproduction is attempted. If the mutation is recessive, it may remain hidden for generations, being added to the genetic load of unfavorable genes for the population. Mutation in somatic cells may result in (1) carcinogenesis in individuals exposed, or by transplacental mechanisms in their offspring (e.g., vaginal cancer in daughters of women who took DES during pregnancy); or (2) structural or functional damage to the developing embryo or fetus, which may not be immediately evident. Somatic mutations may also contribute to aging and heart disease. Of particular concern to the geneticist in recent years is the impact of environmental agents on the genetic makeup of the individual and the long-term effects on the population gene pool. The Environmental Genome Project of the National Institute of Environmental Health Sciences is concerned with how genetic variability influences the effects of environmental exposure in such avenues as cellular receptors, enzymes that modify or activate chemicals or repair DNA damage, and factors that regulate cell cycles, cell division and cell death. They have identified 554 environmentally responsive genes but have focused on a subset of these for immediate research. The Human Proteome Organization also has initiatives for looking at protein polymorphisms and environmental health. Various databases exist for environmental damage including the Developmental and Reproductive Toxicology/Environmental Teratology Information Center (DART/ETIC) available from the National Library of Medicine's Toxicology Data Network (TOXNET).

Some issues that society must consider are how agents with the potential for deleterious genetic, carcinogenic, or teratogenic effects can be identified before release into the environment, whether or not such agents should be used, assessment of the risks and evaluation of the benefits to be gained from their use, and the extent of evidence necessary in order to effect a public health decision on regulation and control. Society must ultimately balance the risks of adverse effects, such as environmental contamination and genetic damage, against utility, economic benefits, and comfort. For example, DDT is restricted in this country, but is considered necessary in other parts of the world to control malaria, which is a major health problem. Persons also look at the utility of such agents differently; the farmer and the wildlife conservationist view the use of pesticides from different perspectives. Society has chosen to use motor vehicles despite the large number of traffic deaths per year. What price will be considered reasonable for the use of genotoxic agents? In this chapter genetic effects from both environmental and workplace exposure are considered.

PROBLEMS IN ASSOCIATING EFFECTS WITH ENVIRONMENTAL AGENTS

There are many difficulties in associating a particular agent with an adverse outcome. These include the following:

- A particular agent may induce a specific genetic change that may be manifested in different phenotypic ways.
- Individual genetic differences can alter susceptibility and resistance.
- Effects may be removed from the obvious impact of the agent. For example, a chemical can change a person's ability to metabolize other substances.
- Chemicals in the environment are rarely present alone; rather they are in mixture and can then interact with other substances.
- Past failure to appreciate that exposure of both males and females can result in germ cell mutations, leading to adverse reproductive outcome as well as risk to future generations.
- Concentrations of a chemical may not reflect its biologic activity.
- There may be difficulty in detecting an increase in a birth defect that is rare or within a small population.
- There may be failure to account for synergistic and additive effects.
- There may be lack of knowledge of a person's past status (e.g., were chromosomes normal before exposure?).
- It is hard to pinpoint an exposure period to a specific agent retrospectively.
- Persons may not know that they were exposed to a particular agent.
- If they know they were exposed to a toxic agent, they may not know what it was.
- Influence of personal habits, such as smoking, on outcome is not always known or accounted for.
- There may be no available confirmatory records of either the exposure or the genotoxic outcome available.
- It is difficult to make an association between common exposures to an agent. For example, if several workers are exposed to one chemical, and all of them developed a certain type

of cancer but were seen by practitioners in towns many miles apart, the connection might not be made.

- There is a dependence on memory recall or incomplete or vague data.
- The duration, dosage, and concentration of the agent to which they were exposed may be unknown.
- The person may be embarrassed, may selectively omit vital information, may fear job loss, may feel an outcome is detrimental to his or her self-image, may have poor recall, or may not be aware of an adverse outcome in his or her spouse, and therefore may not reveal vital information.
- Political and economic pressure is brought to bear by private industry, health departments, the military, and the government because of fear of litigation, expediency, or perceived necessity for the use of a substance.
- Testing systems are insensitive.
- Long-term testing is not done because of high costs and time.
- It is difficult to extrapolate test results from animal studies to humans.
- An outcome that occurs years after exposure may not be associated with it, or if thought to be, may not be able to be proven.
- Information related to compliance with the use of protective measures may not be available.
- Companies may be reluctant to inform workers and others of all substances used in processing because of "trade secrets."

Other difficulties particularly related to teratogenic agents are discussed in chapter 13.

HAZARDOUS EXPOSURES IN THE ENVIRONMENT AND WORKPLACE

Hazardous exposures to genotoxic agents may occur through the release of substances into the environment or through exposure in the workplace. In fact, much of the information about the effects of such substances in humans has been obtained through unintentional exposure. Exposure is usually of two types—that of a low dosage over a long-term period or a short-term intense exposure such as occurs more often in accidents.

There may be overlap in exposures between the workplace and environment, since those exposed to a toxic agent at work may also live near the workplace. Families of those working in certain industries are exposed to certain agents through contact with clothes and other articles of the worker. Sometimes hazardous workplaces, such as university chemistry laboratories, are hard to recognize. As discussed in chapter 13, interindividual differences play a critical role in manifestation of effects after deleterious exposures as does the timing, duration, intensity and other factors relating to the exposure.

Deleterious genetic effects can be manifested by adverse changes in the reproductive capacity or process in both males and females. This may be evidenced by impaired fertility (as seen in menstrual irregularities, abnormal sperm, etc.), infertility, spontaneous abortion, fetal or perinatal death, stillbirth, intrauterine growth retardation, birth defects, or altered sex ratios in offspring. These may be used as endpoints in monitoring exposure effects. A registry of environmental mutagens is maintained at Oak Ridge National Laboratories, and there are other information sources, such as the National Institute for Occupational Safety and Health (NIOSH) hotline and online services, and the Reproductive Toxicology Center which sponsors an information system on environmental hazards to human reproduction and development. The National Human Monitoring Program within the Environmental Protection Agency monitors human tissues for toxic substances. Some agents believed to cause such effects are listed in Table 14.1, but there is a lack of agreement as to most of these in the literature. Selected agents are discussed in the text that follows.

Evidence of environmental contamination by toxic chemicals often comes to light because of the observation of what appears to be a high frequency or clustering of birth defects, spontaneous abortions, or miscarriages, and may be observed by citizens or professionals. One of the first widespread examples was discovered in 1956 in the Minamata Bay area of Japan. Industrial waste containing methylmercury from a fertilizer company was discharged into the bay that was used for fishing. The fish and shellfish were contaminated and concentrated the methylmercury. Many people eating the fish became ill and many died. Many pregnant

TABLE 14.1   Selected Environmental Agents with Reported Genotoxic and Reproductive Effects in Humans

Agents	Reported effects*
Benzene	↑Chromosome aberrations including breaks; leukemia
Carbon disulfide	Sperm abnormalities, impotency, decreased libido (M); menstrual disorders (F); ↑spontaneous abortions; ↑prematurity
Chlordecone (Kepone)	↓Spermatogenesis; ↓libido (M)
Chlorinated hydrocarbon pesticides	↑Blood dyscrasias; ↑childhood neuroblastomas
Chloroprene	↑Spontaneous abortions in wives of male workers; ↑chromosome aberrations, disturbances in spermatogenesis
Dibroomoshloropropane (DBCP)	Low/absent sperm; infertility (M)
Formaldehyde	↑Spontaneous abortions; ↓birth weight in offspring
Hexachlorophene	↑Birth defects
(PCBs)	↓Birth weight in offspring; specific congenital anomalies such as brown pigmentation, gum hyperplasia, skull anomalies; developmental retardation
Nonionizing radiation	↑Perinatal death; ↑congenital malformations; ↓birth weight
Smelter emissions (mixed substances including arsenic, sulfur dioxide, cadmium, lead, mercury)	↑Spontaneous abortions; infertility (M); ↓birth weight; ↑congenital anomalies; ↑frequency of Wilms tumor in offspring
Vinyl chloride	↑Chromosome aberrations; ↑spontaneous abortion in wives of workers; carcinoginesis, ↑birth defects
High temperature exposure	↓spermatogenesis; ↑birth defects (?)

Note. * For most of these agents, research reports vary; some report these effects, others report negative findings.
↑ = increased, ↓ = decreased, M = male, F = female.

women either aborted or gave birth to infants with a congenital neurologic disorder resembling cerebral palsy, although the women often showed no ill effects themselves. Infants also received methylmercury in breast milk. Research studies confirmed the chain of transmission. They also verified that animals had provided an early warning system. As early as 1950, cats became "mad" and died, as did birds, pigs, and dogs. Fish were easy to catch by hand, and many died. Follow-up studies have shown that many who were exposed in utero later showed other developmental deficits and mental deficiency. However, not all who were apparently exposed developed disease, a finding believed due to genetic variation or an unknown factor. In 1964, a similar epidemic occurred in Niigata, Japan, caused by methylmercury in waste from a plastics factory. In Iraq, imported grain from Mexico that was treated with methylmercury as a fungicide was used for bread, instead of planting, by large numbers of individuals. The warning about toxicity was

in Spanish and was not understood. Many of the infants subsequently born to women eating bread made with the grain also showed a cerebral palsy-like illness that included blindness and brain damage. In the United States, a family in New Mexico who ingested pork that had been fed grain contaminated by organic mercury used as a fungicide also became ill, and the pregnant mother gave birth to an infant with features of the disorder. In all these cases, some persons were more susceptible to the mercury, as not all those who ate contaminated products evidenced toxicity. High levels of mercury (>1 ppm) are present in certain fish such as swordfish, shark, tilefish, whale meat, and mackerel in the United States, and that pregnant women, nursing mothers, and young children should minimize the amount of these fish that they eat. Another source of mercury is thimerosal used as a preservative in vaccines. This use has engendered concerns that have been somewhat controversial. Although some have believed that the use of thimerosal in vaccines was associated with the development of autism spectrum disorders the present published research findings do not resolve the issue. In the United States, this use has virtually been eliminated. Use continues in other countries since the World Health Organization (2002) has indicated that thimerosal use in vaccines is safe. Dental amalgam fillings are a source of inorganic mercury exposure, often through inhalation during preparation or removal. Cultural practices such as in religious ceremonies in some sects such as Voodoo and Santaria may also expose segments of the population as may the use of cosmetic creams that contain calomel.

Perhaps the most controversial and widely publicized episode of environmental exposure to hazardous wastes was that of the Love Canal neighborhood of Niagara Falls, New York. In the 1940s, chemical companies filled an abandoned canal with toxic wastes including chlorinated hydrocarbons, amounting to more than 21,000 tons of more than 200 different chemicals. In 1953, Hooker Chemical and Plastics Company sold the property to the Niagara Falls Board of Education for one dollar. Hooker maintains that the board was told the site was not suitable for a school, and the deed apparently contains a clause indicating the presence of the waste with provisions that no claims could be filed. In the late 1950s, about 100 homes were built along the banks of the dirt-covered canal, with a school built in the center. Residents noticed chemicals migrating through the topsoil, children falling in the soil received chemical burns, and there were odors and seepage in basements. Eventually, the anger and fears of the residents became largely directed at the state health department, because the chemical companies were major employers in the area and the state was not perceived as taking adequate actions. Differences also existed within the scientific community as to the handling, analysis, and interpretation of data. For example, data on spontaneous abortions and birth defects could be analyzed by simple proximity to the canal center, or by those homes designated as "wet" (those which were on former stream beds from the canal) versus "dry" homes. A study that was about 15 years old was chosen as the control group for comparing the frequency of spontaneous abortions. This study had a preselected population and bias because it was done on a group of women with previous problem pregnancies. Debate also centered on the methods and results of chromosome studies, including the lack of a contemporary control group. Also controversial was the method of interpretation of data related to cancer development in the Love Canal area. Love Canal has now been deemed safe for occupancy by some, and new homes have been sold in that area.

Toxic exposure to lead has occurred by means of environmental pollution through air and contaminated water and agricultural soil, from substances such as lead-based paint in older homes, and also through the workplace, as people in many occupations are exposed to lead. Exposures from hobbies may also occur. A comparison of pregnancy outcomes was done in two Missouri cities—Rolla, in the lead mining belt, and Columbia, which is not in the belt. In Rolla there was a statistically higher rate of prematurity and molar pregnancies. Other studies have indicated sperm abnormalities and decreased fertility in male lead workers and increased spontaneous abortion rates in their wives. Some workers have found an increased rate of chromosome aberrations, whereas others have not. In adults, presentation may include unexplained neurological symptoms, attention deficit disorder, arthralgias, or headaches. It is believed that the fetus may be sensitive to lead but not manifest such sensitivity until early childhood in the form of impaired intelligence, subtle neurobehavioral changes, growth delay including decreased height and weight, speech, language or attention deficits, behavior abnormalities, and developmental deficits. The effect of lead exposure particularly prenatally and in infancy in regard to future social behavior is a relatively new area of study. This includes aggressive and criminal acts as related to lead exposure. Microcytic anemia may be seen. It can be difficult to sort out prenatal effects from environmental exposure in infancy and childhood. Low birth weight may be associated with lead exposure. Various genetic factors may influence the vulnerability of the brain to lead as well as lead absorption. Recent studies have indicated that higher blood lead concentrations, even below 10 μg per deciliter (the "acceptable" level), are associated with a decline in IQ points in children 3 to 5 years of age (Canfield et al., 2003). Delays in pubertal development have also been associated with environmental lead exposure (Selevan et al., 2003). The definition of "acceptable" lead levels in children has been decreased over time, and it is thought that the current level may be too high.

Prevention of lead exposure is critical, and if children live in areas of exposure, Rogan and Ware (2003) state that this exposure should be interrupted. This is not always easy to accomplish in a short period of time. In areas where the drinking water is high in lead, nurses can advise women planning pregnancy to have their water checked and use an alternate source, such as bottled water, for drinking, if necessary. Additionally, household substances such as paint, dust in contaminated areas, or contamination through employment such as construction work can pose a risk to the worker and the family. It is important to advocate safe environmental lead levels, and to provide the necessary education and resources such as public health departments to make homes and communities safe from lead contamination. Good preconceptional counseling and prenatal care can help the mother reduce lead exposure in pregnancy and after. Of special interest to nurses are the results of many research studies of the toxic effects of waste anesthetic gases. The first such report was in 1967 in which 18 of 31 pregnancies in the Russian anesthetists surveyed terminated in spontaneous abortion. Other small studies led to a large-scale one that involved the American Association of Nurse Anesthetists, the Association of Operating Room Nurses, the Association of Operating Room Technicians, and the American Society of Anesthesiologists. Control groups were sections of the American Nurses Association and the American Academy of Pediatrics. Questionnaires were sent to 49,585 operating room personnel and 23,911 persons in the control group. This study showed a statistically significant increase in spontaneous abortion, congenital anomalies in the live-born infants of both exposed females and the wives of exposed males, and for cancer, hepatic, and renal disease in exposed females when compared with controls. Other researchers have demonstrated an increased rate of stillbirths in exposed females and decreased birth weight. Smoking was associated with higher risks. Other studies have found dentists and dental technicians to be at higher risk for the same problems. Interestingly, the increased rate of anomalies did not return to normal until the person was absent from the operating room for 2 years.

Although these studies have not demonstrated a direct cause-and-effect relationship, one precaution has been the scavenging of waste anesthetic gases and minimal exposure. These procedures have evolved over time to minimize risks. A detailed recent review by Burm (2003) reviews past studies, including directed criticisms of methodology, especially in those that were retrospective. He does note that chronic exposure to nitrous oxide concentrations of 1,000 ppm or higher was teratogenic in animals, and that at higher levels found in today's operating rooms, some inhalational anesthetics can affect perceptual, cognitive, and motor skills. He provides information to limit occupational exposure to anesthetics. Personnel in the operating room should be aware of the risks and make an informed decision as to whether they wish to take such a risk. Hospitals and other places using anesthesia should take appropriate measures to minimize the presence of waste anesthetic gases in the operating room environment. For persons with previous spontaneous abortions or birth defects in their offspring, choosing another work location may be more important than for others.

The largest radiation accident occurred at the Chernobyl nuclear power plant in the Ukraine on April 26, 1986. The most contaminated areas were the Ukraine, Belarus, and the Russian Federation, but other areas of Europe were exposed. At least five million people were exposed to ionizing radiation as a result. One of the major outcomes was the increase in childhood thyroid cancer when compared with pre-Chernobyl figures. In addition, children exposed during early pregnancy in Greece were 2.6 times more likely to develop leukemia than those who were unexposed. Some children exposed in utero were said to exhibit mental retardation and behavioral effects. Excesses in unstable chromosome-type aberrations were seen but not chromatid-type aberrations.

The occurrence of other well-known episodes of toxic exposures include pesticide spraying in Alsea, Oregon and Cape May, New Jersey; ketone exposure in Virginia; the 1976 explosion at a chemical plant in Seveso, Italy, releasing dioxin into the environment; the mass contamination of cooking oil leading to polychlorinated biphenyl (PCB) poisoning in Japan and Taiwan; the contamination of animal feed, animals, and human food by polybrominated biphenyls (PBB) in Michigan; the exposure of Times Beach, Missouri residents to dioxin; the exposure of civilian and military personnel to Agent Orange in Vietnam and the exposure to various agents in Persian Gulf war veterans. The issue of birth defects among Gulf War veterans is not fully settled. A large-scale study found that certain birth defects conceived postwar were at higher prevalence but the study did not determine if the cause was genetic or environmental factors. Children born postwar to Gulf War male veterans had an excess of tricuspid valve insufficiency, aortic valve stenosis, and renal agenesis or hypoplasia, while those born to women veterans had an excess or hypospadias in male infants. Such episodes, plus daily exposure to substances on the job, and by virtue of home location, have impelled members of the scientific community to develop protocols and measurement end points to be used in such investigations and present various study designs, depending on the type of exposure and other factors. Nurses should know that such guidelines are available for use, because poorly conducted research will result in unusable data that will not benefit anyone involved, least of all the exposed population.

There are more than 100,000 waste sites in the United States. Therefore, nurses should be prepared to deal with the types of issues identified by the Love Canal incident. These included inadequate communication among professionals and between professionals and residents, misconceptions about what the research studies could actually show, inadequate attention to the needs and fears of the residents, poor preparation and planning for the research needed to examine the impact of the wastes on the health problems present, and the political issues and legal liabilities that impinged on the entire investigation. Other exposures may occur in communities due to wastewater disposal or even the chlorination disinfection of drinking water, which suggest that by-products such as trihalomethanes and trichloroethylene may be associated with certain birth defects and adverse pregnancy outcomes.

Another important aspect of both environmental and workplace exposures has to do with socioeconomic status. Often it is those in lower socioeconomic groups who experience actual and potential toxic environmental exposures through housing, or because of the type of job available to them. Society is not always willing or able to spend the necessary resources for environmental cleanup and protection activities. The nurse who is involved with potential or actual hazardous exposures in the community or workplace may feel role conflict between responsibility to the employer and to the client. There are some ways in which he or she can participate in the prevention of such hazards and the protection of the client, both as a citizen and as a professional. Some ways involve consideration of the following questions:

1. Which agents are of major concern in causing genetic damage or carcinogenesis?
2. How can they be accurately identified before exposure occurs?
3. What actions should be taken when a potential genotoxic agent is discovered?
4. What are minimum safe levels of exposure?
5. How can exposure be minimized?
6. Are there protective devices and measures that can be taken?
7. What are they?
8. Are they likely to result in nonadherence?
9. Can individuals who are susceptible to damage by a specific agent because of their genetic constitution be identified?
10. If so, how should this information be used?
11. What weight should it have?
12. Does it affect males and females the same way?
13. If not, what special precautions must be taken?
14. What information should be given to workers? Should all workers know their genetic profile in relation to toxic chemicals?
15. How should this information be presented?
16. How can their risks be explained to them in a noncoercive, realistic manner?

Some of these problems are addressed in the next section. It is important for the nurse to have the deserved confidence of the client so that effective protection can take place.

TESTING, SURVEILLANCE, AND GENETIC MONITORING

There are several approaches that can be taken for the minimization of genetic hazards from agents used in the workplace and encountered in the environment. They include:

1. identifying agents with potential mutagenic, teratogenic, and carcinogenic effects before widespread human exposure occurs, by the use of various types of assays including the comet assay which can directly study geno-toxicity in cells exposed to a variety of agents, and through the use of large toxi-cogenomic databases;
2. devising appropriate regulations, controls, standardization, and guidelines for the use of such agents;
3. monitoring the emission of toxic substances and the concentration and levels of toxic agents emitted into the atmosphere, water, food, and so on of the environment and workplace;
4. using protective practices and devices within the workplace;
5. using preemployment screening and testing; and
6. using on-going periodic genetic monitoring of those believed to be exposed to toxic agents.

Various new methods of monitoring and sta-nardization are being developed using DNA and RNA microarray and profiling technology for both detecting genetic variations and gene expression variations leading to risk assessment and monitoring.

WORKPLACE SCREENING AND TESTING

The use of genetic testing and/or screening before or during employment has been controversial. On the one hand, they could be used to minimize the deleterious genetic effects of agents used in the workplace by identifying the genetically predisposed or hypersusceptible individual, before employment in the particular industry or before assignment to a new location where different potentially hazardous substances will be encountered. On the other hand such use could lead to stigmatization and various types of discrimination including job loss. At present, only a small number of individuals who have genetically determined differences in susceptibility to environmental agents found in the workplace can be identified,

but the potential is growing. In addition, the use of such testing to determine possession of genes for susceptibility to diseases such as colon or breast cancer or for the development of a late-onset disorder such as Huntington disease presents dilemmas. What is the potential for discrimination not only in terms of initial employment but also for promotion opportunities? Can a company refuse to hire a qualified individual because testing shows they will eventually develop Huntington disease? Can such discrimination extend to family genetic testing? Genetic screening and testing are discussed in chapter 11.

In one recent case of genetic testing of employees in the workplace, a legal challenge filed in 2001 stated that the Burlington Northern Railway Company was requiring those who claimed work-related carpal tunnel syndrome to undergo DNA testing for a genetic predisposition to this disorder, specifically deletion of the peripheral myelin protein-22 gene. This deletion can result in hereditary neuropathy with a liability to pressure palsies that can result in carpal tunnel syndrome. Brandt-Rauf and Brandt-Rauf (2004) related that at least one person was not told that blood samples requested were for genetic testing, and that one person who refused was threatened with firing if he did not comply. The company agreed to stop such testing. As discussed in chapter 11, not fulfilling informed consent, coercion, and not providing genetic counseling did not fulfill minimum standards for genetic testing or screening.

There may be some justification in determining susceptibility to agents used at the employment site. On one side is the argument that such identification diminishes health hazards, can prevent severe reactions or disease, and allows early diagnosis and ongoing monitoring for the identified individual. On the other side is concern about an approach that may "blame the victim," and decrease the responsibility of the industry to control hazardous environmental conditions. At one point, the Occupational Safety and Health Administration (OSHA) medical surveillance requirements and National Institute for Occupational Safety and Health (NIOSH) bulletin recommendations for preplacement for occupational exposure to certain chemicals required "genetic factors" to be included in the personal, family, and occupational history. In 1997, Andrews estimated that 1 in 20

U.S. companies were using or planning to use routine genetic screening and monitoring along with tests for genetic susceptibility. On the other hand, employers might be expected to protect their employees from hazards in the workplace by use of genetic testing. For example, the Dow Chemical Company was sued by the widow of a worker who had died from leukemia who claimed that cytogenetic testing might have detected early indications of leukemia development secondary to the worker's exposure to benzene in the workplace. It is expected that the use of genetic testing in the workplace will grow and that the issues engendered by such use must be sufficiently addressed before growth occurs.

Some of the known genetically determined differences in susceptibility that manifest problems after certain exposures include the following:

1. Persons with G6PD deficiency may experience hemolysis on exposure to certain chemicals such as aniline, acetanilid, benzene, carbon tetrachloride, chloroprene, lead, nitrites, toluidine, and others;

2. Exposure to respiratory irritants and cigarette smoke aggravates respiratory disease in persons with alpha-l-antitrypsin deficiency;

3. Hypersensitivity on immunologic skin tests can detect sensitivity to organic isocyanates and indicate which individuals are most likely to exhibit an asthma-like syndrome or a delayed hypersensitivity response when exposed;

4. Persons who are slow acetylators of N-acetyltransferase, which inactivates chemical arylamines such as naphthylamine, benzidine, and others, may have higher risks of bladder cancer when exposed to these agents;

5. Persons with the low activity form of the enzyme paraoxinase, which inactivates the pesticide parathion, may be predisposed to developing poisoning at low levels of exposure, either as spray pilots, mixers, field hands, or from general environmental exposure. An interesting example followed the release of sarin, a nerve gas, in Tokyo in 1995. It is believed that those who died were more vulnerable than others because their paraoxanase activity was such that they did not convert the sarin to a less toxic chemical rapidly enough;

6. Those with reduced capacity to metabolize carbon disulfide may develop sensitivities such as polyneuritis.

Regardless of the type of screening used, the meaning of the test and what it actually shows must be understood. An example of widespread misunderstanding was the restriction of persons with sickle cell trait from becoming pilots in the United States Air Force because of the inaccurate belief that high altitudes could not be tolerated. Genetic testing should not be used to discriminate. However, only relatively few states have laws prohibiting employer discrimination on the basis of genetic testing. In a suit that was filed in California, it was alleged that black employees had been tested for the sickle cell gene mutation without their consent. The suit was dismissed on grounds that this did not consitute employee privacy intrusion! Although the Equal Employment Opportunity Commission (EEOC) compliance manual for ADA states that under ADA employers cannot discriminate based on genetic information, how extensive this is and whether full protection is offered is debated. National legislation is needed for protection. The workplace may also be a site for a population screening for genetic disorders or carrier conditions. For example such screening has been conducted for hemochromatosis. However, while the usual standards for genetic screening must be met in such programs, maintaining privacy and confidentiality and protecting workers from any adverse effects on employment are extremely important.

SMOKING IN THE WORKPLACE

Increased evidence of adverse effects of smoking and exposure to environmental agents led to the issuance of a NIOSH bulletin indicating ways in which smoking can interact with occupational exposures to chemical and physical agents, whether genetically susceptible or not.

Nurses can make a real contribution to the promotion of health and disease prevention by the development, initiation, and evaluation of smoking cessation programs for workers and their families. Because such programs benefit both, they usually have the support of worker and company representatives. Some companies now exclude smokers from sites with unavoidable respiratory exposure and are preferentially hiring nonsmokers over smokers. This may provide additional motivation to the worker to stop smoking. Smoking also increases the risk for workers who are genetically susceptible to respiratory disease, as for example in persons with alpha-l-antitrypsin deficiency (see chapter 22).

SHORT-TERM ASSAYS

Ideally agents with the potential for causing mutagenesis, teratogenesis, and carcinogenesis would be identified before human exposure occurs, so that the agent would either not be widely distributed, another less toxic agent could serve as a substitute, or, if the agent was essential for production or use, proper precautions, guidelines, and protective mechanisms could be devised. There is no one short-term test that can detect all classes of chemical mutagens or carcinogens, although more than 100 such assays have been developed. National and international collaborative efforts are seeking to develop a battery of assays that would be valid, reliable, sensitive, nonrepetitive, inexpensive, and test for different types of mutation in a variety of organisms. Some agents show a mutagenic effect in some test assays and not in others, or in certain organisms but not others. It can be difficult to extrapolate results accurately to humans, and to include all types of mutation at the level of DNA, the gene, and the chromosome. In addition, humans usually have the capacity to repair DNA damage. Mechanisms that can result in gene mutation vary. A comprehensive battery of tests must include the possibility that an agent can cause a variety of effects. In addition, some agents do not exhibit a mutagenic or carcinogenic effect unless they are metabolically activated, so that assays may need to include this component. The unique genetic makeup of an individual also influences his/her response. In general, the more long-term the assay is, the more expensive it is. Some effects may be missed in short-term assays and if small numbers of test organisms are used.

GENETIC MONITORING

Periodic genetic monitoring of individuals exposed to toxic agents in the workplace have usually used the following tests: chromosome analysis for sister chromatid exchange (SCE) and chromosome aberrations; body fluid analysis for mutagenic activity; and semen analysis for sperm counts, motility, morphology, and nondisjunction. However, more sophisticated technology using DNA sequencing and gene expression arrays are now available. Many companies use one or more of these tests before employment so that they can compare these results with future findings. Chromosome analysis already is used in workers exposed to radiation and radioactivity. SCE refers to exchanges between homologous sites on two chromatids of the same chromosome. They appear to be a consequence of exposure to mutagens and are detected using special media. Their significance, and the mechanism causing their occurrence, are not currently well understood. The detection of chromosomal abnormalities is directed mainly at breakage and certain structural aberrations. There are differences among cytogeneticists in their scoring of certain aberrations, particularly between chromosome and chromatid gaps and breaks. Many believe that using certain configurations, such as dicentric chromosomes and ring chromosomes, is less ambiguous and are less likely to be caused by the action of other agents. Such studies need to be interpreted in the light of the person's habits and exposures, for example, diagnostic X-rays, drugs, recreation, medications, cigarette smoking, infectious diseases, and history. There is disagreement about the clinical significance and the extrapolation that can be made from the findings of chromosome abnormalities, especially since repair may occur. In addition, different laboratories report varying background levels of chromosomal breakage due to differences in culture techniques, and thus it can be difficult to compare findings between laboratories.

Body fluids such as urine, blood, feces, or breast milk can be used in microbial test systems such as the Ames test to detect mutagenic activity from increased rates of gene mutation. Detection of somatic cell mutation for five genes, hypoxanthine phosphoribosyl transferase, glycophorin A, antigens at the HLA locus, DNA adducts, specific hemoglobin mutations, and the loss of T cell receptors from peripheral T lymphocytes have been used recently as direct mutation measures. Semen analysis in male workers can be used to examine sperm counts, motility, morphology, and the presence of double Y bodies. The presence of the latter infers nondisjunction in other chromosomes as well. Such nondisjunction has some preliminary correlation with exposure to certain drugs and radiation as well as to chemicals. Increased rates of double Y bodies in sperm mandates discussion regarding genetic counseling and continued monitoring if the couple plans conception. If the female is already pregnant, amniocentesis may be advised. Sperm production can be affected directly by agents or indirectly by hormonal interference. Aberrant sperm counts or motility can be related to infertility. Although semen samples are more easily accessible than examining the male gamete in other ways, it may be repugnant to many male workers and needs to be accompanied by discussion and counseling.

PROTECTIVE DEVICES AND PRACTICES

Concern about the effect of certain chemical and physical agents on fertile women has also been a source of some controversy. Regulations have been devised in regard to substances to which the pregnant worker cannot be exposed. In some cases, concern has also been directed as to the employment of fertile women in certain industries or for work with certain agents. This is because, in some cases, the agent in question is not universally recognized as having mutagenic or teratogenic effects and exposure may thus not be regulated; women may choose to work in such areas because of pay advantages and therefore assume risk; or they may even choose sterilization because they perceive the risk of job loss if they become pregnant. Some companies have offered comparable pay at other jobs for fertile or pregnant women when the substance is known to be fetotoxic. Others have instead immorally, and in some circumstances illegally, withheld raises or promotion unless women chose to be sterilized in order to stay at certain jobs with risky exposures. This whole issue is fraught with complexities about sex and job discrimination and legal compensation. Substances can be mutagenic or affect the fetus through the male, directly or indirectly, such as secondary exposure of the wives of such employees through contaminated clothing and other items. Physical protective measures such as the use of respirators and protective clothing may be used to minimize exposure to employees handling some known toxic substances. In these instances, compliance may be an important factor because of the severe discomfort associated with such protection or because of failure to associate danger with substances that are odorless, colorless, and tasteless with no immediately apparent effect. Some employers consider employees also responsible for their own protection in their (a) adherence to safety regulations and (b) relation to personal habits such as cigarette smoking or alcohol consumption, which may increase their risk of carcinogenesis.

SURVEILLANCE

Surveillance for genetic effects of chemical agents may be done in the workplace or in the general environment. For example, monitoring the rates of spontaneous abortions, general or specific birth defects, and an increased incidence of specific cancers are methods that are used to try to detect a change that may be attributed to a specific agent that has been previously undetected. This may be done among specific workers and their spouses, or in specific geographic areas. There can be difficulties because (1) there can be many different etiologies for these outcomes, (2) the exposed populations are too small to readily establish statistical significance, or (3) the effects seen are only apparent years or decades after the event. As one can imagine, how easy would it be to connect a case of neuroblastoma in a child with his father's employment working with chlorinated hydrocarbon pesticides 4 years previously? A long-term study of the occupations of parents of infants with certain birth defects was conducted by the Centers for Disease Control and Prevention. Preliminary results indicated that nurses were found more frequently than expected among the mothers of infants with cleft lip or palate. There was an excess of printing industry employment among mothers of infants with omphalocele (a ventral congenital wall defect with herniation of the abdominal viscera covered by a membrane) and gastroschisis (a defect of the anterior abdominal wall with evisceration of abdominal contents not covered by a membrane. Hewitt's (1992) secondary analysis of nurses working with antineoplastic drugs found a higher relative risk for

TABLE 14.2   Selected Occupations and Potential Exposures to Toxic Agents

Occupation	Possible exposures
Barber, hairdresser, beautician	Aerosol propellants, hair dye, acetone, ethyl alcohol, benzyl alcohol, halogenated hydrocarbons, hair spray resins
Dentist, dental technicians	Mercury, nitrogen dioxide, anesthetics, X-rays, vibration
Farmer	Mercury, arsenic, lead, nitrogen dioxide, silica, pesticides, fertilizers
Dry cleaner	Benzene, contaminated clothing, trichloroethylene, naphtha
Nurse	Anesthetic gases, alcohol, ethylene oxide, carcinogenic agents, radiation, infectious agents, nitrogen dioxide
Photographer	Mercury, bromides, iodides, silver nitrate, caustic agents, iron salts, lead
Printer	Inks, antimony, lead, noise, vibration, benzene, methylene chloride
Textile industry	Cotton dust, synthetic fiber dust, formaldehyde, benzene, toluene, chloroprene, styrene, carbon disulfide, heat

the development of leukemia and other cancers than in the controls. Nurses' risks with these drugs have also been found by many others. Nurses, like workers in any other industry where toxic agents are used, should be aware of specific hazards and take advantage of protective measures. Some states are now acquiring detailed occupational data on birth certificates, but some view this as an invasion of privacy. When taking an occupational or recreational history, the nurse should be sensitive to potential exposures commonly found among certain occupations. Some of these are listed in Table 14.2. Questions pertinent to the histories are discussed in chapter 9.

SUMMARY

Chemical and physical agents in our environment constantly bombard us whether it be at home, at work, at school, or at leisure. Various genes are involved in the metabolism of such chemicals and in mechanisms of repair in response to them. Understanding has increased as to the role that genes play in the manifestation of effects from both short-term and long-term exposures, but there is still not a uniform consensus on the best ways to assess damage or on the interpretation of results. The field of toxicogenomics is addressing many of these issues by new molecular techniques and bioinformatic support. In addition to the projects of the Environmental Genome Project of the National Institute of Environmental Health Sciences, NIH, there is a proposed National Children's

study protocol to examine childhood environmental exposures from prenatal through 21 years of age. Nonetheless, education and prevention remain important components for addressing environmental hazards to health and reproduction.

BIBLIOGRAPHY

Alavanja, M. C. R., Hoppin, J. A., & Kamel, F. (2004). Health effects of chronic pesticide exposure: Cancer and neurotoxicity. *Annual Review of Public Health, 25,* 155–197.

Aleem, A., & Malik, A. (2003). Genotoxic hazards of long-term application of wastewater on agricultural soil. *Mutation Research, 538,* 145–154.

Andrews, L. (1997). Body science. *American Bar Association Journal, 83,* 44–49.

Anwar, W. A. (1997). Biomarkers of human exposure to pesticides. *Environmental Health Perspectives, 105*(Suppl. 4), 801–806.

Araneta, M. R., Schlangen, K. M., Edmonds, L. D., Destiche, D. A., Merz, R. D., Hobbs, C. A., et al. (2003). Prevalence of birth defects among infants of Gulf War veterans in Arkansas, Arizona, California, Georgia, Hawaii, and Iowa, 1989–1993. *Birth Defects Research Part A Clinical and Molecular Teratology, 67*(4), 246–260.

Baden, J. M., & Simmon, V. F. (1980). Mutagenic effects of inhalational anesthetics. *Mutation Research, 75,* 169–189.

Barrett, J. C., Vainio, H., Peakall, D., & Goldstein, B. D. (1997). 12th meeting of the Scientific Group on Methodologies for the Safety Evaluation of

Chemicals: Susceptibility to environmental hazards. *Environmental Health Perspectives, 105*(Suppl. 4), 699–738.

Bellinger, D. C. (2004). Lead. *Pediatrics, 113*, 1016–1022.

Black, C. M., Welsh, K. L., Walker, A. E., Bernstein, R. M., Catoggio, L. J., & McGregor, A. R. (1983). Genetic susceptibility to scleroderma-like syndrome induced by vinyl chloride. *Lancet, 1*, 53–55.

Bolognesi, C. (2003). Genotoxicity of pesticides: A review of human biomonitoring studies. *Mutation Research, 543*, 251–272.

Bove, F., Shim, Y., & Zeitz, P. (2002). Drinking water contaminants and adverse pregnancy outcomes: A review. *Environmental Health Perspectives, 110*(Suppl. 1), 61–74.

Brandt-Rauf, P. W., & Brandt-Rauf, S. I. (2004). Genetic testing in the workplace: Ethical, legal, and social implications. *Annual Review of Public Health, 25*, 139–153.

Brent, R. L. (2004). Utilization of animal studies to determine the effects and human risks of environmental toxicants (drugs, chemicals, and physical agents). *Pediatrics, 113*, 984–995.

Brent, R. L., Tanski, S., & Weitzman, M. (2004). Pediatric perspective on the unique vulnerability and resilience of the embryo and child to environmental toxicants: The importance of rigorous research concerning age and agent. *Pediatrics, 113*, 935–944.

Brent, R. L., & Weitzman, M. (2004). The current state of knowledge about the effects, risks, and science of children's environmental exposures. *Pediatrics, 113*, 1158–1166.

Brown, P., & Clapp, R. (2002). Looking back on Love Canal. *Public Health Reports, 117*, 95–98.

Burm, A. G. L. (2003). Occupational hazards of inhalational anaesthetics. *Best Practice & Research Clinical Anaesthesiology, 17*, 147–161.

Burdorf, A., & Van Tongeren, M. (2003). Commentary: Variability in workplace exposures and the design of efficient measurement and control strategies. *Annals of Occupational Hygiene, 47*, 95–99.

Canfield, R. L., Henderson, C. R., Jr., Cory-Slechta, D. A., Cox, C., Jusko, T. A., & Lanphear, B. P. (2003). Intellectual impairment in children with blood lead concentrations below 10µg per deciliter. *New England Journal of Medicine, 348*, 1517–1526.

Chapin, R. E., Robbins, W. A., Scieve, L. A., Sweeney, A. M., Tabacova, S. A., & Tomashek, K. M. (2004). Off to a good start: The influence of pre- and periconceptional exposures, parental fertility, and nutrition on children's health. *Environmental Health Perspectives, 112*, 69–78.

Clarkson, T. W., Magos, L., & Myers, G. J. (2004). The toxicology of mercury—Current exposures and clinical manifestations. *New England Journal of Medicine, 349*, 1731–1737.

Cohen, E. N., Brown, B. W., Wu, M., et al. (1979). Anesthetic health hazards in the dental operatory. *Anesthesiology, 51*, S254.

Cohen, F. L. (1986.). Paternal contributions to birth defects. *Nursing Clinics of North America, 21*(1), 49–64.

Colburn, T., Dumanoski, D., & Myers, J. P. (1996). *Our stolen future.* New York: Dutton.

Costa, L. G., Cole, T. B., Jarvik, G. P., & Furlong, C. E. (2003). Functional genomics of the paraoxonase (PON1) polymorphisms: Effects on pesticide sensitivity, cardiovascular disease, and drug metabolism. *Annual Review of Medicine, 54*, 371–392.

Culliton, B. J. (1980). Continuing confusion over Love Canal. *Science, 209*, 1002–1003.

da Silva Augusto, L. G., Liber, S. R., Ruiz, M. A., & Deouza, C. A. (1997). Micronucleus monitoring to assess human occupational exposure to organochlorides. *Environmental and Molecular Mutagenesis, 29*, 46–52.

Davidson, P. W., Myers, G. J., & Weiss, B. (2004). Mercury exposure and child development outcomes. *Pediatrics, 113*, 1023–1029.

Dolk, H. (2004). Epidemiologic approaches to identifying environmental causes of birth defects. *American Journal of Medical Genetics, Part C (Seminars in Medical Genetics), 125C*, 4–11.

Emory, E., Ansari, Z., Pattillo, R., Archibold, E., & Chevalier, J. (2003). Maternal blood lead effects on infant intelligence at age 7 months. *American Journal of Obstetrics and Gynecology, 188*, S26–S32.

Garfunkel, A. A., & Galili, D. (1996). Dental health care workers at risk. *Dental Clinics of North America, 40*(2), 277–291.

Greim, H. A. (2004). The endocrine and reproductive system: Adverse effects of hormonally active substances? *Pediatrics, 113*, 1070–1075.

Hartmann, A., Plappert, U., Poetter, F., & Suter, W.

(2003). Comparative study with the alkaline Comet assay and the chromosome aberration test. *Mutation Research, 536,* 27–38.

Hay, A. (1983). Defoliates in Vietnam: The long-term effects. *Nature, 302,* 208–209.

Health Consequences of the Chernobyl Accident. (1996). *World Health Statistics Quarterly, 49*(1), 72.

Hemminki, K. (1997). DNA adducts and mutations in occupational and environmental biomonitoring. *Environmental Health Perspectives, 105*(Suppl. 4), 823–827.

Hewitt, J. B. (1992). *Cancer risks of nurses to assess the carcinogenic potential of antineoplastic drugs.* Unpublished doctoral dissertation. University of Illinois at Chicago.

Holmberg, K., Meijer, A. E., Harms-Ringdahl, M., & Lambert, B. (1998). Chromosomal instability in human lymphocytes after low dose rate gamma-irradiation and delayed mitogen stimulation. *International Journal of Radiation Biology, 73,* 21–34.

Iannaccone, P. M. (2001). Toxicogenomics: "The call of the wild chip." *Environmental Health Perspectives, 109,* A8–A11.

Kaiser, J. (2003). Tying genetics to the risk of environmental diseases. *Science, 300,* 563.

Knill-Jones, R. P., Newman, B. J., & Spence, A. A. (1975). Anaesthetic practice and pregnancy. *Lancet, 2,* 807–809.

Kolata, G. B. (1980). Love Canal: False alarm caused by botched study. *Science, 208,* 1239–1242.

Kramer, D. A. (2005). Commentary: Gene-environment interplay in the context of genetics, epigenetics, and gene expression. *Journal of the American Academy of Child and Adolescent Psychiatry, 44,* 19–27.

Lash, L. H., Hines, R. N., Gonzalez, F. J., Zacharewski, T. R., & Rothstein, M. A. (2003). Genetics and susceptibility to toxic chemicals: Do you (or should you) know your genetic profile? *Journal of Pharmacology and Experimental Therapeutics, 305,* 403–409.

Lidsky, T. I., & Schneider, J. S. (2003). Lead neurotoxicity in children: Basic mechanisms and clinical correlates. *Brain, 126,* 5–19.

Mattingly, C. J., Colby, G. T., Forrest, J. N., & Boyer, J. L. (2003). The Comparative Toxicogenomics Database (CTD). *Environmental Health Perspectives, 111,* 793–795.

Merrick, B. A. (2003). The Human Proteome Organization (HUPO) and environmental health. *Environmental Health Perspectives, 111,* 797–801.

Miller, R. W. (2004). How environmental hazards in childhood have been discovered: Carcinogens, teratogens, neurotoxicants, and others. *Pediatrics, 113,* 945–951.

Nailor, M. G., Tariton, F., & Cassidy, J. J. (Eds.). (1978, September). Love Canal—public health time bomb. A special report to the governor and legislature. Albany, New York: State Department of Health.

Nisselle, A. E., Delatycki, M. B., Collins, V., Metcalfe, S., Aitken, M. A., du Sart, D., et al. (2004). Implementation of HaemScreen, a workplace-based genetic screening program for hemochromatosis. *Clinical Genetics, 65,* 358–367.

Nordström, S., Beckman, L., & Nordenson, I. (1979). Occupational and environmental risks in and around a smelter in northern Sweden. *Hereditas, 90,* 297–302.

Orphanides, G. (2003). Toxicogenomics: Challenges and opportunities. *Toxicology Letters, 140–141,* 145–148.

Paigen, B. (1982). Controversy at Love Canal. *Hastings Center Reports, 12*(3), 29–37.

Petridou, E., Trichopoulos, D., Dessypris, N., Flytzani, V., Haidas, S., Kalmanti, M., et al. (1996). Infant leukemia after in utero exposure to radiation from Chernobyl. *Nature, 382,* 352–353.

Picciano, D. (1980). Love Canal chromosome study. *Science, 209,* 754.

Rabinowitz, P. M., & Poljak, A. (2003). Host-environment medicine. *Journal of General Internal Medicine, 18,* 222–227.

Reich, M. R. (1983). Environmental politics and science: The case of PBB contamination in Michigan. *American Journal of Public Health, 73,* 302–313.

Rogan, W. J. (1982). PCBs and cola-colored babies: Japan, 1968, and Taiwan, 1979. *Teratology, 26,* 259–261.

Rogan, W. J., & Ware, J. H. (2003). Exposure to lead in children—how low is low enough? *New England Journal of Medicine, 348,* 1515–1516.

Rowland, A. D., Baird, D. D., Weinberg, C. R., Shore, D., Shy, C. M., & Wilcox, A. (1992). Reduced fertility among women employed as dental assistants exposed to high levels of nitrous oxide. *New England Journal of Medicine,* *327,* 993–997.

Salomaa, S., Sevan'kaev, A. V., Zhloba, A. A., Kumpusalo, E., Makinen, S., Lindholm, C., et al. (1997). Unstable and stable chromosomal aberrations in lymphocytes of people exposed to Chernobyl fallout in Bryansk, Russia. *International Journal of Radiation Biology, 71,* 51–59.

Samet, J. M., DeMarini, D. M., & Malling, H. V. (2004). Do airborne particles induce heritable mutations? *Science, 304,* 971–972.

Sarna, L., Bialous, S. A., Wewers, M. E., Froelicher, E. S., & Danao, L. (2005). Nurses, smoking, and the workplace. *Research in Nursing and Health, 28,* 79–90.

Savitz, D. A., & Chen, J. (1990). Parental occupation and childhood cancer: Review of epidemiologic studies. *Environmental Health Perspectives, 88,* 325–327.

Schulte, P. A. (2004). Some implications of genetic biomarkers in occupational epidemiology and practice. *Scandinavian Journal of Work and Environmental Health, 30,* 71–79.

Schwartz, J. (2004). Air pollution and children's health. *Pediatrics, 113,* 1037–1043.

Selevan, S. G., Lindbohm, H., Hornung, R. W., & Hemminki, K. (1985). A study of occupational exposure to antineoplastic drugs and fetal loss in nurses. *New England Journal of Medicine, 313,* 1173–1178.

Selevan, S. G., Rice, D. C., Hogan, K. A., Euling, S. Y., Pfahles-Hutchens, A., & Bethel, J. (2003). Blood lead concentration and delayed puberty in girls. *New England Journal of Medicine, 348,* 1527–1536.

Senn, K. M., McGuinness, B. M., Buck, G. M., Vena, J. E., Anderson, S., & Rogers, B. T. (2005). Longitudinal study of babies born to mothers enrolled in a preconception prospective pregnancy study: Study design and methodology, New York State Angler cohort study. *Environmental Research, 97,* 163–169.

Shaw, M. J. (1980). Love Canal chromosome study. *Science, 209,* 751–752.

Shea, K. M., and the Committee on Environmental Health. (2003). Pediatric exposure and potential toxicity of phthalate plasticizers. *Pediatrics, 111,* 1467–1474.

Silbergeld, E. K., & Flaws, J. A. (2002). Environmental exposures and women's health. *Clinical Obstetrics and Gynecology, 45,* 1119–1128.

Skov, T., Maarup, B., Olsen, J., Rørth, M., Winthereik, H., & Lynge, E. (1992). Leukaemia and reproductive outcome among nurses handling antineoplastic drugs. *British Journal of Industrial Medicine, 49,* 855–861

Spence, M., Cohen, E. N., Brown, B. W., Jr., Knill-Jones, R. P., & Himmelberger, D. V. (1977). Occupational hazards for operating room-based physicians. *Journal of American Medical Association, 238,* 955–959.

Stewart, P. A., Stewart, W. F., Siemiatycki, J., Heineman, E. F., & Dosemeci, M. (1998). Questionnaires for collecting detailed occupational information for community-based case control studies. *American Industrial Hygiene Association Journal, 59,* 39–44.

Strobino, B. R., Kline, J., & Stein, Z. (1978). Chemical and physical exposures of parents: Effects on human reproduction and offspring. *Early Human Development, 1,* 371–399.

Stücker, I., Caillard, J-F., Collin, R., Gout, M., Poyen, D., & Hemon, D. (1990). Risk of spontaneous abortion among nurses handling antineoplastic drugs. *Scandanavian Journal of Work and Environmetnal Health, 16,* 102–107.

Sun, M. (1983). Missouri's costly dioxin lesson. *Science, 219,* 367–369.

Sze, J., & Prakash, S. (2004). Human genetics, environment, and communities of color: Ethical and social implications. *Environmental Health Perspectives, 112,* 740–745.

Tariton, F., & Cassidy, J. J. (1981, April). Love Canal—A special report to the governor and legislature. New York: NY State Department of Health.

Wagener, D. K., Selevan, S. G., & Sexton, K. (1995). The importance of human exposure information: A need for exposure-related data bases to protect and promote public health. *Annual Review of Public Health, 16,* 105–121.

Weiss, B., Amler, S., & Amler, R. W. (2004). Pesticides. *Pediatrics, 113,* 1030–1036.

World Health Organization. (2002). Vaccines and biologicals: Recommendations from the Strategic Advisory Group of Experts. *Weekly Epidemiological Record, 77,* 305–312.

15

Therapeutic Modalities

THERAPEUTIC STRATEGIES EMPLOYED IN GENETIC DISORDERS

Although prevention is the ideal goal for genetic disorders, various types of therapeutic management are available. Such management approaches depend on the nature of the defect, how well it is understood at the genetic and biochemical levels, and the practical feasibility of correction. In some conditions certain management is now tailored to the specific genotype. The client being treated may be the fetus, the infant, the child, or the adult. Treatment methods used in genetic disorders may involve surgical, cognitive/behavioral, pharmacologic, dietary, environmental avoidance, transfusion, plasma exchange, enzyme, behavioral, cell, or gene therapy (see Table 15.1). Some have been developed on the basis of knowledge of the defect in the gene and its product, whereas others are empirical or aimed at controlling or mediating signs and symptoms without cure. Different rationales thus underlie the previously described methods (see Table 15.2). They are basically aimed at (1) limiting the intake of a substrate or its precursor; (2) depleting the accumulation or promoting the excretion of a substrate, precursor, or product; (3) directly or indirectly replacing or stimulating production of the enzyme, gene product, or (4) replacing, repairing, or reprogramming the gene itself. For example, diet therapy may be based on the principle of limiting the amount of a specific substrate that cannot be adequately metabolized by the appropriate enzyme, as in phenylketonuria, or it might be aimed at providing a product needed in order to circumvent a metabolic pathway, as in the provision of uridine in orotic aciduria. Gene product replacement might involve the administration of the product

directly (e.g., insulin in type 1 diabetes mellitus) or indirectly by means of bone marrow transplantation (e.g., in severe combined immunodeficiency caused by adenosine deaminase deficiency). Toxic substances can be removed by chelation with drugs, plasmapheresis, or surgical bypass procedures. The administration of pharmacologic doses of vitamins supplies the needed cofactor for holoenzyme function in certain vitamin-responsive disorders.

Pharmacological approaches have taken advantage of underlying genetic mechanisms in certain disorders, most notably in treating certain cardiac conditions and cancers. For example, it is known that for some disorders, multiple combinations of therapies are necessary. In Refsum disease (an autosomal recessive disorder with retinitis pigmentosa, ataxia, peripheral neuropathy, and accumulation of phytanic acid), for example, both dietary restriction of phytanic acid and plasmapheresis at weekly intervals are usual. Correction of birth defects such as craniofacial anomalies or limb anomalies usually involves multiple phases of surgical treatment at various stages of the development of the individual, along with the use of prosthetic devices and a long rehabilitation. Such interventions require a skilled treatment group that is prepared to deal not only with the physical correction by surgery, but with the nursing, psychological, speech, hearing, and rehabilitative measures needed to achieve optimum results. Thus therapeutic approaches may range from a one-time surgical correction of a birth defect to a long-term special diet, to an infant stimulation program to improve maximum potential, to experimental gene replacement. This chapter concentrates on those therapeutic modalities that are unique to, or especially important in, genetic disorders, and those

TABLE 15.1   Treatment Methods Used in Selected Genetic Disorders

Method	Examples
Surgical	Reconstructive surgery in cleft lip and palate; Portacaval shunt in glycogen storage diseases I and III to limit deposition of glycogen. Liver transplant to provide missing enzymes in Wilson disease and hereditary tyrosinemia by replacing defective tissue. Bone marrow transplant to supply missing enzyme in severe combined immune deficiency caused by adenosine deaminase deficiency. Stem cell transplant in β-thalassemia Correct defect in congenital heart disease.
Pharmacological	Danazol (an androgen) in angioedema to prevent acute attacks. Tigason (a synthetic retinoid) in Darier disease (autosomal dominant skin disorder). Growth hormone in pituitary dwarfism. Insulin in type 1 diabetes mellitus. Zinc in acrodermatitis enteropathica (an autosomal recessive disorder) to ameliorate zinc deficiency and bring clinical improvement. Clofibrate in hyperlipoproteinemia III to decrease blood lipids.
Dietary	Limitation of phenylalanine in PKU for substrate restriction. Limitation of lactose and galactose in galactosemia for substrate restriction and prevention of accumulation. Administering uridine in orotic aciduria to inhibit the first enzyme in the metabolic pathway and decrease orotic acid.
Environmental avoidance	Avoiding mechanical stress to prevent fractures in osteogenesis imperfecta. Avoiding halothane and related anesthetics in malignant hyperthermia. Not eating fava (broad) bean in G6PD deficiency to prevent hemolytic anemia. Avoiding sulfonamides in unstable hemoglobins to prevent hemolysis. Avoiding alcohol consumption in acute intermittent porphyria. Avoiding ultraviolet light in xeroderma pigmentosa to minimize skin lesions.
Transfusion	Administration of factor VIII in hemophilia A as a replacement for the lacking circulating serum protein.
Behavioral	Infant stimulation program to maximize potential in Down syndrome and other syndromes that include developmental delay.
Plasmapheresis	In Refsum disease to remove high blood levels of phytanic acid due to defective metabolism.
Enzyme	By administering cofactor such as biotin to allow increased propionyl-CoA carboxylase activity in propionic acidemia. Intravenous administration of α-galactosidase A in Fabry disease.
Gene	Direct gene transfer of β hemoglobin gene copies into bone marrow cells of patients with β-thalassemia. Use of recombinant DNA to produce insulin. Use of ribozymes to inactivate expression of mutant gene.
Preventive	Genetic counseling. Genetic testing and screening. Prenatal detection and diagnosis. Newborn screening.

TABLE 15.2   Selected Approaches to Treatment of Genetic Disorders

Approach	Examples
Restricting or eliminating intake of substrate or precursor.	
Diet therapy	Restricting intake of the branched chain amino acids in MSUD, or phenylalanine in PKU, to prevent the accumulation of these substances and subsequent consequences.
Environmental avoidance	Nonuse of barbiturates in hepatic porphyrias.
Depleting the accumulation or promoting the excretion of a substrate, precursor, or unwanted product.	
Chelation	Using D-penicillamine as a chelating agent to deplete copper in Wilson disease. Using deferoxamine as a chelating agent to promote excretion of ferritin secondary to iron overload in β-thalassemia.
Surgical bypass	Surgical bypass procedures such as portacaval shunt in glycogen storage diseases I and III, and ileal jejunal bypass in hyperlipoproteinemia IIa to decrease cholesterol absorption from the gut.
Enhanced excretion	Enhancing excretion of bile salts to reduce serum cholesterol by giving cholestyramine in familial hypercholesterolemia. Promoting waste nitrogen excretion by giving arginine as a dietary supplement in patients with argininosuccinate synthetase deficiency.
Plasmapheresis (mechanical)	Plasmapheresis in Refsum disease for elimination of phytanic acid.
Metabolic inhibition	Clofibrate in hyperlipoprotenemia III to inhibit glyceride and decrease blood lipid levels.
Replacing or stimulating production of enzyme, gene product, or gene.	
Enzyme induction	Use of phenobarbital in Gilbert and Crigler-Najjar syndromes results in increased glucuronyl transferase.
Cofactor administration (in vitamin responsive forms)	Thiamine (B1) administration is pyruvic acidemia for pyruvate decarboxylase; in MSUD for branched chain ketoacid decarboxylase. Ascorbate administration in Ehler-Danlos syndrome VI for collagen lysyl hydroxylase. Pyridoxine (B6) in gyrate atrophy for ornithine ketoacid aminotransferase; in homo-cystinuria for cystathionine synthetase; in infantile convulsions caused by glutamic acid decarboxylase. Biotin in propionic acidemia for propionyl CoA carboxylase; in mixed carboxylase synthetase. Cobalamin (B12) for methylmalonicaciduria from adenosylcobalamin synthesis and methylmalonic CoA mutase. Folate for homocystinuria caused by methylenetetrahydrofolate reductase.
Enzyme administration (surgical and non-surgical approaches	Organ and tissue transplantation as in the kidney for Fabry disease and cystinosis; Islet cell transplantation for diabetes; liver for hereditary tyrosinemia; fibroblasts in mucopolysaccharide disorders. Transfusion of placental glucocerebrosidase in Gaucher disease (experimental). Intravenous infusion of α-galactosidase A in Fabry disease. Oral pancreatic enzyme supplementation in cystic fibrosis.
Direct administration of gene product	Factor VIII in classic hemophilia. Cortisol in congenital adrenogenital syndrome Thyroxine in congenital hypothyroidism.
Direct gene transfer	Factor IX in hemophilia B (experimental)
Blocking production of a protein.	
Antisense oligonucleotide therapy	Blocks translation of mRNA into protein; for example, in blocking conversion of angiotensinogen to angiotensin to control hypertension (experimental).

requiring understanding and manipulation of the genetic problem at a biochemical level or at the level of the gene itself.

DIET MANIPULATION

One of the most common therapeutic modalities likely to be encountered by the nurse is diet manipulation. Diet manipulation may be used to restrict or eliminate a specific substrate from the diet in order to prevent build-up of the substrate itself, its product in a specific metabolic pathway, or a metabolic byproduct. Such diet manipulations have been applied to several inherited biochemical disorders. Because of their rarity and complexity, specialized and expert team management is required and may be only available in specialized centers. After therapy is initiated, continued management can be accomplished in the person's home community. Often the community health or school nurse becomes the link between the family and a host of other professionals involved in the care. Because PKU is the most frequent among these, this will be discussed in detail as a prototype while others are briefly discussed. Principles that nurses can apply generally to patients on these long-term substrate restricted diets are given later.

Nursing Pointers

• Parents, and the child when old enough, need to understand the relationship of the basic defect in the disorder to the dietary restrictions. This should be explained in simple terms; all information should be culturally congruent at a level the client can understand. Written information should be supplied for them to refer to, understanding should be assessed periodically, and initial teaching should be reinforced. Programmed types of instructional material or videotapes may be an easy way to communicate the essentials. The shock accompanying initial diagnosis may result in the nonretention of factual material that is presented at such a time, and so the information should be repeated again at another time.

• Parents should be told orally and also in written form, the equipment that is necessary to have in the home to implement the diet and where it can be obtained. Some centers provide all necessary equipment.

• Parents must understand the dietary prescription and be able to use it with common household measurements. The importance of accurate measurement should be stressed.

• The dietary prescription should be given in written form and gone over verbally. All information should be in easily understood terms.

• Parents should be able to plan a sample day's diet from a given dietary prescription; the nurse can ask to have them do this while visiting the home.

• For the infant, formula preparation should be demonstrated. A return demonstration by the parents should be observed in their home so that potential problems can be averted and misunderstandings can be corrected.

• The meaning of the specific disorder in the family's cultural context should be determined and used in teaching and long-range planning.

• Consider ways for the dietary implementation and maintenance in the context of different cultural, ethnic, religious, and social eating patterns, so that they can be applied to families in ways appropriate.

• Help may be needed for the parent to get used to the time-consuming routine of a special diet. The nurse may be able to help the parent organize a schedule.

• Financial needs should be recognized. Some states, through health departments or services for children with special needs, provide free formula or food for metabolic disorders, and others pay part of the costs. Groups such as the March of Dimes help with travel costs to the main treatment center in some communities. Nurses should help the family locate all available sources of aid.

• Stress the importance of reading labels in all commercial foods or sending to commercial manufacturers for such ingredient lists if they are not listed on the label.

• Parents should understand the importance of not running out of special necessary foods or formula, and they should have an emergency stockpile on hand at all times.

• Essential products and formulas should be taken with the family on trips and vacations.

• Parents should know what to do in case of illness, refusal to eat prescribed foods, failure to stay on the prescribed diet, or appetite fluctuations. These should be in written form and verbally reviewed.

• Parents should have a telephone number to call where a response is always available whenever they have specific diet-related questions.

• When possible, parents should be encouraged to use foods that are acceptable in the special diet for all family members, provided that a dietary imbalance would not result (e.g., everyone could have fruit ices for dessert instead of just the child with galactosemia while others ate ice cream).

• Neighbors, friends, relatives, babysitters, and teachers should have a clear explanation of foods that the child can and cannot have. If the child is likely to have a snack at a particular friend's, specially prepared or acceptable snacks could be kept there. For example, home-baked cookies from a recipe that is low in phenylalanine can be enjoyed by all.

• Open communication and involvement of school officials and teachers, so that the child is treated as one who is normal, healthy, and on a special diet, is essential. The nurse may help initiate contacts or give a program to teachers to alleviate their concerns.

• Parents may be helped to plan the diet by using some foods from the school lunch menu if it is possible to minimize differences where possible.

• Involving the child in his or her own food choices from approved foods can be done by the age of 3 years or when developmentally appropriate for that child.

• Parent groups are useful for support and sharing coping measures.

Phenylketonuria

Because phenylalanine (phe) is one of the essential amino acids for humans, it cannot be totally eliminated from the diet. The aim in the diet therapy of PKU is to restrict phe in the diet enough to prevent its buildup in the blood, allowing the affected infant to reach its normal intellectual potential and yet provide enough nutrients for normal metabolism and optimum growth. Too little phe from excessive restriction can cause catabolism of body protein, whereas too much can result in mental retardation. A balance must be maintained. Today most infants with PKU are detected by newborn screening programs. It is essential to begin the restricted diet as quickly as possible after diagnosis and optimally before 2 weeks of age. Because of newer information about the effects of hyper-phenylalanemia, often infants who do not have classic PKU but have phe levels of 6–8 mg/dl or above on an unrestricted intake of breast milk or formula may be placed on some form of restricted phe diet, at least in the short term.

The initiation of diet therapy immediately after the detection of PKU is sometimes done as an inpatient at a center experienced in PKU treatment. If the family lives near enough that they can be seen daily for blood phe determination, adjustment of the diet, and participation in the therapeutic process, these adjustments may be accomplished on an outpatient basis. After treatment is established, maintenance may be accomplished by means of linkage among local health professionals, the family, and the PKU treatment center, with periodic revisits to the center. A study of mothers, some of whose children had PKU, indicated varying demands and needs of services (Read, 2003).

The infant is usually begun on the phe-restricted diet with a phe-free formula such as Phenex-1. Its use alone rapidly decreases blood phe levels to the appropriate range. Phe levels are monitored daily, and when they are in the acceptable range, then phe-containing formula is added to maintain this. Recommendations from the British, European, and American communities vary somewhat in what the optimum blood phe levels should be maintained at, but the range is 2–4 mg/dl for some and 2–6 mg/dl for others. A dietary prescription is developed by establishing the infant's phe, protein, and energy needs. The amount of the phe needed varies between individuals and also with growth, weight, and metabolism at different times in the same individual, so that there is no single standard to be used. Adjustments are made based on the blood phe determinations and the dietary intake record, as well as reports of any illness. In the 1st year of life, after the initial diet institution, monitoring of serum phe levels with accompanying adjustment is usually done weekly. Later, after phe levels are stabilized, this may be liberalized to a monthly determination. Parents are taught to take a capillary blood sample and to bring it or mail it to the main treatment center. The center staff usually telephones changes and confirms this in written form. Strict attention to adequate intake of vitamins and trace elements is essential. Building a trust relationship with the family is an essential component of the treatment program. If the mother is breast-feeding the infant, the nurse should ascertain if she wishes to continue and make the treatment team aware of her wishes. The dietary prescription can include breast-feeding, bottle-feeding, or a Lact-Aid device can be used to provide the phe-restricted formula.

There are different ways to implement the actual diet. The diet can be given in values per average serving of phe (in mg) and portions can be weighed, or it can be calculated in a manner similar to diabetic exchange lists where an amount of phe is equal to one exchange (e.g., 15 mg = 1 exchange) and the number of exchanges in the basic food categories are designated as part of the prescription. If a parent is having trouble with the method being used, the nurse can suggest to the treatment team that an alternate approach be attempted.

Several burdens fall on the parents and family in the implementation of the phe-restricted diet. The products used are more expensive than other formula and foods. Keeping a necessary record of all the foods the infant eats, collecting the capillary blood samples, and constantly regulating the diet may be stressful for parents. Physical examinations, EEGs, intelligence testing, and other procedures such as MRIs that may be done periodically throughout childhood at the treatment center add to the parents' stress.

After the initial implementation of the diet, home visits by nurses or nutritionists may be helpful to assess the parents' understanding of the actual implementation of the dietary prescription, and to teach or reinforce the teaching or the collection of the weekly capillary blood samples. At that time nurses can also review the food intake chart and discuss any problems the parents are having. For example, the integration of the phe-restricted diet into the family's cultural and social eating patterns is particularly important in the older infant and young child.

When the child is a little older, he or she is usually switched to a protein-substitute product such as Phenyl-Free which was traditionally used. Newer protein substitutes have been developed that are more palatable and some are concentrated in tablet preparation and as gels or pastes so that palatability is increased. The use of a phe-free flavoring such as Tang, strawberry QUIK powder, or carob

powder can be used to make it more palatable, and new products that are somewhat more acceptable are becoming available. Some believe that the child can exercise some control by choosing the flavoring he or she wishes, while others believe that children should accept the formula as is with flavorings being used only for a special treat. For the older child, Phenyl-Free or other protein substitutes are used to meet protein and energy needs and solid foods are used to meet the phe requirement. An adequate formula intake is required to stabilize blood phe levels. Additional energy needs are met by adding low- or free-phe foods, such as those listed in Table 15.3.

Low-phe products and recipes are available for baking cookies, cakes, etc., and some low-phe ready-made products are also available. A young child can have difficulty in distinguishing these special foods from regular ones (e.g., pasta products, cookies), and may need additional instruction. By 3 years of age, or when developmentally appropriate for that child, he/she should participate in his or her own food selection. Aspartame (NutraSweet) is a sweetener in common use that contains phe, and must be specifically looked for in making appropriate food selections. There are books and coloring books about PKU written for the child, some of which illustrate the dietary choices by use of traffic signals for food—red for things they cannot eat such as eggs, yellow for things that need measuring such as potatoes and

TABLE 15.3   Some Foods with Little or No Phenylalanine

Beverages—carbonated drinks, lemonade, Kool-Aid, Tang

Candy—butterscotch, hard candy, lollipops, jelly beans, gumdrops, cream mints

Corn starch

Cranberries, raw

Cranberry sauce

Danish dessert

Fruit ices and popsicles

Jellies

Juices—apple, apricot, and peach nectar

Rich's toppings

Seasonings—salt, soy sauce

Sweeteners—sugar, corn syrup, molasses, maple syrup

Wheat starch

rice, and green for things that can be eaten without consideration such as tomatoes, pears, and tea. The child can attend preschool or nursery school. The nurse may be a liaison and help teachers with their own concerns, and can help find acceptable foods. Some suggested techniques for help in the schools are found through lay help groups.

Normal infant and child behaviors, especially those related to feeding, may be seen as stemming from the diet restriction rather than from normal developmental processes. On the other hand, the older child may become manipulative about the diet or parents may have misconceptions. Anticipatory guidance for developmental milestones and behavioral stages is one of the important roles for the nurse. Other problems involved may not be immediately obvious until the nurse develops a good relationship with the family and observes carefully in the home. For example, PKU may lead to contradictions between beliefs among the children in the family. If one without PKU is told that he or she should eat meat to be healthy, what does the child with PKU think? Another example is the incident of a younger sibling being born, and the child with PKU asking, "Is Paula like me?," and the mother inadvertently replying, "No, Paula is okay." The child in such a situation may often be confronted with conflicting emotions—on the one hand being happy that the baby is unaffected, while on the other hand examining what is wrong with himself/herself. Parents' and peer support groups located in their home community or region can be a very useful way to help deal with problems and to share recipes or effective techniques. Nurses can start and perhaps lead such groups if they are knowledgeable. Parents can also be helped to deal with behavioral problems encountered by using behavioral modification methods or by being referred for further counseling, if appropriate.

Both too low and high levels of phe must be avoided. Too low serum phe levels can result from (1) increased requirements due to growth; (2) inadequate ingestion of phe due to refusal to eat, vomiting; or (3) inaccuracy in measuring or prescribing the diet. High phe levels can result from (1) fever, infection or illness; (2) inadequate intake of protein or calories; (3) increased intake of phe due to misunderstandings, inaccurate measurement of food portions, or not sticking to the diet or making poor choices; (4) decreased require-

ments caused by decreased growth; and (5) failure to divide the formula evenly over the day, leading to hunger and excessive intake of phe.

At this time, the thinking is that the diet may need to be lifelong, although some believe liberalization may be permitted after 10 years of age with levels remaining under 2–6 mg/dl (1–6 mg/dl recommended by some), and less frequent blood phe monitoring. Adherence is problematic. A review by Walter et al. (2002) found that in the 0 to 4 and 5 to 9 year age groups, about 1/4 had phe levels above the maximum recommended limit. Of those in the 10 to 14 and 15 to 19 years of age groups one-half and three-quarters respectively had phe levels above the maximum recommended limits, illustrating a serious challenge for health care professionals. Pre-adolescent females with PKU should be made cognizant of the problems involved in maternal PKU and the need for adequate contraception. Pregnancy should be planned to avoid damage to the fetus so that the diet can be adjusted before conception and through the pregnancy. If they become pregnant, it is necessary for strict diet implementation which may be as low as 1 to 4 mg/dl, as discussed in chapters 11 and 13, and pregnancies should be monitored carefully, including nutrient intake and weight gain. Although normal intellectual attainment is possible in those maintained on low phe diets from infancy, some studies suggest that there are subtle neurologic consequences in the form of perceptual, cognitive, and behavioral disturbances and some evidence of intellectual impairment in persons with PKU as compared with their normal siblings. Particularly affected are problem solving, abstract reasoning, speed of mental processing, and sustained attention. A study of PKU in adulthood (Koch et al., 2002) found that those who maintained a restricted diet had less problems than those who didn't, especially in relation to eczema, asthma, headache, mental disorders, and hyper- and hypoactivity. Tetrahydrobiopterin has been used in some instances to lower plasma phe concentrations and allow more diet variation to improve adherence. Newer approaches to enzyme replacement therapy have shown promise. Gene therapy for PKU appears possible in the near future, and long-term correction via gene transfer has been demonstrated in mouse models.

Galactosemia

In galactosemia, galactose cannot be metabolized to glucose (see chapter 11). Because most of the dietary galactose comes from lactose intake, all forms of milk are removed from the diet. This includes buttermilk, cream, ice cream, cheese, yogurt, milk sherbet, and nonfat milk solids. Organ meats are also forbidden. Infant formulas such as Nutramigen, Soyalac, Prosobee, or Isomil are used along with supplementary vitamins. In the older infant, flavoring may be added. Specific dietary problems to be watched for are "hidden" sources of lactose that may be present in commercial bakery products, mixes, candy, vegetables, creamed soups, sausages, cold cuts, or commercial pills. Kosher meat products or those marked pareve do not contain lactose. Care must be taken to maintain needed amounts of riboflavin, calcium, and Vitamin D. In addition to other care, similar to that described under PKU and in general, children must be carefully monitored for growth of bones and have frequent eye examinations for early detection of cataract development. The diet is usually maintained for a lifetime, with some liberalization in the teenager and adult. However, the outcome may not be as good as was hoped for. Later complications have included speech defects, reduced intelligence, learning disabilities, neurological deficits, and ovarian failure. It may be that damage occurs in utero, dietary adjustment may not be precise, or that treatment is not instituted early enough in infancy. It is thought by many that stricter control than formerly believed necessary may be desirable throughout life. Thus it is important to periodically assess children with galactosemia for cognitive problems in order to intervene early.

Maple Syrup Urine Disease

In classical maple syrup urine disease (MSUD), the inborn error lies in the metabolism of not one but three branched chain amino acids—leucine, isoleucine, and valine, specifically in decreased or absent activity of branched chain α-ketoacid dehydrogenase. All are essential in humans. The increase in leucine levels have a particularly adverse effect on other amino acid transport in and out of both cells and organs. As in PKU, these must be supplied in adequate amounts for proper growth, energy, and development, but not in amounts that result in elevated blood levels. Because MSUD is very rare, experience with diet therapy is much more limited, but diet therapy may need to be maintained through the individual's lifespan. Some children treated for MSUD have died from unknown causes by early adolescence despite the apparent success of the diet therapy. To prevent mental damage, the diet must be started in the first week of life. At that time the infant is usually acutely ill. To adjust the diet, analysis of the branched chain amino acids is generally done. Leucine, isoleucine, and valine in the diet are calculated by the nutritionist. Parents are taught to monitor leucine intake. Supplements are available that are free of valine, leucine, and isoleucine. They need to be supplemented with vitamins, energy sources, and sources of natural protein. The range of tolerance is very narrow. An early sign of relapsing from control is irritability, followed by ataxia and clumsy walking. Later signs include lethargy, the characteristic maple-syrup-like odor, and convulsions. Folic acid deficiency is common and should be specifically looked for.

INTRAUTERINE AND FETAL THERAPY

The widespread use of prenatal detection has allowed the early identification of fetuses with both biochemical errors and congenital defects. Until recently, such detection allowed for a limited number of choices—(a) selective termination of the pregnancy, (b) choice of a different mode of delivery (e.g., abdominal delivery in a fetus with osteogenesis imperfecta), (c) altering the geographic site of delivery for highly specialized management, (d) specific prevention of premature labor, (e) induced preterm delivery for the earliest possible correction or to prevent further damage (e.g., amniotic band syndrome), and (f) preparation for immediate postnatal treatment at the normal delivery time. Now both direct and indirect therapy are possible. Some types of fetal or intrauterine treatment include the administration of intravenous and oral digoxin to the mother for intrauterine treatment of fetal paroxysmal tachycardia as well as direct injection to the fetus; maternal administration of glucocorticoids for female fetuses with congenital adrenal hyperplasia; maternal administration of vitamin B_{12} to treat a fetus with methylmalonic acidemia; maternal administration of biotin to treat the fetus with multiple carboxylase deficiency; placement of a shunt in the fetus for correction of obstructive hydrocephalus; repair of diaphragmatic hernia involving direct fetal exposure; intrauterine intraperitoneal exchange transfusion for erythroblastosis fetalis; treatment of a fetus with hypothyroidism by the administration of intra-amniotic thyroxine; in utero treatment of urinary tract obstruction by insertion of an indwelling suprapubic catheter for fetal bladder drainage; direct fetal intravenous transfusion for severe hemolytic disease through the fetoscope; ultrasound guided laser treatment to perforate a ureterocele and overcome bladder obstruction; and infusion of genetically altered bone marrow stem cells to treat a fetus with severe combined immunodeficiency. These procedures have had various degrees of success and risk. Experimental techniques such as in utero surgery to correct certain craniofacial anomalies have been suggested. Newer technologies use minimal access as well as lasers through a fetoscope. Placental surgery to correct variants of twin-twin transfusion syndrome in monochorionic twins has been done. In utero hematopoetic stem cell transplantation has been accomplished in a few cases, and may be particularly useful for immunodeficiency disorders such as X-linked agammaglobulinemia, hemoglobinopathies such as β-thalassemia, and inborn errors of metabolism such as Gaucher disease. Umbilical cord blood banking for stem cells for autologous or nonautologous transplant is attractive because of reduced risk of immunological reactions. These present some ethical issues.

Experience with many of the specific modalities used in intrauterine therapy has been limited due to the rarity of many of the individual disorders, technical difficulties, and the hazards that may be involved. For example, in fetal surgery some of the possible undesirable outcomes include hemorrhage, infection, spontaneous abortion, premature labor, serious injury or death to the fetus or mother; the possibility of the need for future abdominal delivery due to the hysterotomy necessary for surgery, that the surgery would not be successful, that it would be successful but the outcome

ultimately could be unsuccessful, the presence of other undetected defects in the fetus, and untoward effects from the anesthesia used.

As opportunities for fetal therapy grow, ethical and moral dilemmas are becoming more apparent. In addition to implications from the risks given previously, others include divergent societal views of the fetus, conflicts between the rights and desires of the parents and the fetus, the weighing of risks and benefits between the mother and the fetus, the lack of information on the chances for successful outcomes, the fact that the mother becomes a patient with the fetus and may possibly be an unwilling participant in fetal therapy, whether the right of a fetus with a treatable defect is the same as the right of a fetus with an untreatable defect, the question of whether or not a fetus can be truly considered a patient, and the interests of the researchers in advancing expertise and knowledge. Dilemmas are increased when twins are present and one is normal and the other has a defect, which has actually occurred in several reported cases. Nurses should make sure that as much information is provided to parents involved in such a decision as is available, help to clarify choices, make sure that the information presented is in terms that are understood, provide an environment that is free from coercion and pressure, and support whatever decision the couple makes. Guidelines for fetal research and therapy supported by federal funds have been developed by various groups. There are concerns by some that fetal treatment can become too aggressive when alternative methods are available. For example, how much advantage is attained by fetal bone marrow transplant as opposed to performing this procedure after birth?

GENE PRODUCT REPLACEMENT

The replacement of the normal gene product may be accomplished in several ways—by simply administering the missing substance (e.g., thyroxin for hypothyroidism, factor VIII for classical hemophilia, or pancreatic supplementation below 10,000 units of lipase per kg in cystic fibrosis) on a periodic basis, by manipulating the defective enzyme by cofactor/coenzyme therapy, by organ or tissue transplantation, or by the direct replacement of the deficient or defective enzyme.

Enzyme Replacement Therapy

Several years ago, it appeared that enzyme replacement therapy would be relatively simple in those disorders in which the enzyme defect was identified at the molecular level. In practice, the administration of enzymes in conventional ways was not effective. A major reason for this was that most enzymes are not normally circulating serum components like factor VIII (a blood-clotting factor deficient in hemophilia A). They need to gain access to cell interiors in specific organs and then reach specific organelles. The enzyme must get there without being destroyed, and it needs an appropriate delivery system. For example, in the lysosomal storage diseases, the cells' normal delivery system must be used to get the enzyme into the lysosome by allowing the enzyme with its carrier to bind to the cell surface receptors as a macromolecule and allowing normal pinocytosis to occur. Replacement with alglucerase in Gaucher disease (see chapter 6) has been relatively successful in type 1 disease, and other approaches such as the potential for using inhibitors of sphingolipid biosynthesis are being examined. Difficulties in the practical implementation of enzyme therapy have included the following:

- Enzyme must remain intact and be transported without being inactivated until it arrives at the tissue where needed.
- Animal models for pretesting are necessary.
- There are difficulties in developing suitable carriers.
- The blood-brain barrier to deliver the enzyme in question to cells of the central nervous system that are involved in many inherited biochemical disorders must be overcome.
- It can be difficult to establish the optimum dosage for enzyme replacement.

Requirements that should be met before enzyme therapy can be effective are as follows:

- The ability to produce large quantities at low cost of purified enzyme.
- The molecular properties of each enzyme must be understood.
- The enzyme preparation must have a high specific activity in the body.
- It must be feasible to target the enzyme to specific tissue.
- A safe way to prevent antibody reaction to the introduced enzyme must be developed.
- The enzyme must be able to function in the specific tissue as it normally would for a substantial period of time.

The intravenous administration of purified enzyme using carrier erythrocytes or liposomes for delivery and slow release, or linking the enzyme to low-density lipoproteins as carriers, are relatively new therapeutic approaches. In the mucopolysaccharide disorders, transplanted HLA-compatible fibroblasts have been used to supply normal enzymes on a longer-term basis, but evidence of clinical success has been limited. The use of renal transplants to supply missing enzymes has been most successful in the treatment of Fabry disease, but now infusion therapy is possible. Bone marrow transplantation has been used to treat a variety of genetic conditions, including severe combined immunodeficiency caused by adenosine deaminase deficiency and Hurler disease (see chapter 6). Liver transplantation has been used to replace enzymes in Nieman-Pick disease and for the correction of the enzymatic defect in Wilson disease (a disorder of copper metabolism) if penicillamine treatment has not been effective.

The evaluation of enzyme therapy has been uneven, and different criteria have been used to judge clinical versus biochemical success. Therefore, it is difficult to realistically evaluate overall effectiveness across disorders. For example, intravenous enzyme therapy for Gaucher disease using a macrophage-targeted enzyme preparation, alglucerase, has been relatively successful—the chief barrier has been cost, which can range from $100,000 to $400,000 per year.

COFACTOR/COENZYME THERAPY

As discussed in chapter 6, many enzymes are holoenzymes; that is, they are composed of an apoenzyme (protein part) plus a cofactor/coenzyme (prosthetic part) that is needed for function. Cofactors are frequently vitamins or metal ions. Many inherited biochemical disorders have both vitamin responsive and nonresponsive subtypes. The replacement of a missing or defective cofactor or supplying it in megadoses allows the formation of a functional holoenzyme or allows binding when large amounts of cofactor are available. In this way they regulate the activity and amounts of apoenzyme. At least 25 vitamin-responsive inherited biochemical disorders are known. Fetal vitamin therapy for certain vitamin responsive disorders has been accomplished, and the potential exists for the feasibility of this approach with the others. Giving vitamins in high doses has been found in some cases to activate other pathways unintentionally, with accompanying ill effects, and this must be watched for during therapy.

RECOMBINANT DNA

Briefly, the process of creating recombinant DNA for use in the manufacture of certain proteins enzymes and hormones is as follows. So-called foreign DNA from a higher biologic organism or human is cut into specific sections containing the normal functioning gene of interest by a type of enzyme called restriction endonucleases and is purified. These enzymes also are used to remove a segment from the DNA of a vector or carrier. Vectors most commonly used are bacteriophages (bacterial viruses) or plasmids (a type of bacterial DNA). The foreign DNA and the DNA from the vector are allowed to unite, thus forming a recombinant DNA molecule that is inserted into a host bacterial cell. This bacterium, with its own DNA plus that of the vector with the foreign DNA, multiplies, making identical copies of the foreign DNA inserted and its product—the protein or enzyme desired. This process is called cloning, and is being used commercially to produce human insulin, growth hormone, interferon factor VIII, and other substances in large quantities. This has made available for wider use substances that were formerly limited in production, and has removed the necessity of extraction from pooled blood, thus making safer (free of infectious organisms such as hepatitis or human immunodeficiency virus) product available. Another use of restriction endonucleases is in the creation of gene "probes" for diagnosis, as discussed in chapter 2.

GENE THERAPY

Gene therapy is the most direct approach to the treatment of genetic diseases and if successful would eliminate the need for all of the other therapeutic modalities previously described. It has long been known that genetic material has been transferred nonpurposefully from one organism or species to another, as in the case of viruses that invade human tissue and become integrated into the cellular DNA. Gene therapy usually consists of inserting a new gene into either somatic or germline cells, but it may also refer to repair or reprogramming of a gene. The new gene must not only be delivered but expressed correctly over time. Among current interests in gene therapy is the understanding of gene regulation and tissue-specific gene expression control that can be manipulated to correct the defect. Gene therapy can be used to (1) replace a missing function, as in the case of absent or deficient gene product that usually occurs in autosomal recessive biochemical disorders; (2) enhance or activate normal functioning; (3) provide a new function, such as resistance to a disease such as influenza; or (4) interfere with an undesired or aberrant function, such as in the case of an abnormal gene product formed in an autosomal dominant disorder. Gene therapy could be used to treat both genetic diseases and common diseases such as cancer and heart disease, and also as a prevention strategy. The idea of using germ cells for correction of a genetic defect has aroused ethical concerns about whether or not it is appropriate to alter the human genome for future generations, and the effect on those future generations. It is technically difficult, but is appealing in that it ideally would correct the genetic defect in all cells and in all descendants. Germline gene therapy is not now actively being pursued in humans. Somatic cell gene therapy corrects the defect only in the person treated and not in his or her descendants. The first human gene therapy trial was the insertion of a functional gene into somatic cells (T-lymphocytes) to correct the defect in adenosine deaminase deficiency (ADA), a type of severe combined immunodeficiency disorder, and the return of these cells by infusion to the affected children. This was not permanent, and infusions every 1–2 months were needed initially followed by 3 to 6 months. Newer approaches involve the insertion of normal ADA genes into bone marrow stem cells. Other examples of conditions in which clinical trials of gene therapy have been done are the introduction of the gene for the low density lipoprotein (LDL) receptor into the liver cells of patients with familial hypercholesterolemia, and the introduction of the *CFTR* gene into lung and airway cells in cystic fibrosis patients. Gene therapy trials received a setback when an 18-year-old male with ornithine transcarbamylase deficiency, who was receiving intravenous infusion of the normal gene via a weakened adenovirus vector, developed multiple organ failure and died. After this the Food and Drug Administration (FDA) and others instituted stricter regulation. In late 2002, the development of leukemia in some children enrolled in a French gene therapy trial, using retroviral vectors to insert genes into stem cells for X-linked severe combined immunodeficiency disease, led to a temporary halt in 2003 of these types of trials by the FDA (Twombly, 2003). It is believed that it was the retrovirus vector used that led to the activation of a T-cell oncogene, *LMO2*, which led to leukemia development (McCormack & Rabbitts, 2004).

The optimal gene therapy would be the replacement of the abnormal gene with a normal copy in the proper location of that gene in every cell with appropriate expression. To this end, attempts to promote homologous recombination between the chromosome with the mutant gene and the one with the altered gene have been tried but have not been successful to date. Gene therapy involves getting the gene to the selected target cells so that they will eventually express the appropriate gene product.

Somatic cell gene therapy could involve gene insertion not only into the infant, child, or adult, but also prenatally. The times for this would be in the zygote before and after fusion of pronuclei (this could be done by the microinjection of DNA into the male pronucleus of the fertilized ovum), in the preimplantation embryo, perhaps in conjunction with embryo transfer, or postimplantation into the embryo or the fetus at an early age of development before damage from the mutant gene has occurred. In some neurologic genetic diseases, damage is detectable by the 3rd month or earlier. Newborn gene therapy also appears promising because of the infant's small size and for other reasons, and ADA has been treated in this way. In one case, in utero stem cell transplantation of bone marrow from the father to the male fetus was accomplished to prevent the X-linked type of severe combined immunodeficiency disease (Bartolomé et al., 2002). Several infusions were necessary using ultrasound-guided intraperitoneal injection, and at 5 months of age the boy appeared well. The Patent and Trademark Office has allowed patents for gene therapy techniques.

Gene-based therapies have been tested for diseases such as cancer and heart disease. In cancer, one approach has been to alter cells to produce substances that alter the host response to cancer cells. In heart disease, angiogenic factors can be delivered into ischemic heart muscle. In HIV, it has been suggested that introducing drug-resistance genes into normal bone marrow cells would allow more aggressive chemotherapy. Genetically engineered islet cells have been transplanted in type 1 diabetes mellitus.

Gene Transfer

Once the normal gene has been cloned, it has to be delivered into the target cell by a vector system. Methods include chemical and physical ones. Various vectors have been used such as liposomes, viruses such as adenoviruses, adeno-associated viruses, Moloney murine leukemia virus (MoMLV), herpes simplex virus, the vaccinia virus, retroviruses; nonviral delivery systems have been used such as lipoplexes, polyplexes, cationic glycopolymers, naked DNA, and others. Each of these vectors has certain advantages and disadvantages and infects, and therefore enters, different types of cells, taking the gene of interest with it. In some cell types, integration into the host genome then occurs and can be passed on to descendents. It is usually desirable to make these vectors replication deficient. A problem can arise if they integrate randomly into chromosomes with the potential to disturb function, and even activate an oncogene. Gene transfer can be done in vivo, or in vitro (although some now use the term, ex vivo). An ex vivo approach is by removing cells such as those in bone marrow, incubating them in a culture with the recombinant DNA containing the normal gene until the cells take it up, and then reintroducing the genetically modified cells back into the patient. This can be accomplished in embryonic cells in culture that were then treated and implanted in the mother. Ex vivo therapy is shown in Figure 15.1. In

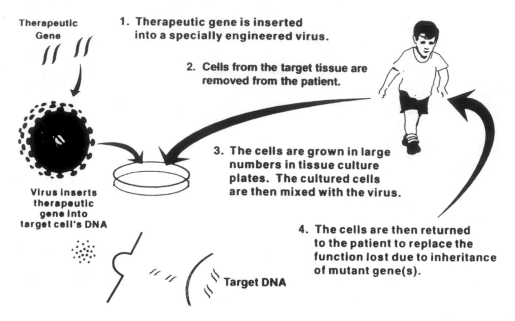

Therapeutic Gene

1. Therapeutic gene is inserted into a specially engineered virus.

2. Cells from the target tissue are removed from the patient.

Virus inserts therapeutic gene into target cell's DNA

3. The cells are grown in large numbers in tissue culture plates. The cultured cells are then mixed with the virus.

4. The cells are then returned to the patient to replace the function lost due to inheritance of mutant gene(s).

Target DNA

FIGURE 15.1   Ex vivo gene therapy.
Courtesy of Karina Boehm, National Human Genome Research Institute, National Institutes of Health.

the in vivo approach, a recombinant gene can be introduced directly. In the simplest approach, the DNA can be delivered by injection into a specific tissue (e.g., the dystrophin gene into muscle cells to treat muscular dystrophy), or in other diseases it can be infused directly into, for example, the liver. Hepatocytes can be cultured, genes inserted, and returned via the portal vein with seeding to the liver and gene expression. Injection of DNA that is contained within liposomes can also be done. Naked DNA gene transfer is becoming more efficient and can be done through intravascular delivery. Alternative delivery modes include transplantation of the cell in question—for example hepatocytes after retroviral transduction. In cystic fibrosis, recombinant *CFTR*-cloned DNA that is expressed by a heterologous constitutive promotor can be delivered to the epithelial cells in the airway via the nasal passages or bronchial epithelium (by bronchoscope) using an adenovirus vector. These have appeared promising.

Problems in Gene Therapy

The problems associated with gene therapy are both ethical and technical, and include the following:

- It is not known how stable the inserted gene might be in the human organism.
- It must go to a desired location in the chromosome.
- The use of tissue-specific promotors may be needed depending on the vector used so that the genes are expressed in the desired cell.
- Insertion must be done in such a way that the inserted gene replicates when the cell divides.
- Only the desired gene segment must be prepared, or else extra unwanted material will be present.
- The inserted gene must be functional.
- It must be able to be controlled and regulated in the usual manner.
- It must respond to the usual physiological and biochemical stimuli.
- It must remain unaltered and stable in the cell.
- It must not cause any harm to the organism, such as an increased incidence of cancer or autoimmune disease.
- It must not present a biohazard.
- The long-term evolutionary effects are unknown.
- There exists a potential for the misuse of genetic engineering.

- There are difficulties in getting the requisite gene inserted in all body cells for effective therapy in those disorders in which active gene product is need in all cells, not just in a select group.

Various federal guidelines and regulations are in place in regard to gene therapy and research, and fetal therapy and research. Other ethical issues are emerging, such as how target diseases are chosen for gene therapy research, the issues involved in germline therapy, and the potential use of gene therapy not just for cure but for genetic enhancement purposes. The latter is generally considered unacceptable at the present time.

EPIGENETIC THERAPIES

Epigenetics refers to changes in gene expression not coded for in DNA. Various genetic disorders are due to inappropriate gene silencing or expression. These may occur through such mechanisms as DNA methylation and modifications in chromosomal histones, and are discussed in chapter 4. Thus it follows that epigenetic therapeutic approaches would be developed. For example, inhibitors of DNA methylation, such as 5-azacytidine, are being examined for their ability to reactivate genes that have been silenced. Applications include in certain cancers such as myeloid dysplastic syndrome and certain hemoglobinopathies. Another approach is through inhibiting histone deacetylases, for example clinical trials of depsipeptide for cutaneous T-cell lymphoma.

BIBLIOGRAPHY

Baker, A. H. (2004). Designing gene delivery vectors for cardiovascular gene therapy. *Progress in Biophysics and Molecular Biology, 84,* 279–299.

Bartolomé, J., Porta, F., Lafranchi, A., Rodríguez-Molina, J. J., Cela, E., Cantalejo, A., et al. (2002). B cell function after haploidentical in utero bone marrow transplantation in a patient with severe combined immunodeficiency. *Bone Marrow Transplantation, 29,* 625–628.

Blau, N. (2003). Tetrahydropbiopterin control in phenylketonuria. *Genetics in Medicine, 5,* 57–58

Blomberg, P., & Smith, C. E. (2003). Gene therapy of monogenic and cardiovascular disorders. *Expert Opinion in Biological Therapeutics, 3,* 941–949.

Bosch, A. M., Grootenhuis, M. A., Bakker, H. D., Heijmans, H. S., Wijburg, F. A., & Last, B. F. (2004). Living with classical galactosemia: Health-related quality of life consequences. *Pediatrics, 113,* e423–e428.

Bottino, R., Lemarchand, P., Trucco, M., & Giannoukakis, N. (2003). Gene- and cell-based therapeutics for type 1 diabetes mellitus. *Gene Therapy, 10,* 875–889.

Cavazzana-Calvo, M., Lagresle, C., Hacein Bey Abina, S., & Fischer, A. (2005). Gene therapy for severe combined immunodeficiency. *Annual Review of Medicine, 56,* 585–602.

Chervenak, F. A., McCullough, L. B., & Birnbach, D. J. (2004). Ethical issues in fetal surgery research. *Best Practices and Research in Clinical Anaesthesiology, 18,* 221–230.

Chinen, J., & Puck, J. M. (2004). Successes and risks of gene therapy in primary immunodeficiencies. *Journal of Allergy and Clinical Immunology, 113,* 595–603.

Cortes, R. A., & Farmer, D. L. (2004). Recent advances in fetal surgery. *Seminars in Perinatology, 29,* 199–211.

Desnick, R. J. (2004). Enzyme replacement and enhancement therapies for lysosomal diseases. *Journal of Inherited and Metabolic Diseases, 27,* 385–410.

Ding, Z., Harding, C. O., & Thöny, B. (2004). State-of-the art 2003 on PKU gene therapy. *Molecular Genetics and Metabolism, 81,* 3–8.

Driskell, R. A., & Engelhardt, J. F. (2003). Current status of gene therapy for inherited lung diseases. *Annual Review of Physiology, 65,* 585–612.

Egger, G., Liang, G., Aparicio, A., & Jones, P. A. (2004). Epigenetics in human disease and prospects for epigenetic therapy. *Nature, 429,* 457–463.

Flake, A. W. (2002). Genetic therapies for the fetus. *Clinical Obstetrics and Gynecology, 45,* 684–696.

Gaziev, J., & Lucarelli, G. (2003). Stem cell transplantation for hemoglobinopathies. *Current Opinion in Pediatrics, 15,* 24–31.

Gruchala, M., Roy, H., Bhardwaj, S., & Yla-Herttuala, S. (2004). Gene therapy for cardiovascular diseases. *Current Pharmaceutical Design, 10,* 407–423.

Hajjar, R. J., Huq, F., Matsui, T., & Rosenzweig, A. (2003). Genetic editing of dysfunctional myocardium. *Medical Clinics of North America, 87,* 553–567.

Harling, R. R., Stelnicki, E. J., Hedrick, M. H., & Longaker, M. T. (2003). In utero models of craniofacial surgery. *World Journal of Surgery, 27,* 108–116.

Herweijer, H., & Wolff, J. A. (2003). Progress and prospects: Naked DNA gene transfer and therapy. *Gene Therapy, 10,* 453–458.

Hildinger, M., & Auricchio, A. (2004). Advances in AAV-mediated gene transfer for the treatment of inherited disorders. *European Journal of Human Genetics, 12,* 263–271.

Hopkin, R. J., Bissler, J., & Grabowski, G. A. (2003). Comparative evaluation of α-galactosidase A infusions for treatment of Fabry disease. *Genetics in Medicine, 5,* 144–153.

Joy, S. D., Rossi, K. Q., Krugh, D., & O'Shaughnessy, R. W. (2005). Management of pregnancies complicated by anti-e alloimmunization. *Obstetrics & Gynecology, 105,* 24–28.

Keswani, S. G., & Crombleholme, T. M. (2004). Gene transfer to the tracheobronchial tree: Implications for fetal gene therapy for cystic fibrosis. *Seminars in Pediatric Surgery, 13,* 44–52.

Kim, W., Erlandson, H., Surendran, S., Stevens, R. C., Gamez, A., Michals-Matalon, K., et al. (2004). Trends in enzyme therapy for phenylketonuria. *Molecular Therapy, 10,* 220–224.

Koch, R., Burton, B., Hoganson, G., Peterson, R., Rhead, W., Rouse, B., et al. (2002). Phenylketonuria in adulthood: A collaborative study. *Journal of Inherited and Metabolic Disease, 25,* 333–346.

Lu, Q. L., Bou-Gharios, G., & Partridge, T. A. (2003). Non-viral gene delivery in skeletal muscle: A protein factory. *Gene Therapy, 10,* 131–142.

Lyerly, A. D., & Mahowald, M. B. (2003). Maternal-fetal surgery for treatment of myelomeningocele. *Clinics in Perinatology, 30,* 155–165.

Miller, H. I. (2000). Gene therapy's trials and tribulations. *Scientist, 14,* 16.

MacDonald, A., Daly, A., Davies, P., Asplin, D., Hall, S. K., Rylance, G., & Chakrapani, A. (2004). Protein substitutes for PKU: What's new? *Journal of Inherited and Metabolic Diseases, 27,* 363–371.

McCormick, M. P., & Rabbitts, T. H. (2004). Activation of the T-cell oncogene *LMO2* after gene therapy for X-linked severe combined immunodeficiency. *New England Journal of Medicine, 350,* 913–922.

Magnaldo, T. (2004). Xeroderma pigmentosum: From genetics to hopes and realities of cutaneous gene therapy. *Expert Opinion on Biolgical Therapy, 4,* 169–179.

Mochizuki, S., Mizukami, H., Ogura, T., Kure, S., Ichinohe, A., Kojima, K., et al. (2004). Long-term correction of hyperphenylalaninemia by AAV-mediated gene transfer leads to behavioral recovery in phenylketonuria mice. *Gene Therapy, 11,* 1081–1086.

Morton, D. H., Strauss, K. A., Robinson, D. L., Puffenberger, E. G., & Kelley, R. I. (2002). Diagnosis and treatment of maple syrup disease: A study of 36 patients. *Pediatrics, 109,* 999–1008.

Muntau, A. C., Roschinger, W., Habich, M., Demmelmair, H., Hoffmann, B., Sommerhoff, C. P., et al. (2002). Tetrahydrobiopterin as an alternative treatment for mild phenylketonuria. *New England Journal of Medicine, 347,* 2122–2132.

Nabel, G. J. (2004). Genetic, cellular and immune approaches to disease therapy: Past and future. *Nature Medicine, 10,* 135–141.

National Institutes of Health. Consensus Development Panel. (2001). National Institutes of Health Consensus Development Conference Statement: Phenylketonuria: Screening and management, October 16-18, 2000. *Pediatrics, 108,* 972–982.

Peek, G. J., & Elliott, M. J. (2004). Fetal surgery for congenital diaphragmatic hernia. *Pediatrics, 113,* 1810–1811.

Phillips, M. I. (2005). Antisense therapeutics: A promise waiting to be fulfilled. *Methods in Molecular Medicine, 106,* 3–10.

Pho, L. T., Zinberg, R. E., Hopkines-Boomer, T. A., Wallenstein, S., & McGovern, M. M. (2004). Attitudes and psychosocial adjustment of unaffected siblings of patients with phenylketonuria. *American Journal of Medical Genetics, 126A,* 156–160.

Prieto, J., Herraiz, M., Sangro, B., Qian, C., Mazzolini, G., Melero, I., et al. (2003). The promise of gene therapy in gastrointestinal and liver diseases. *Gut, 52*(Suppl. II), ii49–ii54.

Rabino, I. (2003). Gene therapy: Ethical issues. *Theoretical Medicine and Bioethics, 24,* 31–58.

Read, C. Y. (2003). The demands of biochemical genetic disorders: A survey of mothers of children with mitochondrial disease or phenylketonuria. *Journal of Pediatric Nursing, 18,* 181–186.

Roche, A. C., Fajac, I., Grosse, S., Frison, N., Rondanino, C., Mayer, R., et al. (2003). Glycofection: Facilitated gene transfer by cationic glycopolymers. *Cellular and Molecular Life Science, 60,* 288–297.

Schiffman, R., Kopp, J. B., Ausin, H. A., III., Sabnis, S., Moore, D. F., Weibel, T., et al. (2001). Enzyme replacement therapy in Fabry disease. *Journal of the American Medical Association, 285,* 2743–2749.

Schrier, S. L., & Angelucci, E. (2005). New strategies in the treatment of the thalassemias. *Annual Review of Medicine, 56,* 157–171.

Silver, A. (2003). Cognitive-behavioural therapy with a Huntington's gene positive patient. *Patient Education and Counseling, 49,* 133–138.

Simoneau-Roy, J., Marti, S., Deal, C., Huot, C., Robaey, P., & Van Vliet, G. (2004). Cognition and behavior at school entry in children with congenital hypothyroidism treated early with high-dose levothyroxine. *Journal of Pediatrics, 144,* 747–752.

Soonawalla, Z. F., Orug, T., Badminton, M. N., Elder, G. H., Rhodes, J. M., Bramhall, S. R., et al. (2004). Liver transplantation as a cure for acute intermittent porphyria. *Lancet, 363,* 705–706.

Soothill, P. W., Bartha, J. L., & Tizard, J. (2003). Ultrasound-guided laser treatment for fetal bladder outlet obstruction resulting from ureterocele. *American Journal of Obstetrics and Gynecology, 188,* 1107–1108.

Srivastrava, I. K., & Liu, M. A. (2003). Gene vaccines. *Annals of Internal Medicine, 138,* 550–559.

Sydorak, R. M., & Albanese, C. T. (2003). Minimal access techniques for fetal surgery. *World Journal of Surgery, 27,* 95–102.

Teitel, J. M., Barnard, D., Israels, S., Lillicrap, D., Poon, M. C., & Sek, J. (2004). Home management of haemophilia. *Haemophilia, 10,* 118–133.

Trahms, C. M. (2004). Medical nutrition therapy for metabolic disorders. In L. K. Mahan, & S. Escott-Stump (Eds.). *Krause's food, nutrition, & diet therapy* (11th ed., pp. 1143–1168). Philadelphia: W.B. Saunders.

Twombly, R. (2003). For gene therapy, now-quantified risks are deemed troubling. *Journal of the National Cancer Institute, 95,* 1032–1033.

Vigushin, D. M., & Coombes, R. C. (2004). Targeted histone deacetylase inhibition for cancer therapy. *Current Cancer Drug Targets, 4,* 205–218.

Walter, J. H., & White, F. J. (2004). Blood phenylalanine control in adolescents with phenylketonuria. *International Journal of Adolescent Medicine and Health, 16,* 41–45.

Walter, J. H., White, F. J., Hall, S. K., MacDonald, A., Rylance, G., Boneh, A., et al. (2002). How practical are recommendations for dietary control in phenylketonuria? *Lancet, 360,* 55–57.

Wilmott, R. W. (2005). Maternal engraftment of T-cells in children with severe combined immune deficiency can lead to long term survival. *Journal of Pediatrics, 146,* A2.

Yenari, M. A., & Sapolsky, R. M. (2005). Gene therapy in neurological disease. *Methods in Molecular Medicine, 106,* 3, 75–88.

Zhang, Y. C., Taylor, M. M., Samson, W. K., & Phillips, M. I. (2005). Antisense inhibition: Oligonucleotides, ribozymes, and siRNAs. *Methods in Molecular Medicine, 106,* 11–34.

IV

The Role of Genetics in Common Situations, Conditions, and Diseases

16

Genetics and the Common Diseases

The common diseases have long been observed to "run in families" and thus have a heritable component. The genetic contribution to the common or complex diseases are of particular interest to medical geneticists because of the potential for early identification of susceptible individuals followed by targeted interventions that might prevent the disease, prevent or ameliorate complications, and/or allow for initiation of early treatment. In general, the common diseases refer to disorders that are frequent in the population and that are not, in large part, attributable to monogenic causes following classic Mendelian inheritance. These may include coronary disease, cerebrovascular disease, diabetes mellitus, mental illness, hypertension, cancer, ulcers, chronic obstructive pulmonary disease, and others. Several of these will be discussed in detail in the following chapters.

The common diseases may be complex in regard to their inheritance because both genetic and environmental factors may play a role; there may be the presence of modifications to the genetic contribution, such as reduced penetrance and variable expression, other factors such as pleiotropy, epistasis, genetic heterogeneity, phenocopy, differential sex expression, epigenetic phenomena, and interaction between and among factors. For the most part, they are considered to be multifactorial in nature—being due to the interaction of several genes with environmental factors, although in each case a small percent of cases may be found to be due to a single-gene mutation. The genetic contribution could be one or two major genes in combination with minor ones, several minor ones with additive effects, several genes, some with protective effects, or other combinations. Environmental factors could include cultural, social, and behavioral aspects as well as physical ones. Environment could refer to internal or external and include dietary components, exposure to infectious agents or toxins, exercise, temperature extremes, sunlight exposure, radiation, and the internal milieu. There may be many susceptibility factors for a given condition and these may vary in different populations. Further, susceptibility may not necessarily mean disease development, so that some persons with the gene mutation may develop the condition and others may not. Such variation exists in disorders thought of as completely genetic. It is known that some persons with the same mutant gene for sickle cell anemia can have such a severe case as to cause childhood death, while another person may go unrecognized into late adulthood, the variation depending on the exact nature of the mutation and on unrevealed other genetic and environmental factors. The precise gene combination resulting in a given common disease could vary considerably. For example, more than 270 factors that could result in coronary heart disease have been identified by Stehbens (1992). An interesting question has been raised in the case of ulcers. What is the genetic contribution to the *susceptibility* to infection by *Helicobacter pylori*, and what is the genetic contribution to the *consequences* of such infection?

In some instances, forms of a multifactorial common disorder may be inherited as a single-gene Mendelian disorder. These tend to have an earlier age of onset, be normally infrequent in younger individuals (an example is the occurrence of an adult-type tumor in a child), or in the case of cancers, present with multiple primary neoplasms. An example is a subtype of type 2 diabetes mellitus, maturity onset diabetes of the young (MODY). Several MODY subtypes are now known and autosomal dominant inheritance is the mode of transmission. The identification of mutations in glucokinase (MODY 2) in the majority of MODY cases have led to investigation of the role of this enzyme in other cases of type 2 diabetes mellitus.

A major problem that plagued early investigations of the genetic component in common disorders was the way in which the disease was defined. For example, when colon cancer was not looked at globally but, for example, was considered as colon cancer with extreme polyposis, then it was possible to identify the *APC* gene on chromosome 5 by positional cloning. When searching for genetic contributions, hypertension could be defined by specified elevations in systolic or diastolic pressure only, or by a more precise pathophysiological definition. When conducting genetic investigations, definition of the disease could include the specification of a certain number of affected relatives. Specific ethnic groups that have been genetically isolated are often useful in identifying specific alleles causing a given disorder, such as the Icelanders, Basques, Finns, and others. Examples of these are the identification of a specific type of insulin defect in a Finnish population that resulted in type 2 diabetes mellitus and the identification of asthma genes in an island population in the South Atlantic Ocean.

In order to look for the genetic components in common disorders, a variety of methods have been used. These may, in some instances, look at the genome of affected persons in specific populations, use mathematical and genetic modeling, or may rely on genetic mapping. These may utilize molecular technology or not and include genome scans, positional cloning, linkage analysis, allele-sharing methods, association studies in human populations, twin studies, sibling studies, haplotype construction adoption studies, and genetic analysis of large numbers in model non-human populations.

Research into genetic causes of certain common diseases has been hampered for many reasons that are shared across the common disorders in most instances, although some may be more important in a given disorder than others. These include:

- the basic disease lesion may be unknown (e.g., schizophrenia);
- the pathophysiology may be complex and not completely understood, thus relevant candidate genes may be missed;
- the age of onset may be variable (type 2 diabetes mellitus (DM);
- the age of onset may be late, so that within a family there may be individuals who will eventually become ill but not until after the time frame for the research study (e.g., type 2 DM);
- diagnostic and classification criteria may vary from study to study;
- criteria may be ambiguous;
- individuals may be reassigned into different diagnostic categories at a later point in time;
- the accepted definition of the disorder may change;
- there may not be medical documentation of the condition;
- genetic markers may not have been available in the past;
- penetrance may be incomplete;
- the familial nature of the disease can represent both shared genetic and environmental factors, and it may be difficult to sort out biologic, environmental, and cultural influences;
- the failure in some studies to have "blind" evaluations of relatives of control and affected individuals (particularly in mental illness studies);
- reported disease cases may be grouped together on the basis of superficial characteristics, so that this "lumping" may obscure real differences;
- there may be lack of agreement on diagnostic standards;
- different forms of the disease may occur within a large family due to chance;
- different gene combinations may segregate in different families;
- generalization of study results between cultures and populations may not be possible;
- in biochemical studies, there may be the use of different substrates and methods;
- there may be failure to take into account the base rate of the disorder in the population studied;
- there may be a long asymptomatic period preceding disease development;
- families may be small and difficult to study while there may be long generation times for the condition to be apparent;

- mate selection in humans is usually random, so that the "appropriate" genetic cross is not possible;
- death may result from other causes;
- few multigenerational families may exist for study of the particular disease;
- varying statistical techniques and power may have been used to determine significance;
- the persons in the study groups may vary on parameters that can influence the study results;
- there may be several factors involved in susceptibility, including gene-gene interaction;
- susceptibility factors may differ in different populations; and
- genetic protective factors may affect susceptibility as well.

Twin and adoption studies have been used as methods for attempting to determine the heritable aspect of the common disorders. In twin studies, identical twins are presumed to be genetically identical, and the concordance rate for a particular disorder is calculated for identical and nonidentical twin pairs (of the same sex). This concordance rate provides a measure of heritability. These, too, are fraught with problems in methodology. For twin studies, in addition to the problems mentioned in chapter 17, these include difficulties in determining zygosity, failure to account for the special intrauterine environment of monozygous (MZ) twins, failure to account for the special external environment and relationship between twins, higher frequency of low birth weight, obstetrical complications, epigenetic phenomena, and other factors.

Studying adopted individuals and both their biologic and adoptive relatives provides a mechanism for the separating out of genetic and environmental factors. These methods have been frequently used in schizophrenia studies and have been done in the following ways: (1) the adopted individual of biologic schizophrenic parent(s) who was raised by normal adoptive parents was ascertained and the degree of illness in his or her biologic relatives was compared to that in the adoptive relatives; (2) adopted children born of schizophrenic parents (and adopted by normal parents) were compared to control adoptees born of normal parents and adopted by normal parents; (3) adopted children with normal biologic parent(s) whose adoptive parents were schizophrenic were compared with adoptees whose biologic parents were schizophrenic but whose adoptive parents were normal. Individuals were ascertained for study through the mechanism of studying all individuals placed for adoption within a certain time period, and studying those admitted to a mental hospital versus a sample selected from those remaining; by surveying the patient population of a given institution and ascertaining those who were adopted; or by ascertaining children born to schizophrenic mothers and adopted by normal parents. In adoption studies some problems have included the possible biologic relationship of the adoptive parents to the affected person, differences in the amount of time between birth and placement in adoptive homes, differences in the age when interviewed, differences in ascertainment, failure to study both biologic parents, and effects of adoptees knowing of the condition being looked for, such as mental illness in their biologic relatives.

SUMMARY

A subset of most of the common or complex diseases may be due to single-gene mutations, especially those cases with an early age of onset, but for most causation appears due to multiple gene mutations and environmental influences. As genetic mapping and molecular techniques, especially for genotyping, have evolved, other approaches for the study of complex traits and diseases have emerged. These have included linkage analysis, including affected sib-pair linkage, association mapping, candidate gene approaches, and the use of animal models of disease. Genome-wide linkage scans have contributed to knowledge by identifying potential genes involved in certain complex diseases so that further study could target these. In summary, the genetic contribution to the common diseases has only begun to be fully elucidated. It can be expected that this will become more defined in the near future and will have importance for more personalized disease prevention and health promotion. For the nurse, taking and recording an appropriate family history, coupled with the ability to think genetically will help to identify those at higher risk for common diseases by virtue of genetic factors.

BIBLIOGRAPHY

Bayat, A., Barton, A., & Ollier, W. E. (2004). Dissection of complex genetic disease: Implications of orthopedics. *Clinical Orthopedics, Feb*(419), 297–305.

Bell, J. (2004). Predicting disease using genomics. *Nature, 429,* 453–456.

Botstein, D., & Risch, N. (2003). Discovering genotypes underlying human phenotypes: Past successes for Mendelian disease, future approaches for complex disease. *Nature Genetics Supplement, 33,* 228–237.

Cardon, L. R., & Bell, J. I. (2001). Association study designs for complex diseases. *Nature Reviews Genetics, 2,* 91–99.

Cardon, L. R., & Palmer, L. J. (2003). Population stratification and spurious allelic association. *Lancet, 361,* 598–604.

Carlson, C. S., Eberle, M. A., Kruglyak, L., & Nickerson, D. A. (2004). Mapping complex disease loci in whole-genome association studies. *Nature, 429,* 446–452.

Chakravarthy, M. V., & Booth, F. W. (2004). Eating, exercise, and "thrifty" genotypes: Connecting the dots toward an evolutionary understanding of modern chronic diseases. *Journal of Applied Physiology, 96,* 3–10.

Colhoun, H. M., McKeigue, P. M., & Davey Smith, G. (2003). Problems of reporting genetic associations with complex outcomes. *Lancet, 361,* 865–872.

Conneally, P. M. (2003). The complexity of complex diseases. *American Journal of Human Genetics, 72,* 229–232.

Crawford, D. C., & Nickerson, D. A. (2005). Definition and clinical importance of haplotypes. *Annual Review of Medicine, 56,* 303–320.

Khoury, M. J., Yang, Q., Gwinn, M., Little, J., & Flanders, W. D. (2004). An epidemiologic assessment of genomic profiling for measuring susceptibility to common diseases and targeting interventions. *Genetics in Medicine, 6,* 38–47.

McKeigue, P. M. (2005). Prospects for admixture mapping of complex traits. *American Journal of Human Genetics, 76,* 1–7.

Moore, J. H., & Ritchie, M. D. (2004). The challenges of whole-genome approaches to common diseases. *Journal of the American Medical Association, 291,* 1642–1643.

Morton, N. E. (1998). Significance levels in complex inheritance. *American Journal of Human Genetics, 62,* 690–697.

Nye, S. H., & Ghosh, S. (2001). Genetics of complex diseases. In W. L. Lowe, Jr. (Ed.), *Genetics of diabetes mellitus* (pp. 1–23). Boston: Kluwer Academic Publishers.

Scheuner, M. T., & Gordon, O. K. (2002). Genetic risk assessment for common disease. In D. L. Rimoin, J. M. Connor, R. E. Pyeritz, & B. R. Korf (Eds.), *Emery and Rimoin's principles and practice of medical genetics* (4th ed., pp. 654–674.). New York: Churchill Livingstone.

Scheuner, M. T., Yoon, P. W., & Khoury, M. J. (2004). Contribution of Mendelian disorders to common chronic disease: Opportunities for recognition, intervention, and prevention. *American Journal of Medical Genetics, Part C, Seminars in Medical Genetics, 125C,* 50–65.

Stefan, M., & Nicholls, R. D. (2004). What have rare genetic syndromes taught us about the pathophysiology of the common forms of obesity? *Current Diabetes Reports, 4,* 143–150.

Stehbens, W. E. (1992). Causality in medical science with particular reference to heart disease and atherosclerosis. *Perspectives in Biology and Medicine, 36,* 97–119.

Wiltshire, S., Morris, A. P., McCarthy, M. I., & Cardon, L. R. (2005). How useful is the fine-scale mapping of complex trait linkage peaks? Evaluating the impact of additional microsatellite genotyping on the posterior probability of kinkage. *Genetic Epidemiology, 28,* 1–10.

17

Twins, Twin Studies, and Multiple Births

Whether positive or negative, twins have had a special significance throughout history that varies among different cultures. In some societies twins have been believed to foretell disaster or indicate infidelity; whereas in others, they were considered a special sign of favor and were thought to bring good fortune. Geneticists have been interested in twins since 1875, when Galton noted that twins afforded the opportunity to study "nature vs. nurture." Some problems associated with this assumption are discussed later in the chapter.

Twins are either monozygotic (MZ, identical) or dizygotic (DZ, fraternal). The incidence of MZ twinning is approximately the same throughout the world—1 in 250 births. The incidence of DZ twinning varies in different populations. In the United States DZ twinning is most frequent in non-Hispanic Blacks followed by non-Hispanic Whites, and least frequent in Asians. In certain Nigerian tribes the twinning rate is as high as 45/1000. Early ultrasound techniques have revealed that about 20% of the twin pregnancies seen early result in the "vanishing" of one fetus, resulting in a singleton birth. The majority of higher order pregnancies results from fertility drugs and techniques such as the implantation of multiple fertilized embryos, but the incidence of twin births is increasing in the United States independent of fertility techniques, especially in white women aged 30 years and older living in the Northeast. It is believed that the use of multivitamin supplements periconceptionally is responsible. This can have repercussions because twin pregnancies and births present greater risk to the mother and the fetuses. Twin and higher order births represent a higher rate of preterm delivery and low birth weight, and

a high contribution to overall infant morbidity and mortality as well as to unfavorable long-term sequelae. In some cases, it is believed that gene mutations that increase receptor site sensitivity for where follicle-stimulating hormone binds with the ovaries lead to multiple egg release during ovulation. Occasionally, selective reduction of multifetal pregnancies is done to reduce the absolute number of fetuses, or in cases where one fetus has a defect, posing the ethical issues associated with chosen pregnancy termination. Because the risk of aneuploidy in at least one twin is about 1 in 190 at 31 years of maternal age, prenatal diagnosis is recommended for women at age 31 years if they are carrying twins instead of the usual age 35 years.

MONOZYGOTIC TWINS

MZ twins have been called the most common human structural defect. They are derived from the cleavage of a single fertilized ovum. Separation can occur as early as the 2-cell stage or as late as 8 to 12 days after conception. The time at which it divides determines the placental and fetal membranes present and the number of arteries in the umbilical cord. The later cleavage occurs, the more likely "mirror imaging" phenomena, such as hair whorls that are clockwise in one twin and counterclockwise in the other, will be present. Conjoined twins are MZ twins in whom division was incomplete, occurring more than 12 days after conception. This occurs in 1 in 33,000 to 165,000 births. All reported cases have been of the same sex, and 70% have been female. About 40% of conjoined twins are stillborn and 34% die soon after birth. The recent case of the failed surgical separation and death of two adult conjoined Iranian twins, Lalah and Laden Bijani, following the successful separation of two Guatemalan toddlers, Maria Teresa and Maria de Jesus Quiej Alvarez, has focused attention on this condition.

Although a genetic etiology is not common for MZ twinning, a type has been described that is compatible with a single-gene effect that can be transmitted to the next generation. It follows an autosomal dominant mode of transmission and shows a variable degree of penetrance. MZ twins are more likely to have structural defects than are singletons or DZ twins. In about 10% of MZ births, at least one twin has a congenital anomaly. Schinzel, Smith, and Miller (1979) and Hall (2002) have grouped them in the following categories: (a) malformations that occurred early in morphogenesis that have been presumed to be of the same etiology that gave rise to the twinning phenomenon. These malformations may include anencephaly, renal agenesis, sirenomelia (fused legs and lower body underdevelopment), and absence of a limb; (b) structural defects secondary to vascular interchange or disruption, or due to death of co-twin in utero, such as hydrocephalus, intestinal atresia, and acardia; (c) structural or mechanically induced deformations caused by in utero crowding, such as foot deformations. Little is known about the etiology of MZ twinning, and both genetic and environmental factors such as mechanical stresses may play a role. In other organisms, MZ twinning has been produced by temperature alterations, changes in oxygen levels, and injections of vincristine at different points in development. Late fertilization of the ovum has led to an increase in MZ twinning in the rabbit. Because mothers of MZ twins may have longer than average menstrual cycles, overripeness of the ovum may be related to MZ twinning in the human as well. Although rare, discordance in the number of chromosomes and other parameters and conditions between MZ twins has been described. For example, one twin may have Down syndrome, Russell-Silver syndrome, or Beckwith-Wiedemann syndrome while it is not present in the other. There are also reports of an excess of twins in the relatives of those with neural tube defects, leading to the speculation that there is some shared causal factor. Reasons for these differences have been speculated to involve X-inactivation, mitochondrial mutations, genomic imprinting, loss of imprinting, different intrauterine environments, differences in DNA methylation, and other epigenetic events.

Nurses should carefully assess the co-twin of any MZ twin with a malformation for overlooked or subtle defects. This is particularly important if early therapeutic intervention is indicated. The nurse should send the placenta and membranes of any apparent singleton born with malformations for analysis for any evidence of a deceased co-twin or an incomplete twin. The presence of a deceased co-twin at birth should alert health personnel to the possibility of thrombosis or emboli in the living twin. Any large growth discrepancies noted between twins should indicate the need to check the placenta for vascular interchanges that could be responsible.

Except for the less usual familial twinning described above, most mothers of MZ twins are not considered at higher risk for recurrence. However, women who are MZ twins have a higher risk of having twins of the same sex (relative risk 1.47, confidence interval 1.10–1.97).

DIZYGOTIC TWINS

DZ twins are derived from the fertilization of two ova that could have originated in the same or different ovaries by two sperm. DZ twins have an average of 50% of their genes in common, as do other siblings; however, they share the intrauterine and extrauterine environment at the same time. They can be of the same or different sexes. Cases have been described in which one twin male was white and the other was black because they were fertilized from sperm from different fathers. Dizygotic twins who share a single placenta (monochorionic) have been described, disproving a previously accepted dogma of a single placenta shared by twins, meaning that the twins were MZ.

In contrast to MZ twins, several parameters have been shown to have an effect on DZ twinning. It rises with maternal age, having a peak at about 37 years of age, and then it rapidly falls. Although in general there is an increased twinning rate with increased parity, it has been found that there is a higher DZ twinning rate among women who conceive in the first 3 months of marriage than in those of comparable age who first conceive later.

Nutrition may also play a role, as evidenced by the fall in DZ twinning rates in those countries suffering from undernutrition during World War II, and by the increased incidence of DZ twinning in women who are tall and obese or of normal weight as opposed to those with smaller and lighter body parameters. DZ twins may also have a higher risk for structural defects than singletons, although this risk is lower than for MZ twins.

DZ may result from both autosomal recessive and autosomal dominant inheritance. In one example, autosomal recessive genes might act by increasing the frequency of double ovulation, perhaps through higher pituitary gonadotropin levels. It appears that these genes are sex-limited, and therefore only express themselves in one sex, in this case the female. The tendency toward twinning appears to come mostly from the female side, but paternally derived inheritance patterns have also been described. Once a woman has had a pair of DZ twins, her chances of having another pair is increased fourfold without correction for age. Women who were DZ twins seem to have a moderate increase for having twins (relative risk 1.30, 95% confidence interval 1.14 to 1.49).

DETERMINATION OF ZYGOSITY

Zygosity is difficult to determine from a casual study of the fetal membranes and the placenta. MZ twins can have a double placenta, double chorion, and double amnion, just as DZ twins may if division in MZ twins occurs early (before the trophoblast differentiates). If division occurs later, from about the 5th to 10th day (before the amnion differentiates), then a single placenta, single chorion, and double amnion are found. If division is after differentiation of the amnion, then there is a single placenta, chorion, and amnion present. Both MZ and DZ twins may have a fusion of the two placentas so that it resembles a single placenta. It is difficult to distinguish between a fused dichorionic placenta and monochorionic, diamniotic placenta, and dizygous monchorionic twins have been reported. To establish zygosity, the simplest criterion has been sex, since DZ twins are almost always of unlike sex. However, exceptions introduce some uncertainty as described above [see Hall (2002) for a list]. Genetic markers such as the red blood cell antigens, HLA antigens, and enzymes can be used to determine zygosity, as can dermal ridge counts, physical similarities, and the mutual acceptance of skin grafts. The more biochemical markers that are the same, the greater the percentage of chance that the twins are identical. The final best evidence is through the use of DNA technology; however, Hall (2003) has noted that DNA in blood cells can seem to be identical even when the twin pair were genetically or epigenetically discordant, since about 70% of monozygotic twins share vascular placental connections. For studies in the fields of psychology and education, researchers have developed questionnaires with a high degree of reported accuracy to use for zygosity determination, because the use of biochemical markers may be too costly and cumbersome. These tools rely on noninvasive criteria such as the pattern of the iris, hair texture, and behavioral characteristics.

TWIN STUDIES IN GENETICS

"A devil, a born devil, on whose nature nurture can never stick. . . ." Wm. Shakespeare, *The Tempest*, Act IV, Scene 1, lines 188 to 189.

For centuries, the problem of "nature vs. nurture" has been of intense interest. The study of twins (gemellology) allows one to study environmental influences in a given disease or condition against a standardized genetic background (such as differential fat intake in hypercholesterolemia) to evaluate the extent of the genetic contribution to the etiology of various traits or disorders, such as in diabetes mellitus (DM); and in those diseases whose genetic component is established, to study the degree of penetrance and the extent of variable expression. In a trait that is entirely genetically determined, one would expect virtually 100% concordance in MZ twins and a lower concordance in DZ twins. However, although the pre- and perinatal environments of co-twins are similar, they cannot be presumed to be identical. Possible sources of variation in prenatal environment between co-twins and other twin pairs include:

- Differences in degree of intrauterine crowding;
- Different implantation locations in the uterus;

- Unequal distribution of cytoplasmic constitutents at cleavage of the zygotes;
- Differential action of maternal medications on twins of unequal size;
- Differential exposure time to anesthesia for second-born twin;
- Differences in placenta, chorion and amnion;
- Differences resulting from artificial reproductive technology;
- Differential birth weight between co-twins;
- May or may not share placental circulation;
- Differences in oxygenation, nutrient intake, hormones, waste disposal, etc.;
- Cord anomalies;
- Vascular connections such as arteriovenous anastomoses in co-twins;
- "Transfusion syndrome" may be present between co-twins;
- Somatic mutations;
- Differences in X-inactivation patterns in female co-twins;
- Differences in the antibody and T-cell receptor repertoire;
- Differences in the numbers of mitochondrial DNA molecules due to epigenetic partitioning; and
- Epigenetic phenomena such as methylation differences.

The extent of the influence of this type of variation is unknown.

There are several ways in which twins are used in genetic studies.

1. Each MZ co-twin can be compared with the other and the extent to which a disease or trait occurs in both members (concordance) can be determined (a variation of this method also uses the co-twin as a control but concentrates on a discordance between the two, for example, if one smokes and one does not, a selected aspect relating to development of lung cancer could be compared).
2. MZ twin pairs can be compared with DZ twin pairs in similar environments and the group percentages of concordance can be compared.
3. Twins reared together can be compared for specific traits to twins reared apart.
4. Twins can be compared to singletons.

5. The children of MZ twin pairs who are related to each other as half siblings can be compared through both male and female twin lines.

Ways of selecting twins for a research study can influence the findings. Some ways that have been used are obtaining data from twin registries, twin lay organizations, disease registries, local hospital and physician records, or appeal through the public media for volunteers to participate. Confounding factors that can influence any of the twin studies include the following:

1. Small sample size. In practice it is difficult to assemble large numbers of twins with the specific disorder desired. For example, if the frequency of a disorder were 1 in 1000, a population of 1,000,000 would have to be searched to find 1000 affected people and, of these, the expected number having a twin would be about 20, approximately 15 DZ and 5 MZ.
2. The occurrence of sporadic cases due to mutation.
3. Ascertainment bias or the method used to find cases for study can lead to error.
4. Variable characteristics of the disorder under study, such as its severity, age of onset, the influence of sex on the trait.
5. Inaccurate determination of zygosity.
6. Genetic-environment interactions.
7. Accuracy of the criteria used to diagnose a disease or check for the presence or absence of the trait under study.
8. The definition of concordance. For example, if IQ is studied, does an IQ score on the chosen test of 110 in one twin and 115 in the other constitute concordance or not?

Possible factors that can influence data in studies of twins reared apart and together are the fact that pre- and perinatal effects remain; the numbers of such twins are very small; the age at which the twins were separated may vary; they may have been reunited at various times; blood relatives may have reared one or both; they may have been in the same school; and the adoptive parents may have been matched or selected on a variety of unknown factors. Possible factors that are unique to twins as opposed to single-child births are the following:

Prenatal and Perinatal

- factors relating to intrauterine crowding
- greater number of malformations and defects
- higher perinatal morbidity, such as damage from anoxia
- greater asymmetry of functions, such as left-handedness
- lower birth weight (usually)
- possible differential in nutrition, oxygenation, etc.

Postnatal

- psychodynamics accompanying the unique social group of twins or "couple"
- development of a private language
- "assigned" role for each twin in the "outside world"
- peculiarities of twins in personality and behavior
- delayed speech and language development
- excessive affection or hostility towards co-twin
- retarded growth
- parents of twins may have less time to devote to twins because of having two "concurrent" children
- each twin may form a strong unbalanced attachment to a different parent
- the presence of someone in the household who is the same age throughout infancy, childhood, and adolescence.

Despite possible pitfalls, twins offer a unique research opportunity to the human geneticist. The development of more sophisticated mathematical methods and computer analyses has allowed for the statistical consideration of many of the possible confounding variables. The Swedish Twin Registry (Lichtenstein et al., 2002) was established in the late 1950s, and it has provided a wealth of data on many topics including factors associated with cancer, cardiovascular disease, and dementia. What is most important is that the researcher be aware of potential problems before collecting data and that the reader keep them in mind when evaluating the results of twin research studies.

The prevalence of child abuse is greater in families with twins and higher order births when compared with comparable control families with single

births. The nurse may be able to act in a preventive manner by telling the family that they can expect greater physical and economic demands from twins. They can then discuss some sources of support and ways to cope with feeding, bathing, and so on. There has been an increase in commitment to breast feeding for multiples, and a declaration of rights statement by the International Society for Twin Studies. Greater periods of chronic stress may leave the family vulnerable, and this also should be discussed. The family can be referred to appropriate community groups and should also be told about the organizations and publications for parents of twins. See Appendix B.

BIBLIOGRAPHY

ACOG Ethics Statement: Multifetal pregnancy reduction and selective fetal termination. The Committee on Ethics, American College of Obstetricians and Gynecologists, Washington, DC, November, 1990.

Arnold, W., & Grady, D. (2003, July 9). Iran twins die trying to live separate lives. *New York Times International.* http://www.nytimes.com/2003/07/09/international/asia/09TWIN.html.

Bamforth, F., Brown, L., Senz, J., & Huntsman, D. (2003). Mechanisms of monozygotic (MZ) twinning: A possible role for the cell adhesion molecule, E-cadherin. *American Journal of Medical Genetics, 120A,* 59–62.

Baor, L., & Blickstein, I. (2005). En route to an "instant" family: Psychosocial considerations. *Obstetrics and Gynecology Clinics of North America, 32,* 127–139.

Basso, O., Nohr, E. A., Christensen, K., & Olsen, J. (2004). Risk of twinning as a function of maternal height and body mass index. *Journal of the American Medical Association, 291,* 1564–1566.

Blakely, E. L., He, L., Taylor, R. W., Chinnery, P. F., Lightowlers, R. Nj., Schaefer, A. M., et al. (2004). Mitochrondrial DNA deletion in "identical" twin brothers. *Journal of Medical Genetics, 41,* e19–e22.

Blickstein, I. (2004). How and why are triplets disadvantaged compared to twins? *Best Practice & Research Clinical Obstetrics and Gynecology, 19,* 631–644.

Boklage, C. E. (1987). Twinning, non-righthandedness, and fusion malformations: Evidence for heritable causal elements held in common. *American Journal of Medical Genetics, 28,* 67–84.

Bouchard, T. J., Jr., & Propping, P. (Eds.). (1993). *Twins as a tool of behavioral genetics.* Chichester, England: John Wiley & Sons.

Czeizel, A., Metnecki, J., & Dudás, I. (1994). Higher rate of multiple births after periconceptual vitamin supplementation. *Lancet, 330,* 23–24.

Evans, M. I., Kaufman, M. I., Urban, A. J., Britt, D. W., & Fletcher, J. C. (2004). Fetal reduction from twins to a singleton: A reasonable consideration? *Obstetrics & Gynecology, 104,* 102–109.

Gedda, L., Parisi, P., & Nance, W. E. (Eds). (1981). *Twin Research 3 Part A, B, C.* New York: Alan R. Liss.

Goodship, J., Carter, J., & Burn, J. (1996). X-inactivation patterns in monozygous and dizygotic female twins. *American Journal of Medical Genetics, 61,* 205–208.

Goodship, J., Cross, I., Scambler, P., & Burn, J. (1995). Monozygotic twins with chromosome 22q11 deletion and discordant phenotype. *Journal of Medical Genetics, 32,* 746–748.

Gringas, P., & Chen, W. (2001). Mechanisms for differences in monozygous twins. *Early Human Development, 64,* 105–117.

Hall, J. G. (2002). Twins and twinning. In D. L. Rimoin, J. M. Connor, R. E. Pyeritz, & B. R. Korf (Eds.), *Emery and Rimoin's principles and practice of medical genetics* (4th ed., pp. 501-513). New York: Churchill Livingstone.

Hall, J. G. (2003). Twinning. *Lancet, 362,* 735–743.

Keith, L. G., & Blickstein, I. (Eds.). (2002). *Triplet pregnancies and their consequences.* CRC Press.

Kurosawa, K., Kuromaru, R., Imaizumi, K., Nakamura, Y., Ishikawa, F., Ueda, K., et al. (1992). Monozygotic twins with discordant sex. *Acta Geneticae Medicae et Gemellologiae, 41,* 301–310.

Lichtenstein, P., De Faire, U., Floderus, B., Svartengren, M., Svedberg, P., & Pedersen, N. L. (2002). The Swedish Twin Registry: A unique resource for clinical, epidemiological and genetic studies. *Journal of Internal Medicine, 252,* 184–205.

Machin, G. A. (1995). Some causes of genotypic and phenotypic discordance in monozygotic twin pairs. *American Journal of Medical Genetics, 61,* 229–236.

Meyers, C., Adam, R., Dungan, J., & Prenger, V. (1997). Aneuploidy in twin gestations: When is maternal age advanced? *Obstetrics & Gynecology, 89,* 248–251.

Nance, W. E. (Ed.). (1978). *Twin Research, Part A, B, C.* New York: Alan R. Liss.

Peterson, S. L., & Rayan, G. M. (2004). Monozygotic twins discordant for thumb polydactyly. *Plastic and Reconstructive Surgery, 113,* 449–451.

Petronis, A., Gottesman, II, Kan, P., Kennedy, J. L., Basile, V. S., Paterson, A. D., et al. (2003). Monozygotic twins exhibit numerous epigenetic differences: Clues to twin discordance? *Schizophrenia Bulletin, 29,* 169–178.

Read, J. A. (2001). Multiple gestation. In F. W. Ling, & P. Duff (Eds.), *Obstetrics and gynecology: Principles for practice* (pp. 273–307). New York: McGraw Hill.

Redline, R. W. (2003). Nonidentical twins with a single placenta—disproving dogma in perinatal pathology. *New England Journal of Medicine, 349,* 111–114.

Reynolds, M. A., Schieve, L. A., Martin, J. A., Jeng, G., & Macaluso, M. (2003). Trends in multiple births conceived using assisted reproductive technology, United States, 1997–2000. *Pediatrics, 111,* 1159–1162.

Rogers, J. G., Voullaire, L., & Gold, H. (1982). Monozygotic twins discordant for trisomy 21. *American Journal of Medical Genetics, 11,* 143–146.

Russell, R. B., Petrini, J., Damus, K., Mattison, D. R., & Schwarz, R. H. (2003). The changing epidemiology of multiple births in the United States. *Obstetrics & Gynecology, 101,* 129–135.

Salihu, H. M., Aliyu, M. H., & Alexander, G. R. (2004). The relationship between paternal age and early mortality of triplets in the United States. *American Journal of Perinatology, 21,* 99–107.

Schinzel, A. A. G. L., Smith, D. W., & Miller, J. R. (1979). Monozygotic twinning and structural defects. *Journal of Pediatrics, 95,* 921–930.

Singh, S. M., Murphy, B., & O'Reilly, R. (2002). Epigenetic contributors to the discordance of monozygotic twins. *Clinical Genetics, 62,* 97–103.

Souter, V. L., Kapur, R. P., Nyholt, D. R. E., Skogerboe, K., Myerson, D., Ton, C. C., et al. (2003). A report of dizygous monochorionic twins. *New England Journal of Medicine, 349,* 154–158.

Wachtel, S. S., Somkuti, S. G., & Schinfeld, J. S. (2000). Monozygotic twins of opposite sex. *Cytogenetic Cell Genetics, 91,* 293–295.

18

Drug Therapy and Genetics: Pharmacogenetics and Pharmacogenomics

Nurses have long observed that different individuals receiving the same dose of the same drug can exhibit different degrees of therapeutic effectiveness and can experience variation in the type and degree of side-effects, for no readily apparent reason. Differences in how individuals respond to drugs can be due to genetic or nongenetic factors. Genetic controls can be operational at any stage of the drug handling process—absorption, distribution, protein binding, metabolism, membrane transport, attachment to membrane receptors, tissue sensitivity, tissue storage, elimination, and in the activation of special responses such as the immune response. Genetic variation in drug metabolism and handling can be quantitative or qualitative. Mutant genes may produce enzyme variants with high, intermediate, low, or absent activity. The mutation may only involve a single nucleotide polymorphism (SNP) as discussed previously. Thus human genetic variation whether occurring in individuals as rare mutations or as a consequence of relatively common interindividual variations or polymorphisms including SNPs are important in increased or decreased effective drug dosage for response, drug toxicity, drug side effects, drug–drug interactions and more. The degree and type of variation in an individual's response may not be apparent if there is no significant therapeutic or clinical consequence. Information about response variation is particularly important in drugs with a narrow therapeutic margin. Many drugs have a wide enough margin of safety so that even with individual response variation, effectiveness and safety are not compromised. However, practitioners must recognize that persons from diverse racial and ethnic groups may respond differently to medications because of genetic differences.

Pharmacogenetics began to develop in the late 1950s and is concerned with the consequences of genetic differences in drug handling that affect individual response. These differences can be one feature of a person's genetic disorder such as in the porphyrias or may be the only known abnormality present, such as in pseudocholinesterase variation. Differences may involve variation to the point at which it is a polymorphism, and is therefore relatively common in certain populations, or it may be relatively rare. A single strategically placed defect such as in the enzyme-controlling acetylation of drugs in the liver can have far reaching effects, affecting the metabolism of all the drugs processed along that pathway. Such variation may provide clues to cancer development through understanding of variation and defects in the detoxification of chemicals, and for alcoholism due to differential metabolism.

The terms "pharmacogenetics" and "pharmacogenomics" are increasingly used interchangeably. Various authors define the terms differently. Traditionally, pharmacogenetics has been most concerned with single-gene variations and refers to the effect of genotype on pharmacodynamics, pharmacokinetics, drug absorption, distribution, metabolism, excretion, receptor target affinity, and overall, the response to drugs. Pharmacogenomics has been coined more recently and has been variously described as determination of the genome and products in relation to drug response, often for developing and customizing drugs based on knowledge of the human genome and genetic profiles in patients (Nebert & Jorge-Nebert, 2002; Tsai & Hoyme, 2002). Pharmacogenomics is seen by some as having a broader scope, including genes that cause disease which can be manipulated by drugs (Mukherjee & Topol, 2002). This genome-wide approach also considers the interaction of multiple genes. Another aspect of genetics in regard to drug therapy is the exploitation of genetic knowledge in regard to genetic changes in microorganisms rather than in the human host and in transformed cancer cells to formulate therapeutic approaches. Toxicogenomics, which may be defined as the study of genes and their products important in adaptive responses to toxic exposures, is discussed in chapter 14. In this chapter, both rare pharmacogenetic disorders and common polymorphisms leading to altered response to drugs are discussed, as are pharmacogenomic applications and the ethical problems engendered.

POLYMORPHISMS AFFECTING DRUG METABOLISM

In this section, a polymorphic enzyme variation that has as one component an effect on drug metabolism (glucose-6-phosphate dehydrogenase deficiency) will be discussed as well as selected examples of enzyme families that are important in drug metabolism because of genetic variation.

Glucose-6-Phosphate Dehydrogenase Deficiency

Glucose-6-phosphate dehydrogenase (G6PD) deficiency is the most common enzyme abnormality and affects millions of people throughout the world, especially those of Mediterranean, African, Middle Eastern, Near Eastern, and Southeast Asian origin. G6PD deficiency as a polymorphism is discussed in chapter 3. It is transmitted by a mutant gene on the X chromosome, and thus males are hemizygous. Approximately 10% to 15% of Black males in the United States have G6PD deficiency. In the Middle East, G6PD deficiency may be as

high as 35% of males. Because of this high frequency, more homozygous females are found for G6PD deficiency than are found for other X-linked recessive disorders. Females who are heterozygous for the mutant gene have two types of red cells, those that are normal and those that are deficient. Although the two red cell populations are usually approximately equal as a consequence of X inactivation (see chapter 4), a preponderance of cells with deficient enzyme can result. Therefore, such females are subject to hemolysis on encountering specific drugs and are known as manifesting heterozygotes. For G6PD deficiency, the populations that may show effects are hemizygous males, homozygous deficient females and some heterozygous females.

G6PD is found in all cells where G6PD is necessary in order to catalyze an important oxidation/reduction reaction in the pentose phosphate pathway and also maintains adequate levels of NADPH in cells. In most cells, other metabolic pathways can provide the needed end products from the above reaction. The G6PD deficient red cell usually functions well, but hemolytic anemia can occur when oxidant- or peroxide-producing drugs are taken up, when infection occurs, when exposed to naphthalene in moth balls, or with ingestion of the fava (broad) bean. The severity of the hemolysis varies with the percent of active enzyme present in the specific G6PD variant. There are more than 400 identified G6PD variants, not all of which are clinically significant. Among them are G6PD A- (most prevalent in Africa, the Americas, and West Indies) with 5–15% of normal enzyme activity and associated with mild or moderate hemolysis, and G6PD Mediterranean (most prevalent in the Mediterranean, North Africa, and the Middle East) with 0% to 7% of the normal enzyme activity. Various classifications exist and the WHO classifies G6PD variants are as follows:

Class 1: Severe enzyme deficiency with chronic nonspherocytic hemolytic anemia

Class 2: Severe enzyme deficiency with intermittent hemolysis (less than 10%)

Class 3: Moderate enzyme deficiency with intermittent hemolysis

Class 4: Very mild or no enzyme deficiency (60–100%)

Most persons with G6PD deficiency never demonstrate clinical manifestations. Clinical outcomes of G6PD deficiency include hemolysis from drugs, infection, or the fava bean (favism); neonatal jaundice and chronic nonspherocytic hemolytic anemia. Only those related to drugs will be discussed here.

Hemolysis following the intake of certain drugs in persons with G6PD deficiency was first identified with the use of the antimalarial drug, primaquine. Since the original work, some drugs have been classified by the World Health Organization (WHO) as those to be avoided by all, those to be avoided by those G6PD-deficient persons of Mediterranean, Middle Eastern, and Asian origin and those to be avoided only by those with the African (A-) variant. Still others categorize drugs by degree of certainty of association with hemolysis. In some cases, the decision to use a particular drug depends on the need for that drug and the dosage used. Other factors that influence response include genetic differences, the severity of the G6PD deficiency, the hemoglobin level, factors relating to the red cell, as well as the age of the person and the presence of other sources of oxidative stress such as infection. Drugs and chemicals with a definite association with hemolysis in persons with G6PD deficiency include: acetanilide, doxorubicin, dapsone, methylene blue, nalidixic acid, naphthalene, niridazole, nitrites, nitrofurans including furazolidone, nitrofurantoin, nitrofurazone, pamaquine, pentaquine, phenazopyridine, phenylhydrazine, primaquine, sulfacetamide, sulfamethoxazole, sulfanilamide, sulfapyridine, toluidine blue, triazolesulfone, and trinitroluene (Beutler, 1994; Luzzetto, Mehta, & Vulliamy, 2001; WHO Working Group, 1989). Drugs possibly associated with significant hemolysis include chloramphenicol, ciprofloxacin, chloroquine, norfloxacin, sulfamethoxypyridazine, sulfadimidine, and sulfamerizine (Luzzetto et al., 2001). Debated are such drugs as aspirin, ascorbic acid, vitamin K analogues, probenecid, and others.

Drug-induced hemolysis typically begins within one or a few days of starting the drug, and includes a fall in Hb, Heinz bodies in the red cells, eventual hemolytic anemia, and when severe includes dark urine and back pain. Hemolysis can also result from infections, particularly infectious hepatitis, pneumonia, typhoid fever, and other viral, bacterial,

and rickettsial infections. Acute renal failure often follows hepatitis or urinary tract infections in G6PD-deficient persons. Hemolysis may also follow the ingestion of the fava or broad bean (favism), a common dietary component in the Mediterranean, Middle and Far East, and North Africa. The response occurs suddenly within 24 to 48 hours with acute hemolytic anemia manifested by pallor, hemoglobinuria, and jaundice. Hemolysis has occurred in breast feeding G6PD-deficient infants whose mothers ate fava beans. Chronic nonspherocytic hemolytic anemia accompanies certain variants and may be made worse by stress, infection, or drug intake. They may have a history of neonatal jaundice, and may have gallstones, splenomegaly, decreased stamina, weakness, iron overload, and progressive hepatic damage.

Some researchers believe that all individuals in population groups at risk should be screened for G6PD deficiency before any of the drugs listed are prescribed. Awareness of G6PD deficiency has become important in administering drugs such as dapsone used to treat many patients with HIV infection. In some instances the need for the drug outweighs the risk of hemolytic anemia. Nurses should review the patient's prior drug exposure history with the individual at the time of treatment, inquire about any drug reactions in blood relatives, and consider whether further testing for G6PD deficiency is merited. Once an individual is known to have G6PD deficiency, agents that can precipitate hemolytic anemia should be listed and reviewed with the person, who should be counseled to avoid them. Avoidance of the fava bean should be included as well as discussion of breast feeding risks if the infant is deficient in G6PD. The individual should be advised that family members may be at risk and should be screened for the deficiency in order to identify them. Persons should be advised to wear some type of medical information.

Acetylator Status and Drug Metabolism

The ability to metabolize and eliminate certain drugs depends on acetylation in the liver by the enzyme N-acetyltransferase with two functional genes, *NAT1* and *NAT2*, located on chromosome 8. Each gene has multiple alleles. Further descriptors are designated by an asterisk and the allele designation, for example *NAT2*5B*. Both drug efficacy and toxicity are linked to the functioning of this enzyme, which has genetically determined polymorphic variation. In North American and European populations, between 50% and 70% are slow acetylators, as are about 90% of some Mediterranean populations such as Egyptians and Moroccans. In eastern Pacific populations such as Chinese, Koreans, Japanese, and Thais, about 10% to 30% are slow acetylators, as are about 4% of Alaskan natives. Individuals can be categorized into the following basic phenotypic groups—slow or poor, rapid, and ultrarapid acetylators.

The importance of acetylator status was first recognized during therapy for tuberculosis with isoniazid (INH). Drug therapy for which acetylator status is known to have clinical relevance includes INH; dapsone, a sulfone; hydralazine (Apresoline), an antihypertensive; procainamide (Pronestyl), an antiarrhythmic; phenelzine (Nardil), an antidepressant; nitrazepam (Mogadon), a sedative; and sulfasalazine (Azulfidine), a sulfonamide derivative. Caffeine metabolism is also mediated by this system. Slow acetylators maintain higher serum levels of these drugs than do rapid acetylators. In general, slow acetylators are more likely to experience greater therapeutic responses but also a higher incidence of side-effects than rapid acetylators when the same medication regime is used for the drugs mentioned above. Slow acetylators are also at greater risk for the development of spontaneous SLE (systemic lupus erythmatosis) with certain drugs such as hydralazine and procainamide. Roberts-Thomson et al. (1996) found that fast acetylators who ate meat were at higher risk for colorectal cancer, and slow acetylators had a higher risk for bladder cancer when exposed to arylamines and cigarette smoke.

Isoniazid

Daily therapy for tuberculosis with INH is not influenced by acetylator status, but it is significant for weekly and semi-weekly regimens. Slow acetylators are at significantly greater risk for developing isoniazid-induced peripheral neuropathy because they maintain higher serum levels of INH. The concurrent administration of pyridoxine prevents this. Slow acetylators show a better therapeutic response to weekly INH therapy than do rapid acetylators, but rapid acetylators are more likely to develop isoniazid-induced hepatitis, especially in

those persons of Chinese and Japanese heritage. When individuals with both tuberculosis and epilepsy are taking INH and phenytoin (Dilantin) together, high INH concentrations that develop in slow acetylators inhibit phenytoin metabolism, thus allowing toxic levels and severe side effects to occur. When considering long-term INH therapy, it is useful for the nurse to recommend the determination of the person's acetylator status. If it is not feasible to do this, the regimen can be begun by empirically adjusting therapy according to the patient's ethnic group and carefully observing for side effects.

Cytochrome P-450 Polymorphisms

The hepatic cytochrome P450 enzyme system is comprised of a group of related enzymes known as a superfamily. These enzymes are responsible for oxidizing many chemicals and drugs. A separate gene codes for each isozyme and more than 200 have been identified, some of which have multiple allelic forms. They are named according to the following system: CYP followed by a family number, a subfamily letter, and a number for the individual form. One of the important polymorphisms in this system is the CYP2D6 gene polymorphism, sometimes referred to as the debrisoquine-sparteine type because it was first identified in the oxidation of debrisoquine (Declinax), an antihypertensive agent, and sparteine, an antiarrhythmic drug. Although debrisoquine and sparteine are no longer clinically important drugs, many other drugs also use this pathway. The CYP2D6 gene is located on chromosome 22. As mentioned above, a number of allelic variants are known (more than 75), designated by an asterisk and number, for example CYP2D6 *18. The significance of these are that differing mutations may lead to similar but not identical phenotypic outcomes, a finding which may have future implications for drug therapy and response. Ingelman-Sundberg (2004) identifies four basic phenotypes in this system: (1) poor metabolizers who lack the functional enzyme; (2) intermediate metabolizers who may either be heterozygous for one deficient allele or carry two alleles causing reduced activity; (3) extensive metabolizers who have two normal alleles; and (4) ultrarapid metabolizers who have multiple gene copies. About 6% to 20% of Whites, 5% to 8% of

African Blacks, and only about 1% to 2% of Arabs and Asian populations are poor metabolizers. Others are either extensive metabolizers or ultrarapid metabolizers (a recently identified state due to gene amplification). As a result, for one type of allele, there is a mild poor metabolizer that has a frequency of 50% in Asian populations. Those who are poor metabolizers of debrisoquine also have impaired metabolism of other drugs using the same pathway, and this may be important in up to 20% of commonly prescribed drugs. These include beta blockers and antihypertensive drugs such as metoprolol (Lopressor), timolol (Blockadren), propranolol (Inderal); antiarrhythmic and antianginal drugs such as flecainide (Tambocor), encainide (Enkaid), perhexiline, propafenone; tricyclic antidepressants such as nortriptyline (Pamelor), clomipramine (Anafranil), desipramine (Norpramin); neuroleptic drugs such as haloperidol; and other drugs such as phenacetin, phenformin, and codeine. Poor metabolizers of the beta blockers need only a daily dose, whereas extensive hydroxylators need the same dose two or three times a day for effectiveness. Poor metabolizers show more intense and prolonged beta blockade if the dose is not adjusted, leading to side-effects such as bradycardia. Those with ultrarapid metabolism may not show the expected therapeutic effectiveness, and thus demonstrate treatment failure due to low blood concentrations of the drug. A specific mutation found extensively in certain Chinese populations renders them more sensitive to desipramine and haloperidol. Both genotyping and phenotyping are available for detection of these mutations.

Of particular interest to nurses is the inhibited metabolism of codeine in poor metabolizers. These poor metabolizers do not demethylate codeine to morphine and thus receive no analgesic effect from codeine. Thus, when a patient is not getting the expected pain relief from codeine the reason may be a genetic one, and the nurse needs to believe the patient's response and find appropriate analgesic relief, not increase the dose of codeine.

Another polymorphism in the system is the CYP2C19 enzyme, which metabolizes S-mephenytoin, an anticonvulsant. Approximately 2% to 6% of Whites and 14% to 30% of Asians are poor metabolizers of mephenytoin. Among the drugs using this pathway are diazepam, proguanil, omeprasole, and mephenytoin. Little clinical data are available to show that the genetic variations influence success or failure of malaria treatment or prevention with proguanil. Those who are poor metabolizers of omeprazole (a proton pump inhibitor) appear to have higher rates of *Helicobacter pylori* eradication, better acid suppression and faster healing of both gastric and duodenal ulcers. Those who are poor metabolizers of diazepam have longer half-lives of the drug which can lead to prolonged sedation. Persons who are poor metabolizers who take mephenytoin may experience severe toxicity. CYP2C9 is a major enzyme involved in the metabolism of the anticoagulant, warfarin, that is prescribed for more than one million persons in the United States each year. Specific polymorphisms of CYP2C9 include CYP2C9*2 (R144C) and CYP2C9*3 (I359L), which have frequencies of 11% and 7% respectively. These result in varying decreased enzymatic activity of 30% and 80% respectively. In Chinese patients, a different polymorphism may reduce warfarin requirements. Those who are poor metabolizers of warfarin may experience greater toxicity than others. CYP2E1 variants may be associated with nasopharyngeal cancer in Chinese populations, and there may be an association with alcoholic liver disease. This enzyme may metabolize various tobacco-related nitrosoamines, and some genotypes may play a role in susceptibility to smoking-induced bladder cancers.

Other polymorphisms are beginning to be recognized as important, such as those in the CYP1A subfamily, CYP1B1 which has a role in steroid metabolism, CYP2B6, CYP2A6 which has a role in nicotine metabolism, and CYP3A variations which may affect quinidine metabolism.

Thiopurine-s-Methyltransferase

Identified genetic polymorphisms in this system include those heterozygotes with intermediate enzyme levels (11%); and very low or absent levels in about 0.4% of persons homozygous for the deficient allele, while the rest (about 89%) have high activities not related to ethnic or racial groups. Thiopurine-s-methyltransferase (TPMT) is involved in the metabolism of azathioprine, an immunosuppressant, used widely in dermatology and to treat systemic lupus erythematosis, the anticancer drug, thioguanine, used to treat acute non-lymphocytic leukemia, and the anticancer drug, mercaptopurine (6-MP), used often for acute lymphocytic leukemia. When the metabolic pathway is not functioning properly, these drugs are directed to another pathway and form toxic thioguanine nucleotide concentrations that are reciprocally related to leukocyte counts. Persons with low TPMT levels who are treated with the usual doses of azathioprine, thioguanine or 6MP are at high risk for hematopoetic toxicity such as profound neutropenia, while those with higher levels might be able to tolerate a dose-intensive treatment and could have relapses due to undertreatment with the usual doses. Before beginning therapy with these drugs, patients may be tested for TPMT activity or genotyped for allelic variants of the *TPMT* gene. The *TPMT* gene has at least 11 variant alleles known. Those who have high metabolic inactivation can be given a larger dose, and those who have low inactivation of 6MP may be given a dose that is 10 to 15 times smaller. Those with defective TPMT may also be prone to an increased risk of secondary malignancy after acute lymphocytic leukemia.

Paraoxonases

Three paraoxonase genes located on chromosome 7, *PON1, PON2,* and *PON3*, code for paraoxonases, also known as calcium-dependent A-esterases. PON1 is an high-density-lipoprotein associated enzyme, playing a role in coronary heart disease and also hydrolyzing organophosphates such as parathion, an insecticide, and sarin, a nerve gas. Various variant alleles are known that essentially divide people into those with low, intermediate, and high activity. Those with low activity are sensitive to organophosphate poisoning, especially parathion, an insecticide. The Q192R polymorphism is important in the quality of PON1. It has been suggested that Gulf War veterans with low PON1 activity may have been more protected against organophosphates possibly used deliberately and/or prophylactic pyridostigmine than those with other profiles, thus not showing evidence of the "Gulf War Syndrome" (Nebert & Jorge-Nebert, 2002). An interesting finding has been the low paraoxonase activity in those with very reduced HDL cholesterol levels such as in Tangier disease.

POLYMORPHISMS AFFECTING OTHER ASPECTS OF DRUG ACTIVITY AND RESPONSE

As indicated above, other aspects of drug activity are influenced by genetic factors. For example, certain variations in the gene, *KCNE2*, which encodes the MinK-related peptide subunit of the cardiac potassium channel I_{Kr}, result in susceptibility for long QT syndrome and drug-induced torsades de pointes after exposure to clarithromycin and also to trimethoprim/sulfamethoxazole. Certain polymorphisms (TT) of the bradykinin B(2) receptor gene result in the appearance of cough when taking angiotensin-converting enzyme (ACE) inhibitors, commonly used to treat essential hypertension. Thymidylate synthase expression in colorectal tumors has been noted to be a predictor of response to 5-fluorouracil therapy, where those with lower expression had a greater response and longer survival. In the treatment of congestive heart failure, responsiveness to therapy with beta blockers such as carvedilol was dependent on the genotype of the β_2-adrenergic receptor, thus explaining, in some cases, clinical variation in response to therapy. In about one-third of patients with epilepsy, seizures persist despite drug therapy. In one study (Siddiqui et al., 2003), a specific polymorphism (C to T at position 3435) in the ATP-binding cassette subfamily B member 1 (ABCB1), also known as MDR1, which is a multidrug transporter, was associated with drug-resistance in epilepsy. These results suggest that by genotyping, other drugs that are not ABCB1 substrates, or drugs that inhibit ABCB1 or evade ABCB1, it could be predicted what agents might be more effective in certain people. People with a certain mutation of the mitochondrial 12S ribosomal RNA gene (1555A>G mutation) are susceptible to aminoglycoside-induced ototoxicity. Persons with HIV disease possessing *HLA-B*5701* may have a severe hypersensitivity reaction to abacavir (a nucleoside-analogue reverse transcriptase inhibitor). Persons with cancer who take methotrexate and who have the C677T variant of the gene that encodes methylenetetrahdrofolate reductase have greater toxicity and may have reduced efficacy. Other examples abound. These areas are a source of intensive pharmaceutical research. The exploitation of genetic knowledge for therapy is illustrated by the use of irinotecan for colorectal cancer, gefinitib for nonsmall cell lung cancer, and imatinib for CML and is discussed in chapter 23.

LESS COMMON SINGLE-GENE DISORDERS

Malignant Hyperthermia

Malignant hyperthermia (MH) occurs in about 1:10,000 to 1:15,000 anesthetized pediatric and 1:50,000 anesthetized adult patients. There are pockets of higher incidence of gene mutations in north central Wisconsin, and some populations in North Carolina, Austria, and Quebec. MH has been cited as the most common cause of death due to anesthesia. The mortality rate formerly was 60% to 70%, but improved recognition and management have lowered it to about 10%. The first recognized case was published by Denborough and Lovell (1960) and contained features that are often present. A 21-year-old male student with a fractured leg was brought to the hospital, where he turned out to be less concerned about the fracture than he was about having general anesthesia. Since 1922, 10 of his relatives had died as a direct consequence of having general anesthesia. Halothane was used to anesthetize the student, but nonetheless MH occurred. His recovery, and the subsequent publication of the incident, led to awareness of the previously unrecognized problem.

The symptoms of MH include tachycardia, progressive muscle rigidity especially in the masseters with rhabdomyolysis (muscle breakdown), tachypnea, hypercarbia, cardiac arrhythmias, a rapid rise in body temperature that may reach 42° to 44°C, the darkening of blood on the operative field with the later development of metabolic imbalances such as hyperkalemia and respiratory and metabolic acidosis. Cardiac arrest can occur before the rise in temperature. Treatment includes IV dantrolene, hyperventilation with 100% oxygen through an endotracheal tube, and cooling. Myoglobinuria may appear 4 to 8 hours later. After the initial episode there is a risk of acute recurrence hours later and of disseminated intravascular coagulation.

The underlying defect is a pre-existing defect in skeletal muscle affecting the concentration and release of calcium that is manifested after exposure to certain halogenated inhalation anesthetics and depolarizing muscle relaxants such as succinylcholine. Anesthetics triggering MH include inhalation agents such as halothane, halogenated ethers such as ethrane, sevoflurane, desflurane, isoflurane, and enflurane, and ether and cyclopropane which are not used today. In some, but not all, cases of MH, the mutation(s) responsible are in the ryanodine receptor gene (RYR1) (a skeletal-muscle calcium-release channel gene) on chromosome 19q13.1. Allelic mutations in RYR1 and other implicated defective genes (on chromosomes 1, 3, 7, and 17) have been identified. About 50 allelic mutations in RYR1 are known. The mode of transmission is autosomal dominant with varying penetrance. Among the other implicated genes are CACNA1S (chromosome 1) and CACNA2D1 (chromosome 7) which encode subunits of a voltage-gated calcium channel (VDCC) of skeletal muscle (known as the dihydropyridine receptor). The model may be that of a major gene with the effect of modifying genes. MH may be one end of a spectrum of muscle susceptibility, which may even change within one individual with age, trauma, or exercise. Although no definitive noninvasive population screening test is currently available, elevated creatine phosphokinase (CPK) levels in close relatives of known susceptible individuals is usually strong enough evidence of that person's susceptibility. The caffeine/halothane muscle contracture test known as the in vitro halothane contracture test (IVCT) requires 500 mg of fresh skeletal muscle tissue to perform, and thus is only used in certain circumstances. Another test proposed is measurement of local carbon dioxide pressure stimulated by caffeine. In some cases, molecular screening may be done but to date this detects a small percentage of affected families. It is expected this will become more useful in the future.

RYR1 gene mutations also occur in several myopathies such as central core disease (CCD) or minicore myopathy. These are closely associated with MH. CCD is considered in Online Mendelian Inheritance of Man to be an autosomal dominant disorder but in some of the other MH associated myopathies, inheritance is less clear. The person with MH usually appears well, as the myopathy associated with it in the absence of an already identified myopathy is subclinical until exposure to a volatile depolarizing anesthetic. In about one third, there may be complaints or signs of mild ptosis, strabismus, muscle cramps, muscle weakness, recurrent dislocations, hernia, back problems such as kyphosis or scoliosis, short stature, unusual muscle bulk, other musculoskeletal complaints and sometimes presence of a cleft palate, before exposure to a volatile depolarizing anesthetic. A preponderance of heavily muscled young males have been noted to be susceptible to MH. Because the heart is a muscle, it may also be affected. Major stress, strenuous exercise, or trauma may also induce MH. It is possible that fatal episodes of heat stroke and death from unknown causes in athletes may really be caused by MH, as may some cases of sudden infant death syndrome. Persons with other hereditary muscle disorders such as myotonia congenita, and Duchenne muscular dystrophy are also at risk for MH when given anesthesia. In the Online Mendelian Inheritance in Man (2005), the syndrome formerly called King-Denborough is incorporated under MH. Family members of the person with CCD may be susceptible to MH even though they have no evidence of CCD themselves. Other factors such as drugs, including local anesthetics (lidocaine), atropine, calcium gluconate, digoxin, norepinephrine, succinylcholine, decamethonium, and isoprotorenol; muscle injury; extreme emotional agitation or anxiety; and high environmental temperatures may also precipitate MH reactions in susceptible individuals. The combination of succinylcholine and the administration of halogenated inhalation anesthesia is especially provocative, although MH can occur after succinylcholine administration alone. Hyperkalemia, sudden general muscle rigidity, and/or isolated contraction of the jaw muscles can occur following succinylcholine administration, usually after inhalation induction. This type is frequent in children.

Nursing Considerations

The following are particularly pertinent to nurses who are working with clients before, during, and after surgery, in obstetrics, and the schools, especially certified registered nurse anesthetists.

The discussion of MH in a wide variety of professional journals has led to a legal agreement of a minimum standard of practice. *Items marked with an asterisk represent the minimum standards.* Preoperative prophylactic doses of dantrolene (Dantrium) have been believed to protect the susceptible person from an episode of MH, even with inhalation anesthesia, but a recent case of MH that occurred in a patient so treated may mean that such protection is not universal. Nurses and nurse anesthetists are in an ideal position to help minimize morbidity and mortality from MH.

• Before either surgical or obstetric anesthesia is given to any patient, a thorough family and personal history should be taken that includes the following questions: Have you ever had anesthesia? If so, what type? Have you ever had surgery? Was there any difficulty or problem with surgery or anesthesia? Dental surgery should be included, and specific complications such as fever, rigidity, dark urine, or any unexpected reactions should be asked about. The nurse should also ask about any musculoskeletal complaints, any history of heat intolerance or fevers of unknown origin, or any unusual drug reaction (some MH patients have been reported to exhibit cramps or fever when taking alcohol, caffeine, or aspirin). The same questions should be asked about all family members, including any sudden or unexplained deaths, particularly while participating in an athletic event. The nurse should review this family history with the person, going back two or three generations and including cousins. Any answers indicating sudden death or fever while receiving anesthesia should be further investigated before the individual receives anesthesia.* Perhaps the same information should be collected before a student participates in strenuous school sports.

• Anesthesia for the MH susceptible person can be planned before surgery. Planning may include prophylactic dantrolene administration, although this is somewhat controversial and can cause muscle weakness. Choice of anesthetic is based on avoiding the use of triggering agents. Regional anesthesia is a better choice for procedures that can be accomplished with its use. Special preparation of the anesthesia machine should be done. The best situation is the availability of a machine whose components have never been exposed to volatile triggering agents or, if not, the removal of vaporizers from the machine and the replacement of components such as the tubing, ventilator bellows, CO_2 absorption canisters, and reservoir bag with unused parts and the flushing of the machine with oxygen for more than 10 minutes and usually one hour to remove trace amounts of volatile agents. A safe muscle relaxant such as pancuronium (Pavulon), atracurium (Tracrium), or mivacurium (Mivacron) should be used.

• A high index of suspicion should be maintained for an individual with any or all of the following characteristics, particularly young males with short stature, cryptorchidism, ptosis, low-set ears, lordosis, kyphosis, pes cavus, strabismus, weak serrati muscles, antimongolian slant of the palpebral fissures. Cases of MH have followed corrective surgery for strabismus.

• Abnormal electrocardiograms or unexplained cardiomyopathy in young patients may represent a person susceptible to MH and should be investigated.

• Any preoperative or preanesthetic physical examination should include a search for subclinical muscle weakness and the presence of any physical signs previously described, especially related to the muscular system.

• If succinylcholine (Anectine, Quelicin) is administered, the nurse or anesthetist should be alert for any abnormal reaction such as failure to relax as expected, masseter stiffness, or muscle fasciculations that are greater than usual. Such a response should prompt consideration of postponing the surgical procedure pending further investigation and preparation. About half of children who develop this are later found to be MH susceptible.

• During surgery, the temperature and pulse should be continually monitored.* Unexplained tachycardia is often the first sign, but this may be preceded by a rising end tidal CO_2 as shown by capnography. The development of any symptoms described earlier should mean the immediate institution of emergency procedures,* the cessation of anesthesia, and the conclusion of surgery, unless some other reason can account for a rapid rise in body temperature, such as excessive draping in a hot operating room, which would be rare today.

• Any rapid rise in body temperature or myoglobinuria, as evidenced by dark red urine occurring in the first 24 hours after surgery, should be considered as possibly caused by MH and should be investigated further.*

• Resuscitation equipment and drugs necessary for treating an MH crisis should be standard equipment in all operating rooms.*

• Patients known to be susceptible to MH must be cautioned to avoid potent inhalation anesthetics such as those mentioned earlier. None is considered completely safe. Depolarizing muscle relaxants such as succinylcholine and decamethonium should also be avoided.

• Information regarding MH should be put into written form for the susceptible person. One should be in professional language for his or her personal health care provider, and the other should be in the language that the patient and family can understand.

• Genetic counseling in MH includes discussing with the patient the necessity for informing relatives of the potential risk for them, and urging them to seek further evaluation. This may include the use of CPK levels and, in some cases, even muscle biopsy. Molecular genetic testing for MH has become available and is moving into clinical practice with appropriate guidelines. It is anticipated that in the future, proponents may suggest MH as a candidate condition for population screening. The written information mentioned above can be used for that purpose. Referral should be made to a support group such as the Malignant Hyperthermia Association of the United States (MHAUS), which maintains a hotline (see Appendix B).

• Patients who are susceptible to MH should be advised to wear a Medic-Alert bracelet or similar medical alert identification with this information and told how to get one.

The Porphyrias

The porphyrias are a group of errors in the pathway for heme biosynthesis leading to excessive porphyrins or their precursors. Most of them are inherited. Each type of porphyria is due to a specific defect in a different enzyme in a step on this pathway, and is located at a distinct chromosomal site. Specific symptoms and features vary, but the two major classifications are hepatic and erythropoietic or erythroid. The more common hepatic group includes acute intermittent porphyria (AIP), varigate porphyria, hereditary coproporphyria, ALA dehydratase deficiency porphyria (ADP, very rare), and porphyria cutanea tarda. The erythropoietic group includes erythropoietic protoporphyria (EPP), and erythropoietic porphyria (EP). Others classify the porphyrias as acute (characterized by acute attacks with neurological symptoms) and nonacute (characterized by photosensitivity); as cutaneous or noncutaneous; or by type of inheritance. Most of the porphyrias are inherited in an autosomal dominant manner, which is unusual for disorders of enzyme metabolism. Depending on the type, symptoms can vary. Clients with acute intermittent porphyria, the most common hepatic, acute porphyria, are often first seen by the nurse during or following an acute attack that results from the exposure to alcohol, certain drugs (including oral contraceptives), or because of infection, fever, reduced caloric intake, or hormonal changes especially during menses or pregnancy, all of which can precipitate attacks. Only the most common porphyrias precipitated by drugs will be discussed.

AIP is the most common genetic type, occurring in all races. It is an autosomal dominant disorder caused by deficiency of porphobilinogen deaminase (hydroxymethylbilane synthase). AIP is genetically heterogenous, with multiple mutations found in the responsible genes, a few of which are most prevalent. It has an incidence of approximately 1:50,000 to 60,000 worldwide and an incidence in Scandinavia approaching 1:1,500. The prevalence of latent AIP is higher, and many cases never come to attention. AIP is usually latent until puberty or early adulthood, with few cases presenting after menopause. Clinical expression appears more frequent in females, perhaps because of contributing hormonal factors. In AIP, the most common symptoms during acute attacks include severe abdominal pain, which may be mistaken for an acute surgical abdomen such as appendicitis, nausea, vomiting, constipation. Symptoms can also include abdominal distention with paralytic ileus, urinary retention, tachycardia, hypertension, neuropathy; motor symptoms which include muscle weakness (especially of the extremities), sensory disturbances including the loss of pain and touch sensation; mental symptoms including anxiety, insomnia, depression, disorientation, hallucinations, and paranoia. Respiratory paralysis may occur. No skin manifestations are seen. Patients may become violent, and are often treated with drugs such as narcotic analgesics that worsen the symptoms. The urine may become the color of port wine during an attack. Some cases of AIP present as respiratory failure. The acute attack can last several days to weeks, and can become chronic at a low level. Early onset chronic renal failure may occur perhaps because of increased susceptibility to analgesic nephropathy, the effects of the porphyrins, or because of the hypertension.

A case eventually diagnosed as AIP known to the author was that of a college student who was admitted to the emergency room after a party at which she drank alcoholic beverages that precipitated an acute attack, and resulted in confusion and hallucinations. Her initial diagnosis was acute psychosis, and it was not until later that the diagnosis of AIP was made.

Porphyria variegata (PV) is particularly frequent in South Africa (for an example of founder effect, see chapter 3) and in Finland, and is an AD trait usually manifesting after puberty. Among white South Africans, expecially the Dutch Afrikaaners, the prevalence may be as high as 1:300–400, and elsewhere is about 1:50,000 to 100,000. The defective enzyme is protoporphyrinogen oxidase. Like AIP, those with PV suffer from acute attacks precipitated by essentially the same factors. Lead from moonshine alcohol and other sources may precipitate attacks. However, the clinical picture also includes skin manifestations including severe photosensitivity, skin fragility, milia, erosions, blisters, and bulla with eventual scarring. Hypertrichosis and hyperpigmentation may be seen. Skin manifestations are prominent on the face, ears, neck, and back of the hands. Porphyria cutanea tarda (PCT) is the most common type and can be either sporadic or inherited; it has an incidence of 1:25,000 in North America and is more common in the Czech Republic and Slovakia. Some cases appear acquired. Hepatitis C has been observed frequently in PCT. In the inherited form (type II), the autosomal disorder usually appears in adulthood but can appear earlier, and is due to deficiency of uroporphyrinogen decarboxylase. Men seem to be more frequently affected. Cutaneous findings are similar to PV but acute attacks are not seen. However, PCT may be precipitated by alcohol, estrogens (including oral

contraceptives), iron exposure, and polyhalo-
genated hydrocarbons.

After AIP is identified, a primary preventive
effort is the avoidance of precipitating drugs, substances, and events. Drugs known to cause attacks
in AIP include alcohol, aminoglutethamide,
antipyrine, barbituates, carbamezepine, carbromal,
chloramphenicol, chlorpropamide, danazol, dapsone, diphenylhydantoin, ergot preparations, estrogens, glutethamide, griseofulvin, halothane,
meprobamate, methyldopa, novobiocin, oral contraceptives, phenylbutazone, phenytoin, progesterone, pyrozolone, sulfonamides, theophylline,
tolbutamide, and valproic acid. A detailed listing of
these drugs may be found in the reference by
Desnick, Astrin, and Anderson (2002). The nurse
should question the prescription of these for a
patient with known or suspected porphyria. Family
members should be screened for the enzyme deficiency. Smoking may also precipitate attacks.
Those with a deficiency should be warned to avoid
the drugs and agents mentioned above; instructed
as to the association between their use and acute
attacks; advised to wear a medical identification
bracelet indicating that they have porphyria; and
instructed to avoid alcohol ingestion, oral contraceptives, and low calorie diets. If planning surgery,
the person with porphyria needs to talk with the
surgeon and anesthetist regarding porphyria as
both long periods of NPO and certain drugs can be
dangerous. In some types of porphyrias, anti-
seizure medication may be needed and in other
types phlebotomy may be useful. For those with
skin manifestations, care should be taken to avoid
the sun and to use opaque sunscreens such as those
with titanium dioxide. Topical antibiotics and beta
carotene may also be useful. Patients may be seen
in pre-or postoperative periods; during severe illness, infection or fever; or during pregnancy. Support and encouragement are especially important
in the care of these patients because the very
uniqueness of their symptoms may cause health
professionals to think that they are faking or may
result in misdiagnosis.

Methemoglobin Reductase Deficiency

Deficiency of the enzyme methemoglobin reductase (cytochrome-b5 reductase deficiency) is a rare
inherited autosomal recessive disease. that may

occur in erythrocytes only (type I), in all tissues
(type II), or be limited to hemopoietic cells without neurologic effects (type III). Deficiency of
cytochrome b5 reductase can result in methemoglobinemia also (type IV), that has as one of its
effects a sensitivity to methemoglobin-forming
oxidizing drugs, and results in a dark blue skin
color. The frequency of heterozygote carriers in the
general population is estimated at about 1%, and
they have enzyme levels that are about 50% of normal. Such heterozygotes (as well as homozygotes)
are more likely than normal individuals to develop
methemoglobinemia, cyanosis, headache, vomiting, dyspnea, or fatigue when exposed to drugs or
chemicals such as chloroquine, dapsone, primaquine, nitrites, nitrates, and aniline derivatives.
Increases in acute attacks have been seen in recent
years due to nitrite compounds in commercial
products such as room deodorizers. Infant formulas made with nitrate-rich water have caused toxic
methemoglobinemia in nurseries, with a 10%
mortality. The disorder is most frequent in native
Alaskans, Puerto Ricans, Mediterranean populations, and the Navaho people. However, a large
interesting family, the Fugates, from Troublesome
Creek, Kentucky, with methemoglobulinemia is
described (Trost, 1982). Somewhat isolated, they
intermarried and had large families, many of
whom were blue. Methylene blue will clear the
cyanosis seen.

Unstable Hemoglobins

Many hemoglobins (Hb) variants that involve an
amino acid substitution in the Hb molecule are
known. There are many that alter the stability of
the molecule and are therefore known as unstable
hemoglobins. Some examples are Hb Zurich, Hb
Torino, Hb Shepherd's Bush, Hb Saskatoon, and
Hb Peterborough. Such individuals are often clinically asymptomatic unless they are exposed to
certain drugs, infection, severe stress, or fever.
Hemolytic anemia can then occur. Drugs that cause
the hemolysis are oxidants, and the sulfonamides
are most often responsible. Primaquine and nitrites
also cause hemolysis. A woman treated for a urinary tract infection in an emergency room suffered
severe hemolysis after taking the prescribed sulfa
drug. She was later found to have Hb Zurich. The
true frequency in the population is unknown, as

most are neither uncovered nor tested for. In Maryland, Dickerman estimated that the frequency of Hb Zurich is 1:100,000. Before administering drugs known to precipitate anemia in such individuals, patients should be questioned regarding their past drug history, as they may have had a prior episode, and about any such reactions in relatives. Also, once an individual is identified as having an unstable Hb, his or her blood relatives should be tested for the Hb variant, so that an episode of hemolytic anemia can be prevented. Teaching should include instruction on which drugs are implicated in precipitating hemolysis including over-the-counter preparations containing those agents. Persons with Hb M disease, an autosomal dominant condition, also suffer from methemoglobinemia and milder cyanosis. They are also sensitive to the same chemicals and drugs listed above.

Succinylcholine Sensitivity or Pseudocholinesterase Variation

Succinylcholine (Anectine) is a common short-acting muscle relaxant often used during surgery. Normally, the enzyme pseudocholinesterase rapidly inactivates the drug. Genetically determined variants (polymorphisms) can result in little or no enzyme activity or in defective enzyme function, depending on which alleles are present. It is estimated that about 3% to 4% of populations of European origin are heterozygotes for this condition, especially U.S. Whites, Greeks, Yugoslavs, and East Indians; 1:2,500 to 1:3,500 are homozygous and are at risk for prolonged apnea due to depression of respiration when given succinylcholine. It is estimated that approximately 1.5% of Alaskan Eskimos are homozygous for this autosomal recessive condition that is located at 3q26.1-q26.2. Before succinylcholine is administered, a complete personal and family history that includes both sensitivity and any episodes of apnea in either the individual or blood relatives should be obtained. Equipment for resuscitation and purified enzyme preparation should be standard emergency equipment available for anyone receiving the drug. Some believe that before receiving succinylcholine, individuals should be tested for pseudocholinesterase variation; this is not routinely done in most hospitals due to cost-benefit, rather than ethical, considerations. The nurse should pursue such testing for those in the population groups in whom the risk is higher, and in any individual with a positive or suspicious history.

OTHER PHARMACOGENETIC DISORDERS

Other genetic disorders are known to have, as one component, altered responses to therapeutic agents. Some pharmacogenetic traits are quite rare or of limited therapeutic significance, or have complicated heredity. These are summarized in Table 18.1.

ETHICAL, LEGAL, AND SOCIAL ISSUES RELATED TO PHARMACOGENOMICS

As the field of pharmacogenomics has evolved, various ethical concerns have been raised. Some concerns override many of the applications of genetics—confidentiality and the potential for misuse of genetic information, with the potential for stigmatization for various groups. This is because the genotype of an individual specifically pertaining to their disease and treatment would be known to the practitioner perhaps just by the drug they were receiving. Further the potential for selective drug development to benefit specific ethnic groups with a particular frequency of a certain genotype related to disease and treatment might exist at the expense of other ethnic groups or genotypes, as it might for those who can afford tailored treatments.

END NOTES

Pharmacogenetics and pharmacogenomics are still young. However, it is clear that the genetic contribution to drug metabolism, transport, and genetic variation in drug receptors is recognized as extremely important. Eventually information about differences in the metabolism of alcohol and illicit drugs will lead to new information about the genetic role in drug dependence and addiction. Entire journals such as *Pharmacogenomics, Pharmacogenomics Journal, Current Pharmacogenomics,*

TABLE 18.1   Selected Inherited Disorders with Altered Response to Therapeutic Agents

Condition or disorder	Examples of agents	Response or effect
Acatalasia	Hydrogen peroxide	Tissue ulceration
Arene oxide metabolism defect	Phenytoin (Dilantin)	Hepatotoxicity
Crigler-Najjar syndrome	Salicylates, tetrahydrocortisone, menthol	Jaundice, drug toxicity
Down syndrome	Atropine	Increased response
Dubin-Johnson syndrome	Oral contraceptives	Jaundice
Familial dysautonomia	Norepinephrine	Increased pressor response
Gilbert syndrome	Oral contraceptives, alcohol, cholecystographic agents	Increased blood bilirubin, jaundice
Glaucoma (open-angle)	Corticosteroids	Increased intraocular pressure
Glaucoma (narrow-angle)	Atropine, mydriatics	Increased intraocular pressure
Lesch-Nyhan syndrome	Allopurinol, 6-mercaptopurine, azathioprine, azaguanine	Drug not metabolized to active form, resistance Formation of xanthine stones (allopurinol)
Hydantoin hydroxylation defect	Hydantoin (Dilantin)	Toxic plasma concentrations with severe side effects
Methylenetetrahydrofolate reductase deficiency	Nitrous oxide	An infant with a severe form of this defect in folate metabolism died after being anesthetized with nitrous oxide
Osteogenesis imperfecta	General anesthesia	Elevation of body temperature
PKU	Catecholamines	Increased pressor response
Warfarin resistance	Warfarin	Decreased response to warfarin, so 20–25 times usual dose is needed for therapeutic effect; increased requirement for vitamin K

and *Pharmacogenetics,* are devoted to this topic. Different individuals may require different doses of the same drug in order to achieve maximum effectiveness, others may not respond at all to certain drugs, and different adverse reactions may be manifested. This variability is largely genetic, and some families may be at greater risk for the rare single-gene disorders than the population at large. The well-known and recently discovered polymorphisms in the genes coding for many enzymes affecting drug metabolism, transport, disposition, excretion, and drug receptors affect large numbers of persons worldwide. The clinical significance depends on a variety of factors, some of which are not directly genetic, such as the condition of organs such as the liver, including the therapeutic index of the drug. For the most part, persons taking drugs with broad therapeutic ranges and safety profiles will not usually show significant clinical consequences even if they are poor metabolizers. However, when taking drugs with a narrow therapeutic index, such as many antidepressants or isoniazid, the genetic polymorphism becomes clinically important. These polymorphisms are also important in regard to unfavorable drug-drug interactions, and the patient's relevant genotype and phenotype may need to be considered in multiple drug prescribing. Knowledge about genetic influences in metabolism is being used to tailor the administration and plan for cancer drug therapy including amonafide and fluouracil. The occurrence of mental changes as side-effects in drug therapy with agents such as the corticosteroids, reserpine, amphetamines, methyidopa, and others that occur in some, but not all, of patients receiving them, may uncover further information about the etiology of mental disorders, and also identify susceptible subgroups in the population. Nurses are in an excellent position to observe interindividual differences in response to drugs that can lead to further research. These will add to the knowledge of the inborn errors of drug metabolism and also to the further delineation of genetic diversity of metabolic functions that have both theoretical interest and clinical importance.

Receptor mutations are known to cause functional changes causing disease. An application of this research is in regard to opiate receptor variability and drug dependence. Inherited drug receptor variants leading to resistance to vasopressin, estrogen, insulin, the steroid hormones, and others are known.

Important pharmacogenetic and pharmacogenomic implications in testing new therapeutic agents are for testing the agent in populations of different ethnic backgrounds, as the information obtained regarding metabolism, effectiveness, and side-effects cannot be wholly transferred from one population to another. Information regarding polymorhisms and genetic variability is beginning to be incorporated into drug-development trials. It is important to remember that the usual effective dose of a drug when given to any individual patient may be effective, ineffective, or even toxic depending on his/her genetic makeup, and that the drug itself may be ineffective, as in the 6% to 10% of those who are unresponsive to codeine. Thus, in regard to drug therapy, one size does not fit all. Recent moves to reduce costs by limiting hospital formularies can have unintended pharmacogenetic consequences. In the future, one can envision designer medications tailored to specific genotypes and labelled as such while others will need to be avoided by certain genotypes. The marketing of DNA chips for both *CYP2C6* and *CYP2C19* to identify poor drug metabolizers is just the beginning of the application of this technology to clinical drug therapy.

Eventually the field of pharmacogenomics will allow the determination of a genetic profile for pharmacological treatment of a specific disease. This will allow drug therapy not only to be tailored to genetic profile for maximum effectiveness, but will also determine the best dosage and allow the withholding of drugs which might be ineffective or result in side-effects. Another advantage would be that fewer medications might be needed for a given condition and therefore patient adherence would be enhanced. Eventually gene therapy will also consider pharmacogenomic profile. Many of these uses have already begun; they will be expanded rapidly. Other pharmacological approaches to treatment are discussed in chapter 23.

BIBLIOGRAPHY

Almarsdottir, A. B., Bjornsdottir, I., & Traulsen, J. M. (2005). A lay prescription for tailor-made drugs—focus group reflections on pharacogenomics. *Health Policy, 71,* 233–241.

Anstey, A. (1995). Azathioprine in dermatology: A review in the light of advances in understanding methylation pharmacogenetics. *Journal of the Royal Society of Medicine, 88,* 155P–160P.

Austin, C. P. (2004). The impact of the completed human genome sequence on the development of novel therapeutics for human disease. *Annual Review of Medicine, 55,* 1–13.

Baliga, R., & Narula, J. (2003). Pharmacogenomics of congestive heart failure. *Medical Clinics of North America, 87,* 569–578.

Benkusky, N. A., Farrell, E. F., & Valdivia, H. H. (2004). Ryanodine receptor channelopathies. *Biochemical and Biophysical Research Communications, 322,* 1280–1285.

Beutler, E. (1994). G6PD deficiency. *Blood, 84,* 3612–3636.

Beutler, E. (2001). Hemoglobinopathies associated with unstable hemoglobin. In E. Beutler, B. S. Coller, M. A. Lichtman, T. J. Kipps, & U. Seligsohn (Eds.), *Williams hematology* (6th ed., pp. 607–610). New York: McGraw-Hill.

Blackledge, G., & Averbuch, S. (2004). Gefitinib ('Iressa,' ZD1839) and new epidermal growth factor receptor inhibitors. *British Journal of Cancer, 90,* 566–572.

Brini, M. (2004). Ryanodine receptor defects in muscle genetic diseases. *Biochemical and Biophysical Research Communications, 322,* 1245–1255.

Choi, J-Y., Lee, K-M., Cho, S-H., Kim, S-W., Choi, H-Y., Lee, S-Y., et al. *CYP2E1* and *NQO1* genotypes, smoking and bladder cancer. *Pharmacogenetics, 13,* 349–355.

Clunie, G. P. R., & Lennard, L. (2004). Relevance of thiopurine methyltransferase status in rheumatology patients receiving azathioprine. *Rheumatology, 43,* 13–18.

Costa, L. G., Cole, T. B., Jarvik, G. P., & Furlong, C. E. (2003). Functional genomics of the paraoxonase (PON1) polymorphisms: Effects on pesticide sensitivity, cardiovascular disease, and drug metabolism. *Annual Review of Medicine, 54,* 371–392.

Crentsil, V. (2004). The pharmacogenomics of Alzheimer's disease. *Aging Research Reviews, 3,* 153–169.

Daly, A. K. (2003). Pharmacogenetics of the major polymorphic metabolizing enzymes. *Fundamental & Clinical Pharmacology, 17,* 27–41.

Daly, A. K., Brockmöller, J., Brody, F., Eichelbaum, M., Evans, W. E., Gonzalez, F. J., et al. (1996). Nomenclature for human *CYP2D6* alleles. *Pharmacogenetics, 6,* 193–201.

Denborough, M. A., & Lovell, R. R. H. (1960). Anaesthetic deaths in a family. *Lancet, 2,* 45.

Desnick, R. J., Astrin, K. H., & Anderson, K. E. (2002). Inherited porphyrias. In D. L. Rimoin, J. M. Connor, R. E. Pyeritz, & B. R. Korf (Eds.), *Emery and Rimoin's principles and practice of medical genetics* (4th ed., pp. 2586–2623). New York: Churchill Livingstone.

Dickerman, J. D. (1981). A familial hemolytic anemia associated with sulfa administration. *Hospital Practice, 16*(9), 41, 44, 47.

Erbe, R. W., & Salis, R. J. (2003). Severe methylenetetrahydrofolate reductase deficiency, methionine synthase, and nitrous oxide—a cautionary tale. *New England Journal of Medicine, 349,* 5–6.

Erichsen, H. C., & Chanock, S. J. (2004). SNPs in cancer research and treatment. *British Journal of Cancer, 90,* 747–751.

Evans, E. E., & McLeod, H. L. (2003). Pharmacogenomics—drug disposition, drug targets, and side effects. *New England Journal of Medicine, 348,* 538–549.

Evans, W. E. (2003). Pharmacogenomics: Marshalling the human genome to individualise drug therapy. *Gut, 52*(Suppl. II), ii10–ii18.

Evans, W. E. (2004). Pharmacogenetics of thiopurine S-methyltransferase and thiopurine therapy. *Therapeutic Drug Monitoring, 26,* 186–191.

Evans, W. E., & Relling, M. V. (2004). Moving toward individualized medicine with pharmacogenomics. *Nature, 429,* 464–468.

Freeman, B. D., & McLeod, H. L. (2004). Challenges of implementing pharmacogenetics in the critical care environment. *Nature Reviews Drug Discovery, 3,* 88–93.

Girard, T., Treves, S., Voronkov, E., Siegemund, M., & Urwyler, A. (2004). Molecular genetic testing for malignant hyperthermia susceptibility. *Anesthesiology, 100,* 1076–1080,

Haga, S. B., & Burke, W. (2004). Using pharmacogenetics to improve drug safety and efficacy. *Journal of the American Medical Association, 291,* 2869–2871.

Hajjar, R. J., Huq, F., Matsui, T., & Rosenzweig, A. (2003). Genetic editing of dysfunctional myocardium. *Medical Clinics of North America, 87,* 553–567.

Hetherington, S., Hughes, A. R., Mosteller, M., Shortino, D., Baker, K. L., Spreen, W., et al. (2002). Genetic variations in HLA-B region and hypersensitivity reactions to abacavir. *Lancet, 359,* 1121–1122.

Higashi, M. K., Veenstra, D. L., Kondo, L. M., Wittkowsky, A. K., Srinouanprachah, S. L., Farin, F. M., et al. (2002). Association between CYP2C9 genetic variants and anticoagulation-related outcomes during warfarin therapy. *Journal of the American Medical Association, 287,* 1690–1698.

Hillman, R. S., & Ault, K. A. (2002). *Hematology in clinical practice* (3rd ed.). New York: McGraw-Hill.

Hosford, D. A., Lai, E. H., Riley, J. H., Xu, C. F., Danoff, T. M., & Roses, A. D. (2004). Pharmacogenetics to predict drug-related adverse events. *Toxicologic Pathology, 32*(Suppl. 1), 9–12.

Hughes, D. A., Vilar, F. J., Ward, C. C., Alfirevic, A., Park, B. K., & Pirmohamed, M. (2004). Cost-effectiveness analysis of *HLA B*5701* genotyping in preventing abacavir hypersensitivity. *Pharmacogenetics, 14,* 335–342.

Ingelman-Sundberg, M. (2004). Pharmacogenetics of cytochrome P450 and its applications in drug therapy: The past, present and future. *Trends in Pharmacological Sciences, 25,* 193–200.

Innocenti, F., Undevia, S. V., Iyer, L., Chen, P. X., Das, S., Kocherinsky, M., et al. (2004). Genetic variants in the *UDP-glucuronosyltransferase 1A1* gene predict the risk of severe neutropenia of Irinotecan. *Journal of Clinical Oncology, 22,* 1382–1388.

Iqbal, S., & Lenz, H. J. (2003). Targeted therapy and pharmacogenomic programs. *Cancer, 97*(Suppl. 8), 2076–2082.

Jaffé, E. R., & Hultquist, D. E. (2001). Cytochrome b$_5$ reductase deficiency and enzymopenic hereditary methemoglobinemia. In C. R. Scriver, A. L. Beaudet, W. S. Sly, & D. Valle (Eds.), *The metabolic and molecular bases of inherited disease* (8th ed., pp. 4555–4570). New York: McGraw-Hill.

Jensen, J. D., & Resnick, S. D. (1995). Porphyria in childhood. *Seminars in Dermatology, 14,* 33–39.

Johansson, I., Lundqvist, E., Bertilsson, L., Dahl, M-L., Sjoqvist, F., & Ingelman-Sundberg, M. (1993). Inherited amplification of an active gene in in the cytochrome P450 CYP2D locus as a cause of ultrarapid metabolism of debrisoquine. *Proceedings of the National Academy of Science, USA, 90,* 11825–11829.

Johnson, J. A. (2003). β-blockers in heart failure: Will we someday select therapy based on genetics? *Pharmacogenetics, 13,* 375–377.

Kalow, W., & Grant, D. M. (2001). Pharmacogenetics. In C. R. Scriver, A. L. Beaudet, W. S. Sly, & D. Valle (Eds.), *The metabolic and molecular bases of inherited disease* (8th ed., pp. 225–255). New York: McGraw-Hill.

Kauppinen, R. (2005). Porphyrias. *Lancet, 365,* 241–252.

Kaye, D. M., Smirk, B., Williams, C., Jennings, G., Ester, M., & Holst, D. (2003). β-adrenoceptor genotype influences the response to carvedilol in patients with congestive heart failure. *Pharmacogenetics, 13,* 379–382.

Keating, K. E., Quane, K. A., Manning, B. M., Lehane, M., Hartung, K., Censier, A., et al. (1994). Detection of a novel RYR1 mutation in four malignant hyperthermia pedigrees. *Human Molecular Genetics, 3,* 1855–1858.

Kirschheiner, J., & Brockmoller, J. (2005). Clinical consequences of cytochrome P450 2C9 polymorphisms. *Clinical Pharmacology & Therapeutics, 77,* 1–16.

Lammer, E. J., Shaw, G. M., Iovannisci, D. M., Van Waes, J., & Finnell, R. H. (2004). Maternal smoking and the risk of orofacial clefts: Suscep-

tibility with *NAT1* and *NAT2* polymorphisms. *Epidemiology, 15,* 150–156.

Li Wan Po, A. (2005). Drug evaluation, drug development and pharmacogenetics: Celebrating 30 years of progress. *Journal of Clinical Pharmacy and Therapeutics, 30,* 1–4.

Luzzetto, L., Mehta, A., & Vulliamy, T. (2001). Glucose 6-phosphate dehydrogenase deficiency. In C. R. Scriver, A. L. Beaudet, W. S. Sly, & D. Valle (Eds.), *The metabolic and molecular bases of inherited disease* (8th ed., pp. 4517–4553). New York: McGraw-Hill.

Lynch, T. J., Bell, D. W., Sordella, R., Gurubhagavatula, S., Okimoto, R. A., Brannigan, B. W., et al. (2004). Activating mutations in the epidermal growth factor receptor underlying responsiveness of non-small-cell lung cancer to gefitinib. *New England Journal of Medicine, 350,* 2129–2139.

Marsh, S., & McLeod, H. L. (2004). Cancer pharmacogenetics. *British Journal of Cancer, 90,* 8–11.

Miranda, S. R., Kimura, E. M., Saad, S. T., & Costa, F. F. (1994). Identification of Hb Zurich [alpha 2 beta 2(63)(E7)His–>Arg] by DNA analysis in a Brazilian family. *Hemoglobin, 18*(4–5), 337–341.

Mukae, S., Aoki, S., Iroh, S., Iwata, T., Ueda, H., & Katagiri, T. (2000). Bradykinin B(2) receptor gene polymorphism is associated wtih angiotensin-converting enzyme inhibitor-related cough. *Hypertension, 36,* 127–131.

Mukherjee, D., & Topol, E. J. (2002). Pharmacogenomics in cardiovascular diseases. *Progress in Cardiovascular Diseases, 44,* 479–498.

Nadal, E., & Olavarria, E. (2004). Imatinib mesylate (Gleevec/Glivec) a molecular-targeted therapy for chronic myeloid leukemia and other malignancies. *International Journal of Clinical Practice, 58,* 511–516.

Nebert, D. W., & Jorge-Nebert, L. F. (2002). Pharmacogenetics and pharmacogenomics. In D. L. Rimoin, J. M. Connor, R. E. Pyeritz, & B. R. Korf (Eds.), *Emery and Rimoin's principles and practice of medical genetics* (4th ed., pp. 590–631). London: Churchill Livingstone.

Nelson, T. E., Rosenberg, H., & Muldoon, S. M. (2004). Genetic testing for maligant hyperthermia in North America. *Anesthesiology, 100,* 212–214.

Nordmann, Y., & Puy, H. (2002). Human hereditary hepatic porphyrias. *Clinica Chimica Acta, 325,* 17–37.

Online Mendelian Inheritance in Man, OMIM (TM). (2005). Center for Medical Genetics, Johns Hopkins University (Baltimore, MD) and National Center for Biotechnology Information, National Library of Medicine (Bethesda, MD). Retrieved from http://www.nebi.nlm,nih.gov/omim/

Palmieri, C., Vigushin, D. M., & Peters, T. J. (2004). Managing malignant disease in patients with porphyria. *Quarterly Journal of Medicine, 97,* 115–126.

Pedley, T. A., & Hirano, M. (2003). Is refractory epilepsy due to genetically determined resistance to antiepileptic drugs? *New England Journal of Medicine, 348,* 1480–1482.

Petros, W. P., & Evans, W. E. (2004). Pharmacogenomics in cancer therapy: Is host genome variability important? *Trends in Pharmacological Sciences, 25,* 457–464.

Roberts-Thomson, I. C., Ryan, P., Khoo, K. K., Hart, W. J., McMichael, A. J., & Butler, R. N. (1996). Diet, acetylator phenotype and risk of colorectal neoplasia. *Lancet, 347,* 1372–1374.

Robinson, R., Hopkins, P., Carsana, A., Gilly, H., Halsall, J., Heytens, L., et al. (2003). Several interacting genes influence the malignant hyperthermia phenotype. *Human Genetics, 112,* 217–218.

Ross, D. M., & Hughes, T. P. (2004). Cancer treatment with kinase inhibitors: What have we learned from imatinib? *British Journal of Cancer, 90,* 12–19.

Rothstein, M. A. (Ed.). (2003). *Pharmacogenetics: Social, ethical, and clinical dimensions.* Hoboken, NJ: John Wiley.

Rueffert, H., Olthoff, D., Deutrich, C., Schober, R., & Froster, U. G. (2004). A new mutation in the skeletal ryanodine receptor gene *(RYR1)* is potentially causative of maligant hyperthermia, central core disease, and severe skeletal malformation. *American Journal of Medical Genetics, 124A,* 248–254.

Sei, Y., Sambuughin, N., & Muldoon, S. (2004). Malignant Hyperthermia Genetic Testing in North American Working Group Meeting. *Anesthesiology, 100,* 464–466.

Sesti, F., Abbott, G. W., Wei, J., Murray, K. T., Saksena, S., Schwartz, P. J., et al. (2000). A common polymorphism associated with antibiotic-induced cardiac arrhythmia. *Proceedings of the National Academy of Sciences, USA, 97,* 10613–10618.

Siddiqui, A., Kerb, R., Weale, M. E., Brinkmann, U., Smith, A., Goldstein, D. B., et al. (2003). Association of multidrug resistance in epilepsy with a polymorphism in the drug-transporter gene ABCB1. *New England Journal of Medicine, 348,* 1442–1448.

Sindrup, S. H., & Brøsen, K. (1995). The pharmacogenetics of codeine hypoanalgesia. *Pharmacogenetics, 5,* 335–346.

Smith, M. W., & Mendoza, R. P. (1996). Ethnicity and pharmacogenetics. *Mount Sinai Journal of Medicine, 63,* 285–290.

Spitz, J. L. (1996). *Genodermatoses.* Baltimore: Williams & Wilkins.

Trost, C. (1982, November). The blue people of Troublesome Creek. *Science, 82,* 34–39.

Tsai, Y. J., & Hoyme, H. E. (2002). Pharmacogenomics: The future of drug therapy. *Clinical Genetics, 62,* 257–264.

Wojnowski, L. (2004). Genetics of the variable expression of CYP3A in humans. *Therapeutic Drug Monitoring, 26,* 192–199.

Working Group. World Health Organization. (1989). Glucose-6-phosphate dehydrogenase deficiency. *Bulletin of the World Health Organization, 67*(6), 601–611.

Weinshilboum, R. (2003). Inheritance and drug response. *New England Journal of Medicine, 348,* 529–537.

Wrensch, M. R., Sison, J. D., Kelsey, K. T., Liu, M., McMillan, A., et al. (2005). CYP1A1 variants and smoking-related lung cancer in San Francisco Bay area Latinos and African Americans. *International Journal of Cancer, 113,* 141–147.

Ziegler, D. S., Dalla Pozza, L., Waters, K. D., & Marshall, G. M. (2005). Advances in childhood leukaemia: Successful clinical-trials research leads to individualised therapy. *Medical Journal of Australia, 182,* 78–81.

19

Genetics and the Immune System

The immune system is extremely complex, with many interactions that determine its function and effectiveness, including both antibody (B cell) and cellular (T cell) responses. The four major components of the immune system are the cellular, humoral, complement, and phagocytic mechanisms. Genetic control of the immune response is both structural and regulatory. Examples of the diverse mechanisms known to be under genetic control are the determination of the structure, function, and amounts of immunoglobulins (Ig) or antibodies; complement components, human leukocyte antigen (HLA) system, ABO antigens, the control of receptor sites on cell membranes, the modulation of the degree of immune responsiveness, the way in which macrophages handle antigens; B and T cell proliferation and differentiation; the interactions between B and T cells; the production of enzymes responsible for bacteriocidal action; and the factors necessary for chemotaxis and macrophage mobilization. A complete discussion of the immune system is beyond the scope of this chapter. The blood group systems, the HLA system, immunodeficiency diseases, and transplantation are discussed below.

BLOOD GROUP SYSTEMS

Immunogenetics began in 1900 when Landsteiner discovered the ABO blood group system. At this time, 26 such systems plus 5 collections and 2 series are known in man, but all are not necessarily clinically significant. A 6-digit number is given to every blood group antigen in which the first 3 digits represent the system, collection or series and the second 3 digits represent the antigen. The International Society of Blood Transfusion (ISBT) pub-

lished an international terminology (Daniels et al., 2003) and maintains a Web site at http://www.iccbba.com/. The systems that are best characterized and most important include ABO, Rhesus, Kell, Lewis, Duffy, MNSs, Lutheran, P, Kidd, Diego, Yt, Xg, Dombrock, Chido/Rogers, and Scianna. The application of these to human variability is discussed in chapter 3. The functions of the products coded for by some of these genes are not yet completely elucidated, and therefore the full understanding of their importance is not known. For example, it is relatively recently that the Kidd gene locus was recognized as coding for the urea transporter of the erythrocyte.

ABO System

The ABO system is the most clinically important. The major alleles present at the ABO locus on chromosome 9 are A, B, and O. Both the A and B alleles are dominant to the O, but codominant to each other. The A and B alleles code for certain enzymes, glycosyltransferases, that add sugar groups to the H substance precursor to form the A and B glycoprotein antigens. The O allele does not produce an enzyme. These A and B antigens are not confined to the red cell but are widely distributed throughout the body. There are various subtypes of the A, B, and O alleles with more polymorphisms being revealed by newer DNA techniques, but only A1 and A2 appear to have any antigenic importance. The relationship between genotype and blood group is shown in Table 19.1, and examples of the inheritance of the ABO blood groups are illustrated in Figure 19.1 (top). Persons with blood group O are sometimes said to have a "null" phenotype. Independent of the ABO system are the H and secretor systems.

TABLE 19.1   Relationships in the ABO Blood Group System

Blood group (phenotype)	Genotype(s)	Red cell antigen(s)	Antibodies in serum
A	AO, AA	A (+H)	Anti-B
B	BO, BB	B (+H)	Anti-A
AB	AB	A, B (+H)	none
O	OO	H	Anti-A Anti-B

Persons with the genotype HH or Hh produce the H substance, which is the precursor for the A and B antigens, and is modified by the enzymes produced by the A and B alleles. Thus, individuals with A, B, or AB blood groups use up some or all of the H substance. Because the O allele does not produce a transferase, it exerts no effect on this pathway, the H substance is unmodified, and more H antigen remains present. The allele h is a rare silent allele recessive to H. Persons with hh who have the A or B allele do not express them due to the absence of the H substrate. The secretor (Se, se) locus determines whether or not the ABH antigens will be secreted in body fluids, such as saliva. Individuals who are nonsecretors (sese) do not secrete ABH antigens. Approximately 80% of the White population are secretors. The secretor gene appears to have a regulatory function on the H gene.

The clinical significance of these relationships is illustrated by the case of a woman who contacted a genetic counseling center. She was believed to have blood group O, her husband was A, and her child was AB. She had been told by local health professionals that this was not possible unless the child had a different father than her husband. The situation was causing considerable stress in their marital relationship. Investigation demonstrated that she, in fact, had the B allele, but was homozygous for the rare Bombay phenotype known as hh. B antigen production was blocked by the two h alleles, even though she actually had at least one B gene. This client had contacted the genetic counseling center on her own. The health professionals involved in this case had simply accepted what they considered to be the most likely explanation, without further investigation or consultation. Rare cases of other variance are known.

The frequency of the ABO blood group varies in different population groups, and has been used in human genetics to study diversity, migration, and selection.

The Rhesus System

It was not until 1940 that Landsteiner and Wiener discovered the rhesus (Rh) system. This system has become increasingly more complex. Many variants and about 45 antigens are known, and various symbols have been used to describe the major components. The most common is the one proposed by Fisher, Race, and Sanger that reflects the existence of three very closely linked loci: C or c, D or d (no d antiserum for the d antigen has been found and those who are RhD negative actually lack the gene; however "d" is used here for convenience), E or e that are written together as cDe. The C and E alleles are much less antigenic than the D. The D allele is considered responsible for determining Rh positivity (+) in a dominant relationship to d. This inheritance pattern is illustrated in Figure 19.1 (bottom). The percentage of Rh negative individuals in the White population is approximately 15%. Few Native Americans or Asians are Rh negative. In the Black population approximately 7% are Rh negative, and about 25% of all Blacks carry VS, a Rh-system allele that is rarely seen in other groups. Its significance is unknown.

MATERNAL–FETAL INCOMPATIBILITY

The major importance of the Rh system lies in its application to maternal–fetal incompatibility. When a father is Rh (+) and the mother is Rh (−), a

ABO system*

Parents	AO x BO ↓	AB x OO ↓	AA x BB ↓	AA x BO ↓	AB x BB ↓	BB x OO ↓
Offspring genotype	AB,AO,BO,OO	AO,BO	AB	AB,AO	AB,BB	BO
Theoretical proportion for each pregnancy	$^1/_4$ $^1/_4$ $^1/_4$ $^1/_4$	$^1/_2$ $^1/_2$	all	$^1/_2$ $^1/_2$	$^1/_2$ $^1/_2$	all
Blood group phenotype	AB, A, B, O	A, B	AB	AB, A	AB, B	B

Rh system

Parents	DD x dd	Dd x dd	Dd x Dd
Offspring	Dd	Dd, dd	DD, Dd, dd
Theoretical proportion for each pregnancy	all	$^1/_2$ $^1/_2$	$^1/_4$, $^1/_2$, $^1/_4$
Rh type	Rh(+)	Rh(+), Rh(–)	Rh(+), Rh(+), Rh(–)

FIGURE 19.1   Examples of transmission of blood group genes. *Top:* ABO system. *Bottom:* Rh system.
*Not all possible combinations are shown.

fetus that is Rh (+) induces antibodies in the mother that can readily cross the placenta and cause hemolytic disease of the newborn (erythroblastosis fetalis). Such sensitization can occur through fetomaternal blood exchange in utero or at the time of delivery. Hemolytic disease of the newborn is not usually seen until the second or later pregnancies. An Rh (–) (dd) woman and an Rh (+) man are more likely to have an Rh (+) child if the father is homozygous (DD) than if he is heterozygous (Dd). In the latter case, the chance that the child would be Rh (+) at each pregnancy is 50% as opposed to 100%.

Since the availability of Rh (D) immunoglobulin in 1968, the incidence of hemolytic disease of the newborn has markedly decreased. However, not all women who should be receiving Rh immunoglobulin are actually receiving it. Therefore, nurses need to be aware of events that can cause sensitization and thus require Rh immunoglobulin administration. These include any fetomaternal hemorrhage, spontaneous or induced abortion even in early pregnancy, any previous blood transfusion that was or might have been Rh incompatible, amniocentesis, chorionic villus sampling, fetal blood sampling, and fetoscopy. The nurse should also be aware of events that are associated with an increased risk of fetomaternal hemorrhage such as

abdominal trauma, Cesarean section, and others. Other factors influence Rh immunization, such as ABO compatibility between the fetus and mother. Other major reasons for failure to prevent Rh immunization include the giving of an inadequate dose of Rh immunoglobulin postpartum, especially if there was severe transplacental hemorrhage during delivery; giving it later than recommended and after Rh immunization has already begun; and failure of the responsible health professional to recognize the need for immunization or give an adequate dose. A review of birth certificates conducted by the Centers for Disease Control and Prevention in 2000 and reported by Moise (2002) identified Rh sensitization complicating 6.8 pregnancies per 1,000 live births. The current recommendation is to administer 300 µg of Rh immunoglobulin to nonsensitized Rh negative women at 28 weeks gestation, thus reducing the incidence of antenatal alloimmunization to about 0.1%. This same dose should be given after birth if the infant is RhD-positive as soon as possible, but within 72 hours after delivery. However, it can be given up to the 14th day. The Rh status of every pregnant woman should be determined, and if she is Rh (–), then antibody status must be done. If the Rh of the father of the child is unknown, and other conditions indicate the possibility of incompatibility [e.g., mother Rh (−), second pregnancy], Rh immunoglobulin should be administered. Detailed guidelines for various situations are given by Moise. Rh incompatibility can be diagnosed through genotyping of amniocytes using PCR.

Although incompatibility in the Rh system is the most important, ABO incompatibility can also cause injury. This occurs when the mother is blood group O, the father is A, B, or AB, and the child is A or B. Even though this reaction is not usually too severe in the newborn, the incompatibility is now believed to lead to early embryonic deaths and is often not recognized as a cause. ABO incompatibility may cause severe fetal anemia as well as fetal ascites and polyhydramnios. Erythroblastosis caused by ABO incompatibility may be observed in the first pregnancy in contrast to the usual situation existing for Rh. It is interesting to note that ABO incompatibility is somewhat protective against Rh immunization. These relationships are shown in Figure 19.2. Incompatibilities in the Kell system have also been shown to be responsible for hemolytic disease.

BLOOD GROUPS AND DISEASE

The first association between the ABO blood groups and disease was made in the case of stomach cancer. Persons having blood group A were 1.26 times more likely to develop stomach cancer than persons with other blood types. Other associations were subsequently determined that linked pernicious anemia with type A; rheumatic fever with type A, B, or AB; smallpox with type A or AB; and duodenal or gastric ulcer with type O. The risk of duodenal ulcer in nonsecretors with type O blood is $2\frac{1}{2}$ times that of types A, B, and AB secretors. Nonsecretors appear to have increased oral carriage of *Candida albicans* and increased susceptibility to increased urinary tract infection with *Escherichia coli*. The Duffy (Fy) blood group has three alleles. In Africa, the null allele Fy (a-b-) is found in almost 100% of African Blacks, and it is found in about 85% of American Blacks. The Duffy antigenic sites on red cells are the receptors for *Plasmodium vivax*, one of the malarial parasites. Those who are Fy negative thus do not bind the parasite and do not develop malaria. They have a considerably selective advantage over individuals with the other Fy alleles in malarial areas. Other associations between blood groups and diseases are known.

THE HLA SYSTEM

Characteristics and Inheritance

The HLA (human leukocyte antigen) system is the major histocompatibility complex (MHC) in humans. Major normal functions of the HLA system include acting as a marker of self and the presentation of antigen, particularly to T helper cells. There are three MHC regions located close together on the short arm of chromosome 6 (6p). These include the class I and II HLA genes and the class III genes that code for non-HLA products that are often involved with immune function. The most clinically important antigen groups at this time are the class I loci: HLA-A, HLA-B, HLA-C, and the classical class II loci: HLA-DR, HLA-DP, and HLA-DQ, although the roles of others are emerging. The HLA system is the most polymorphic system known. This allows for a tremendous amount of human variability, especially ensuring resistance to a wide variety of pathogens.

The HLA system is defined either serologically or by nucleotide sequence analysis. An international committee determines and updates standardized nomenclature, and accepts new designations. The older serologic definitions use the locus specificity such as HLA-A followed by a number, as in the following examples: HLA-A2, HLA-B27, HLA-DR4, or HLA-Cw2. Much of the classic work in this area defined HLA specificity in this way. Those defined by sequence analysis use the gene name followed by an asterisk and a four digit number, such as *B*2703* where the locus is HLA-B, the first two numbers (27) are the specificity, and the last two numbers (03) are the unique nucleotide sequence for that specificity. Thus HLA-B*2701 through HLA-B*2707 are related alleles that encode different HLA molecules but which all type serologically as HLA-B27. In the case of the class II antigens, some of which consist of one or more alpha and beta chains that are coded for by α and β genes, there is a more precise designation. An example is *DRB1*0401* in which it is shown that the reference is to the HLA-DR locus, the first beta chain, with the specificity being 04 and the

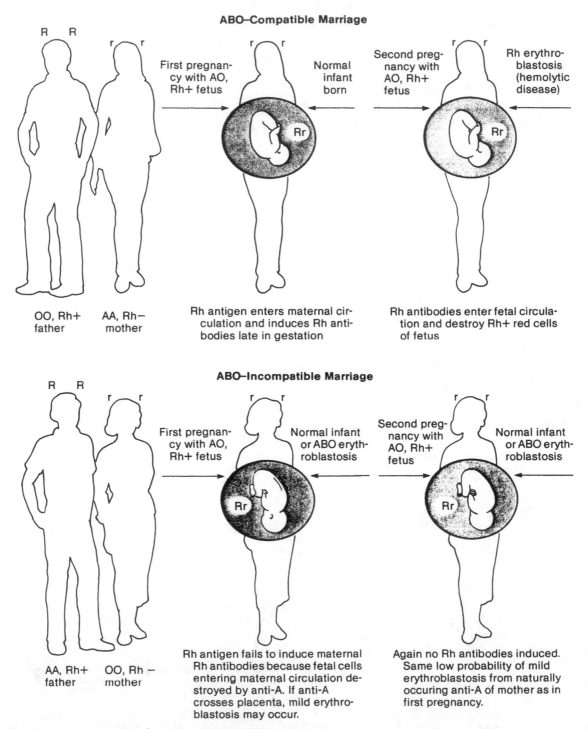

FIGURE 19.2   Second or later Rh-positive children of Rh-negative mothers may be severely anemic or die of Rh antibodies induced by passage of fetal blood cells into maternal circulation in the absence of ABO incompatibility. Usually, milder ABO erythroblastosis may occur in first or later pregnancies mainly in O type mothers with A- or B-positive fetuses, irrespective of presence or absence of Rh incompatibility. (Reprinted with permission. Hildemann WH, Clark EA, Raison RL: Comprehensive Immunogenetics. New York, Elsevier Science Publishing Co., 1981).

nucleotide sequence being 01. In discussing the antigens that are coded for by the HLA alleles, "w" has also been retained to distinguish HLA-Cw8. It also is used in T-cell defined specificity which is designated by Dw (for HLA-D-associated) followed by a number such as Dw13.

The major class I antigens are HLA-A, HLA-B, and HLA-C. Other genes in that region are non-classic class I genes, HLA-E, -F, -G, and the class I pseudogenes, HLA-H, -J, -K, -L. More than 210 Class I alleles are known. HLA-A, HLA-B, and HLA-C antigens are present on the cell membrane of almost all cells, although somewhat weakly on erythrocytes and spermatozoa. A small amount is in the serum. HLA-A, HLA-B, and HLA-C are associated with beta microglobulin on the cell membranes. Class I antigens present antigenic peptide to CD8+ T cells and determine the response of natural killer cells.

Class II includes the classic HLA-DR, -DQ, and -DP antigens along with the less polymorphic -DM and -DO antigens. These glycoproteins consist of an alpha and a beta chain which are coded for by α and β genes. For example, the DQ alpha and beta chains could be coded for by *DQA1* and *DQB1*. More than 225 class II alleles are recognized and new ones are continually added. The transporters associated with antigen processing genes, *TAP1* and *2*, whose importance has been recognized relatively recently, have been located in the class II region. HLA-DQ, -DP, and -DR are somewhat more restricted in their distribution because they are primarily expressed on the surfaces of immuno-competent cells such as B-lymphocytes, monocytes, endothelial cells, dendritic cells, activated T-lymphocytes, and macrophages. However, when stimulated by interferon γ, they are now believed to be expressed by almost all cells. Class II molecules present antigenic peptide to CD4+ T cells.

The class III region includes certain complement components such as C2, Bf, C4A, and C4B, other genes with immune-related function, as well as products unrelated to the immune system, such as steroid 21-hydroxylase, the major heat shock protein, and tumor necrosis factors (TNF).

Because letters were assigned to the HLA loci in the order of their discovery, they do not reflect their order on the chromosome. Because of the close proximity of each locus to the other HLA loci on the chromosome, the genes are tightly linked and are usually inherited together, with infrequent (less than 1%) recombination occurring. The segment of each chromosome with its set of HLA genes is known as a haplotype, whereas the two haplotypes together comprise the HLA genotype. Thus, multiple HLA specificities are present in each individual. Inheritance is codominant, and the phenotypic expression of the genes as evidenced by the specific antigens they produce can be demonstrated by HLA typing procedures. Other haplotypes are used to study linkage and recombination.

Linkage Disequilibrium and Population Distribution of HLA

The phenomenon of linkage disequilibrium occurs when two or more of the alleles in the HLA system occur together in a haplotype significantly more frequently than would be expected by chance alone. In European populations, HLA-A1 and HLA-B8 occur together with an observed frequency that far exceeds the expected frequency. The frequency of individual HLA antigens varies according to different populations, for example, HLA-A9 is present in 65% of Asian populations but only 17% of European Caucasian population. HLA-B8 is common in White populations and rare in Asians.

Disease Associations

Intense interest in the HLA system was originally generated because of the realization of its role in grafts and transplant success. That interest now includes the relationship between specific HLA antigens and certain diseases. Many diseases have been studied in the hope of finding a significant association with a specific HLA antigen or haplotype. Some of the strongest associations have been with autoimmune diseases or disorders with an immunologic defect. This association has led to the search for an autoimmune or immunological association with disorders originally not known to be so associated, such as in type 1 diabetes mellitus and in narcolepsy. Estimates of the strength of the association can be made. Relative risk refers to how much more frequently a specific disease develops in an individual carrying a specific HLA antigen compared to the frequency of disease in individuals who are not carrying the HLA antigen. In addition, not all who have a particular HLA type may develop a given disorder despite the strong association. The etiologic fraction for a positive association in which the relative risk exceeds one, in a broad sense, indicates how much of the disease is due to the HLA factor. Formulas for these calculations may be obtained. In addition to disease susceptibility, HLA-related protective effects have also been noted. For example, HLA-DR2 and the associated *HLA-DQB1*0602* allele is associated with resistance to type 1 diabetes mellitus, and HLA-B*53 is protective against severe malaria in west Africa. *HLA-DQB1*0601* protects against the development of narcolepsy.

Two of the most striking and undisputed associations are between HLA-B27 and ankylosing spondylitis (an inflammatory joint disease often resulting in vertebral fusion) and of *HLA-DQB1*0602* and narcolepsy [a primary sleep disorder characterized by excessive daytime sleepiness and disturbances of rapid eye movement (REM) sleep due to deficiency of the neuropeptide, hypocretin]. HLA-B27 is found in 90% to 95% of patients with idiopathic ankylosing spondylitis regardless of ethnic group. In populations without the disorder, HLA-B27 is found in 6% to 8% of European and North American Whites, 2% of Chinese and Black Americans, and 0.2% of Japanese populations. In Australian aborigines, neither HLA-B27 nor ankylosing spondylitis are found. It is estimated that a male with the B27 antigen has a relative risk of developing the disorder that is 90 to 100 times greater than a male not possessing this antigen. The chance for a person who has HLA-B27 to develop ankylosing spondylitis is estimated at 5% to 20%. Thus, not all those with HLA-B27 develop ankylosing spondylitis, although some may have subtle symptoms that never develop into disease and are thus overlooked unless carefully looked for. HLA-B27 is also associated with other seronegative inflammatory types of arthritis (often called HLA-B27-associated rhematoid diseases) and is found in 75% of persons with Reiters disease and up to 90% of persons who develop arthritis after enteric infection due to *Shigella, Salmonella,* and certain *Yersinia* species. One theory proposed to explain the association is that the configuration of the B27 antigen resembles certain infective microorganisms such as the above plus *Klebsiella,* leading to an inadequate, inappropriate, or delayed host response. If the microorganism persists in the host, it may lead to antibody production that turns into autoimmune disease production. This is known as the molecular mimicry hypothesis. The application of DNA techniques has revealed that HLA-B27 includes at least 9 subtypes *(B*2701-B*2709)*. Some of these subtypes, such as *B*2702, B*2704,* and *B*2705,* are more frequently associated with disease than the others. Recently, HLA-B27 has been associated with a cardiac syndrome of conduction system abnormalities and aortic regurgitation as well as other possible cardiac associations.

In narcolepsy, *HLA DQB1*0602* is present in 90% to 100% of persons with narcolepsy and cataplexy (present as part of the classic group of symptoms in narcolepsy in the majority of patients. It is a brief sudden episode of weakness in voluntary muscles that may be triggered by emotion such as laughing or anger). In contrast, *HLA DQB1*0602* is present in 12% to 38% of the general population. Hypocretin genes are located in this HLA vicinity although how they interact is not known. There has also been an association between HIV-1 disease and various HLA genotypes. For example both HLA-B27 and HLA-B57 have been associated with slow progression, while certain HLA-B35 alleles *(HLAB*3502, *3503,* and *3504)* have been associated with rapid progression. HLA class I homozygosity has been associated with rapid progression to AIDS. For details see Carrington and O'Brien (2003).

Clinical Uses of HLA

Currently the largest single use for HLA typing is in tissue and organ transplantation, including blood products. In some institutions, typing of the HLA-A, HLA-B, and HLA-C loci is used to screen donors for platelet and leukocyte transfusions because of the problem of sensitivity for those persons already having such multiple transfusions.

In some instances, HLA typing is used in genetic counseling. For example, in one counseling case, a mother with narcolepsy was concerned about the chances of her two adolescent daughters developing narcolepsy. One of them was showing signs of excessive sleepiness (not uncommon in adolescents!). HLA typing was done, and the "sleepy" daughter was found to have HLA-DR2 (this case was before more precise definition in this kind of typing was available) as was her mother, while the other child had an HLA type not known to be related to narcolepsy development. Thus, it seemed that one daughter was in fact developing narcolepsy, while the risk for the other to do so was extremely low. HLA typing is also useful for counseling in other disorders such as families with ankylosing spondylitis, but it is not yet clinically useful for disorders with weak associations. This may change as specific nucleotide sequences are noted to have stronger associations with certain diseases.

Pharmacologic applications for HLA have also been noted. In the investigation of all patients with systemic lupus erythematosus (SLE) induced by hydralazine, those most prone to developing SLE were those who were both slow acetylators (see chapter 18) and were also HLA-DR4. Thus, individuals who possess HLA-DR4 should not be treated with hydralazine for hypertension if other therapy can be used. Similarly, when treating rheumatoid arthritis patients with gold, nephropathy is associated with patients who have HLA-DR3, and mouth ulcers are associated with patients who have HLA-DR2. HLA-B27 is associated with an increased risk of adverse reactions to levamisole in patients with rheumatoid arthritis. Thus, knowing an individual's HLA type in certain instances may prevent toxic drug reactions.

Knowledge of HLA type may also be used to prevent illness. For example, individuals with HLA-DR3 and HLA-DR4 might avoid precipitating diabetes mellitus if they avoid steroids, oral contraceptives, and obesity. Because persons with myasthenia gravis who do not have HLA-DR3 are more prone to develop thymomas than those who do possess HLA-DR3, clinicians should be very careful in their assessment of the patient in order to avoid missing such a tumor. A child with mouth ulcers who has HLA-B5 might be treated with systemic steroids in order to prevent the onset or ameliorate the course of the rare Behçets disease. HLA-B27 males who have back pain should be helped to choose a career that will not be adversely affected by the limitations of ankylosing spondylitis. Idiopathic hemochromatosis is an autosomal recessive disorder closely linked to the HLA-II region in certain cases, and the HFE gene has been found in that area which, when mutated, causes some cases. By studying the effected person in a family, those siblings who are HLA identical to the patient can be identified as having a genetically susceptible background. Therefore, their iron status can be followed, and preventive measures can be instituted before organ damage occurs. Many of the clinical applications are in the beginning stages. HLA has been used in prenatal diagnosis to detect congenital adrenal hyperplasia in certain appropriate cases, as the 21-hydroxylase deficient gene and HLA are linked.

HLA also offers a chance for research with clinical applications. Some of these are the investigation of:

1. whether similar diseases have similar or different HLA associations;
2. further defining the HLA association with specific syndrome components, for example, if within certain diseases one HLA type has a different clinical course or different age of onset;
3. investigating the association of HLA types with responses to treatment or survival rates; and
4. delineating the association between HLA, immunity, microorganisms, and inheritance.

IMMUNODEFICIENCY DISORDERS

The relatively rare primary immunodeficiency diseases have been instrumental in developing knowledge of the functions and interactions of the immune system. They have also been leading candidates for treatment through gene therapy strategies. They occur in 1:2,000 to 1:10,000 live births.

Types

A variety of classifications exist. In one, disorders are classified into five groups—defects in stem cell development that usually lead to a combined immunodeficiency of both the cellular and humoral components (30%), T-cell defects leading to defective cellular immunity (50%), B-cell defects leading to defective Igs and impaired humoral immunity (10%), complement component disorders (4%), and phagocytic functional defects, both qualitative and quantitative (6%). Selected examples of immunodeficiency diseases and their inheritance patterns follow.

Combined Deficiencies or Stem Cell Defects

Examples of stem cell defects include severe combined immune deficiencies (SCID), which include several disorders with functional deficiency in both cellular and humoral immunity and different inheritance patterns depending on the type. Mutations in at least 10 genes can cause SCID. One type, with autosomal recessive (AR) inheritance is due to adenosine deaminase (ADA) deficiency arising from various mutant alleles. This disorder results in both cellular and humoral deficiency with recurrent infections and skeletal dysplasia. Another example is Wiskott-Aldrich syndrome that shows selective defects in cellular and humoral immunity, with functional defects in monocytes, granulocytes, and platelets. Of note is the inability to produce antibodies to polysaccharide antigens. The major features are thrombocytopenia manifested by purpura and bleeding, susceptibility to infection with all classes of microbes, eczema, bloody diarrhea, and the development of autoimmune disease such as juvenile rheumatoid arthritis, and malignancy, with death usual before age 10 years. While usually an X-linked recessive disorder, it now appears that there may be autosomally transmitted variants. The basic defect is in the Wiskott-Aldrich syndrome protein which may be needed to bind a family of protein-tyrosine kinases that are needed in signalling pathways. An allelic variant of mutation in the Wiskott-Aldrich syndrome protein gene is X-linked thrombocytopenia, a milder congenital disorder characterized by thrombocytopenia and small platelets but not the other features of Wiskott-Aldrich syndrome.

T-Cell or Cellular Defects

Examples include purine nucleoside phosphorylase deficiency (PNP), an autosomal dominant disorder, which causes an immunodeficiency characterized by abnormal T-cell function resulting from the cessation of purine catabolism leading to deficient uric acid excretion, but increases in other purines and an accumulation of substrates in the pathway. Other findings include neurological abnormalities and lymphoma development.

B-Cell or Antibody Defects

Examples include Bruton agammaglobulinemia, an X-linked recessive disorder with agammaglobulinemia but intact cell-mediated immunity due to a defect in Bruton tyrosine kinase. These individuals are prone to bacterial infections and infection with

Giardia lamblia and are at increased risk for the development of rheumatoid arthritis.

Complement Defects

Examples include hereditary angioedema (HAE), which results from C1 esterase inhibitor deficiency. The incidence is between 1:10,000 to 1:50,000. About 25% of affected people have no family history and have new mutations. There are three variants. HAEI and II are transmitted in an autosomal dominant manner while the third appears transmitted in an X-linked dominant manner or possibly an autosomal dominant manner that is sex-limited or has reduced penetrance. HAE is characterized by recurrent swelling of the extremities, face, upper respiratory tract or gastrointestinal tract. The latter may cause abdominal pain, vomiting and diarrhea. Laryngeal edema can result in death. Onset may be in childhood with worsening in adolescence but can begin in adulthood. HAE can be triggered by trauma, stress, knfection or hormones such as in birth control pills and hormone replacement therapy. Attacks of angioedema may be preceded by a nonpruritic erythematous rash. Prophylaxis consists of synthetic anabolic androgens such as danazol, anti-fibrinolytic drugs such as aminocaproic acid (Amicar), and replacement therapy with purified C1 inhibitor concentrate or treatment with a recombinant plasma kallikrein inhibitor. Support groups are listed in Appendix B.

Phagocytic Defects

Examples may include myeloperoxidase deficiency, inherited in an AR manner that results in defective cellular immunity. Disseminated candidiasis is a major feature. Another disorder is Chediak-Higashi syndrome (AR inheritance) which affects the lysosomal transport protein LYST, resulting in defective mobility and bacteriocidal activity in the neutrophils leading to recurrent infections. Partial oculocutaneous albinism is a distinguishing feature along with photophobia and nystagmus. Malignant lymphoma and leukemia often develop and death often occurs by seven years of age.

Assessment Points Leading to Suspicion of Immunodeficiency

An increased susceptibility to infections is characteristic of the immunodeficiencies. Although this includes increased frequency, severity, and prolonged duration of infection, the former, particularly of the respiratory tract, is the most common finding. The development of complications, rare disease manifestations, or infections with organisms that are generally weak pathogens such as *Pneumocystis carinii* should evoke suspicion of immune system compromise. Some of the primary immunodeficiencies have milder forms that become evident in later childhood rather than earlier.

The following points are ones that should alert the nurse to consider the possibility of immune dysfunction or deficiency in an infant or child (although no one point is diagnostic by itself, and may occur in other disorders as well):

- Frequent and severe upper respiratory infections in excess of the normal 6 to 8 per year
- Bronchitis, purulent otitis, tonsillitis, or sinusitis eventually resulting in mastoiditis, draining ears, pneumonitis, bronchiectasis, or pneumonia
- Osteomyelitis or meningitis
- History of unusually severe childhood illnesses such as chicken pox
- Distended abdomen
- Chronic diarrhea, with *Giardia lamblia* often being isolated from the stool
- Skin rashes such as eczema and lesions
- Malabsorption and vomiting
- Persistent *Candida* infections of mouth, anal area, or mucous membranes
- A family history of early deaths or severe courses of infection or consanguinity
- An altered response to immunization. A normal response to live-virus vaccines usually indicates a normal cellular immune system.

In addition, the following may also be seen: failure to thrive leading to growth retardation, delay of developmental milestones, paleness, listlessness, and irritability. In humoral deficiencies, the gram-positive bacteria are usually responsible for infection, whereas in cellular immune deficiencies, the gram-negative bacteria, fungi, viruses, protozoa, and mycobacteria are found more often.

The time of the development of symptoms can be suggestive. In SCID, symptoms such as diarrhea, pneumonia, and unresponsive candidiasis are evident within the first 3 months of life. In contrast, males with X-linked agammaglobulinemia may appear healthy for the first 6 to 12 months, until recurrent severe bacterial infections develop. Males with chronic granulomatous disease may develop skin infections, draining lymph nodes, or osteomyelitis when they are toddlers. Thus, the nurse must be alert for immunodeficiencies at various stages of early childhood. Several of the known immunodeficiencies have distinctive features present in addition to the general ones described. For example, Job (hyperimmunoglobulin E) syndrome is known to occur most frequently in females with red hair, fair skin, hyperextendible joints, with eczema and recurrent cold staphylococcal abscesses occurring along with defects in neutrophil chemotaxis and high serum IgE levels, along with susceptibility to respiratory infections, pneumatocele formation, dentition abnormalities, and candidiasis that is typically inherited in an autosomal dominant manner. Recently an autosomal recessive form has been identified which has slightly different features including vasculitis and central nervous system manifestations.

Once the particular immunodeficiency is determined, genetic counseling services should be sought. Some types of deficiency are detectable through prenatal diagnosis. If the disease is detected in one sibling, the others should be screened in order to prevent complications that otherwise could be avoided and to detect siblings who are heterozygotes so that, when appropriate, they can benefit from genetic counseling and reproductive planning, and also because some may have subtle immune system alterations.

Therapy varies according to the disorder. Infusions of purified human immunoglobulin (IVIG) may be used for certain combined immunodeficiencies, and for agammaglobulinemias for example. Because the mortality rate is very high for disorders such as SCID, bone marrow transplantation may be a viable alternative. One of the first trials of gene therapy was for ADA deficiency and this promised hope for treatment in other conditions (see chapter 15). However, gene therapy complications, such as leukemia in some children receiving gene therapy for SCID, and deaths have led to restrictions. One preventive measure is the widespread use of rubella vaccination to eliminate those immunodeficiencies that develop secondary to in utero rubella infection.

TRANSPLANTATION

Interest in transplantation accelerated with the increased interest in skin grafting during WW II and Medawar's realization of the importance of leukocyte associated antigens in acceptance or rejection. Terminology currently related to grafting and transplantation include the following:

Allograft—Graft between members of the same species with different genotypes, that is, between humans.

Autograft—Tissue grafted back to the person donating it; a self graft

Isograft—Graft between individuals with the same genotype (syngeneic), that is, identical twins.

Xenograft—Graft between individuals of different species, such as between a human and a pig.

Allogeneic—Members of the same species with different genotypes

Syngeneic—Members of the same species with identical genotypes.

Transplantation can be used for solid organs such as kidney, liver, pancreas, lungs, and heart, or for bone marrow, corneas, and skin. Renal transplants have enjoyed the greatest success of all solid organs transplanted. The major problem limiting success has been immunologic rejection due to incompatibility, but technical surgical problems, poor recipient condition, and properties unique to the specific type of tissue being transplanted have also played a role that has varied in importance with the type of transplant. Corneal transplants have generally been considered to be immunologically privileged, which has meant that rejection phenomena are rare unless vascularization has taken place. Nonetheless, success is improved by matching the donor and recipient. Among the red cell antigens, the ABO is the most important. The sex of the donor and recipient should be the same, as the H-Y antigen can play a role in rejection. The genes within the HLA system are the most important in determining the histocompatibility between the donor and the recipient. The best matches come from siblings who have HLA haplotypes identical to those of the recipient. For all donors, including unrelated ones and cadavers, the better the HLA type matching, the more successful the graft tends to be. The newer techniques may lead to better typing at the DNA level that will improve success.

Bone marrow transplantation is an accepted form of therapy in some immunodeficiency diseases and in diseases in which aplastic anemia is a feature, such as Fanconi anemia. The main complications of bone marrow transplantation are graft rejection, interstitial pneumonia, and graft-versus-host disease (GVHD). It is estimated that GVHD occurs in more than half of the patients with bone marrow transplantation. For this to occur the patient must have a very depressed cellular immune system, have received a sufficient quantity of foreign (donor) immunocompetent cells, and there must be some histocompatibility difference between the donor and recipient, even if it is a minor one. The occurrence of GVHD in cases of identical HLA matching indicates the importance of other immune response genes or failure to match HLA at the DNA level. Clinical signs of acute GVHD occur 7 to 30 days after the graft. Often a skin rash is seen first, which may be maculopapular or erythematic, followed by fever, hepatic abnormalities, and jaundice, diarrhea, abdominal pain, and ileus. The mortality rate after acquiring GVHD is high. The use of laminar-air flow rooms increases survival. Because early symptoms of GVHD may mimic other illnesses, any of these symptoms must be thoroughly investigated so that immunosuppressive treatment can be given to halt progression. Chronic GVHD does not usually develop until 3 to 15 months after the transplant. A variation (A/A) in a certain section of the interleukin-10 gene has been associated with low risk for GVHD. Typing patients will provide information that can be used clinically including such factors as influencing the optimal immunosuppressive drug regimen to be used (Cooke & Ferrara, 2003).

Some centers, such as the bone marrow transplantation program at Children's Hospital in Philadelphia, have developed a child advocate system to avoid the potential conflict of interest that can arise when parents are asked to give informed consent for both the donor and recipient. The advocate seeks to determine that the risks to the donor are minimal, that the donor is eager to help the sibling, that the participants are fully informed about the risks, that consent if fully and voluntarily given both by the parents and donor, and that the bone marrow transplant is necessary for treatment. This is the final step of an extensive procedure geared at preparing the family both physically and psychologically. Nurses often play an active role in working with such families.

GENETIC INFLUENCES ON INFECTIOUS DISEASE SUSCEPTIBILITY AND RESISTANCE

Typically, not every person exposed to an infectious disease becomes infected. Various examples have been given earlier in this chapter and in chapters 1 and 3. Some genetic variations in both agents and hosts are associated with susceptibility and resistance to infectious diseases. Obvious ones are due to primary immunodeficiency diseases but less obvious ones are becoming known. Some of the evidence comes from twin and adoption studies; studies from linkage studies of a variety of loci, many involved in immune response such as HLA, ABO blood group, and other blood group associations as well as others such as the vitamin D receptor polymorphisms; and from heterozygous advantages of certain genotypes in the presence of infectious diseases, such as that which is known for sickle cell disease and malaria (see chapter 3). Some types of gene variations involve those that allow the entry of a microorganism into the cell and its replication, those that regulate the type and strength of various components that result in the host immune response to the microorganism, sequelae of complications after infectious disease, and those that influence response to antimicrobial drugs. In the microorganism, gene variations in structure and expression influence virulence and pathogenicity, allow elucidation of pathogenesis, ability to become resistant to antimicrobial agents, identify drug targets, and allow vaccine approaches, as well as identify contacts and trace outbreaks. Some examples of genetically determined susceptibility and resistance to infectious disease are given in Table 19.2.

As an example, leprosy is a disease due to infection with *Mycobacterium leprae* that still affects about 700,000 people each year. The clinical manifestations can range from limited self-healing disease to disseminated lesions (lepromatous). Genetic variations have been found to affect both susceptibility to disease and modification of the clinical form it will take. Gene expression profiling has been used to discern the classification of the clinical form in an infected person. The leukocyte immune globulin receptor family genes were upregulated in lesions of patients with the disseminated form, and appeared to depress certain innate host defense mechanisms in one study (Bleharski et al., 2003). In examining sequelae after Epstein-Barr virus (EBV) infection, patients who progressed to X-linked lymphoproliferative disease, a fatal immunologic disorder, had an altered gene *(SAP)* that resulted in B and T cell proliferation during EBV infection. This is an example of how genetic variation can lead to various consequences of infection. In another example, those who have a gene alteration in the terminal component of complement or properdin have increased susceptibility to meningococcal infection. Homozygous mutations in the mannose-binding lectin *(MBL)* pathway of complement activiation appear important for susceptibility to infection in persons with malignancies and with cystic fibrosis as well as susceptibility to meningococcal infection. Among persons infected with the same type of *Streptococcus pyogenes* causing invasive disease, those with the DRB*1501/DRB1*0602 HLA haplotype were less likely to develop severe systemic disease.

Genetic studies have also been used in regard to studying the pathogenesis and resistance of microorganisms and in epidemiological studies of transmission. These types of studies allow further understanding of pathogenesis and the development of new drugs based on identified targets. For example, in regard to tuberculosis, genotyping of *Mycobacterium tuberculosis* has been used to identify pseudo-cases due to cross-contamination in the lab, distinguish between the reasons for developed drug resistance, determine if a second episode of disease is due to relapse or reinfection, investigate and delineate an outbreak, improve the investigation of contacts, and guide measures to reduce transmission, evaluate tuberculosis control efforts, determine reasons for variation in strain virulence and spread, and select effective drug treatments, vector controls, and diagnosis. Understandings of gene variations and expression in

TABLE 19.2   Selected Examples of Genetically Determined Susceptibility and Resistance in Infectious Diseases

Genes/Variants	Comments
ABO blood group O	Susceptibility to cholera observed
Cystic fibrosis transmembrane conductance regulator *(CFTR)* mutation	Results in cystic fibrosis and in defects in clearing *Pseudomonas aeroginosa* from respiratory tract. Certain mutations may be associated with sinusitis
Duffy blood group negative	Resistance to *Plasmodium vivax* malaria
Fucosyltransferase *(FUT2)* mutation, nonsecretors	Susceptibility to recurrent urinary tract infections
Galactose-1 phosphate-uridyltransferase *(GALT)* mutation	Susceptibility to neonatal gram negative bacterial sepsis
*HLA-DRB1*11*	Associated with resistance to persistent hepatitis C infections in some European populations
*HLA-DRB1*1302*	Associated with resistance to persisent hepatitis B infections in West African populations
*HLA-DQB1*0501*	Susceptibility to *Onchocerca volvulus* infection which causes river blindness
Interleukin 12 Receptor, Beta-1 *(IL12Rβ1)*	Homozygous mutations are associated with both *Salmonella* and *Mycobacterium* infections
Microsomal epoxide hydrolase deficiency	Associated with chronic hepatitis C liver disease severity and hepatocellular carcinoma risk
Human prion protein gene *(PRPN)* homozygous at position 129	Associated with greater susceptibility to Creutzfeldt-Jakob disease
Plasminogene activator inhibitor-1 *4G/4G* genotype	Associated with poor outcome from sepsis in meningococcal disease

malaria in humans, the malarial parasite, and the mosquito vector are leading to new approaches to treatment and vaccines.

BIBLIOGRAPHY

Barnes, P. F., & Cave, M. D. (2003). Molecular epidemiology of tuberculosis. *New England Journal of Medicine, 349,* 1149–1156.

Bleharski, J. R., Li, H., Meinken, C., Graeber, T. G., Ochoa, M-T., Yamamura, M., et al. (2003). Use of genetic profiling in leprosy to discriminate clinical forms of the disease. *Science, 301,* 1527–1530.

Bodmer, J. (1996). World distribution of HLA alleles and implications for disease. *Ciba Foundation Symposium, 197,* 233–258.

Bonilla, F. A., & Geha, R. S. (2003). Primary immunodeficiency diseases. *Journal of Allergy and Clinical Immunology, 111,* S571–S581.

Buckley, R. H. (2003). 27. Transplanation immunology: Organ and bone marrow. *Journal of Allergy and Clinical Immunology, 111*(Suppl. 2), S733–S744.

Buckley, R. H. (2004). Pulmonary complications of primary immunodeficiencies. *Paediatric Respiratory Review, 5*(Suppl. A), S225–S233.

Burgner, D., & Levin, M. (2003). Genetic susceptibility to infectious diseases. *Pediatric Infectious Disease Journal, 22,* 1–6.

Carrington, M., & O'Brien, S. J. (2003). The influence of *HLA* genotype on AIDS. *Annual Review of Medicine, 54,* 535–551.

Cavazzana-Calvo, M., Lagresle, C., Hacein-Bey-Abina, S., & Fischer, A. (2005). Gene therapy for severe combined immunodeficiency. *Annual Review of Medicine, 56,* 585–602.

Chabas, D., Taheri, S., Renier, C., & Mignot, E. (2003). The genetics of narcolepsy. *Annual Review of Genomics and Human Genetics, 4,* 459–483.

Chapel, H., Geha, R., & Rosen, F. for the IUIS PID Classification Committee. (2003). Primary immunodeficiency diseases: An update. *Clinical and Exploratory Immunology, 132,* 9–15.

Conley, M. E. (2005). Molecular basis of immunodeficiency. *Immunological Reviews, 203,* 5–9.

Cooke, K. R., & Ferrara, J. L. M. (2003). A protective gene for graft-versus-host disease. *New England Journal of Medicine, 349,* 2183–2184.

Crawford, D. C., & Nickerson, D. A. (2005). Definition and clinical importance of haplotypes. *Annual Review of Medicine, 56,* 303–320.

Daniels, G. (2002). *Human blood groups* (2nd ed.). Oxford, England: Blackwell Science.

Daniels, G. L., Cartron, J. P., Fletcher, A., Garratty, G., Henry, S., Jørgensen, J., et al. (2003). ISBT Committee on Terminology for Red Cell Surface Antigens. Vancouver Report. *Vox Sanguinis, 84,* 244–247.

De Maio, A., Torres, M. B., & Reeves, R. H. (2005). Genetic determinants influencing the response to injury, inflammation, and sepsis. *Shock, 23,* 11–17.

Faas, B. H., Beckers, E. A., Wildoer, P., Ligthart, P. C., Overbeeke, M. A., Zondervan, H. A., et al. (1997). Molecular background of VS and weak C expression in blacks. *Transfusion, 37,* 38–44.

Fugger, L., Tisch, R., Libau, R., van Endert, P., & Devitt, H. O. (2001). The role of human major histocompatibility complex (HLA) genes in disease. In C. R. Scriver, A. L. Beaudet, W. S. Sly, & D. Valle (Eds.), *The metabolic and molecular bases of inherited disease* (8th ed., pp. 311–341). New York: McGraw-Hill.

Hemingway, J., & Craig, A. (2004). New ways to control malaria. *Science, 303,* 1984–1985.

Hill, A. V. S. (2001). Genes and susceptibility to infectious diseases. In C. R. Scriver, A. L. Beaudet, W. S. Sly, & D. Valle (Eds.), *The metabolic and molecular bases of inherited disease* (8th ed., pp. 203–214). New York: McGraw-Hill.

Hosseini-Maaf, B., Irshaid, N. M., Hellberg, A., Wagner, T., Levene, C., Hustinx, H., et al. (2005). New and unusual O alleles at the ABO locus are implicated in unexpected blood group phenotypes. *Transfusion, 45,* 70–81.

Howard, H., Martlew, V., McFadyen, I., Clarke, C., Duguid, J., Bromilow, I., et al. (1998). Consequences for fetus and neonate of maternal red cell allo-immunisation. *Archives of Disease in Childhood Fetal & Neonatal Edition, 78,* F62–F66.

Hughes, D. (2003). Exploiting genomics, genetics and chemistry to combat antibiotic resistance. *Nature Reviews Genetics, 4,* 432–441.

Imai, K., Morio, T., Zhu, Y., Jon, Y., Itoh, S., Kajiwara, M., et al. (2004). Clinical course of patients with WASP gene mutations. *Blood, 103,* 456–464.

Joy, S. D., Rossi, K. Q., Krugh, D., & O'Shaughnessy, R. W. (2005). Management of pregnancies complicated by anti-e alloimmunization. *Obstetrics & Gynecology, 105,* 24–28.

Kalman, L., Lindegren, M. L., Kobrynski, L., Vogt, R., Hannon, H., Howard, J. T., et al. (2004). Mutations in genes required for T-cell development: *IL7R, CD45, IL2RG, JAK3, RAG1, RAG2, ARTEMIS,* and *ADA* and severe combined immunodeficiency: HuGE review. *Genetics in Medicine, 6,* 16–26.

Kaslow, R. A., Dorak, T., & Tang, J. J. (2005). Influence of host genetic variation on susceptibility to HIV type 1 infection. *Journal of Infectious Diseases, 191*(Suppl. 1), S68–S77.

Kotb, M., Norrby-Tegland, A., McGeer, A., El-Sherbini, H., Dorak, M. T., Khurshid, A., et al. (2002). An immunogenetic and molecular basis for differences in outcomes of invasive group A streptococcal infections. *Nature Medicine, 8,* 1398–1404.

Lebedeva, T. V., Ohashi, M., Huang, A., Vasconcellos, S., Flesch, S., & Yu, N. (2005). Emerging new alleles suggest high diversity of HLA-C locus. *Tissue Antigens, 65,* 101–106.

Le Roch, K. G., Zhou, Y., Blair, P. L., Grainger, M., Moch, J. K., Haynes, J. D., et al. (2003). Discovery of gene function by expression profiling of the malaria parasite life cycle. *Science, 301,* 1503–1508.

Lin, M. T., & Albertson, T. E. (2004). Genomic polymorphisms in sepsis. *Critical Care Medicine, 32,* 569–579.

Marsh, S. G., Albert, E. D., Bodmer, W. F., Bontrop, R. E., Dupont, B., Erlich, H. A., et al. (2002). Nomenclature for factors of the HLA system, 2002. *European Journal of Immunogenetics, 29,* 463–515.

Mignot, E. (1998). Genetic and familial aspects of narcolepsy. *Neurology, 50*(Suppl. 1), S16–S22.

Moise, K. J., Jr. (2002). Management of Rhesus

alloimmunization in pregnancy. *Obstetrics & Gynecology, 100,* 600–611.

Murray, M. F., & Versalovic, J. (2002). Susceptibility and response to infection. In D. L. Rimoin, J. M. Connor, R. E Pyeritz, & B. R. Korf (Eds.), *Emery and Rimoin's principles and practice of medical genetics* (4th ed., pp. 1083–1100). New York: Churchill Livingstone.

Nuki, G. (1998). Ankylosing spondylitis, HLA B27, and beyond. *Lancet, 351,* 767–769.

Olives, B., Mattei, M-G., Huet, M., Neau, P., Martial, S. Cartron, J-P., et al. (1995). Kidd blood group and urea transport function of human erythrocytes are carried by the same protein. *Journal of Biological Chemistry, 270,* 1507–1561.

Olsson, M. L., & Chester, M. A. (1996). Frequent occurrence of a variant O1 gene at the blood group ABO locus. *Vox Sanguinis, 70,* 26–30.

Online Mendelian Inheritance in Man, OMIM (TM). (2005). Center for Medical Genetics, Johns Hopkins University (Baltimore, MD) and National Center for Biotechnology Information, National Library of Medicine (Bethesda, MD). Retrieved from http://www.ncbi.nlm.nih.gov/omim.

Parkman, R. (2004). Getting a handle on graft-versus-host disease. *New England Journal of Medicine, 350,* 614–615.

Primary immunodeficiency diseases. Report of a WHO Scientific Group. (1995). *Clinical and Experimental Immunology, 99*(Suppl. 1), 1–24.

Relman, D. A. (2004). Shedding light on microbial detection. *New England Journal of Medicine, 349,* 2162–2163.

Renner, E. D., Puck, J. M., Holland, S. M., Schmitt, M., Weiss, M., Frosch, M., et al. (2004). Autosomal recessive hyperimmunoglobulin E syndrome: A distinct disease entity. *Journal of Pediatrics, 144,* 93–99.

Reveille, J. D. (2004). The genetic basis of spondyloarthritis. *Current Rheumatology Reports, 6,* 117–125.

Siebold, C., Hansen, B. E., Wyer, J. R., Harlos, K., Esnouf, R. E., Svejgaard, A., et al. (2004). Crystal structure of HLA-DQ0602 that protects against type 1 diabetes and confers strong susceptibility to narcolepsy. *Proceedings of the National Academy of Sciences, 101,* 1999–2004.

Simpson, J. L., & Elias, S. (2003). *Genetics in obstetrics and gynecology* (3rd ed.). Philadelphia: W.B. Saunders.

Somech, R., Amariglio, N., Spirer, Z., & Rechavi, G. (2003). Genetic predisposition to infectious pathogens: A review of less familiar variants. *Pediatric Infectious Disease Journal, 22,* 457–461.

Tiwari, J. L., & Terasaki, P. (1985). *HLA and disease associations.* New York: Springer-Verlag.

Trucco, M., & Bias, W. B. (2002). Transplantation genetics. In D. L. Rimoin, J. M. Connor, R. E. Pyeritz, & B. R. Korf (Eds.), *Emery and Rimoin's principles and practice of medical genetics* (4th ed., pp. 1101–1124). New York: Churchill Livingstone.

Twombly, R. (2003). For gene therapy, now-quantified risks are deemed troubling. *Journal of the National Cancer Institute, 95,* 1032–1033.

Vogel, F., & Motulsky, A. G. (1997). *Human genetics: Problems and approaches* (3rd ed.). Berlin: Springer-Verlag.

Wilmott, R. W. (2005). Maternal engraftment of T-cells in children with severe combined immune deficiency can lead to long term survival. *Journal of Pediatrics, 146,* A2.

Zago, M. A., Tavella, M. H., Simoes, B. P., Franco, R. F., Guerreiro, J. F., & Santos, S. B. (1996). Racial heterogeneity of DNA polymorphisms linked to the A and the O alleles of the ABO blood group gene. *Annals of Human Genetics, 60*(Pt. 1), 67–72.

Zuraw, B. L. (2003). Diagnosis and management of hereditary angioedema: An American approach. *Transfusion and Apheresis Science, 29,* 239–245.

20

Mental Retardation

The prevalence of all degrees of mental retardation (MR) is about 3% in the United States, with more affected males than females. Today terminology for mental retardation varies and includes the terms mentally challenged and mentally limited as well as intellectually disabled. About 1 in 10 Americans has a relative who is mentally retarded. MR is costly, both in tangible and nontangible costs. Accurate current national data are difficult to assemble as appropriations and expenditures specifically earmarked for mental retardation involve at least eight different federal agencies as well as state and local funds. Measures directed at prevention, such as screening, immunization, and other programs, have generally been found to be cost effective.

DEFINITION AND ETIOLOGY

Intelligence is believed to be multifactorial and derived from both genetic and environmental factors, with a normal or bell-shaped distribution in the general population. If a normal curve based on IQ scores in the population is plotted, scores below an arbitrary threshold of about 70–75 are considered to denote MR. Degrees of MR have been distinguished as shown in Table 20.1 and some subdivide MR into mild (IQ of 50 to 70–75) and severe (below 50). Definition and criteria by *DSM-IV TR* (2000) includes significantly subaverage intellectual functioning existing concurrently with deficits in present adaptive functioning in at least two of the following areas: communication, self-care, home living, social/interpersonal skills, use of community resources, self-direction, functional academic skills, work, leisure, health, and safety with onset before 18 years of age. The American Psychological Association (2000) uses 22 years instead of 18 years in defining MR consistent with the federal definition of developmental disability (DD), and the American Association of Mental Retardation (AAMR) does not use IQ classifications. Among assumptions that accompany the definition is the notion that valid assessment includes consideration of differences in communication, behavioral factors, support systems, and cultural and linguistic diversity that may be evaluated in the context of the individual's community. AAMR defines mental retardation as ". . . a disability characterized by significant limitations both in intellectual functioning and in adaptive behavior as expressed in conceptual, social, and practical adaptive skills. This disability originates before age 18" (Luckasson et al., 2002, p. 8).

MR may result from diverse causes. In the past, idiopathic MR, particularly of the mild type, was believed to be transmitted in a multifactorial manner and to represent the lower end of the bell-shaped curve of IQ. Often mild MR was considered to be due to social or cultural causes while severe MR was believed to be due to biological and genetic causes. Newer diagnostic techniques have identified specific genetic causes such as microdeletions for up to 25% of cases of mild MR, and it is possible that this will increase with the advent of even more sophisticated tools. MR is also known to be a component of about 1,000 known inherited single-gene and chromosome disorders including Down syndrome, phenylketonuria, and fragile X syndrome. Single gene disorders that include MR may be transmitted in an autosomal recessive, autosomal dominant, X-linked recessive, or X-linked dominant manner or by mitochondrial inheritance. Changes in gene dosage due to cryptic cytogenetic rearrangements including subtelomeric

TABLE 20.1   Classification and Terms Used to Describe Mental Retardation**

Degree retardation present classification	SD below mean*	IQ test scores	Educational
Mild	2–3	50–54 to 70–75	Educable
Moderate	3–4	36–40 to 50–54	Trainable
Severe	4–5	20–25 to 35–39	Dependent retarded
Profound	above 5	below 20–25	Custodial

*SD = standard deviation.
**Note: These terms are less frequently used currently in health care.
Sources: American Psychiatric Association (2000), Jacobson & Mulick (1996).

rearrangements are being identified using newer technologies such as multiplex amplifiable probe hybridization, multiplex ligation dependent probe amplification and array based comparative genomic hybridization. A comprehensive listing of human mental retardation genes may be found in Inlow and Restifo, 2004. Data on etiology are difficult to extrapolate depending on the population used to ascertain the cause, definitions of MR, and differing definitions of causes. Older studies are more likely to list a greater percentage of cases in the unknown category than recent ones. An estimated distribution of causes of MR by the time period in which the causative event is thought to have occurred is given in Table 20.2.

The degree of actual functional impairment is important, and various risk factors may act independently or together to result in impaired functioning in the person with MR. These are biomedical, social, behavioral, and educational.

THE FRAGILE X SYNDROME AND OTHER FRAGILE SITES

There is an overall excess of mentally retarded males. In some families nonspecific mental retardation was noted to follow an X-linked pattern of transmission and some early researchers referred to these cases as Martin-Bell syndrome or Renpenning syndrome. In 1969, Lubs studied a family in which the males with mental retardation had a certain "marker" X chromosome described as having a secondary constriction. Its significance was not fully appreciated until later. Further reports in the late 1970s elucidated the connection between the

fragile site on the X chromosome and mental retardation in males. The fragile sites on the metaphase X chromosome were demonstrated in a percentage of cells using culture-medium deficient in folic acid or thymidine. These chromosomes appeared to have nonstaining gaps. However, observations regarding the transmission of the fragile X syndrome did not fit with known X-linked inheritance.

It was not until 1991 that the fragile X syndrome fragile site was shown to result from a tandem trinucleotide repeat expansion of the nucleotides cytidine, guanosine, guanosine (CGG) located on the long arm of the X chromosome (Xq27.3) in the FMR1 (fragile X mental retardation) gene (Verkerk et al., 1991). One result is triggering of CpG methylation, essentially stopping transcription. Normal individuals possess approximately 29–30 CGG repeats with a range of 7 to about 54. Persons with more than approximately 200–230 repeats are said to carry the full mutation which can contain hundreds to thousands of copies. There is a "gray zone" also called intermediate, inconclusive, or borderline of 45 to 54 repeats. This refers to the fact that there is not a clear delineation between the upper limit of normal and the lower limit of the premutation. Some individuals have approximately 55 repeats as a lower limit and 200 repeats as the upper limit and are said to carry a premutation. The prevalence of premutation expansions of the FMR1 gene are estimated at 1 in 259 females and 1 in 813 males (Jacquemont et al., 2004). Persons with the premutation were originally thought to be unaffected; however recent research has shown that about 20% of adult carrier females may develop premature ovarian failure

TABLE 20.2   Estimated Distribution of Causes of Severe Mental Retardation

Cause	Range (in percentage)
Prenatal	56–73
Known genetic etiology including chromosome and single-gene defects	36–52
Multifactorial conditions and syndromes whose etiology is unknown	12–30
Acquired including infection, anoxia, defective maternal environment (e.g., maternal diabetes mellitus, maternal PKU), alcohol, drugs, etc.	8–10
Perinatal	
Hypoxia, infection, hyperbilirubinemia, intracranial hemorrhage, birth trauma, etc.	7–13
Postnatal	
Severe malnutrition, trauma, infection, etc.	1–12
Unknown	12–22

defined as cessation of menses before 40 years of age. Elderly male premutation carriers may manifest the fragile-X-associated tremor/ataxia syndrome (FXTAS) which consists of parkinsonism, intention tremors, cerebellar ataxia, autonomic dysfunction, peripheral neuropathy and weakness in the legs and cognitive decline including short-term memory loss and executive function deficits. Female premutation carriers have also been identified and it is believed that effects in these older women may be more subtle. It is believed that about one-third or more of all male carriers will develop FXTAS over time. Progression is variable. An implication of the identification of FXTAS is that those older people who manifest ataxia and intension tremor should be screened for the *FMR1* mutation even in the absence of a positive family history. Hagermann et al. (2004) describe that FXTAS came to be identified when mothers of children with fragile X syndrome spoke about their own fathers (premutation carriers) who were experiencing tremors and gait problems. Premutation carriers (especially males) may also have emotional or learning problems, some of which respond to psychological or pharmacological interventions. Thus, as part of genetic counseling, DNA testing for *FMR1* in at-risk family members, especially siblings, of a person with fragile X syndrome should be recommended. Developmental testing may also be indicated if a premutation is present.

In general, when a male with a premutation passes it to his daughters, they are unaffected but their children are at risk. The premutation must pass through the female in order for it to expand to a full mutation and be expressed clinically. This expansion is believed to occur during early development of the embryo. There can be mosaicism or somatic heterogeneity, with some persons having both a premutation and a full mutation. When there are more than 200 repeats present, methylation of the promotor region occurs and the *FMR1* gene is not expressed. The *FMR1* gene encodes a protein (FMRP) which is expressed most in the brain and testes. There appears to be a linear relationship between the extent of FMRP deficit and the degree of connective tissue involvement. To sum up inheritance, an unaffected transmitting male may pass on a premutation to all of his daughters (sons do not normally inherit their father's X chromosome). The daughters will be unaffected carriers themselves as there has been no amplification of the premutation from their father during spermatogenesis. But, during oogenesis, amplification of the repeats occurs to more than 200. The daughter's sons will therefore inherit a full mutation and be affected; their daughters inherit a full mutation and may show a spectrum of clinical expression because of X-inactivation. This can be modified. For example, if the premutation is at the lower end of the range, there may be less of an increase in the size of the unstable sequence as it is passed through oogenesis. Thus, somatic features tend to be less noticeable than in males but they can have full expression with characteristic features and profound mental retardation.

The fragile X syndrome is now considered the most common inherited cause of MR and the second most common genetic cause after Down syndrome. Males with the fragile X syndrome generally have one or more of the following: macroorchidism (enlarged testes which may not be seen until 8 or 9 years of age but is seen in 90%

after puberty), large, prominent jaw and forehead, low-set ears, a large head circumference, hypotonia, flat feet, soft skin which may become callused with biting, a self-injurious behavior sometimes seen, hyperextendible joints, mitral valve prolapse, hyperactivity, and 85% or more have some degree of mental retardation. Autism may occur. It is often the behavioral aspects that are most striking. These include attentional deficits, sensitivity to sensations, mood lability, and tantrums. Language and speech difficulties occur and include echolalia, repetition of words continuously at the end of the phrase, and talking inappropriately and incessantly about a single topic. In females with the full mutation, approximately 50% to 67% have some mental impairment; approximately 1/3 are mentally retarded. About 1/3 have normal intelligence. Females with full fragile X often have learning difficulties and behavior problems that might suggest the diagnosis such as attentional deficits, language problems, mathematical difficulty, excessive shyness, and social anxiety. Facial features are similar to males. Fragile X premutation carrier females have a median age of menopause that is 6 to 8 years earlier than other women, and about 20% have ovarian failure before 40 years of age. She may be at increased risk for lower bone mineral density. The facial features begin to appear in childhood, but are not prominent until adolescence or adulthood. A man with fragile X syndrome is shown in Figure 20.1. Males with fragile X may have a high birth weight. The prevalence of fragile X has been revised downward and may be approximately 1 in 4,000 males and 1 in 6,000 females, but some believe it is more common. In a few cases, the fragile X syndrome is due to deletions or point mutations.

In those who are not mentally retarded there is usually a variant pattern of methylation so that the FMR1 gene is not completely turned off and some product is produced. Molecular diagnosis is possible for diagnostic testing and prenatal diagnosis but has not been recommended for population screening at this time, although in a study by McConkie-Rosell et al. (1997) obligate carriers favored early carrier testing. Testing for fragile X syndrome should be considered for persons with MR, developmental delay, autism, individuals with a family history of fragile X, or undiagnosed MR. Prenatal diagnosis is indicated if the mother is a carrier. All testing should be accompanied by

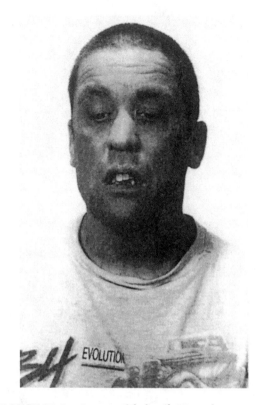

FIGURE 20.1   A man with fragile X syndrome.
Courtesy of Louise Gane, The Fragile X Treatment & Research Center. The Children's Hospital. Denver, CO.

appropriate counseling as discussed in chapters 10 and 11. Testing for older men and women for premutations may be indicated in those showing neurological symptoms as described earlier in this section as well as for women with premature ovarian failure. The siblings of persons with fragile X syndrome may benefit from testing for premutation since many manifest emotional problems or learning or behavioral difficulties, and thus could be appropriately assisted if warranted. Because this inheritance is complex, it is essential that the testing and counseling be done in such a way as to be understood by the client and the family. In a study of family experiences with diagnosis, the average age of concern regarding development was at 13 months with confirmation of a fragile X diagnosis at an average of about 32 months. Future reproductive risks for families was not always provided during counseling (Bailey, Skinner, & Sparkman, 2003). In a CDC study, children with fragile X syndrome were almost always diagnosed after birth, and 50% of the sample reported having another child before diagnosis was made. Early identification allows for providing a diagnosis, participation in intervention programs, genetic counseling, for all family members, and family planning, and allows affected children to receive publicly funded developmental services under Part C of the Individuals with Disabilities Education Act (Centers for Disease Control and Prevention, 2002).

Other cytogenetic fragile sites have been identified on the X chromosome. *FRAXE* is associated with a milder MR with a prevalence of about 1 in 50,000 males. *FRAXF* and *FRAXD* have also been identified. In addition, fragile sites on autosomes such as 16 and 11 have been identified. All of these conditions have been proposed for newborn screening programs, but are debatable because no curative treatment is available and the benefits would be mostly in terms of anticipatory guidance for the individual and genetic counseling, prenatal diagnosis, and reproductive options for the family (see chapter 11 for discussion). Organizations for patients and families include the National Fragile X Foundation. See Appendix B.

REPRODUCTION AND STERILIZATION IN MENTAL RETARDATION

A legacy from the activities of the eugenicists are varying state regulations on the involuntary and compulsory sterilization of the institutionalized mentally incompetent and retarded. The famous quote from Justice Holmes in the 1927 case of Buck versus Bell that "three generations of imbeciles is enough" supported the genetic basis for the state eugenic sterilization statutes. In some states these laws remain on the books, although they are not usually invoked. In some states it is often difficult to obtain the procedure. In Oregon, recently, Governor Kitzhaber apologized for past abuses of sterilization, occuring from 1923 to 1981 (Josephson, 2002).

The fundamental right of an individual to procreate and to choose whether or not to "bear or beget a child" has been recognized in other Supreme Court decisions, but states can override fundamental rights in instances where a compelling state interest can be demonstrated. The exercise of the police power in the state's interest is evidenced by laws regarding marriage to relatives,

premarital blood tests for sexually transmitted disease, and newborn screening programs. Amid this concern for the protection of the procreative rights of the person with MR is also concern for the protection of their right to choose not to procreate. For some persons with MR, sterilization is the most reliable contraceptive measure, and thus may be protective (at least reproduction-wise) in certain situations, such as sexual exploitation. However, the availability of long-term pharmacological contraception means that this will usually be the preferred method.

Issues to consider in contemplating sterilization are as follows: (a) the extent of increased risk for MR in the offspring, (b) the capability of the person to care for a child, (c) the capacity for making reproductive decisions, and (d) whether or not a person with MR can give informed consent for what is a medical procedure. Persons with mental retardation cannot be considered as one population either in capability or in the cause of the MR. Thus, a person with severe retardation may not be capable of child care, but a person with mild retardation may be able to provide a warm and loving environment. A person who could act in the best interest of the person with MR may need to be designated by the court, as the parent or legal guardian is not always seen as able to fulfill this role. In some states, the procedure is a complex one because of the potential for liability for the physician, hospital, and even the judge who is ruling on the sterilization request. Both the American Academy of Pediatrics (1990) and the American College of Obstetricians and Gynecologists (ACOG Committee Opinion, 1999) have made statements regarding sterilization that affirm the need for the person with MR to participate in decision-making when possible, and using the least permanent and intrusive methods with the lowest patient risk.

PREVENTION

Methods of achieving prevention of MR include public and professional education; research; delivery of health care services, both preventive and therapeutic; and the identification of environmental hazards. These methods must always be planned with careful consideration of the culture, values, habits, and developmental level, and through gaining the trust of the clientele at whom they are aimed, in order to maximize success. Preventive measures for reducing the risk for MR can be applied in the period prior to conception, beginning in school health programs, as well as the prenatal, perinatal, and postnatal periods. The following are some components of prevention for nurses to consider in each period that are ultimately aimed at the prevention of MR.

Preconception

1. Educational programs in the schools, community and media that emphasize
   a. the importance of maternal health and care before and during pregnancy, including good nutrition and avoidance of food faddism, as well as risks of smoking, alcohol consumption, radiation exposure, drug use, potential occupational hazards, sexually transmitted and other infectious disease
   b. the importance of family planning, avoidance of rapid, consecutive pregnancies, optimal ages for reducing risks in pregnancy (unfavorable outcome more often associated with those younger than 18 years of age and over 35 years of age)
   c. use of contraceptive techniques
   d. teaching good parenting skills and child development
   e. development of personal coping and decision-making skills
   f. knowledge of risk factors in pregnancy
   g. basic child health and safety and the importance of preventive health maintenance such as immunization programs
   h. the need for seeking early prenatal care, and
   i. assessment of environment for risks such as lead (see chapters 13 and 14)
2. Taking good family, occupational, social, reproductive, and health histories to determine those at increased risk
3. Stabilize diseases that alter maternal metabolism such as in those with diabetes mellitus, PKU
4. Laboratory tests for establishment of rubella antibody titers, syphilis, and blood type determinations of both parents

5. Immunization programs in childhood and beyond to prevent intrauterine infection (e.g, rubella)
6. Treatment of known maternal diseases before pregnancy
7. Genetic testing and/or screening programs for those known to be at risk for genetic disorders by virtue of history, ethnic group, etc., coupled with genetic counseling.

Prenatal

1. Items 1 through 4 above and 7 are also appropriate here
2. Early prenatal history screening should be done on an outreach or regional basis for identifying those at high risk for genetic disorders who would be candidates for prenatal diagnosis (see chapter 12)
3. Minimization of exposure to infectious agents and other risk factors such as alcohol, drugs, etc. (see chapter 13)
4. Assess nutritional status; plan diet in pregnancy with client including folic acid and multivitamin supplementation, coupled with education and referral to programs such as the Special Supplemental Nutrition Program for Women, Infants, and Children (WIC), if needed (this should be ongoing during the pregnancy)
5. Detect susceptibility to disease in pregnancy such as hypertension and diabetes; watch for the exacerbation of any known chronic diseases and seek effective therapy
6. Monitor fetal growth during pregnancy, assess for any unfavorable signs or symptoms, watch for multiple pregnancy
7. Identify those clients at high risk due to any items mentioned above and arrange for appropriate care
8. Refer to prenatal classes
9. Begin promotion of parent-child bonding
10. Arrange with parents and facilities for delivery in hospital with high risk obstetrical facilities if it appears warranted.

Perinatal

1. Be alert for abnormal features of labor and avoid prolonged labor

2. Avoid the administration of excess medication during labor
3. Monitor fetal response to labor
4. Clinicians should aim for a normal, spontaneous, vaginal delivery at term
5. Arrange for transfer to a hospital with high-risk nursery and obstetric facilities if indicated early enough in labor, or immediately after delivery, if warranted

Postnatal

1. Item 1 and item 5 under Preconception, if not accomplished prenatally, and item 7 under Preconception.
2. All high-risk infants should be followed-up, preferably with home visits
3. The institution of special programming aimed at specific groups in the community
4. Newborn genetic screening programs should also be accompanied with follow-up for specimens needed later in infancy, or for confirmation of a presumptive result accompanied by appropriate education, treatment (if needed), support, and counseling
5. Home visits and community resource identification, as well as clinic facilities, should be part of the program for any infant who is high risk or identified as MR or having a genetic disorder that is being treated
6. Community case finding
7. The promotion of parent–child bonding
8. The availability of classes with provision for infants to accompany parents that emphasize child feeding and nutritional needs, growth and development, care, parenting skills, and prevention of child abuse
9. Child safety programs geared to the reduction and prevention of motor vehicle and home accidents (this may be educational and may also include infant seat loan programs, etc.)
10. Programs for the detection of lead poisoning
11. Intensive nursing care for premature and low birth-weight infants
12. Provision of Home Start-type programs and home and community-based interdisciplinary early intervention programs for children with or at risk of MR and for those who can benefit from infant stimulation and development programs, progressing to "head-start" type programs at an older age
13. Developmental assessment programs including vision, hearing, and other screening tests
14. Immunization programs
15. Provision of genetic counseling for those with an unfavorable pregnancy outcome.

Although it is not currently possible to prevent all cases of mental retardation because of the occurrence of new mutations and the unknown etiology of many, reduction by prevention and amelioration by maximum stimulation and therapy are reasonable goals.

ENCOUNTERING THE CLIENT WITH MENTAL RETARDATION

Nurses, particularly those in acute care or office settings, may not be accustomed to clients who are mentally retarded or developmentally delayed, whether children or adults. Many pointers about such clients are covered in chapter 8. Adults with MR usually receive primary care in the community. Even though they may have guardians, it is important to involve the person in his/her own care to the degree possible. Preferences and meaningful choices are part of person-centered planning and client independence. It is also important to not let the diagnosis of MR overshadow all other symptoms or conditions. For example, depression may be due to MR or could be from another cause. When clients need care, it is important not to skimp on the usual assessment or treatment because of the nurse's own feelings of insecurity or possible negative reaction. Language problems are common, and become handicapping in and of themselves, if the person cannot make himself/herself understood. Sometimes persons with MR can use words that they have heard but do not really understand. Therefore, the nurse must clarify what is said, perhaps by asking questions. She/he should act in a calm, unhurried manner to increase the client's comfort. It may be prudent to allow extra time for such a client. The nurse may need to acquire assistive technology such as communication and mobility devices or personnel (such as an interpreter for the deaf) for help in communication and teaching. The nurse should not forget to ascertain the needs and problems of other members of the family, particularly the major caregiver of the mentally retarded person as well as their siblings.

Before hospitalization, or during an episode of acute illness, parents or caregivers should be asked ways in which the person usually asks for essential items such as food and bathroom facilities, how he/she expresses emotions such as pain or distress, and for information on positioning, handling, issues around eating, and so on. These should be clearly communicated both verbally and in writing to all involved in the patient's care. Pictures may be used to facilitate communication. Those who are profoundly retarded, with little speech, still need calm soothing voices, to be treated with respect, positioned with attention to comfort, pain anticipated, and relief provided. Close cooperation with the usual caregivers is essential.

GENETIC COUNSELING IN MENTAL RETARDATION

As indicated earlier, many genetic disorders as well as non-genetic ones have MR as a feature. Careful diagnosis is therefore a prelude to effective and accurate counseling in MR. Benefits of diagnosis include identification of appropriate therapeutic strategies, educational planning, anticipatory guidance, prenatal diagnosis, genetic testing for family, genetic counseling, reproductive planning, and referral for appropriate social services. Attempts to accurately diagnose persons with MR who are institutionalized or in long-term facilities so that genetic counseling could be offered to their families have not always been vigorous, and many remain undiagnosed. Those with nonspecific mild mental retardation that is often called "familial," and who have no detectable congenital anomalies, are often assumed to have MR due to multifactorial or environmental factors. However various cytogenetic abnormalites which may be subtle, and gene variants associated with nonspecific MR are being increasingly identified. Thus diagnosis should be actively sought in order to provide accurate counseling. If no cause or inheritance pattern can be determined for the specific family, the

recurrence risk for two normal parents to have a second child with MR is about 3% to 6%. The risk for two persons with mild MR of unknown etiology to have a child with MR is 40% to 50%, a considerable risk figure. Further detail on risk figures for MR are available in Crow and Tolmie (1998).

BIBLIOGRAPHY

ACOG Committee Opinion. (1999). Sterilization of women, including those with mental disabilities. Number 216, April 1999 (replaces number 63, September 1988, and number 73, September 1989). Committee on Ethics, The American College of Obstetricians and Gynecologists. *International Journal of Gynecology and Obstetrics, 65,* 317–320.

American Academy of Pediatrics. Committee on Bioethics. (1990). Sterilization of women who are mentally handicapped. *Pediatrics, 85,* 868–871.

American College of Obstetricians and Gynecologists. Committee Opinion. (1995, October). *Fragile X syndrome. No. 161.*

American Psychiatric Association. (2000). *Diagnostic and statistical manual of mental disorders* (4th ed.). Washington, DC: American Psychiatric Press.

Bailey, D. B., Jr., Skinner, D., & Sparkman, K. L. (2003). Discovering fragile X syndrome: Family experiences and perceptions. *Pediatrics, 111,* 407–416.

Berry-Kravis, E., Potanos, K., Weinberg, D., Zhou, L., & Goetz, C. G. (2005). Fragile X-associated tremor/ataxia syndrome in sisters related to X-inactivation. *Annals of Neurology, 57,* 144–147.

Brussino, A., Gellera, C., Saluto, A., Mariotti, C., Arduino, C., Castellotti, B., et al. (2005). FMR1 gene premutation is a frequent genetic cause of late-onset sporadic cerebellar ataxia. *Neurology, 64,* 145–147.

Centers for Disease Control and Prevention. (2002). Delayed diagnosis of fragile X syndrome—United States, 1990–1999. *Morbidity and Mortality Weekly Report, 51,* 740–742.

Cornish, K., Kogan, C., Turk, J., Manly, T., James, N., Mills, A., et al. (2005). The emerging fragile X premutation phenotype: Evidence from the domain of social cognition. *Brain and Cognition, 57,* 53–60.

Crow, Y. J., & Tolmie, J. L. (1998). Recurrence risks in mental retardation. *Journal of Medical Genetics, 35*, 177–182.

Diekema, D. S. (2003). Involuntary sterilization of persons with mental retardation: An ethical analysis. *Mental Retardation and Developmental Disability Research Reviews, 9*, 21–26.

Dosen, A. (2005). Applying the developmental perspective in the psychiatric assessment and diagnosis of persons with intellectual disability: Part I—assessment. *Journal of Intellectual and Developmental Disabilities Research, 49*(Pt. 1), 1–8.

Finucane, B., Haas-Givler, B., & Simon, E. W. (2003). Genetics, mental retardation, and the forging of new alliances. *American Journal of Medical Genetics, Part C. (Seminars in Medical Genetics), 117C*, 66–72.

Hagerman, R. J., & Hagerman, P. J. (2002). *Fragile X syndrome: Diagnosis, treatment, and research.* Baltimore: Johns Hopkins University Press.

Hagerman, R. J., Hagerman, P. J. (2004). The fragile-X premutation: A maturing perspective. *American Journal of Human Genetics, 74*, 805–816.

Hagerman, R. J., Leavitt, B. R., Farzin, F., Jacquemont, S., Greco, C. M., Brunberg, J. A., et al. (2004). Fragile-X-associated tremor/ataxia syndrome (FXTAS) in females with the *FMR1* premutation. *American Journal of Human Genetics, 74*, 1051–1056.

Hundscheid, R. D. L., Smits, A. P. T., Thomas, C. M. G., Kiemeney, L. A. L. M., & Braat, D. D. M. (2003). Female carriers of fragile X premutations have no increased risk for additional diseases other than premature ovarian failure. *American Journal of Medical Genetics, 117A*, 6–9.

Inlow, J. K., & Restifo, L. L. (2004). Molecular and comparative genetics of mental retardation. *Genetics, 166*, 835–881.

Jacobson, J. W., & Mulick, J. A. (1996). *Manual of diagnosis and professional practice in mental retardation.* Washington, DC: American Psychological Association.

Jacquemont, S., Hagerman, R. J., Leehey, M. A., Hall, D. A., Levine, R. A., Brunberg, J. A., et al. (2004). Penetrance of the fragile X-associated tremor/ataxia syndrome in a premutation carrier population. *Journal of the American Medical Association, 291*, 460–469.

Jin, P., & Warren, S. T. (2003). New insights into fragile X syndrome: From molecules to neuro- behaviors. *Trends in Biochemical Sciences, 28,* 152–158.

Josephson, D. (2002). Oregon's governor apologises for forced sterilisations. *British Medical Journal, 325*, 1380.

Kahler, S. G., & Fahey, M. C. (2003). Metabolic disorders and mental retardation. *American Journal of Medicial Genetics, Part C, 117C*, 31–41.

Kriek, M. J., White, S. J., Bouma, M. C., Dauwerse, H. G., Hansson, K. B. M., Nijhuis, J. V., et al. (2004). Genomic imbalances in mental retardation. *Journal of Medical Genetics, 41*, 249–255.

Loesch, D. Z., Huggins, R. M., Bui, Q. M., Taylor, A K., & Hagerman, R. J. (2003). Relationship of deficits of *FMR1* gene specific protein with physical phenotype of fragile X males and females in pedigrees: A new perspective. *American Journal of Medical Genetics, 118A*, 127–134.

Lubs, H. A. (1969). A marker X chromosome. *American Journal of Human Genetics, 21*, 231–244.

Luckasson, R., Borthwick-Duffy, S., Buntinx, W. H. E., Coulter, D. L., Craig, E. M., Reeve, A., et al. (2002). *Mental retardation: Definition, classification and systems of supports* (10th ed.). Washington, DC: American Association on Mental Retardation.

Maddalena, A., Richards, C. S., McGinniss, M. J., Brothman, A., Desnick, R. J., Grier, R. E., et al. (2001). Technical standards and guidelines for Fragile X: The first of a series of disease-specific supplements to the Standards and Guidelines for Clinical Genetics Laboratories of the American College of Medical Genetics. Genetics in Medicine, 3, 200–205.

Matheson, E., & Jahoda, A. (2005). Emotional understanding in aggressive and nonaggressive individuals with mild or moderate mental retardation. *American Journal of Mental Retardation, 110*, 57–67.

McConkle-Rosell, A., Spiridigliozzi, G. A., Iafolla, T., Tarleton, J., & Lachiewiez, A. M. (1997). Carrier testing in the fragile X syndrome: Attitudes and opinions of obligate carriers. *American Journal of Medical Genetics, 68*, 62–69.

O'Donnell, W. T., & Warren, S. T. (2002). A decade of molecular studies of fragile X syndrome. *Annual Review of Neuroscience, 25*, 315–338.

Oberle, I., Rousseau, F., Heitz, D., Kretz, C., Devys, D., Hanauer, A., et al. (1991). Instability of a 550-base pair DNA segment and abnormal methylation in Fragile X syndrome. *Science, 252,* 1097–1102.

Patterson-Keels, L., Quint, E., Brown, D., Larson, D., & Elkins, T. E. (1994). Family views on sterilization for their mentally retarded children. *Journal of Reproductive Medicine, 39,* 701–706.

Philips, G. F., & Parry, J. (2002). *The handbook on mental disability law.* ABA Commission on Mental Disability Law.

Reed, S. C. (1980). *Counseling in medical genetics* (3rd ed.). New York: Alan R. Liss.

Ropers, H. H., & Hamel, B. C. (2005). X-linked mental retardation. *Nature Reviews Genetics, 6,* 46–57.

Santoro, N. (2003). Mechanisms of premature ovarian failure. *Annals of Endocrinology, 64,* 87–92.

Shevell, M., Ashwal, S., Donley, D., Flint, J., Gingold, M., Hirtz, D., et al. (2003). Practice parameter: Evaluation of the child with global developmental delay: Report of the quality standards subcommittee of the American Academy of Neurology and The Practice Committee of the Child Neurology Society. *Neurology, 60,* 367–380.

Symons, F. J., Clark, R. D., Hatton, D. D., Skinner, M., & Bailey, D. B., Jr. (2003). Self-injurious behavior in young boys with fragile X syndrome. *American Journal of Medical Genetics, 118A,* 115–121.

van Karnebeek, C. D., Jansweijer, M. C., Leenders, A. G., Offringa, M., & Hennekam, R. C. (2005). Diagnostic investigations in individuals with mental retardation: A systematic literature review of their usefulness. *European Journal of Human Genetics, 13,* 6–25.

Verkerk, A. J. M. H., Pieretti, M., Sutcliffe, J. S., Fu, Y-H., Kuhl, D. P. A., Pizzuti, A., et al. (1991). Identification of a gene (FMR-1) containing a CGG repeat coincident with a breakpoint cluster region exhibiting length variation in Fragile X syndrome. *Cell, 65,* 905–914.

Wald, N. J., & Morris, J. K. (2003). A new approach to antenatal screening for Fragile X syndrome. *Prenatal Diagnosis, 23,* 345–351.

Warren, S. T., & Sherman, S. L. (2001). The fragile X syndrome. In C. R. Scriver, A. L. Beaudet, W. S. Sly, & D. Valle (Eds.), *The metabolic and molecular bases of inherited disease* (8th ed., pp. 1257–1289). New York: McGraw-Hill.

Wenstrom, K. D. (2002). Fragile X and other trinucleotide repeat diseases. *Obstetrics and Gynecology Clinics of North America, 29,* 367–388.

Xu, J., & Chen, Z. (2003). Advances in molecular genetics for the evaluation of mental retardation. *American Journal of Medical Genetics, Part C, 117C,* 15–24.

Yu, S., Pritchard, M., Kremer, E., Lynch, M., Nancarrow, J., Baker, E., et al. (1991). Fragile X genotype characterised by an unstable region of DNA. *Science, 252,* 1179–1181.

21

Aging, Longevity, and Alzheimer Disease

With the rapid growth of the population that is 85 years and above, the study of aging has intensified. The influence of genetics on biologic aging can be considered in relationship to length of life or longevity, patterns of aging, senescence or the aging process, and maximum life span in different species. The search for specific aging genes has resulted in interest in disorders with a known genetic basis that have some of the characteristics of aging. The latter are often caused by mutation in structural genes, although it is possible that aging and longevity are under the control of regulatory genes. It appears likely that a relationship similar to that of the genetic control of embryonic and fetal development could also be operative in aging. Aging could be one of the last phases in a continuum of growth, development, and differentiation. This may involve precisely timed repression and derepression of different genes that involve the switching on and off of certain genes, along with control and modification of their activity. Martin (2001) estimates that thousands of genes are involved in aging in some way. For example, many physical, behavioral, and functional phenotypic changes occur with aging such as changes in skin, hair, susceptibility to age-related diseases such as cataracts, and the processing of various substances. Martin believes that biologically speaking, there is no reason to keep us alive for long past our reproductive potential.

Various molecular defects in aging have been identified by many different researchers, such as impaired capability of DNA repair mechanisms, decreased RNA synthesis, production of abnormal proteins through error, alterations in chromatin structure, impaired cell target receptors, impaired immunorecognition systems, failure to inactivate mutagens, ribosomal errors in protein synthesis, the accumulation of amyloid in Alzheimer disease, and many more. For those who believe that fewer genes determine longevity, research strategies in nonhuman experimental systems for candidate genes that influence longevity include searching for genes whose regulation changes later in life, induction of mutations and then screening for life span extension, and the mapping of existing variation. The term "longevity assurance genes" refer to genes that promote longevity and extend the health span. The production of free radicals is thought to play a role in aging. Antioxidants reduce their effects, and so superoxide dismutase and vitamin E are the subjects of research. The accumulation of somatic mutations in both nuclear and mitochondrial (mt) genes are believed associated with aging and with cancer. Respiratory complex activities in the mitochondria decline with age and the decline is correlated with the accumulation of somatic mtDNA mutations. Other candidate genes that influence aging might involve susceptibility and resistance to stress or ultraviolet light. One or more alleles of the apolipoprotein E gene may be associated with longevity. In one study (Barzilai et al., 2003) of a group of people with exceptional longevity and controls, those who had exceptional longevity had increased homozygosity for the variation of isoleucine to valine (I405V) also known as the VV genotype in the cholesteryl ester transfer protein (CETP) gene as well as increased high density lipoprotein and low density lipoprotein particle sizes, and less cardiovascular disease prevalence. Thus, for longevity, persons may have longevity-enabling genes, have genetic variations that confer resistance to age-related illnesses and conditions, and lack genetic variations that contribute to various diseases. Environmental influences will interact with this genetic background. This chapter considers aspects of the relationship of genetics to aging and length of life as well as specific genetic disorders associated with features of premature aging. Although Alzheimer disease does not necessarily accompany aging, genetic aspects of Alzheimer disease are considered in this chapter.

MAXIMUM LIFE SPAN POTENTIAL

It is generally agreed that the species-specific maximum life span potential (MLP) for all organisms is genetically determined. MLP is defined as the maximum life span possible for an organism under optimal nutritional conditions with detrimental environmental factors kept at a minimum. In some organisms (e.g., annual plants, some insects), death occurs in a relatively short time period without a slow progressive loss of function and appears to be genetically programmed. It is thought that this may occur either by switching on a lethal gene, or by switching off genes needed for maintenance of life and metabolism.

Because the genetic constitution determines whether an organism is in one species or another, it follows that genetic differences are responsible for MLP. Species-specific life span characteristics may be a consequence of evolution. However, genes favorable to a species in early life may be detrimental to it later, so selection must play a role. Within a species, individuals with varying natural life spans are common. It is unknown how much MLP can be deliberately modified by the environment. In some organisms, restricting calorie intake to a certain level increases the life span. In nature, where conditions tend to be more hazardous, longer levels may not be achieved. In a controlled environment, it might be possible to extend the normally observed maximum life span, but it is believed that each species has a point beyond which life cannot be extended.

GENETICS AND THE LENGTH OF LIFE

The association between heredity and longevity in the mind of the lay person can be summarized by the following statement: "If you want to live long, choose long-lived parents." Studies may approach the problem in a negative way—looking at how genes shorten life span, or in a positive way—looking for genetic influences that appear to lengthen it. Inherited longevity may involve the lack of a predisposition to die from a specific cause and also "vigor," a well-known phenomenon in hybrid plants and animals.

There are many difficulties that are inherent in studying human longevity at the present time. The long life span of humans means that the research has to be passed on from one researcher to another; records may be poor, so that verification of ages may be difficult; many environmental factors, such as nutrition, exposure to ionizing radiation, disease, temperature, occupation, place of birth, etc., may influence aging; there may be data ascertainment bias; the possibility of cultural inheritance; the possibility that events that favor the acceleration of the aging process and a shortening of life may be balanced by those that have the opposite effect (e.g., impaired molecules in cells may be repaired, removed, or replaced); and various methodological problems such as attrition, differential fertility, and weighting.

Nevertheless, many researchers beginning in the 1940s have found a familial component in longevity. Kallman and co-workers (1948) found greater concordance for longevity in monozygous twins than in dizygous twins, indicating that genetic factors played a role. In early studies of nonagenarians and centenarians, Pearl and Pearl (1943) computed an index of ancestral longevity that included the ages of their six immediate ancestors and found them to be significantly greater than the control group. Of the nonagenarians and centenarians, 48.5% and 53.4%, respectively, had two long-lived (over 70) parents. In a study of long-lived subjects, 86.6% had at least one long-lived parent. Parental age may be more important for sons rather than daughters, and the maternal contribution may be more important than the paternal one, fitting in with the potential role of mitochondrial mutations in aging. To date the oldest verified human was a female who died at age 122 years. Interest in the exceptionally old has also focused on the concept of genetic resistance to certain cardiovascular disorders and Alzheimer disease as well as survivor advantage.

MOLECULAR CHANGES ASSOCIATED WITH THE AGING PROCESS

Investigation of the effect of age on the chromosomes in peripheral lymphocytes was reported as early as 1961. Researchers have found that there is increased aneuploidy (changes in the number of individual chromosomes) in aging, due both to chromosome loss (hypodiploidy) and chromosome gain (hyperdiploidy). These include X-chromosome loss in females over 60 years of age, and Y-chromosome loss in males over 70 years of age, and loss of chromosomes 21 and 22 may occur in both. Nonrandom trisomy 2 has also been noted. The nature of the association of aging and chromosome changes is not known. Shortening of the telomeres on the end of the chromosomes has been noted to occur in some normal tissues with cellular aging, and this might compromise some cell sets by reducing the number of times lost cells could be replaced and also result in genomic instability, rearrangements, cell senescence, and even death.

KNOWN GENETIC DISORDERS AND AGING

Many genetic syndromes have as one or more of their features characteristics that are like those found in aging. Three genetic syndromes (progeria, Werner syndrome, Cockayne syndrome) were formerly thought to represent actual premature aging syndromes, but on closer study this proved not to be true. How well a syndrome can be used as a model for overall premature onset of aging or its accelerated progression depends on what criteria one uses to define phenotypic parameters of aging. Some syndromes may have a few of these, whereas others may have many, but none are known to have all. Additionally, there may be differences in their severity, morphology, or distribution when compared with "normal" aging criteria. Martin (2001) identified that in the listings included in McKusick's *Mendelian Inheritance in Man,* nearly 7% of the loci could modulate the pathobiology of aging. If one looks at various characteristics of aging such as premature graying or loss of hair or both, many disorders can be identified that have these characteristics. Down syndrome has many of the criteria of aging in addition to the ones that were classically

thought of in this way (progeria, Cockayne and Werner syndromes). Other syndromes said to resemble aging in four or more of aging features were ataxia telangiectasia, Berardinelli-Seip syndrome (an autosomal recessive disorder featuring generalized lipodystrophy, hypertrichosis, diabetes mellitus, mental retardation, hyperlipidemia, and other features) familial cervical lipodysplasia, Klinefelter syndrome, Turner syndrome, myotonic dystrophy, and Rothmund-Thomson syndrome (an autosomal recessive disorder characterized by skin atrophy, hyperpigmentation, hypogonadism, short stature, and juvenile cataract).

Progeria (Hutchinson-Gilford Syndrome)

First described in 1754, progeria is such an extremely rare disorder that, although it is believed to be inherited in an autosomal dominant manner, there is some uncertainty because a family with affected siblings has been described, suggesting autosomal recessive inheritance. However, this may be the result of germinal mosaicism. In the *Online Mendelian Inheritance in Man* (2004) it is classified under autosomal dominant, usually sporadic, and related to increased paternal age, with the note that there may be families with autosomal recessive transmission. A mutation in the *LMNA* gene which encodes Lamin A, a component of nuclear laminae appears responsible for progeria. The affected infant's weight and height are normal at birth with growth retardation, senile skin changes, prominent superficial blood vessels, and hair loss typically becoming evident between 6 and 12 months of age. Dwarfism, skeletal dysplasia, dental abnormalities, loss of subcutaneous fat, and the appearance of premature aging occurs. Atherosclerosis may occur as early as 5 years of age. Intelligence is not affected, and nurses should encourage families to try to allow as normal a life as possible, although fatigue is common. Death usually occurs between 7 and 27 years with a mean of about 14 years of age, usually caused by coronary occlusion.

Cockayne Syndrome

This extremely rare autosomal recessive condition is characterized by dwarfism, microcephaly, dysmorphic features, hearing loss, and mental retardation with loss of adipose tissue beginning in infancy. At least two complementation groups are known, with corresponding genes of *CSA* and *CSB*. Clinically, two major types are described, "classical" or type I, which has an onset around age 2 years with progression over a few years usually due to *CSA* on chromosome 5, and type II usually due to *CSB* on chromosome 10q11, which appears either prenatally or during the first few weeks with congenital or infantile cataracts and rapid progression. Ocular findings are prominent, including salt and pepper retinal pigmentation, cataract, and strabismus as well as photosensitivity with dermatitis. The risk to develop various cancers especially of the skin is increased. The phenotype is that of premature aging. Various phenotypic variability has been described and it is difficult to fully elucidate the syndrome because of the small number of affected persons identified. Cockayne syndrome is a DNA repair disorder in one of the pathways, known as transcription-coupled repair, which removes lesions in DNA that are on the transcribed strand of active genes. Overlap between Cockayne syndrome complementation groups and xeroderma pigmentosum complementation groups in other than the classic syndromes has been described but will be sorted out with molecular identification. Death usually occurs by early adolescence.

Werner Syndrome

In contrast to the first two disorders mentioned, Werner syndrome is not usually diagnosed until early adulthood, and the appearance of gray hair in late adolescence may be the first sign that leads to the diagnosis. It is inherited in an autosomal recessive manner. The gene mutated in Werner syndrome is *WRN*, located on chromosome 8. This gene codes for the RecQ family of DNA helicases, involved in the unwinding of DNA before replication. Other features of the disease include scleroderma-like skin changes, short stature (no adolescent growth spurt occurs), hair loss, cataracts, premature osteoarthritis, premature osteoporosis, premature aged facies, diabetes mellitus, hypercholesterolemia, and frequent malignancy, especially osteosarcoma. Death usually occurs between 45 and 60 years.

ALZHEIMER DISEASE

Alzheimer disease (AD) is the fourth leading cause of death in the United States, and the most common cause of dementia in older persons. There are other types of dementia, and Picks disease (frontal lobe atrophy) is believed due to a single AD gene in about 20% of cases. The lifetime risk of developing AD is 15% in the general population. AD is characterized by dementia involving personality changes, memory loss, deterioration of cognitive functions such as language, motor skills, perception, and attention with neuronal cell loss, deposition of senile plaques and neurofibrillary tangles in the cerebral cortex. There may also be associated symptoms such as depression, emotional outbursts, gait disorder, seizures, incontinence, sexual disorders, and others. The deposition of plaques and tangles also occurs in normal aging but not in the number and extent seen in AD. The plaques are largely composed of β-amyloid, a peptide derived from the β-amyloid precursor protein (APP). AD is genetically heterogenous. Cases of AD may be early onset (60–65 years of age or below) or late (above 60–65 years). To date, four gene defects have been associated with AD, three genes whose defects cause familial AD, and one that appears to be a susceptibility gene. These are shown in Table 21.1.

The amyloid percursor protein *(APP)* gene mutations on chromosome 21 are interesting because Down syndrome involves an extra chromosome 21 and people with Down syndrome have a cognitive decline similar to AD. There are various *APP* mutations which may result in familial AD (FAD), but they account for less than 10% of all FAD cases. Commercial genetic testing is not yet available. AD3 is also a directly inherited form with the defect in presenilin-1 or the *PS1* gene. This category may represent 30% to 60% of the early onset familial AD cases. More than 70 types of mutations in *PS1* are known and can cause FAD. Mutations in the *PS2* gene appear extremely rare, and only a few variants have been described. Relatively few families have been identified. This group was initially identified in a group of Volga German families. All of these three types are inherited in an autosomal dominant fashion, and predictive testing is possible for these groups.

The association between a specific genotype for apolipoprotein E *(APOE)*, a lipoprotein involved in

TABLE 21.1   Genes Associated with Alzheimer Disease

Type	Chromosome	Defective gene	Approximate age of onset
AD1—Early onset, familial	21	*APP*	43–62 yrs.
AD2—Late onset familial and sporadic susceptibility	19	*APOE ε4*	Over 55 yrs.
AD3—Early onset familial	14	*PS1* (presenilin-1)	29–62 yrs.
AD4—Early onset familial	1	*PS2* (presenilin-2)	40–88 yrs.

cholesterol metabolism and synthesized in the brain, and susceptibility to late onset AD is potentially important because it is believed that between 15% and 50% of all cases of AD may be accounted for by this ε4/ε4 genotype. The *APOE* gene has at least 7 allelic forms, ε1–ε7. The most important appears to be ε4. Persons with 2 alleles of ε4 have a higher risk (5- to 10-fold or more) of developing amyloid deposition and AD than those with 1 or no alleles. Farlow (1997), Ashford (2004), and Raber, Huang, and Ashford (2004), estimate that the ε4 allele is a susceptibility gene for as many as 50% of cases of AD in the general population. Lahiri, Sambamurti, and Bennett (2004) believe that although the ε4 allele is important, it may account for a lesser proportion. People with the ε4 allele have an increased risk of developing AD after head trauma. The ε4 allele may also be associated with a faster progression to AD and an earlier age of onset. The ε2 allele may actually have a protective effect by lowering the risk and increasing the age of onset. These findings have implications for genetic susceptibility testing, drug treatment, and preventive drug compounds that might mimic the action of *APOE* ε2. This is not necessarily a direct relationship since persons without the ε4 allele may develop AD, and those with it may not. Thus it is a risk factor. The effect of the APOE genotype on age of onset and AD symptoms is shown in the reference by Clark and Karlawish (2003).

More than 50 other genes have been implicated in late onset AD, including candidate genes on chromosomes 10 and 12. More recently APOE promotor polymorphisms have been implicated in susceptibility to AD. Mitochondrial dysfunction in AD has also been postulated. Tang et al. (1998) found that African Americans and Hispanics have a higher risk for AD apart from that conferred by *APOE* ε4. They speculate that an additional gene(s)

is associated with AD in these ethnic groups. An approach to therapy using the genetic information has been suggested. Since presenilin-1 is key for beta-amyloid formation in AD, silencing the presenilin-1 gene by S-adenosylmethionine by using methylation might prevent beta-amyloid production.

Testing for the *APOE* genotype could be for diagnosis of a person who already has symptoms of dementia, or for those who are asymptomatic and at-risk (predictive or presymptomatic testing). The issue of clinical testing for the *APOE* genotype has provoked various statements from groups such as the American College of Medical Genetics/American Society of Human Genetics (1995), Alzheimer disease groups, the National Institute on Aging (1996), and the Alzheimer's Disease and Related Disorders Association. The American Association for Geriatric Psychiatry, the Alzheimer's Association, and the American Geriatrics Society in 1997 released a statement that did not recommend genetic testing for APOE for predictive screening in asymptomatic persons because the *APOE* ε4 allele is also found in persons without AD and is not found in many with AD. Opinions vary on the utility of genetic testing for those who are already symptomatic. Some believe that it might be a valuable adjunct to diagnosis while others recommend conservatism in such use. In a study by Roberts et al. (2003) of adult children with a parent with Alzheimer disease (AD), nearly 78% sought presymptomatic testing. Among the reasons for doing so were for future research, to arrange personal affairs, and hoping for effective treatment development. The best predictor for seeking testing was their belief that other family members would need to be prepared for AD. The same issues of genetic testing that have been presented in connection with Huntington disease (see chapter 11) and in cancer testing (see chapter 23) apply here. In a study by Roberts et al. (2004), after family history was taken and risk assessment information was given, persons most likely to seek predictive testing for AD had the following attributes: below 60 years of age, female gender and college education. Major concerns revolve around the risk magnitude, especially across ethnic and racial groups, diagnostic accuracy, patient understanding of the meaning of the results, unnecessary anxiety, stigmatization, confidentiality, disclosure, emotional impact, financial, job, and insurance implications. Essential to any predictive testing for AD is appropriate education by a person knowledgeable in this area of genetics and the appropriate accompanying genetic counseling availability. Post et al. (1997) give the example of the person who undergoes predictive testing and who has one ε4 allele who might be a little forgetful and make life plan adjustments based on the belief that he/she had already developed AD. Tracy (1997) believes that asymptomatic people who request testing and who are at increased risk should be offered testing. Consent for testing in those who are already symptomatic is also an issue. Thus there are questions about who should be offered the test, handling the potentially large demand for such a test, and standards that govern the confidentiality and disclosure of test results as well as the necessary support services such as education and counseling. It is difficult to predict demand for genetic testing if available. In one early onset, *APP* autosomal dominant AD family in Sweden only three asymptomatic persons wanted to be tested (Lannfelt et al., 1995). Those who did not have the mutant allele were greatly relieved, but the one who did reacted with depression and suicidal thoughts. A major issue with susceptibility testing for late onset AD disease is the associated uncertainty of the meaning of the results. Even if the individual in question learns that they do not possess the ε4 allele, they may still eventually develop AD and if they are at higher risk for the development of AD because they do possess the ε4 allele this still does not mean that AD will develop in their lifetime. In an ethical case study involving a child at risk for AD, the mother wished to have him tested. She has decided that if he carried the *APOE ε4* allele, she will not allow him to pursue football but will direct him instead to musical pursuits, given the described impact of head injury on persons with that allele and the future

development of AD ("Susceptibility testing for children," 2003). Another issue will revolve around prenatal testing. If it becomes available would mothers choose to terminate pregnancy if the fetus were diagnosed with a genotype predictive of AD? This question and other ethical questions surrounding prenatal diagnosis are discussed in chapter 12.

NOTES

Interest in the contribution of genetics to the normal aging process and to the potential for increasing longevity has increased. Studies of exceptional longevity are revealing new information, some of which revolves around genetic determinants that may contribute to healthy aging and less susceptibility to conditions such as cardiovascular disease and diabetes mellitus that typically can contribute to morbidity and mortality. Information from genetic diseases that show premature aging will continue to provide new insights into the aging process. The further identification of genetic contributions to Alzheimer disease will not only suggest new therapeutic approaches but will also raise issues of identification of persons at risk and the options of predictive or susceptibility testing. As testing becomes more widely available, there must be professionals with the knowledge in genetics to provide the appropriate initial risk assessment, educaiton, and genetic counseling that will be needed.

BIBLIOGRAPHY

Alzheimer's Disease International. Medical and Scientific Advisory Committee. (1995). Consensus statement on predictive testing for Alzheimer disease. *Alzheimer Disease and Associated Disorders, 9*, 182–187.

American College of Medical Genetics/American Society of Human Genetics. Working Group on ApoE and Alzheimer Disease. (1995). Statement on use of apolipoprotein E testing for Alzheimer disease. *Journal of the American Medical Association, 274*, 1627–1629.

Ashford, J. W. (2004). APOE genotype effects on Alzheimer's disease onset and epidemiology. *Journal of Molecular Neuroscience, 23*, 157–165.

Barber, M., & Whitehouse, P. J. (2003). Susceptibility testing for Alzheimer's disease: Race for the future. *Lancet Neurology, 1,* 10.

Barzilai, N., Atzmon, G., Schechter, C., Schaefer, E. J., Cupples, A. L., Lipton, R., et al. (2004). Unique lipoprotein phenotype and genotype associated with exceptional longevity. *Journal of the American Medical Association, 290,* 2030–2040.

Bertoli-Avella, A. M., Oostra, B. A., & Heutink, P. (2004). Chasing genes in Alzheimer's and Parkinson's disease. *Human Genetics, 114,* 413–438.

Busson-Le Coniat, M., Boucher, N., Blanche, H., Thomas, G., & Berger, R. (2002). Chromosome studies of in vitro senescent lymphocytes: Nonrandom trisomy 2. *Annals of Genetics, 45,* 193–196.

Castellani, R., Hirai, K., Aliev, G., Drew, K. L., Nunomura, A., Takeda, A., et al. (2003). Role of mitochondrial dysfunction in Alzheimer's disease. *Journal of Neuroscience Research, 70,* 357–360.

Chen, L., Lee, L., Kudlow, B. A., Dos Santos, H. G., Sletvold, O., Shafeghati, Y., et al. (2003). LMNA mutations in atypical Werner's syndrome. *Lancet, 362,* 440–445.

Chomyn, A., & Attardi, G. (2003). MtDNA mutations in aging and apoptosis. *Biochemical and Biophysical Research Communications, 304,* 519–529.

Chong, L., McDonald, & Strauss, E. (2004). Deconstructing aging. *Science, 305,* 1419.

Clark, C. M., & Karlawish, J. H. T. (2003). Alzheimer disease: Current concepts and emerging diagnostic and therapeutic strategies. *Annals of Internal Medicine, 138,* 400–410.

Clark, W. R. (Ed.). (2003). *The means to an end: The biological basis of aging.* Oxford, UK: Oxford University Press.

Cooke, M. S., Evans, M. D., Dizdaroglu, M., & Lunec, J. (2003). Oxidative DNA damage: Mechanisms, mutation, and disease. *FASEB Journal, 17,* 1195–1214.

Crentsil, V. (2004). The pharmacogenomics of Alzheimer's disease. *Aging Research Reviews, 3,* 153–169.

Cupples, L. A., Farrer, L. A., Sadovnick, A. D., Relkin, N., Whitehouse, P., & Green, R. C. (2004). Estimating risk curves for first-degree relatives of patients with Alzheimer's disease: The REVEAL study. *Genetics in Medicine, 6,* 192–196.

De Sandre-Giovannoli, A., Bernard, R., Cau, P., Navarro, C., Amiel, J., Boccaccio, I., et al. (2003). Lamin A truncation in Hutchinson-Gilford progeria. *Science, 300,* 2055.

Farlow, M. R. (1997). Alzheimer's disease: Clinical implications of the apolipoprotein E genotype. *Neurology, 48*(Suppl. 6), S30–S34.

Fernandez-Capetillo, & Nussenzweig, A. (2004). Aging counts on chromosomes. *Nature Genetics, 36,* 672–674.

Green, B. C., Cupples, A., Go, R., Benke, K. S., Edeki, T., Coriffitia, P. A., et al. (2002). Risk of dementia among white and African-American relatives of patients with Alzheimer's disease. *Journal of the American Medical Association, 287,* 329–336.

Hardy, J. (2004). Toward Alzheimer therapies based on genetic knowledge. *Annual Review of Medicine, 55,* 15–25.

Hasty, P., Campisi, J., Hoeijmakers, J., van Steeg, H., & Vijg, J. (2003). Aging and genome maintenance: Lessons from the mouse? *Science, 299,* 1355–1359.

Hayflick, L. (1980). Cell aging. *Annual Review of Gerontology and Geriatrics, 1,* 26–67.

Hekimi, S., & Guarente, L. (2003). Genetics and the specificity of the aging process. *Science, 299,* 1351–1354.

Hodes, R. J., McCormick, A. M., & Pruzan, M. (1996). Longevity assurance genes: How do they influence aging and life span? *Journal of the American Geriatrics Society, 44,* 988–991.

Janssen, J. C., Beck, J. A., Campbell, T. A., Dickinson, A., Fox, N. C., Harvey, R. J., et al. (2003). Early onset familial Alzheimer's disease: Mutation frequency in 31 families. *Neurology, 60,* 235–239.

Jones, K. L. (1997). *Smith's recognizable patterns of human malformation* (5th ed.). Philadelphia: W.B. Saunders.

Kallman, F. J., & Sander, G. (1948). Twin studies on aging and longevity. *Journal of Heredity, 39,* 349–357.

Kawas, C. H. (2003). Early Alzheimer's disease. *New England Journal of Medicine, 349,* 1056–1063.

Kipling, D., Davis, T., Ostler, E. L., & Faragher, R. G. A. (2004). What can progeroid syndromes tell us about human aging. *Science, 305,* 1426–1431.

Lahiri, D. K., Sambamurti, K., & Bennett, D. A. (2004). Apolipoprotein gene and its interaction with the environmentally driven risk factors: Molecular, genetic and epidemiological studies of Alzheimer's disease. *Neurobiology of Aging, 25,* 651–660.

Lannfelt, L, Axelman, K., Lilius, L., & Basum, H. (1995). Genetic counseling of a Swedish Alzheimer family with amyloid precursor protein mutation. *American Journal of Human Genetics, 56,* 332–335.

LeRoy, B. S. (2004). Alzheimer's disease and testing. *Genetics in Medicine, 6,* 173–174.

Lleo, A., Berezovska, O., Growdon, J. H., & Hyman, B. T. (2004). Clinical, pathological, and biochemical spectrum of Alzheimer disease associated with PS-1 mutations. *American Journal of Geriatric Psychiatry, 12,* 146–156.

Lopera, F., Ardilla, A., Martinez, A., Madrigal, L., Arango-Viana, J. C., Lemere, C. A., et al. (1997). Clinical features of early-onset Alzheimer disease in a large kindred with an E280A presenilin-1 mutation. *Journal of the American Medical Association, 277,* 793–799.

Lott, I. T., & Head, E. (2005). Alzheimer disease and Down syndrome: Factors in pathogenesis. *Neurobiology of Aging, 26,* 383–389.

Marjaux, E., Hartmann, D., & De Strooper, B. (2004). Presenilins in memory, Alzheimer's disease, and therapy. *Neuron, 42,* 189–192.

Martin, G. M. (2002). The biologic basis of aging: Implications for medical genetics. In D. L. Rimoin, J. M. Connor, R. E. Pyeritz, & B. R. Korf (Eds.), *Emery and Rimoin's principles and practice of medical genetics* (4th ed., pp. 571–589). New York: Churchill Livingstone.

Martin, G. M. (2001). Genetics and aging. In C. R. Scriver, A. L. Beaudet, W. S. Sly, & D. Valle (Eds.), *The metabolic and molecular bases of inherited disease* (8th ed., pp. 215–223). New York: McGraw-Hill.

Martins, R. N., & Hallmayer, J. (2004). Age at onset: Important marker of genetic heterogeneity in Alzheimer's disease. *Pharamcogenomics Journal, 4,* 138–140.

Nath, J., Tucker, J. D., & Hando, J. C. (1995). Y chromosome aneuploidy, micronuclei, kinetochores and aging in men. *Chromosoma, 103,* 725–731.

National Institute on Aging. Alzheimer's Association Working Group. (1996). Apolipoprotein E genotyping in Alzheimer's disease. *Lancet, 347,* 1091–1095.

National Institute on Aging. Progress Report on Alzheimer's Disease, 1996. Washington, DC: National Institute on Aging, National Institutes of Health, US Dept. of Health and Human Services, NIH publication 96-4137.

Nee, L. E., Tierney, M. C., & Lippa, C. F. (2004). Genetic aspects of Alzheimer's disease, Pick's disease, and other dementias. *American Journal of Alzheimer's Disease and Other Dementias, 19,* 219–225.

O'Neill, M., Núñez, F., & Melton, D. W. (2003). p53 and a human premature ageing disorder. *Mechanisms of Ageing and Development, 124,* 599–603.

Online Mendelian Inheritance in Man, OMIM(tm). (2005). National Center for Biotechnology Information, National Library of Medicine, Bethesda, MD. Online at http://www.ncbi.nlm.nih.gov/omim

Pearl, R., & Pearl, E. de W. (1943). Studies on human longevity. *Human Biology, 6,* 98–222.

Perls, T., Kunkel, L., & Puca, A. (2002a). The genetics of aging. *Current Opinion in Genetics & Development, 12,* 362–369.

Perls, T., Kunkel, L., & Puca, A. (2002b). The genetics of exceptional human longevity. *Journal of the American Geriatrics Society, 50,* 359–368.

Popp, D. M. (1982). An analysis of genetic factors regulating life span in congeneic mice. *Mechanisms of Ageing and Development, 18,* 125–134.

Post, S. G., Whitehouse, P. J., Binstock, R. H., Bird, T. D., Eckert, S. K., Farrer, L. A., et al. (1997). The clinical introduction of genetic testing for Alzheimer disease. *Journal of the American Medical Association, 277,* 832–836.

Raber, J., Huang, Y., & Ashford, J. W. (2004). ApoE genotype accounts for the vast majority of AD risk and AD pathology. *Neurobiology of Aging, 25,* 641–650.

Raji, N. S., & Rao, K. S. (1998). Trisomy 21 and accelerated aging: DNA-repair parameters in peripheral lymphocytes of Down's syndrome patients. *Mechanisms of Ageing and Development, 100,* 85–101.

Reiman, E. M., Chen, K., Alexander, G. E., Caselli, R. J., Bandy, D., Osborne, D., et al. (2004). Functional brain abnormalities in young adults at genetic risk for late-onset Alzheimer's dementia. *Proceedings of the National Academy of Sciences, USA, 101,* 284–289.

Ren, Y., Saijo, M., Nakatsu, Y., Nakai, H., Yamaizumi, T., & Tanaka K. (2003). Three novel mutations responsible for Cockayne syndrome group A. *Genes and Genetic Systems, 78,* 93–102.

Richard, F., Muleris, M., & Dutrillaux, B. (1994). The frequency of micronculei with X chromosome increases with age in human females. *Mutation Research, 316,* 1–7.

Roberts, J. S., Barber, M., Brown, T. M., Cupples, L. A., Farrer, L. A., LaRusse, S. A., et al. (2004). Who seeks genetic susceptibility testing for Alzheimer's disease? Findings from a multisite randomized clinical trials. *Genetics in Medicine, 6,* 197–203.

Roberts, J. S., LaRusse, S. A., Katzen, H., Whitehouse, P. J., Barber, M., Post, S. G., et al. (2003). Reasons for seeking genetic susceptibility testing among first-degree relatives of people with Alzheimer disease. *Alzheimer Disease and Associated Disorders, 17,* 86–92.

Roses, A. D. (1997). Genetic testing for Alzheimer disease. Practical and ethical issues. *Archives of Neurology, 54,* 1226–1229.

Sakamoto, S., Matsuda, H., Asada, T., Ohnishi, T., Nakano, S., Kanetaka, H., et al. (2003). Apolipoprotein E genotype and early Alzheimer's disease: A longitudinal SPECT study. *Journal of Neuroimaging, 13,* 113–123.

Samuels, D. C. (2004). Mitochondrial DNA repeats constrain the life span of mammals. *Trends in Genetics, 20,* 226–229.

Scarpa, S., Fuso, A., D'Anselmi, F. & Cavallaro, R. A. (2003). Presenilin 1 gene silencing by S-adenosylmethionine: A treatment for Alzheimer disease. *FEBS Letters, 541,* 145–148.

Schellenberg, G. D., Miki, T., Yu, C-E., & Nakura, J. (2001). Werner syndrome. In C. R. Scriver, A. L. Beaudet, W. S. Sly, & D. Valle (Eds.), *The metabolic and molecular bases of inherited disease* (8th ed., pp. 785–791). New York: McGraw-Hill.

Schmitt, F. A., & Estus, S. (2004). Alzheimer's disease genetic susceptibility and causality: What is ApoE's impact. *Neurobiology of Aging, 25,* 661–662.

Selkoe, D. J. (2004). Alzheimer disease: Mechanistic understanding predicts novel therapies. *Annals of Internal Medicine, 140,* 627–638.

Stone, J. F., & Sandberg, A. A. (1995). Sex chromosome aneuploidy and aging. *Mutation Research, 338,* 107–113.

Selkoe, D. J., & Podlisny, M. B. (2002). Deciphering the genetic basis of Alzheimer's disease. *Annual Review of Genomics and Human Genetics, 3,* 67–99.

Silverman, J. M., Smith, C. J., Marin, D. B., Mohs R. C., & Propper, C. B. (2003). Familial patterns of risk in very late-onset Alzheimer disease. *Archives of General Psychiatry, 60,* 190–197.

Susceptibility testing for children. (2003). *Health Progress, 84*(3), 11–12.

Tang, M-X., Stern, Y., Marder, K., Bell, K., Gurland, B., Lantigua, R., et al. (1998). The *APOE*-ε4 allele and the risk of Alzheimer disease among African Americans, whites and Hispanics. *Journal of the American Medical Association, 279,* 751–755.

Tracy, K. B. (1997). Genetic testing for Alzheimer disease. *Journal of the American Medical Association, 278,* 978–979.

Vijg, J., & Suh, Y. (2005). Genetics of longevity and aging. *Annual Review of Medicine, 56,* 193–212.

Wijsman, E. M., Daw, E. W., Yu, X., Steinhart, E. J., Nochlin, D., Bird, T. D., et al. (2005). APOE and other loci affect age-at-onset in Alzheimer's disease families with PS2 mutation. *American Journal of Medical Genetics Part B (Neuropsychiatric Genetics), 132B,* 14–20.

Worman, H., & Courvalin, J-C. (2004). How do mutations in lamins A and C cause disease? *Journal of Clinical Investigation, 113,* 349–351.

Yu, C-E., Oshima, J., Fu, Y-H., Wijsman, E. M., Hisama, F., Alisch, R., et al. (1996). Positional cloning of the Werner's syndrome gene. *Science, 272,* 258–262.

Zhu, Z., Raina, A. K., Perry, G., & Smith, M. A. (2004). Alzheimer's disease: The two-hit hypothesis. *Lancet Neurology, 3,* 219–226.

22

Emphysema, Liver Disease, and Alpha-1 Antitrypsin Deficiency

Alpha-1 antitrypsin (AAT) deficiency is the most frequent genetic cause of liver disease in infants and children and the most common genetic cause of emphysema in adults. Interest in AAT deficiency was initially stimulated by the serendipitous discovery made by Laurell and Eriksson in 1963 of an association between AAT deficiency and an inherited form of emphysema. In 1969, Sharp, Bridges, Krivit, and Freier linked AAT deficiency with childhood cirrhosis. Since then, AAT research has proliferated, elucidating its normal functions, studying its genetic variation, and exploring its association with disease.

AAT is a *serine proteinase inhibitor* (serpin) that is mainly synthesized by the liver and is rapidly released into the plasma, but there is also some local production within the lung. The small molecular size of AAT allows it to leave the plasma and easily enter other body tissues and fluids, where it is widely distributed. Its chief function is as a protease inhibitor, particularly of elastase, although it has inhibitory activity against trypsin, chymotrypsin, thrombin, tissue kallikrein, renin, bacterial proteases, and others. When proteolytic enzymes such as elastase are released from cells after events such as tissue injury, AAT inhibits their activity and therefore protects organs such as the liver and lungs against damage. The normal serum level ranges from 150 to 350 mg/dl. AAT serum levels vary in response to conditions such as inflammation, trauma, infection, pregnancy, cancer, burns, smoking, estrogen therapy, oral contraceptives, and corticosteroid administration. AAT is known to be inactivated by bacteria such as

Pseudomonas aeruginosa, Proteus mirabilis, and cigarette smoke condensate.

AAT is synthesized under the direction of a gene, known as PI for protease inhibitor as defined previously, that is located on chromosome 14 (14q32.1). The PI system demonstrates much genetic variability and more than 100 alleles coding for different molecular variants have been identified, many of which are common enough that they are polymorphic in some populations (see chapter 3 for a discussion of polymorphisms). The various variants were named according to their migration on an electrical field. Techniques such as electrophoresis or isoelectric focusing separate components of the AAT molecule according to their electrophoretic mobility, and DNA restriction enzyme techniques have been used to reveal greater variation.

The following designations are commonly used although some use Pi instead of PI:

1. PI*M, PI*S, PI*Z etc. for alleles at the PI locus
2. PI*MM, PI*MS, etc. or simply PIMM or PIMS or MM, MS for phenotypes
3. PI*M/PI*S, PI*M/PI*Z etc. or PI*MS or PI*MZ for genotypes

AAT variants may be classified as normal, deficient, null, and dysfunctional. The most common normal allele is PI*M. The most common normal phenotype is PI MM and is associated with a 100% serum level of AAT. There are subtype variants of M such as M1, M2, M3, and others which differ in amino acid sequence but appear to function normally, and there are other normal non-M variants. There are two important deficient variant alleles—PI*Z and PI*S. These may be present in the heterozygous state (PI MS, PI MZ, PI SZ) or in the homozygous state (PI SS or PI ZZ). Thus, there are varying degrees of AAT deficiency. The PI*Z allele is the one most commonly associated with clinically significant effects of low serum AAT levels. The percent of normal AAT activity in the plasma in regard to PI phenotype is shown in Table 22.1. The serum concentration of AAT for the PI ZZ person is 1% to 15% of normal. A person who is PI MZ would have a serum level approximately midway between the two alleles. The null variants are very rare and produce virtually no AAT. These are designated as PI*Q0, which can be followed by the name of the place of discovery of the allele.

AAT deficiency occurs in 1 in 1,600 to 1 in 5,000 live births in white North American and northern European populations and less frequently in southern European and other populations. It is particularly frequent in Sweden, where it is included in newborn screening programs. It is estimated that PI ZZ is present in 1 in 40,000 to 1 in 100,000 black Americans and was originally thought to be infrequent in Asian populations. More recent epidemiological studies among various geographic and ethnic groups in 58 countries indicate that there are at least 3.4 million persons with deficiency alleles (i.e., PI SS, PI SZ, PI ZZ), and 116 million carriers (i.e., PI MS and PI MZ) worldwide, and that AAT deficiency affects persons in all racial subgroups (de Serres, 2002). Stoller (1997) estimates that

80,000–100,000 persons have severe AAT. Even so, AAT deficiency is under-recognized and only about 5% of persons with some degree of deficiency are identified. The inheritance mechanism is autosomal recessive with co-dominant expression of each gene on the basis of both the quantity and activity of the enzyme present.

Clinical expression of AAT deficiency commonly occurs bimodally in relation to age: in infancy or childhood manifested by symptoms of liver disease, or in early adulthood manifested by pulmonary symptoms and more rarely liver disease. Clinical expression also depends on the genotype, the degree of AAT deficiency, and modulating factors such as cigarette smoke exposure. The most information is known about PI ZZ and that will be the major focus of this section. It has been estimated that of all infants born with PI ZZ, 80% will eventually develop emphysema, 10% will suffer from childhood cirrhosis, and the rest will not show any overt clinical disease. AAT deficiency is under-recognized—only about 5% are identified.

LIVER DISORDERS AND ALPHA-1 ANTITRYPSIN DEFICIENCY

Liver disease due to AAT deficiency can be noted in infancy, childhood, adolescence, or adulthood. Liver disease in PI*ZZ deficiency is thought to result from accumulation of mutant protein in the hepatocytes. In infancy, liver involvement is noted in about 10% to 20% of those who are PI ZZ. Typically, this consists of obstructive or cholestatic jaundice in the first 1–4 months of life that may be

TABLE 22.1   Plasma Concentration and Population Frequencies of Selected PI Phenotypes

Phenotype	Percentage of normal AAT activity in plasma	Prevalence of phenotype in United States and Northern Europe (given in %)
MM	100	81–90
MS	79–83	6.5–9
SS	60–65	0.09–0.30
MZ	55–60	1.5–5
SZ	37–45	0.10–0.50
ZZ	1–15	0.04–0.10

Sources: de Serres (2002), Silverman (2002), Pierce (1997), Cox (2001), Sveger (1976), Sharp (1976), and Eriksson, Moestrup, and Hägerstrand (1975).

diagnosed as neonatal hepatitis. The PI ZZ infant accounts for 40% to 50% of all such cases of jaundice in the first 2 months. In most infants, this abates and they become clinically asymptomatic until the development of cirrhosis in later childhood (usually at about 8 years of age) or in early adulthood. In some infants, the jaundice progresses rapidly to ascites, cirrhosis, septicemia, or death. It is estimated that 50% to 75% of PI ZZ infants may have abnormal liver function tests such as elevated transaminase levels. Hepatomegaly or biochemical abnormalities may be present in infants who possess the PI ZZ phenotype but who have never been tested. Occasionally a PI ZZ infant has a bleeding episode such as from the umbilicus or gastrointestinal tract or from bruising. The diagnosis is eventually made when liver dysfunction is found. Breast-feeding during the first year of life may reduce the symptoms of the liver disease. Although Pi ZZ infants with a history of neonatal jaundice are at greater risk for developing cirrhosis later in life than those without symptoms, the eventual course and outcome is not established and approximately 10% of PI ZZ infants with no clinical evidence of childhood liver disease later develop cirrhosis possibly associated with hepatocellular carcinoma. Children with PI ZZ and no evidence of eventual liver disease have also been reported, and cases of childhood cirrhosis have been reported in SS, SZ, and MZ individuals. The prevalence of cirrhosis among all PI ZZ adults is 10%, rising to almost 20% in those over 50 years of age. Children with chronic liver disease should be tested for AAT deficiency.

In some AAT deficient individuals, liver disease may not be found until late childhood or adolescence, when they present with abdominal distention caused by hepatosplenomegaly or portal hypertension and esophageal variceal hemorrhage. Latent hepatic dysfunction in middle-aged and older adults has been found to be due to AAT deficiency. The older adult may present with hepatitis, cryptogenic cirrhosis, and/or hepatocellular carcinoma. Patients in older age groups with liver disease should be tested for AAT deficiency. Patients over 40 years of age with AAT deficiency should have periodic liver function assessment.

All of those patients with the PI*Z allele, and some who are PI MS and PI SS, have abnormal AAT globules in the liver that accumulate in the hepatocytes, but not all develop liver disease. Thus, some other event, such as exposure to alcohol, a hepatitis virus, or some other factor may be necessary for disease expression. Of all infants who develop clinical liver disease, two-thirds are male. Thus, another genetic or hormonal factor may be needed for full expression in the PI ZZ individual.

PULMONARY DISEASE AND ALPHA-1 ANTITRYPSIN DEFICIENCY

The association of AAT deficiency with chronic obstructive pulmonary disease (COPD), particularly emphysema, has been extensively validated. Emphysema caused by AAT deficiency usually involves the basal regions of the lung. Onset is early, often beginning in the late 20s or early 30s. Before age 40, 39–60% of PI ZZ individuals develop COPD, as do 85–90% by 50 years of age. Even in clinically asymptomatic individuals, abnormalities in lung function can be detected early. The first symptom is usually dyspnea on exertion, followed by cough and recurrent pulmonary infections, with severe expiratory airflow limitation and findings typically associated with emphysema. The risk for developing COPD in infancy and childhood is low, but it has been reported, as has an excess of asthma in AAT-deficient infants. By adulthood, it is possible for a PI ZZ individual to have both liver abnormalities and COPD. The detrimental effects of smoking in the PI ZZ individual have been established beyond a shadow of a doubt. The onset of COPD occurs approximately 15 years earlier in those PI ZZ individuals who smoke, and decreases life expectancy. Smoking also leads to an early permanent loss of tolerance for exercise. As in liver disease, gender plays a yet unknown type of protective role. Adult PI ZZ females who are non-smokers are the least likely to develop pulmonary disease, while adult PI ZZ males who smoke are the most likely.

The extent of the risk for heterozygous PI MZ individuals to develop emphysema has been of interest because of their greater frequency in the population. PI MZ individuals who smoke may show greater deterioration than those who do not, and PI MZ heterozygotes as a group appear to run a risk slightly higher than the normal (PI MM) population for developing COPD. However, the

Z allele is responsible for only a small percent of all individuals with COPD. Persons with emphysema, in the absence of other risk factors, especially under 45 years of age, should be tested for AAT deficiency.

ASSOCIATION WITH OTHER DISORDERS

Reports of associations between AAT deficiency and other disorders have appeared in the literature. The strongest associations have been between AAT deficiency and immune or autoimmune disorders. It may be possible that low levels of AAT decreases the ability to combat inflammation or promote the formation of immune complexes. Specific association with disorders are for an increased proportion of PI*MZ and PI*SZ heterozygotes among persons with certain types of rheumatoid arthritis, anterior uveitis and various collagen vascular diseases. A strong relationship has been noted between PI*Z deficiency and vasculitis especially Wegener's granulomatosis. Panniculitis, an inflammatory skin and subcutaneous tissue disorder which may show ulceration, is associated with the PI*Z allele or PI*ZZ phenotype. Heterozygotes for PI*Z allele may be more susceptible to chronic urticaria and to developing acquired angioedema. Islet cell hyperplasia occurs with AAT deficiency. Other associations such as with aneurysms, celiac disease, and glomerculonephritis have been suggested but not confirmed. It has been postulated that a normal function of AAT may be in preventing inflammation and tissue destruction once the disease process has begun, and that the heterozygote does not have an enzyme level that can adequately perform this function. Women with AAT deficiency are at risk for intrauterine growth retardation in their infants, often because of compromised maternal respiratory function.

SCREENING AND TESTING

The American Thoracic Society/European Respiratory Society Statement (2003) delineates those persons for whom genetic testing might or might not be offered, and provides a range of recommendations from A through D as follows (p. 892):

Description	Recommendation designation
Testing is recommended	A
Testing should be discussed; could be accepted or declined	B
Testing is not recommended; should not be encouraged	C
Recommended that testing should not be done; should be discouraged	D

The following summarizes The American Thoracic Society and European Respiratory Society Statement (2003) recommendations in: a) diagnostic testing, b) predispositional testing, c) carrier testing in the reproductive setting for individuals at high risk of having AAT-deficiency related diseases who are planning pregnancy or who are pregnant or their partners; and d) screening situations at different age groups and situations. Each option should be accompanied by appropriate support services such as education and counseling as detailed in chapters 11, 12, and 23.

1. They (pp. 893–894) recommend testing (designation A) in the following situations:
   - For diagnosis in symptomatic adults with emphysema, COPD, asthma with incompletely reversible airflow obstruction; asymptomatic persons with persistent obstructive pulmonary dysfunction due to smoking or occupational exposure; adults, children and newborns with unexplained liver disease; and adults with necrotizing panniculitis.
   - For predispositional testing in adult/adolescent siblings who have a family member who is homozygous of AAT deficiency;
2. They recommend that testing be discussed (designation B) in the following situations:
   - For diagnosis in adults with bronchiectasis of unknown cause and asymptomatic persons with persistent obstructive pulmonary dysfunction without risk factors for AAT deficiency; adults with multisystemic vasculitis
   - For predispositional testing in adults/adolescents for offspring, parents and distant relatives of a family member who is

homozygous for ATT deficiency; and predispositional testing for siblings, offspring, parents and distant relatives of a family member who is heterozygous for AAT deficiency; persons with a family history of obstructive lung disease or liver disease.

- For carrier testing in the reproductive setting individuals at high risk of having AAT deficiency-related diseases who are planning pregnancy or who are in the prenatal period and partners of persons with either AAT deficiency or carrier status who are at high risk themselves.
- For screening in adults and adolescents in countries where the prevalence of AAT deficiency is high (about 1/1,500 or more).

3. They do not recommend testing, and state it should not be encouraged (designation C) in the following situations:
- For diagnostic testing in asthma with completely reversible airflow obstruction.
- For screening in smokers with normal spirometry.

4. They recommend testing not be performed, and state that it should be discouraged (designation D) in the following situations:
- For predispositional testing: Fetal testing for AAT deficiency. The rationale given is that AAT deficiency diseases are not serious enough to warrant prenatal genetic testing; however, they state the family should be informed if they have had a previous child with severe progressive liver disease in the neonatal period. This view is not universally shared and risk figures for various situations are available in Cox (2004).
- For screening in newborns, and in adults and adolescents where there is not a high prevalence of AAT deficiency defined as about 1/1,500 or less frequent.

TREATMENT

Various approaches to treatment have been tried. In most infants, the initial hepatic symptoms spontaneously abate while others may progress to hepatic failure. Advances in liver transplantation techniques appear to offer the best current long-term prognosis for children who have severe end-stage cirrhotic disease, replacing portacaval shunt as a treatment. After such transplantation, conversion of the phenotype is expected. For those with severe damage from emphysema, lung transplantation may be an option. In less severe circumstances, therapy may be directed at treating the symptoms of emphysema or liver disease. Antioxidant therapy may be useful. Augmentation therapy of weekly intravenous infusions of exogenous AAT (Prolastin) can have side effects but generally shows good results. Use of recombinant AAT preparations are also possible and avoid risks of plasma-derived product. Gene therapy aimed at either the lung or liver to correct AAT deficiency may be a future option, and various approaches are being examined, for example using knowledge about the basis for AAT deficiency to block polymerization through small peptide binding to the defective AAT. Administering AAT by inhalation of aerosolized AAT is still considered experimental, but it holds promise.

NURSING PRACTICE APPLICATIONS AND PREVENTIVE MEASURES

The nurse should be clinically alert for the possibility of AAT deficiency in adults and children with COPD and liver disease, as some cases will have this genetic cause. It is not possible to predict along what path a specific individual with AAT deficiency will develop or how severe their disorder will be. All individuals with neonatal jaundice or childhood liver disease should have their AAT status determined by PI typing. Those with AAT deficiency may have their condition ameliorated by a lifetime plan. The nurse should begin with counseling and educating the family, and the child if old enough, about the meaning of AAT deficiency and the desirability of minimizing liver and pulmonary damage. Others in the family should have PI typing done. Contact should be maintained over a long period of time with such families to reinforce counseling and answer questions. Before performing testing, the person, or parents in the case of an infant or child, should be informed about the potential risks and benefits as discussed in chapter 11. For example, Stoller (1997) and Stoller, Smith, Yang, and Spray (1994) reported that diagnosis of severe AAT deficiency in adults led to early retirement for 44%, job loss for 16%, job change for

19%, and loss of health insurance for 11%. The plan with appropriate education should include the following:

- emphasis on never smoking for both the individual and for those living with the affected person because of the danger of second-hand smoke;
- reinforcement of avoiding smoking as the child enters late childhood and early adolescence;
- the avoidance of alcohol and other agents toxic to the liver, including certain medications;
- avoidance of respiratory irritants at home and on the job;
- at the appropriate time, teach affected females to avoid oral contraceptive agents, and provide information on other contraceptive measures;
- emphasize the need for early recognition and treatment of any respiratory infection, including vaccination for pneumococcal infections and other respiratory pathogens as indicated;
- the need for maintaining physical activity to promote cardiovascular fitness without exhausting the individual;
- alertness for symptoms of COPD, liver disease, and glomerulonephritis;
- the need for maintaining good nutritional status and its relationship to immunocompetence and health (what constitutes good nutrition and elements of any special diet should be included);
- eventual career guidance and planning to select a job in which the individual will not be exposed to such known lung irritants as grain, cotton and other fibers, coal dust, wood dust (as in sawmills), hair sprays, or in any chemical industry where they might be exposed to hepatotoxins or noxious chemical irritants;
- the desirability of choosing a permanent place of residence that is low in pollution and grain dust can be discussed with the family or with the nurse, understanding that a family cannot usually make such a major move, and that it is not expected of them (however, the child may wish to consider this factor in his/her eventual choice of locale as a young adult);

- genetic counseling, including the risk for other children with AAT deficiency or for the offspring of the affected person. This can include the availability of prenatal detection for future pregnancies; and
- awareness of the WHO recommendations in regard to those who might be tested for AAT deficiency.

The practice of industrial or preemployment screening for AAT deficient individuals has positive and negative points for the occupational health nurse to consider. Although current employees may benefit from placement in a position that is of lower risk, and from the institution of other health promoting measures as previously described, job discrimination can also result, thus limiting their advancement and even costing them their jobs. As a preemployment measure it may be discriminatory (see chapter 14). A major problem lies in the uncertainty of the magnitude of the risk of clinical disease for heterozygous or even homozygous individuals. At the present time, widespread general population screening is not recommended. All the points specifically relating to screening as discussed in chapter 11 also apply here.

Prenatal detection is possible by amniocentesis and chorion villi sampling for most variants through the application of DNA analysis and by fetal blood sampling. The risk for two heterozygotes for the PI*Z allele to have a PI ZZ child with congenital liver disease progressing to cirrhosis is currently estimated at 1% to 2%. Therefore, this option can be discussed with families known to be at risk, especially those who have already had a child with childhood cirrhosis. Risk estimates vary for other outcomes.

BIBLIOGRAPHY

α_1-antitrypsin deficiency: Memorandum from a WHO meeting. (1997). *Bulletin of the World Health Organization, 75,* 397–415.

American Thoracic Society. (1989). Guidelines for the approach to the patient with severe hereditary alpha-1-antitrypsin deficiency. *American Review of Respiratory Disease, 140,* 1494–1496.

American Thoracic Society/European Respiratory

Society Statement: Standards for the diagnosis and management of individuals with alpha-1 antitrypsin deficiency. (2003). *American Journal of Respiratory and Critical Care Medicine, 168,* 818–900.

Carrell, R. W., & Lomas, D. A. (2002). Alpha$_1$-antitrypsin deficiency—a model for conformational diseases. *New England Journal of Medicine, 346,* 45–53.

Cox, D. W. (2001). α_1-antitrypsin deficiency. In C. R. Scriver, A. L. Beaudet, W. S. Sly, & D. Valle (Eds.), *The metabolic and molecular bases of inherited disease* (8th ed., pp. 5559–5584). New York: McGraw-Hill.

Cox, D. W. (2004). Prenatal diagnosis for alpha 1-antitrypsin deficiency. *Prenatal Diagnosis, 24,* 468–470.

DeMeo, D. L., & Silverman, E. K. (2004). α_1-antitrypsin deficiency. 2: Genetic aspects of α_1-antitrypsin deficiency: Phenotypes and genetic modifiers of emphysema risk. *Thorax, 59,* 259–264.

de Serres, F. J. (2002). Worldwide racial and ethnic distribution of α_1-antitrypsin deficiency. *Chest, 122,* 1818–1829.

de Serres, F. J., Blanco, I., & Fernández-Bustillo, E. (2003).Genetic epidemiology of alpha-1 antitrypsin deficiency in southern Europe: France, Italy, Portugal and Spain. *Clinical Genetics, 63,* 490–509.

de Serres, F. J., Blanco, I., & Fernández-Bustillo, E. (2003). Genetic epidemiology of alpha-1 antitrypsin deficiency in North America and Australia/New Zealand: Australia, Canada, New Zealand, and the United States of America. *Clinical Genetics, 64,* 382–397.

Dhandha, S. (2002, February). Alpha-1-antitrypsin deficiency. *Contemporary OB/GYN.*

Driskell, R. A., & Engelhardt, J. F. (2003). Current status of gene therapy for inherited lung diseases. *Annual Review of Physiology, 65,* 585–612.

Eden, E., Hammel, J., Rouhani, F. N., Brantley, M. L., Barker, A. F., Buist, A. S., et al. (2003). Asthma features in severe alpha (1)-antitrypsin deficiency: Experience of the National Heart, Lung, and Blood Institute Registry. *Chest, 123,* 765–771.

Eriksson, S., Moestrup, T., & Hägerstrand, I. (1975). Liver, lung and malignant disease in heterozygous (PI MZ) α_1-antitrypsin deficiency. *Acta Medica Scandinavica, 198,* 243–247.

Gautam, A., Waldrep, J. C., & Densmore, C. L. (2003). Aerosol gene therapy. *Molecular Biotechnology, 23,* 51–60.

Kleeberger, S. R., & Peden, D. (2005). Gene-environment interactions in asthma and other respiratory diseases. *Annual Review of Medicine, 56,* 383–400.

Larsson, C. (1978). Natural history and life expectancy in severe alpha$_1$-antitrypsin deficiency, PI Z. *Acta Medica Scandinavica, 204,* 345–351.

Laurell, C. B., & Eriksson, S. (1963). The electrophoretic α-1-globulin pattern of serum in α-1-antitrypsin deficiency. *Scandinavian Journal of Clinical and Laboratory Investigation, 15,* 132–140.

Lomas, D. A., & Parfrey, H. (2004). α_1-antitrypsin deficiency. 4: Molecular pathophysiology. *Thorax, 59* 529–535.

Luisetti, M., & Seersholm, N. (2004). α_1-antitrypsin deficiency. 1: Epidemiology of α_1-antitrypsin deficiency. *Thorax, 29,* 164–169.

McElvaney, N. G., Stoller, J. K., Buist, A. S., Prakash, U. B., Brantley, M. L., Schluchter, M. D., et al. (1997). Baseline characteristics of enrollees in the National Heart, Lung and Blood Institute Registry of alpha 1-antitrypsin deficiency. Alpha 1-Antitrypsin Deficiency Registry Study Group. *Chest, 111,* 394–403.

Needham, M., & Stockley, R. A. (2004). α_1-antitrypsin deficiency. 3: Clinical manifestations and natural history. *Thorax, 29,* 441–445.

Parfrey, H., Mahadeva, R., & Lomas, D. A. (2003). α_1-antitrypsin deficiency, liver disease and emphysema. *International Journal of Biochemistry & Cell Biology, 35,* 1009–1014.

Perlmutter, D. H. (1995). Clinical manifestations of alpha-1-antitrypsin deficiency. *Gastroenterology Clinics of North America, 24,* 27–43.

Piitulainen, E., Torling, G., & Eriksson, S. (1997). Effect of age and occupational exposure to airway irritants on lung function in non-smoking individuals with alpha-1-antitrypsin deficiency (PiZZ). *Thorax, 52,* 244–248.

Qu, D., Teckman, J. H., & Perlmutter, D. H. (1997). Review: α_1-antitrypsin deficiency associated liver disease. *Journal of Gastroenterology and Hepatology, 12,* 404–416.

Sharp, H. L. (1976). The current status of α-1-antitrypsin, a protease inhibitor, in gastrointestinal disease. *Gastroenterology, 70,* 611–621.

Sharp, H. L, Bridges, R. A., Krivit, W., & Freier, E. F. L. (1969). Cirrhosis associated with alpha-1-antitrypsin deficiency: A previously unrecognized inherited disorder. *Journal of Laboratory and Clinical Medicine, 73,* 934–939.

Silverman, E. K. (2002). Hereditary pulmonary emphysema. In D. L. Rimoin, J. M. Connor, R. E. Pyeritz, & B. R. Korf (Eds.), *Emery and Rimoin's principles and practice of medical genetics* (4th ed., pp. 1617–1642). New York: Churchill Livingstone.

Sipahi, T., Kara, C., Tavil, B., Inci, A., & Oksal, A. (2003). Alpha-1 antitrypsin deficiency: An overlooked cause of late hemorrhagic disease of the newborn. *Journal of Pediatric Hematology and Oncology, 25,* 274–275.

Stecenko, A. A., & Brigham, K. L. (2003). Gene therapy progress and prospects: Alpha-1 antitrypsin. *Gene Therapy, 10,* 95–99.

Stoller, J. K. (1997). Clinical features and natural history of severe α_1-antitrypsin deficiency. *Chest, 111*(Suppl.), 123S–128S.

Stoller, J. K., Fallat, R., Schluchter, M. D., O'Brien, R. G., Connor, J. T., et al. (2003). Augmentation therapy with α_1-antitrypsin: Patterns of use and adverse events. *Chest, 123,* 1425–1434.

Stoller, J. K., Smith, P., Yang, P., & Spray, J. (1994). Physical and social impact of alpha-1-antitrypsin deficiency: Results of a survey. *Cleveland Clinic Journal of Medicine, 61,* 461–467.

Sveger, T. (1976). Liver disease in alpha$_1$-antitrypsin deficiency detected by screening of 200,000 infants. *New England Journal of Medicine, 294,* 1316–1321.

Sveger, T., Piitulainen, E., & Arborelius, M., Jr. (1994). Lung function in adolescents with alpha-1-antitrypsin deficiency. *Acta Paediatrica, 83,* 1170–1173.

Zhou, H., & Fischer, H. P. (1998). Liver carcinoma in PiZ alpha-1-antitrypsin deficiency. *American Journal of Surgical Pathology, 22,* 742–748.

23

Cancer

The contribution of genetic mechanisms to cancer development and metastasis continues to be elucidated. About 10% of all cancers are believed to be inherited directly. However, genetically determined individual differences that can determine susceptibility to cancer when exposed to a given environmental "trigger" may be important in whether or not cancer eventually develops in a much larger proportion of individuals. The genetic component can be through a gene directly causing cancer, a pre-cancerous condition or a susceptibility to environmental agents that can result in cancer. As an illustration of the latter, there are many polymorphisms in the cytochrome p450 enzymes (see chapter 18). These enzymes metabolize polycyclic aromatic hydrocarbon compounds found in cigarette smoke. Persons with specific polymorphic variants of the cytochrome p450 enzymes metabolize these compounds differently from others and have increased lung cancer rates. Thus, some people are more susceptible to lung cancer when exposed to cigarette smoke because of their different genetic makeup.

In the current understanding of cancer, some change in genetic material occurs causing normal function to go awry. This can be a germline or somatic mutation (see chapters 2, 4). Therefore, all cancer is a genetic disease in one sense although the genetic change may not be heritable or passed to another generation. The understanding of cancer development has been difficult because the term cancer really includes at least 100 different forms of disease that we collectively call cancer. Further, a particular cancer may exist in both a hereditary and non-hereditary form with the basic causative processes being similar. Cancer continues to be a leading cause of death worldwide and is second in the United States. More than 500,000 deaths per year are from cancer. The National Cancer Institute has a Cancer Genome Anatomy Project (see chapter 1) that will eventually define genetic changes in cancer cells, hopefully resulting in ideas for both preventative and therapeutic approaches. In this chapter, mutation of genetic material leading to cancer, single-gene disorders associated with cancer, chromosome abnormalities and cancer, inherited childhood cancers, cancer in families, selected specific cancers with a genetic base, *BRCA1* and *BRCA2* mutations, genetic testing, prevention, and counseling in cancer, including ethical issues, will be discussed.

The development of cancer is thought to be a multi-step process with a necessary first step being a mutation in the genetic material. This first mutation could be a hereditary one occurring in all germline cells, in which case the mutation would be in all body cells, or the mutation could be somatically acquired in one or more cells, and passed to descendants of that cell(s) but not inherited by the next vertical generation (from parent to child) through the gonads. As a second step, an environmental agent could then cause mutations again in one or more somatic cells. In some cases, somatic mutations might accumulate until neoplastic cells arose, divided, and maintained a clone (a population of cells derived from one cell). This might be sufficient to produce malignancy, or other genes could be involved in the steps from hyperplasia to neoplasm to malignancy to metastasis. The model for retinoblastoma is discussed later in this chapter.

At the present time, mutations in three classes of genes appear to be the most important in triggering cancer. These are (1) proto-oncogenes, (2) tumor suppressor genes, and (3) DNA damage recognition and repair genes including DNA mismatch genes. It is also possible that other mutations might predispose individuals to cancer. For example, genes that alter the metabolism of potentially carcinogenic agents in the environment or food, that impact upon a cell-binding site for oncogenic viruses, or that alter the tissue response to hormones or drugs might provide the initial susceptibility for another cancer-causing event to act upon. Mutant genes may also allow tumor cells to attract and develop a blood supply, thus influencing metastasis. Knowledge of these can suggest treatment approaches that interfere with this process. Some known inherited rare single-gene disorders result in cancer, and some forms of cancer are directly inherited.

The three classes of genes mentioned previously, proto-oncogenes, tumor suppressor genes, and DNA repair genes have normal cellular functions. Proto-oncogenes are normally concerned with the regulation of cell growth, differentiation, division, senescence, and apoptosis. Each oncogene appears to code for a protein that is involved in signal transduction from the cell membrane receptors to the nucleus, or has a function in growth factors and their receptors or nuclear proto-oncogenes (such as in the MYC family) and transcription factors.When allelic mutations generate variant oncogenic forms of proto-oncogenes, these become known as oncogenes. Oncogenic alleles can be activated as a result of specific chromosome abnormalities as discussed below or by other mechanisms. The activation of oncogenes has been likened to a jammed accelerator in a car. Tumor suppressor genes (formerly known as anti-oncogenes) are inhibitory to cell growth and division. These genes are involved in complex interactions that integrate stimulatory and inhibitory messages, both internally and externally, and govern the regulation of the cell cycle that includes protein synthesis, rest, DNA replication, and mitosis. Less is known about tumor suppressor genes than oncogenes. The best known tumor suppressor gene is p53 (sometimes known as TP53), which is the most common mutated cancer gene known so far. When functioning normally, p53 suppresses genes that are involved in the stimulation of growth and activates genes involved in the control of growth, differentiation and, apoptosis (the process of

programmed cell death). Another is p16 (also known as CDKNZA) which, when mutated, is associated with multiple primary melanomas and pancreatic cancer in some families. DNA damage repair genes normally do just that—act in ways to repair damage that occurs to DNA either during replication or because of external mutational events. These are also known as DNA mismatch repair genes because they detect DNA sections that do not match. When a mutation in DNA damage repair genes causes a loss of function, the rate of mutation increases generally in affected cells, and may affect tumor suppressor genes and oncogenes.

Events influencing metastasis are also controlled, at least partly, through genetic alterations. NME1 is the gene that encodes Nm23H1, which acts as a metastasis suppressor. When mutated, aggressive metastatic growth has been observed in melanomas, breast cancer, and other tumors.

Cells possess back-up systems that come into play when damage occurs to their structure or control systems. One back-up system is the destruction of a damaged cell by apoptosis. Tumors may occur when a developing cancer cell evades apoptosis. Another theory is one in which the number of times a cell can reproduce itself is limited through the telomeres, a structure at the end of each chromosome, acting like a plastic tip on a shoelace. Telomeres get shorter and shorter as the cell ages. This mechanism eventually instructs the cell to enter senescence. Telomerase is an enzyme that stops telomeres from shortening in the embryo. It is rarely seen in adults except in certain cancers. One theory is that cancer develops because of activation of a gene coding for telomerase in tumor cells, allowing cells to keep replicating and allowing tumors to grow larger. This role of telomerase has been disputed by some. However, the development of agents that can block telomerase and allow cells to die normally is a potential treatment strategy.

Cancer in animals has been shown to arise because of infection with tumor viruses. An example is the Rous sarcoma virus which causes soft tissue tumors in chickens. The viral genes implicated in cancer causation often are altered forms of human oncogenes. Examples are MYC, the avian myelocytomatosis virus, and RAS, the rat sarcoma virus. In humans, acute T-cell leukemia is caused by a retrovirus, HTLV-I. The human papillomaviruses contribute to cervical cancer, probably through interference with tumor suppressor proteins. Primary hepatocellular carcinoma is often associated with chronic viral hepatitis caused by infection with hepatitis virus B or C, and may not appear until 40 or 50 years after initial infection.

Cancer may result because of changes in structure or expression of specific genes by a variety of mechanisms such as gene mutation, gene amplification, chromosomal loss or rearrangement, altered methylation of certain genes, somatic recombination, and others. Once those occur, oncogenes may be activated or tumor suppressor genes inactivated. The result is cell deregulation of cell growth and differentiation that results in a tumor which undergoes genetic changes to become malignant, and eventually, metastatic. A tumor suppressor gene called *PTEN* by one group and *MMAC1* (mutated in multiple advanced cancers 1) by another, when inactivated or lost, allows progression of certain prostate, brain (especially gliomas), and other cancers. Other genes, such as *AIB1,* may enhance tumor growth.

Nurses should be alert for suggestions that a person with cancer may have an inherited form. These include any of the following:

- the occurrence of adult-type tumors in a child,
- occurrence of the cancer at an unusually young age for that cancer (germline tumors generally appear earlier than those due to sporadic causes),
- two or more unusual cancers in the same person or close relative,
- cancer occurring in the less usually affected sex (e.g., breast cancer in the male),
- recognition of syndrome or genetic disease in a person that may predispose to cancer,
- bilateral tumors in paired organs or multiple tumor presentations, and
- multiply affected family members.

For specific diseases, such as breast cancer, bilateral appearance of premalignant lesions, or for colon cancer, the appearance of multiple polyps, may also suggest an inherited predisposition. In addition, for breast and ovarian cancer, some referral guidelines modify guidelines according to the ethnicity of the client. For example, those of Eastern European Jewish descent may be referred for genetic evaluation of breast cancer if was diagnosed at an older age than if the person were not of Jewish descent.

SINGLE-GENE DISORDERS AND CANCER

At least 200 of the known single gene disorders are associated with neoplasia development. A few are shown in Table 23.1. This number might even be larger if the affected person always lived long enough to allow the malignancy to manifest itself. The single-gene disorders can be divided into those in which the cancer itself is considered to be an inherited trait and those genetic syndromes that predispose to malignancy. In the preneoplastic conditions, the initial abnormality is not malignant itself, but the risk of cancer development is greatly increased because of the inherited predisposition. Certain disruptive disorders of tissue organization can predispose to tumor development such as Cowden syndrome, neurofibromatosis (see chapter 6), tylosis (a rare autosomal dominant disorder with keratosis of the palms and feet and esophageal cancer), and others. Albinism and tyrosinemia (see chapter 11) are associated with increased risk for skin cancer and hepatoma respectively.

DNA Repair and Xeroderma Pigmentosa

DNA is constantly being repaired and replicated in the body to counteract damage from both internal and external sources, such as damage resulting from ultraviolet light. DNA damage results in interference with normal transcription and replication and can also result in mutation and chromosome aberrations. Damage can lead to genetic instability with progression to cancer, aging, and cell and tissue degeneration. Various systems repair changed bases, DNA adducts (products formed when carcinogens form bonds with DNA), crosslinks (unwanted connections between strands of DNA or bases), double-strand breaks, and other damage. There are several mechanisms of DNA repair that may involve multiple steps: direct repair, base and nucleotide excision (removal), postreplication repair, and others. In nucleotide excision repair, recognition of damage must first

TABLE 23.1   Some Hereditary Disorders Associated with Cancer

Disorder	Inheritance mode	Other features
Peutz-Jeghers syndrome	AD	Melanin pigmentation of oral mucosa, face, lips, fingers, and toes; diffuse polyposis and cancer of any region of GI tract, especially the small intestine, ovary, testes
Turcot syndrome (many are FAP variants, some are not)	AD	Primary nervous system tumors such as cerebral gliomas, colon adenomatous polyps of colon, carcinoma
von-Hippel-Lindau syndrome	AD	Development of multiple tumors including pancreatic cysts and cancer, renal cell cysts and carcinomas, pheochromocytomas, retinal angiomas, cerebellar hemangioblastomas, carcinoma, pancreatic cysts, and adrenal tumors
Multiple endocrine neoplasia (MEN)	AD	
Type 1 (Wermer syndrome)		Parathyroid hyperplasia, pituitary tumors, pancreatic islet cell tumors, peptic ulcer disease
Type 2A (Sipple syndrome)		Parathyroid hyperplasia, pheochromocytomas, medullary thyroid cancer
Type 2B		Pheochromocytoma, mucosal neuromas, medullary thyroid cancer, characteristic facial appearance with hypertrophied lips, Marfanoid appearance, enlarged nerves of GI tract and megacolon, skeletal abnormalities
Cowden disease (multiple hamartoma syndrome)	AD	Breast fibrocystic disease and cancer, goiters and thyroid cancer, meningioma. Papules on face, especially nose, eyes, mouth; other skin lesions such as vitiligo and café-au-lait spots, polyposis in GI tract
Juvenile polyposis	AD	Multiple juvenile polyps of GI tract, adenocarcinoma of colons, and other GI lesions may be seen. Usually present under 10 years of age, but can be seen into early adulthood.
Hereditary mixed polyposis syndrome	AD	Colorectal polyps including atypical juvenile polyps, adenomas with early adenocarcinoma of the colon and/or rectum. Not firmly established.
XY gonadal dysgenesis	X-linked recessive	Dysgerminoma
Muir-Torre syndrome	AD	Adenocarcinoma of gastrointestinal tract such as colon, duodenum, genitourinary sites, and skin lesions including basal and sebaceous cell carcinoma and adenoma. Rare

AD = autosomal dominant transmission, AR = autosomal recessive transmission, GI = gastrointestinal.

occur, followed by incision of the damaged DNA strand on both sides of the lesion, excision of the damaged part, DNA synthesis, and ligation. Many proteins and enzymes participate in the repair process.

Xeroderma pigmentosa (XP) most often results from defects in nucleotide excision repair and is genetically heterogenous. Several complementation groups have been identified and are known as XP-A to XP-G as well as a variant XP-V. In this variant, excision repair is normal but postreplication repair is defective. Within each group, genetic and clinical heterogeneity may occur. For example in the XP-D group, those with a certain glutamine variant are at increased risk of developing AML after chemotherapy. XP is relatively rare in the population, with a frequency of 1 in 65,000 to 1 in 1,000,000, and is inherited in an autosomal recessive manner. From early infancy, children with XP are extremely sensitive to the sun and UV light. Without protection, their skin develops freckles, dryness, and scaling. Burning with blistering, atrophy, and scarring occurs, and areas of depigmentation may be seen. Various lesions such as keratoses develop, and basal and squamous cell carcinomas arise, in either childhood or early adolescence, followed by malignant melanomas that are usually at multiple sites. The chance for these individuals to develop skin cancer and melanomas is generally considered to be near 100% and 50%, respectively. Damage to the eye is frequent, with corneal damage and eyelid contractures occurring. Death often occurs by 30 years of age. Some cases of XP (about 20%) have neurologic abnormalities such as microcephaly, hearing loss, intellectual impairment, ataxia, and spastic quadriplegia (DeSanctis-Cacchione Syndrome), in addition to the other features. The story of a family with two children with XP was the subject of a 1997 television movie called *Children of Darkness.*

Prototype of Long-Term Nursing Plan

XP is an excellent example of how the nurse can develop a preventative long-term plan to attempt to modify the environment to minimize the severity of effects. Such a plan can be done for any of the rare genetic diseases. The whole family must be involved with the entire approach, which is geared to minimizing the affected person's exposure to UV light and thus preventing its consequences. Much of the prevention of exposure to UV light has been made more reasonable by the availability of products to block UV light, including "frogskin" (available through dermatologists). Some aspects of such a plan, which can also be used as appropriate in albinism and other UV-sensitive disorders, include the following:

- If the breadwinner in the family is mobile, geographic relocation to an area of lower UV exposure, such as the northwest corner of the United States where it is misty, will be a great help, particularly if the area the family presently lives in is a very sunny one.
- Protective clothing with long pants, long-sleeved shirts with a high neck, the use of sunglasses with side panels, and the wearing of a broad-brimmed hat are suggested, but sun blockers may modify the need for some of this.

- Hair should be worn long to protect the neck.
- True sunscreens and blockers, such as titanium dioxide or material such as frogskin, can be used on any exposed skin areas.
- Standard incandescent light bulbs should be used in the home rather than fluorescent fixtures. If the affected individual must frequently be in a location, such as school, where fluorescent lighting is used, covers can be used.
- When riding in a bus, train, or car, the affected person should be away from open windows.
- Physical activity should be encouraged and maintained. Outdoor activities such as tennis, swimming, and track can be done indoors, with adequate protection, or at night.
- As the child with XP begins school, the incorporation of the school administrators, school nurse, and teachers into the protection plan is essential. Potential hazards in the school environment need to be identified and evaluated. In the classroom the child should not be seated near the windows.
- Unnecessary radiation should be avoided.
- Medications should be evaluated for their ability to increase the impact of UV light, and those that do so should not be used if at all possible.
- Chemotherapeutic agents for the treatment of any cancers that may develop can aggravate the basic defect and must be carefully chosen.
- Frequent whole body examinations by a qualified dermatologist should be routine.

Because both parents are usually heterozygous carriers of the gene for XP, referral for genetic counseling should be done. Prenatal diagnosis is available for XP and can allow the parents options in their future reproductive plans.

Reports of an increased rate of malignancy (especially skin cancer) among the carriers of the XP gene should alert the nurse to encourage the entire family to maintain a routine physical examination at regular intervals without arousing unnecessary anxiety. Ongoing emotional support and counseling should be provided from the time of diagnosis for the affected person and all family members in order to avoid potential problems and maintain morale. Extreme commitment and motivation is required to adhere to this type of plan.

The vigilance necessary can lead to behavioral problems in the child and conflicting feelings in the parents, especially when the child "forgets" some aspect of it. Adolescence, with its concerns about self-image and peer group approval, can be a particularly trying time. While much of the treatment is based on manifestations or on prevention as detailed, recently a DNA repair enzyme has been applied topically. Gene therapy would open new possibilities.

Disorders of Chromosome Instability

There are three classic disorders associated with some type of chromosome instability such as breaks, rearrangements, or fragility that predispose to malignancy. These are ataxia telangiectasia, Bloom syndrome, and Fanconi anemia. Another, Nijmegen breakage syndrome (a rare chromosomal instability disorder that includes immune deficiency, microcephaly, hypersensitivity to ionizing radiation, and an increased incidence of lymphoid malignancies), was thought to be a variant of ataxia telangiectasia, but subsequently the defective gene, *NBS-1*, was identified. All are inherited in an autosomal recessive manner and are individually rare in the population.

Ataxia Telangiectasia

Ataxia telangiectasia (AT), also known as the Louis-Bar syndrome, has a prevalence of about 1 in 40,000 in the United States and is more common in some Mediterranean populations. The mutant gene is *ATM*, located at 11q22-23 which encodes a protein kinase that plays a role in DNA damage repair. It appears that this mutation causes effects in gene expression of apparently unrelated genes located downstream from the gene mutation, which may contribute to a phenotype of AT carriers that vary from controls and may contribute to less efficiency in repair of ionizing radiation damage. The affected child usually appears normal at birth, but progressive cerebellar ataxia usually becomes noticeable when the child begins to walk and experiences difficulty. Oculocutaneous telangiectases, appearing as bloodshot eyes, and a butterfly rash on the face become evident in early childhood. The rash worsens on exposure to sunlight. The facial appearance is often sad, with a slow smile. Growth retardation, drooling, and defective speech may

occur. In about one-third, there is mild mental retardation. Humoral and cellular immune dysfunction are present. The immune defects lead to severe and progressive sinopulmonary infections that can lead to early death before malignancies become evident. Lymphoreticular malignancies, especially lymphosarcomas and leukemias, are most common and develop at an early age. Insulin-resistant diabetes mellitus is common. Spontaneous chromosome breakage occurs and cells are extremely sensitive to ionizing radiation. By adolescence these children are usually confined to a wheelchair and the median age of death has been estimated in the mid-20s. AT heterozygotes, who may have a population frequency as high as 1.0% to 1.4%, are at an increased risk of developing breast cancer and may account for 7% to 8% of all breast cancer cases, although there is some debate about this connection. Given this frequency, testing for AT heterozygosity should be done for persons with breast cancer, because they are more sensitive to certain anti-neoplastic regimens than to others (for example radiation), and so a regimen appropriate for them needs to be designed.

Bloom Syndrome

Bloom syndrome (BS) results from a mutation affecting an enzyme needed for genomic stability in somatic cells that is manifested by sister chromatid exchanges and various structural chromosome anomalies and rearrangements called quadriradial patterns. The mutated gene is *BLM* which maps to chromosome 15q26.1. It encodes a RecQ helicase, which is an unwinding enzyme that functions in DNA repair pathways. The affected individual suffers severe growth retardation that begins in utero. The adult height attained is usually under 5 feet. Its frequency is 1:60,000 to 1:1,000,000 depending on the population. It is most frequent among Ashkenazi Jews, and in this group is believed due to a founder mutation with a carrier frequency of about 1% in this population. Sun sensitivity with development of characteristic telangiectasias in a butterfly pattern on the nose and cheeks, malar hypoplasia, and long pointed faces are seen. Exposure to UV light leads to scarring and atrophy. Intelligence is not impaired. Decreased levels of immunoglobulins lead to frequent infections. Primary malignancies develop, with leukemia being most common followed by lymphoma and gastrointestinal adenocarcinomas. Sun protection is essential and premature death, often in the third decade, is usually due to malignancy.

Fanconi Anemia

Fanconi anemia (FA) is manifested by pancytopenic anemia with eventual bone marrow failure (usually before age 40 years), skin pigmentation abnormalities, cafe-au-lait spots, growth retardation, hearing loss, increased cancer risk, and multiple congenital malformations. The most common are defects in the radius or thumbs, gastrointestinal malformations, congenital hip dislocation, scoliosis, vertebral abnormalities, central nervous system malformations, renal malformations, and gonadal abnormalities with decreased fertility. There are at least 8 complementation groups (FA-A-G) and several of the genes have been cloned. Heterogeneity exists. It appears that one of the FA genes, *FANCD1*, may actually be *BRCA2*. Recognition of the interaction between FA proteins and others involved in DNA repair, such as ATM, BRCA1, and BRCA2, are elucidating the consequences of defective DNA repair. Chromosome abnormalities including gaps, breaks, and rearrangements are seen in the cells. People with FA are at increased risk for acute myelogenous leukemia, squamous cell carcinomas, and solid tumors of the liver and gastrointestinal tract. Care must be taken in selecting chemotherapy because of extreme sensitivity to cross-linking agents such as mitomycin C and others. Stem cell transplantation from bone marrow or umbilical cord blood is used for bone marrow failure and in treating leukemia.

Immunodeficiency Diseases

Other immunodeficiency diseases have an increased rate of oncogenesis associated with them, perhaps because there is impairment of the ability to suppress any spontaneous tumor cells that arise, blunting the immunologic response to viruses, allowing activation of latent viral sequences, or for another reason. Many of these individuals have an incidence of malignancy that is 100 to 10,000 times that of the general population when matched for age. Immunodeficiency diseases known to be associated with the development of cancer include Wiskott-Aldrich syndrome, IgA deficiency, severe combined immunodeficiency, and Di George syndrome (see chapter 19). The cancers seen are mostly leukemia, lymphomas, or epithelial.

CONSTITUTIONAL CHROMOSOME DISORDERS AND CANCER

Constitutional chromosome disorders are those in which chromosome abnormalities are present throughout the body cells, not just in one or a few types of tissue. A few are known to be associated with an increased risk of cancer. The best known of these is Down syndrome. The rate of acute leukemia in patients with Down syndrome is 16 to 30 times the rate found in normal individuals of the same age, and its onset is earlier. Acute non-lymphocytic leukemia (ANLL) predominates in children with Down syndrome, in contrast to other types of leukemia in children without Down syndrome in the same age group. A form of megakaryoblastic leukemia develops in about 10% of newborns with Down syndrome and, of those that recover, about 25% will develop acute megakaryoblastic leukemia, usually by 4 years of age. The reason for the association of leukemia and Down syndrome remains unknown, but one speculation is that a general cell sensitivity to transformation or induction into malignancy may be present.

In Klinefelter syndrome (47,XXY), the incidence of breast cancer is increased to approximately 66 times that of normal males. The reason for this is not known, but may be related to disturbances in hormonal balance produced by the presence of the extra X chromosome. There have been reports of an apparent predisposition to the development of ANLL. There is also an increased association between Klinefelter syndrome and both gonadal and extragonadal germ cell tumors. In Turner syndrome, there may be mosaicism with both a 45,X and a 46,XY cell line. In those individuals with the Y chromosome line, the risk of the development of a gonadal malignancy such as dysgerminoma or gonadalblastoma ranges from 15% to 30%. Thus, it is important to identify those patients with a Y chromosome cell line. Periodic examination and monitoring to detect early malignant changes is vital.

CONGENITAL ANOMALIES

The cancer most associated with anomalies appears to be Wilms tumor (often associated with WAGR [Wilms tumor, aniridia, genitourinary anomalies, mental retardation] syndrome and Beckwith-Wiedemann syndrome), which is discussed below. An example of a congenital anomaly that is associated with malignancy is cryptorchidism (undescended testes), which is found at birth in about 2% to 4% of full-term male infants and about 30% of premature infants. They may spontaneously descend by one year of age. The risk of malignancy in cryptorchidism is estimated at about 22 times that for normal testes, and about 10% of all males with testicular malignancy are or have had cryptorchidism. The risk for development of malignancy is about 6 times greater for abdominal than for inguinal testis, and if repair is done before 11 years of age, the risk for malignant development may return to normal. If not, increased risk continues, and about 50% of these males have testicular dysgenesis. Interestingly, about 25% of tumors in patients with unilateral cryptorchidism develop in the descended one. Approximately 4% of males with cryptorchidism have close relatives who are also affected, and it is believed that the disorder is inherited in a multifactorial way. Nurses should stress to the parents the importance of early repair in order to prevent cancer development.

INHERITED CANCERS OF CHILDHOOD

While cancers are relatively rare in childhood, malignancies develop in about 1 in 600 children, and inherited tumors are part of the picture. Two of these, retinoblastoma and Wilms tumor, are discussed below. Another sequela of treatment for childhood cancer has been the risk of development of second cancers, particularly when treated with radiation. Those who have survived germline mutational cancers appear more likely to develop second neoplasms in adulthood. In a study of the outcomes of pregnancy in female partners of childhood cancer survivors, the proportion of pregnancies resulting in a liveborn infant was lower than for a comparison group, and there was a sex ratio

reversal (Green et al., 2003). In contrast to many of the genetic syndromes that predispose to malignancy and often follow a recessive form of inheritance, most of the directly inherited neoplasias follow an autosomal dominant (AD) mode.

Retinoblastoma

In 1971, Knudson proposed a "two-hit" model for retinoblastoma development. Persons with the inherited form of retinoblastoma had a germline mutation that was present in all body cells. A second mutation (somatic) occurring in any developing retinoblasts leads to development of a retinoblastoma (see Figure 23.1). Thus, in some patients with the predisposing germline mutation, a second somatic mutation might never occur, and they would never develop retinoblastoma. In others, bilateral or multifocal tumors might arise due to one or more "hits." In the sporadic type of retinoblastoma, both of the mutational events are somatic and occur in the same retinoblast. This type of event is very infrequent. Each of these two mutational events affects the RB1 gene (a tumor suppressor gene) on a different parental chromosome so that the result is the inactivation of *RB1* within the cell. In some cases the loss of function or loss of heterozygosity (LOH) results from a subsequent, often sub-microscopic, deletion of the chromosome that includes the region of the *RB1* gene, 13q14, or from events such as mitotic recombination followed by nondisjunction. Other tumors may be associated with mutations in both *RB1* alleles such as osteosarcoma, soft tissue sarcomas, breast cancer, bladder cancer, and others. In addition, hypermethylation of part of *RB1* appears significant in nonhereditary unilateral retinoblastoma. In some cases, a parent of origin effect has also been described due to imprinting (see chapter 4).

Retinoblastoma results from loss of function (LOF) in the gene *RB1*, a growth suppressor. In the inherited type, a germline mutation results in every body cell containing a mutant and normal gene, RB1+/RB1−. At this point there is a genetic predisposition for retinoblastoma. For a retinoblastoma to actually occur, a second somatic mutation of the remaining normal allele must occur within the retinal cell, and it does in about 90–95% of those with germline mutations. Thus, about 90–95% of children with a germline *RB1* mutation develop

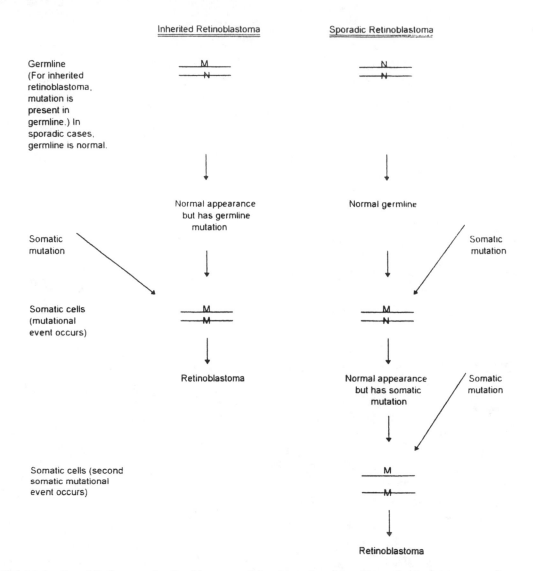

FIGURE 23.1   Two-hit theory of retinoblastoma. (M = Mutation; N = Normal; Mutation can refer to alteration in gene or a deletion.)

retinoblastoma before 5 years of age. They are also at risks approaching 2,000 times that of the general population for developing osteosarcoma.

Retinoblastoma is a childhood tumor formed from the precursors of retinal rod and cone cells. In the United States it occurs in approximately 1 in 15,000–20,000 births. As more individuals survive and reproduce, this frequency should increase. In general, persons with non-hereditary retinoblastoma have only one eye affected by one tumor. Persons with the hereditary type usually are affected bilaterally, but in about 15% of cases, only a unilat-

eral tumor is seen due to either chance alone or because another tumor has not yet developed. Hereditary tumors generally appear earlier than non-hereditary ones (mean ages of 12–15 and 24–30 months, respectively). Detection can be difficult because of early development. Parents may be the ones to report a "glint, gleam, glow, glare, flash, or reflection" in the child's eye or call it a "cat's" or "animal" eye. On ophthalmoscopic examination, a white or yellow-white pupillary reflex (leukocoria) suggests retinoblastoma, and must be further investigated. Infants born to families in which there is a history of retinoblastoma should have a full retinal examination a few weeks after birth and then every two months. Strabismus is another common presenting sign. Treatment of unilateral tumors in particular is generally by enucleation, possibly followed by chemotherapy. Sometimes radiation is used. Diagnosis of retinoblastoma is a devastating experience for parents and family and should be done in a caring, confidential, and sensitive manner with more than one discussion taking place and with the availability of support.

Nurses should realize that lack of a family history of retinoblastoma does not indicate that the tumor in that family is non-hereditary or due to a new mutation because of the possibility of non-penetrance. Thus, careful evaluation of family members including careful history, chromosome analysis, DNA testing in appropriate cases, and clinical indicators will be components of genetic counseling. Murphree and Clark (2002) give the following empirical risk estimates for development of retinoblastoma: in inherited cases, 45% recurrence risk for both siblings and offspring; for nonhereditary cases, about 1% risk for both siblings and offspring; and for cases in which a new mutation occurred in the germline of the affected person, about a 2% recurrence risk for siblings and 45% for offspring. For offspring of familial retinoblastoma where the person is unilaterally affected, Murphree and Clark believe that the risk in both siblings and offspring is less than 45%. Children who have recovered from retinoblastoma should be followed to detect the occurrence of primary tumors developing in later childhood or even adulthood.

Wilms Tumor

Wilms tumor, an embryonal renal malignancy, represents about 6% of all pediatric cancers in the United States, and has a frequency of about 1 in 10,000 children. It occurs in both hereditary and sporadic forms. About 4–5% have bilateral tumors and 1–2% have a family history of Wilms tumors. The first Wilms tumor mutant gene, *WT1*, encoding a zinc finger protein (see chapter 2), is located on chromosome 11p13. It is expressed only in certain tissues. In some cases, there is an association with aniridia, genitourinary anomalies, and mental retardation (WAGR syndrome) associated with deletions of chromosome 11p13, and also with hamartomas and hemihypertrophy. Certain germline mutations in zinc fingers of *WT1* occur in Denys-Drash syndrome (Wilms tumor, male pseudohermaphroditism, congenital nephropathy). Other gene sites exist, including a *WT2* locus, and in a few families, it appears that there may be two familial Wilms tumor loci, *FWT1* (chromosome 17q) and *FWT2* (chromosome 19q). Gene expression studies may eventually lead to targeted treatments and improved prognostic indicators. Those with Beckwith-Wiedemann syndrome (an overgrowth syndrome with gigantism, macroglossia, endocrine problems, and other anomalies) are at increased risk for Wilms tumor. These groups need careful evaluation, screening with ultrasound, and monitoring for early detection. In about half the cases, activation of the silent maternal *IGF2* (insulin growth factor) allele occurs, relaxing imprinting. Increased expression of *IGF2* leads to somatic overgrowth in Beckwith-Wiedemann syndrome and tumor predisposition. The familial forms (usually bilateral, possible family history) are inherited in an autosomal dominant manner with about 60% penetrance. For those with the sporadic form (usually unilateral tumors with no family history, associated defects, or malformations) the recurrence risk for offspring is less than 1–2%. Harper (1998) estimates the risk for subsequent children of a parent with bilateral tumors, parent with unilateral tumor and affected relative, and an unaffected parent with 2 affected children as 30%. For a parent with a unilateral tumor or a sibling with bilateral tumors, the risk for subsequent children is estimated at 10%. When molecular studies are available, these should be reassessed. These children are also prone to develop second tumors after treatment. Firstline chemotherapy is generally with dactinomycin, vincristine and doxorubicin as well as surgical resection and defined radiotherapy in some cases. Survival rates tend to be good, about 90% in localized disease.

CANCER IN FAMILIES

The aggregation of cancer in families has long been a subject of interest. The reasons for such aggregation are not always clear, apart from the known inherited syndromes and tumors previously discussed. The significance of much of Lynch's early work in the area of cancer families was not recognized for its importance at the time. The occurrence of more than one neoplasm in a family can occur simply by chance because of the frequency of neoplasias in the population; it could represent common exposure to environmental factors, either chemical or infectious; or inherited genetic susceptibility can be the cause. Genetic factors can contribute both to familial susceptibility and also to the single occurrences of cancer in smaller families. Nurses should suspect genetic influences when they observe the onset of a common cancer earlier than is usual (for example, 10 to 20 years or more earlier in colon cancer), the occurrence of adult type tumors in a child, bilateral tumor development in paired organs, the occurrence of multiple primary neoplasms, recognition of a genetic condition predisposing to cancer, occurrence of a rare tumor such as adrenocortical carcinomas, or a history of cancer in several family members.

"Cancer families" are particularly interesting because they offer the opportunity for the identification of physical, cytogenetic, or biochemical markers, and because extensive family and personal histories may help to pinpoint the underlying disease mechanism. Additionally, cancer detection measures can be applied to other family members who may be at high risk, especially where screening tests are useful. Various families may show a specific inheritance pattern for certain cancers that are not shown to be heritable in the population at large. Careful family evaluation of each patient presenting with a cancer may help to clarify contributing genetic factors. The formation of a National Cancer Registry with regional centers that would keep track of individuals with familial predispositions to various cancers has been implemented in some places to promote medical counseling as well as surveillance, and individual tumor registries exist. However, some see this as an invasion of privacy and violation of confidentiality.

Li-Fraumeni Syndrome

One of the primary ways to collect information about families can be through a detailed family history. This should include a history of benign neoplasms and birth defects. When meticulously followed up by someone who is trained in the specific information to collect, this can result in identification not only of the type of genetic transmission operating for that family but also of new relationships and understandings. An example is the circumstances that led to the eventual elucidation of the Li-Fraumeni syndrome. Li and Fraumeni (1969) described the investigation of a family that began in Massachusetts with the hospital admission of a child with rhabdomyosarcoma. A family history revealed acute leukemia in the father and unknown cancers in other relatives. Interviews with parents led first to Arizona, where a high frequency of cancers was noted in relatives of the father. Relatives lost to contact were located by means of old family and courthouse records, and family members in Ohio were located. In this branch of the family, 5 of 10 persons had died with cancer. Hospital pathology and mortality records were used to establish and confirm diagnoses. A high proportion of this family's neoplasms were sarcomas and breast cancer, most cases being diagnosed before age 35 years. This experience led these investigators to review the histories of children treated for rhabdomyosarcoma nationally, and ultimately led to the uncovering of excessive soft tissue sarcomas, breast cancers, and multiple primary neoplasms occurring together in several families.

Li-Fraumeni syndrome is a rare autosomal dominant inherited disorder occurring in about 1 in 50,000 in which the affected person develops tumors by young adulthood. The most common are breast cancer, soft tissue sarcoma, brain tumors, osteosarcoma, leukemia, and adrenocortical carcinoma. In later life they may develop lung, prostate, pancreatic, colon, and stomach cancer, melanoma, and lymphomas. Multiple and successive tumors often occur. Thus, this should be looked for during health evaluations. Most affected individuals have germline mutations in the p53 tumor suppressor gene (TP53), located on chromosome 17p13, or the Checkpoint kinase 2 gene (hCHK2) which is located on chromosome 22q12.1. The latter activates protein kinase in response to DNA damage, preventing cell cycle progression. Genetic heterogeneity is present. Observations of the Li-Fraumeni families allowed some elucidation of the effects of p53 inactivation and of involvement in a variety of human cancers.

BREAST AND OVARIAN CANCER

More than 200,000 new cases of breast cancer are diagnosed each year in the United States, and about one million worldwide. Breast cancer was one of the cancers in which a hereditary component had been postulated early and its presence in blood relatives cited as a factor increasing risk, particularly if it occurred in a woman's mother, sisters, or aunts. A family history of breast cancer in a close blood relative such as a mother, sister, or aunt, and breast cancer in the family occurring before age 50 years, denote increased risk. Breast cancer may be associated with another syndrome such as Cowden syndrome, be associated in syndromes with other cancers, or occur alone. Gene mutations conferring breast cancer susceptibility have been suggested to interfere with a variety of functions such as genome integrity, DNA damage repair, cell cycle progression, control of cell growth and differentiation, detoxification of arylamines and other environmental carcinogens, estrogen metabolism, growth factor transcription, and others. Two genes that, when mutated, can result in breast cancer (as well as some others) have been identified and are known as *BRCA1* and *BRCA2*. It is believed that *BRCA1* and *BRCA2* mutations are each responsible for about 20% of the hereditary breast cancers. The rest are attributable to other gene mutations, such as a possible *BRCA3* on chromosome 8p, *p53* mutations in Li-Fraumeni syndrome, alterations in the *PTEN* gene for Cowden disease on chromosome 10q, the *LKB1* gene mutation on chromosome 19p associated with Peutz-Jeghers syndrome, the *ATM* mutation associated with ataxia telangiectasia, the *CHEK2*1100del C variant (which may account for as many as 5% of all cases of familial breast cancer), a putative *TSG101* tumor susceptibility gene, heterozygosity for AT, androgen receptor mutations in males, and others as well as interactions among various mutational variants. There is also a relationship with the Fanconi anemia gene mutation. Thus, *BRCA1* and *BRCA2* mutations are believed to be responsible for about 5–10% of all breast cancer. Other genes as described above, some with low penetrance, may confer susceptibility to breast cancer. Some of the genes involved in breast cancer development are still unknown. Birth prevalence of *BRCA1, BRCA2,* and *p53* mutations have been estimated at 1 in 476,

1 in 667, and 1 in 5,000 respectively. Issues of testing for cancer are discussed later in this chapter. The National Cancer Institute has prepared pamphlets and a videotape for patients on genetic testing for breast cancer risk. DNA microarray testing for gene expression in breast cancer is being used to guide treatment approaches and examine prognosis.

Ovarian cancer is the fifth most common cancer and the most common cause of death from gynecological malignancy in women. At least 90% are sporadic; however, the rest are believed due to inherited susceptibility. Hereditary ovarian cancer is often associated with hereditary breast cancer as part of a syndrome or together. There are at least three known AD syndromes such as familial site-specific ovarian cancer, familial breast and ovarian cancer, and the hereditary nonpolyposis colon cancer discussed later in this chapter. The association of ovarian cancer with *BRCA1* and *BRCA2* mutations is discussed in the following section. As is seen in breast cancer, some of the gene mutations resulting in susceptibility to ovarian cancer are as yet unknown.

BRCA1 and *BRCA2*

BRCA1 and 2 normally function as tumor suppressor genes. Germline mutations of *BRCA1* are associated most with breast and ovarian cancer, but both male and female carriers have elevated risks for colon cancer, and males are at increased risk of prostate cancer. Over 900 mutations are known in the *BRCA1* gene on chromosome 17q12-21. Within families, usually the same alteration in *BRCA1* occurs. Both *BRCA1* and *BRCA2* mutations are particularly prevalent in certain population groups, especially Ashkenazi women, and among those women with ovarian cancer, the hereditary proportion may approach 50%. In *BRCA1* mutations, a particular alteration, 185delAG (deletion of an adenine and guanine) is particularly prevalent in Ashkenazi Jewish women. Approximately 1% of them carry this mutation. Another alteration, 5382insC (insertion of a cytosine), is also prevalent. *BRCA2* is located on chromosome 13q12-13. Multiple mutations are also seen in *BRCA2*. More than 900 different mutations are known. There may be an association between the risk and the mutation location. For example, risk appears higher for *BRCA2* mutations within the ovarian cancer cluster region in exon 11. Further studies will add to this information and make counseling more accurate. For females carrying the mutated *BRCA1*, the lifetime risk of developing breast and ovarian cancer has been variously estimated. These estimates have changed with experience and because of differences in populations studied. It is expected that these risks will be altered as new information is forthcoming, and so recent information should be consulted. The risks in the general population for breast cancer and ovarian cancer are about 11% and 1.6% respectively. Different alleles are associated with different risks of both breast and ovarian cancer, but at this time information is incomplete. Familial breast cancer in males is associated with mutations in this susceptibility gene, and surveillance should be instituted. The lifetime risk for a woman with a germline *BRCA1* mutation to develop ovarian cancer is approximately 16% to 44%. The lifetime risk for a woman with a *BRCA1* or *BRCA2* mutated gene to develop breast cancer has been variously estimated at 50% to 85%. More recent studies tend to the lower end of these ranges. The risk of prostate cancer in male carriers of *BRCA1* mutations is increased fourfold to about 8–16%, and the risk of colorectal cancer is increased fourfold for both males and females. Men with *BRCA2* mutations have an estimated 6% risk of developing breast cancer. For woman with *BRCA2* mutations, the lifetime risk of ovarian cancer is estimated at 10% to 27%. *BRCA1* appears to be involved in some way in X-chromosome inactivation (see chapter 4), and in the offspring of those who had *BRCA1* mutations and breast and/or ovarian cancer, one study noted a sex ratio skewed against male births (de la Hoya et al., 2003). At this time, genetic testing can be done for the major known mutated alleles but not for 100% of all possible mutations. Other genetic factors appear to influence risk and may be additive.

In Iceland, most familial breast and ovarian cancers are associated with *BRCA2* rather than *BRCA1* mutations. In Ashkenazi Jewish women, a particular *BRCA2* mutation, 6174delT, occurs excessively, while 999del5 excessively occurs in Icelanders. About 40–50% of all Ashkenazi Jewish women with ovarian cancer have a germline *BRCA* mutation compared with 5% to 6% of non-Ashkenazi Jewish women. The *BRCA1* and *2* genes are inherited in an autosomal dominant manner. Thus, a daughter of a man or woman with a mutated gene has a 50% chance of inheriting that gene mutation. However, just inheriting the mutant gene does not mean that they will definitely develop cancer although currently it is not possible to predict which gene carriers will develop cancer, and if so, which types, and which will not. In looking for *BRCA1* mutations in the general population of women with breast cancer, Newman, Butler, Millikan, Moorman, and King (1998) found that the best predictors were familial history of both breast and ovarian cancer with at least four affected relatives, followed by family history of ovarian cancer alone. Findings by Newman et al. and by Malone et al. (1998) indicate that some women who have early breast cancer, even with a positive family history, do not have a *BRCA1* mutation, and some do have this mutation without a strong family history. Developing cancer at a young age was found to be important in prediction by Lalloo et al. (2003). Other genetic and nongenetic risk factors also play a role and should be accounted for in individual risk assessments, such as young age at menarche, a body mass index >35, high intake of dietary fat, and others. Thus, developing appropriate guidelines for which women should be offered population-based genetic screening and testing for *BRCA1* or *BRCA2* mutations remains challenging.

COLORECTAL CANCER

Colorectal cancers are another malignancy in which familial clustering has been commonly observed. Several of the rarer Mendelian syndromes have been connected with colorectal cancer. Some have polyps as a feature while others do not, and the number of these polyps can vary considerably and may be linked to genotype or modifying genes. The most frequent directly inherited conditions with colorectal cancer are familial adenomatous polyposis (FAP) and hereditary nonpolyposis colorectal cancer (HNPCC), also known as Lynch syndrome (I and II). FAP is a relatively rare type of autosomal dominant condition caused by germline mutation leading to inactivation of the adenomatous polyposis coli *(APC)* gene located on chromosome 5q. This is a tumor suppressor gene that functions as a regulatory gatekeeper for colorectal epithelial cells and thus, when mutated, hundreds of colon tumors develop and can progress to malignancy. It accounts for about 1% of all colon cancers. A variety of mutations at different *APC* gene locations may occur. A particular *APC* mutation, 11307K, has been found in about 6% of Ashkenazi Jews tested, thus indicating one population in which testing and screening would be useful at this time. Genetic and environmental modifiers are believed to act on the mutated gene because persons with the identical mutation may show diverse FAP phenotypes. Multiple colon polyps are common and are shown in Figure 23.2. Congenital hypertrophy of the retinal pigment epithelium (CHRPE) is a common extracolonic manifestation in FAP, although the CHRPE lesions themselves are not harmful. Somatic mutations of *APC* can occur in sporadic colorectal cancers, and there are other somatic mutated genes associated with a high percentage of colorectal cancers including *p53*, *DCC*, *SAMD4/DPC4*, and *SMAD2*.

HNPCC is more common, represents up to 10% of all colon cancers, and is believed to have a frequency of 1 in 200 to 1 in 2,000. Five different gene mutations have been implicated that account for about three-quarters of HNPCC. These are inactivating germline mutations in various DNA mismatch repair genes. The chromosome location is in parentheses: *MLH1* (3p21), *MSH2* (2p16), *MSH6* or *GTBP* (2p16), *PMS1* (2q31), and *PMS2* (7p). The first two account for most of the cases whereas *MSH6* mutations account for 5% to 10%. Other gene mutations associated with HNPCC include *MLH3*, *EXO1*, and *MSH3*, but at present their significance is unknown. Various mutations in these genes may occur. These genes are involved in DNA mismatch repair—they recognize, excise, and repair mismatched sequences on newly replicated DNA. Some affected persons may have mutations in more than one of these genes. After the initial germline mutation that is inherited, in some cells, the other gene copy is inactivated by a somatic mutation and the result is genetic instability that allows initiated cells to progress rapidly to cancer. Penetrance is about 70% to 80% so that 20% to 30% of those with the mutation may not manifest cancer. HNPCC is autosomal dominant, with a predilection for a proximal colon cancer location and an early age of onset. Type I is limited to colorectal cancer, while individuals with type II (cancer family syndrome) are also at increased cancer risk in other organs, especially the endometrium of the uterus, ovarian, gastric, small intestine, kidney, urinary tract, and hepatobiliary system. The lifetime risk for women with HNPCC is estimated at a 20% to 60% lifetime risk. An observed alteration has been microsatellite instability (MSI), and over 90% of persons with HNPCC-associated colon cancers have MSI. About 15% of persons with colorectal cancer but not HNPCC show MSI. The MSI-H phenotype is present when two of five microsatellite markers are unstable and the MSI-L phenotype is present when one of the five diplays instability. There are various clinical criteria for HNPCC that were developed after the original, more stringent Amsterdam criteria, especially to be used in small families that are known as the Amsterdam II criteria, the Modified Amsterdam criteria, and the Bethesda criteria (Chung & Rustgi, 2003; Vasen, Mecklin, Khan, Lynch, 1991; Vasen, Watson, Mecklin, & Lynch, 1999).

Other patients who have at least two first-degree relatives with colon cancer but who do not appear to have a specific inheritance pattern or gene mutation are often classified as "familial colon cancer." Other genes are involved in colon cancer, such as *BRCA1* discussed above. In some colon cancers, a multistage model has been proposed. For example, beginning with a mutation that results in early adenoma, with *K-RAS* oncogene activation, intermediate disease results; with *DCC* tumor suppressor inactivation, late adenoma occurs; with *p53* tumor suppressor inactivation, colon carcinoma develops; and other mutations contribute to the occurrence of metastasis.

PROSTATE CANCER

Prostate cancer is the most common cancer in men in the United States and accounts for about 40,000 deaths per year. Black males appear to have a higher rate than White, Hispanic, or Asian males in the United States. About 10% to 15% of cases are believed to result from mutated genes. *BRCA1* and *BRCA2* mutations have been discussed above. *BRCA2* mutations have been shown to be responsible for an increased risk for early onset prostate cancer, and 2% of men with early onset prostate

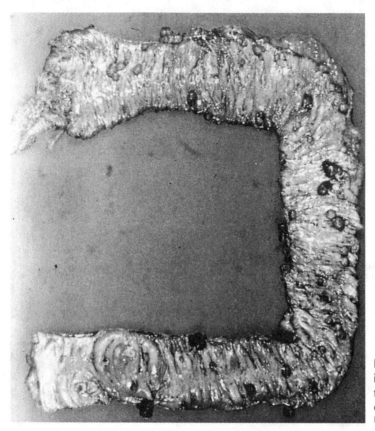

FIGURE 23.2   A section of colon showing the carpeting of polyps as seen in familial adenomatous polyposis.
Courtesy of Dr. John Murphy, Southern Illinois University School of Medicine, Springfield, IL.

cancer were found to harbor germline *BRCA2* gene mutations in one study (Edwards et al., 2003). Another potential susceptibility gene is the hereditary prostate cancer 1 locus *(HPC1)* on chromosome 1q24-25, but other candidate genes are known to be at this location. The major putative susceptibility genes of interest for prostate cancer currently are *ELAC2*, a candidate for the hereditary prostate cancer 2 locus; MSR1, on chromosome 8p; and *RNASEL*, a candidate for *HPC1*, which is a ribonuclease. Mutations of the latter appear more frequent in Ashkenazi Jewish men with prostate cancer than in those without prostate cancer. Other genes proposed to be involved include those that influence cell proliferation and metastasis. For a review, see DeMarzo, Nelson, Isaacs, and Epstein (2003). Genetic polymorphisms such as in the cytochrome P450 gene family such as *CYP3A4*, which is involved in androgen metabolism may also play roles in susceptibility to prostate cancer. At this time, no associated gene mutations are

identified that have as direct and strong association as *BRCA1* does with breast cancer. In persons at risk for this gene mutation by virtue of family history of prostate cancer, it would be beneficial to institute screening for prostate cancer at an earlier age than among the general population, probably at age 40 years, using a serum prostate-specific antigen test in addition to digital rectal examination.

MALIGNANT MELANOMA

Familial malignant melanoma is believed to account for about 10% of all cases of malignant melanoma. The following susceptibility germline gene mutations have been identified—*CDKN2A* (cyclin-dependent kinase inhibitor 2a) or *p16* on chromosome 9p21, *CDK4* on chromosome 12q14, and *P14ARF*, the alternate reading frame protein product of *CDKN2A*. Another gene, *MC1R*, modifies melanoma risk in those with identified

CDKN2A mutations, and may be a low penetrance melanoma gene on its own. The lifetime risk for developing melanoma if the person possesses a susceptibility gene has been estimated by Hansen et al. (2004) at up to 58% in the United Kingdom, 76% in the United States and 92% in Australia, but is influenced by exposure to ultraviolet radiation including sunlight and by modifying genes. Host characteristics such as red hair, freckling, and fair skin are associated with melanoma risk and certain variants of *MC1R* are most prevalent in individuals with those characteristics, while, for example, individuals with dark skin do not usually have those variant alleles. A subset of families with germline *CDKN2A* mutations have an increased risk of other cancers, especially pancreatic cancer, but the American Society of Clinical Oncology [ASCO (2003)] considers genetic testing for these variants to still be in the clinical research realm. Nonetheless genetic testing for *CDNK2A* has been developed and is said by some to be ready for the clinical setting since it meets ASCO criteria (Hansen et al., 2004) but those desiring to have such testing face the benefits and problems associated with other genetic susceptibility tests for cancer discussed later in this chapter.

CHROMOSOME CHANGES AND GENETIC INFLUENCES IN THE LEUKEMIAS, LYMPHOMAS, AND OTHER CANCERS

Specific nonrandom chromosome changes have been reported in most of the leukemias and lymphomas. In the case of the solid tumors, this information has been slower to emerge due to technical problems. The chromosome changes may involve gain or loss of a whole or part of a chromosome, translocations, inversions, or other changes alone or in combination. In many cases, the genes associated with these chromosome changes and their expression profiles are now being elucidated. The major result of chromosome aberrations is usually proto-oncogene activation, often because the gene for a T-cell receptor or antigen receptor gene or immunoglobulin is relocated near it or because a fusion gene is created that may encode and affect transcription factors. The fusion proteins created appear to be particularly important in solid tumor

development. These fusion proteins are considered tumor-specific antigens and may eventually be therapeutic targets.

Chromosome aberrations in relation to leukemia and lymphoproliferative disorders can be used as follows:

1. in diagnosis (for example, demonstrating a clonal chromosome aberration in a myeloproliferative disorder such as polycythemia vera can aid in distinguishing it from a nonneoplastic reactive proliferation);
2. in following the natural history of a disorder (for example, to predict blast crisis in chronic myelogenous leukemia [CML]);
3. establishing a prognosis (for example in AML, a chromosome 16 inversion or a t(8;21) translocation is associated with a relatively good prognosis while the t(9;22) translocation appears to carry a poorer outcome);
4. selecting and monitoring chemotherapy for efficacy and resistance (for example, in adult acute lymphoblastic leukemia (ALL), t(1;9) carries a poor prognosis and also in ALL, patients with t(15;17) are being treated with retinoic acid while those with t(8;21) and inv 16 are being treated with high- dose cytarabine); and
5. predict or establish remission or exacerbation (early relapses can be detected by looking for certain cytogenetic abnormalities and additional therapies can be begun).

A full discussion of cytogenetic changes in cancer are beyond the scope of this chapter. The reader is referred to the reference by Vogelstein and Kinzler (2002). A few examples are discussed below and Table 23.2 illustrates some common cytogenetic abnormalities in cancer.

More than 90% of patients with CML have a specific chromosome marker in bone marrow cells which is known as the Philadelphia (Ph) chromosome. Ph represents a translocation of genetic material from chromosome 22 to chromosome 9, noted as t(9;22). The shorter chromosome 22 is referred to as the Ph chromosome. As a consequence of this translocation, the proto-oncogene, *ABL* (Abelson murine leukemia virus) normally on chromosome 9 is moved to chromosome 22 within the breakpoint cluster region, *BCR,* forming a *BCR-ABL* fusion gene and product that has increased

TABLE 23.2   Nonrandom Chromosome Changes Reported Most Frequently in Selected Neoplasias

Neoplasia	Chromosome abnormalities
Chronic myeloid leukemia	t(9;22), +8, +19, i(17q)
Acute promyelocytic leukemia	t(15;17), t(11;17)
Burkitt's lymphoma	t(8;14), t(2;8), t(8;22)
Small-cell carcinoma of the lung	del (3) (p12 p14)
Melanoma	t(12;22)
Meningioma	−22
Glioma	Double minutes
Ewing's sarcoma	t(11;22), t(7;22)
Testicular teratoma	i(12p)

Note: For explanation of chromosome abnormality abbreviations see chapter 5.

tyrosine kinase activity. The new gene relationship is detected even in CML without detectable cytogenetic rearrangement. The t(9;22) is also seen in about 15% of cases of acute lymphocytic leukemia (ALL), rarely in acute myelogenous leukemia, and in about 5% of cases of acute nonlymphocytic leukemia (ANLL). This molecular information about CML led to the development of a pharmacological treatment, imatinib mesylate, which is a *BCR-ABL* tyrosine protein kinase inhibitor. Detailed information may be found in the reference by Kurzrock, Kantarjian, Druker and Talpaz (2003). In chronic lymphocyte leukemia (CLL), gene expression profiling revealed that expression of a gene *ZAP-70* distinguished with 93% accuracy those who had relatively stable disease from those with progressive disease requiring early treatment (Staudt, 2003). Recently certain *HOX* genes, which are recognized for their roles in development (see chapter 2), have been implicated for various roles in cancer. For example, *HOXA9* over-expression correlates with poor response to treatment in acute myeloid leukemia, and interacts with certain transcription factors.

Another example of well-described chromosomal rearrangement is in Burkitt's lymphoma, a B cell malignancy. Three major translocations are seen. One, t(8;14)(q24;q32) is found in 75%–90% of cases. Two others, t(2;8)(p12;q32) and t(8;22)(q24;q11), account for most of the rest. The result of the t(8;14) translocation is to move the *MYC* gene to the site of the gene for the heavy chain of immunoglobin (Ig), resulting in activation of the oncogene. In t(2;8) and t(8;22),

there is a juxtaposition of the kappa light Ig chain to *MYC* and the lambda light Ig chain to *MYC*, respectively.

ASSESSMENT OF RISK, DETECTION, GENETIC TESTING, PREVENTION, AND COUNSELING IN CANCER

The major significance of inherited types of cancer or cancer susceptibility lies in the possibility of prevention, early detection, and diagnosis, but treatment plans may be affected as well. For example, persons who have *BRCA1* and who have cancer in one breast need to consider the appropriate detection and/or prophylactic strategies, because of the tendency for multifocal tumors and the development of cancer in the contralateral breast. Initial assessment for those who might be at increased risk for hereditary susceptibility for ovarian, breast or colon cancer may take place at the site of the primary care provider. The family history, discussed in chapter 9, is often a source for identifying those who should be referred for more expert risk assessment and/or genetic counseling. Various guidelines are in place in various health provider groups to help the clinician determine who should be referred. These guidelines are discussed in detail in Mouchawar et al. (2003). Criteria that support referral are discussed in this chapter. Genetic testing and counseling may take place within the genetics clinic, the cancer clinic, the familial cancer clinic, or within cancer site specific clinics. The primary risk assessment, education, and counseling is often done by a cancer nurse specialist trained in genetics or by a genetic counselor trained in familial cancer. Probabilities of carrying the mutant *BRCA1* gene under varying histories and findings have been developed. The risk for actually developing cancer when carrying a mutant gene such as *BRCA1* or *BRCA2* is not yet fully elucidated, as discussed above.

Genetic Testing for Cancer

Genetic testing for cancer should, like other genetic testing, take place within the context of adequate and appropriate culturally competent education, counseling, and access to prevention, surveillance, and treatment options. It may begin with the identification of an at-risk person or family, found because of careful history taken over three generations and clarification of findings (for example an aunt's "female" cancer may be cervical and not ovarian) that necessitate medical records and pathology reports if obtainable. The nurse should be able to explain, clarify, and interpret the information at a level that the client can understand, and that is culturally sensitive and appropriate, free from any coercion, and to evaluate that understanding. All persons have the right not to choose genetic testing. If likely to be informative, clients should also have the right to choose to be tested without being coerced into a clinical trial or mandated follow-up, although some recommend this as a protective measure for the individual. Some cancer genetics programs calculate the risk for a person to carry a gene mutation for cancer before recommending testing based on clinical examination, pathology if relevant, family history, and so on. All this may occur in the context of a cancer risk assessment or evaluation program including physical examination, education, psychological assessment, cancer risk assessment and/or risk of being a carrier of a mutant gene, and genetic counseling.

Some of the elements that should be addressed, and could be included in informed consent, before a person decides to participate in genetic testing for cancer are essentially the same as those discussed in chapters 10 and 11, and not all will be repeated here. The person may also want to ascertain the extent of insurance coverage for the laboratory, counseling, education, and medical services including prophylactic tests and surgery, if desired and indicated. These elements include:

1. the reason that testing is appropriate for this person/family and why they have decided to have testing;
2. what is being tested for (for example, a mutation in a cancer susceptibility gene(s);
3. what estimation of risk and recommendations for surveillance can be done without genetic testing;
4. what the procedure for the specific test being considered entails, including description and exactly what will be analyzed, total cost including counseling, length of time, where it is to be done;
5. what can and cannot be tested for—this should include the information that while some mutations will be looked for and detected, other rare ones might not be;
6. what would both positive and negative results mean, including that negative results do not necessarily translate to a zero risk for the particular type of cancer or other cancers, and a positive test may indicate susceptibility for cancer with a percentage below 100% with a precise estimate unknown;
7. the accuracy, validity, and reliability of the test, including the likelihood of false negative or false positive results and the suitability of this test for the desired information;
8. the possibility that testing will not yield additional risk information and thus not be informative;
9. the length of time between the procedure and when the results are obtained;
10. how the results will be communicated to them;
11. a discussion of the risks of medical and life insurance and for adverse effects related to present and future coverage;
12. a discussion of possible adverse effects on employment including limitations on promotions, raises, and opportunities as well as educational opportunities.
13. the level of confidentiality of results and what this means (who can know or find out the results);

14. risks of psychological distress and impact on family including stigmatization (with both positive and negative findings), altered self-image, and guilt;
15. risks of passing on the mutation to children and the meaning of the risks;
16. what disclosure might they consider for other family members, why this can be important, and whom will they tell (if anyone) about the test results;
17. provision for referral for periodic surveillance, testing, and/or treatment after testing; and
18. what these options and limitations are in the context of both positive and negative results.

As in other genetic testing, a negative test result can have several meanings including: that the individual is truly free of the disease, that the result is "false negative" due to laboratory error, that the case is sporadic, or indicate the possession of alternate alleles than what could be or was tested for.

Who should be tested for cancer predisposition? Uncertainties also exist in who is a candidate for testing. A woman with a mother who developed breast cancer at age 70 years may seek testing but is not very likely to be a carrier of *BRCA1* (although she could be). Likewise, the absence of one particular gene mutation does not mean that there is no susceptibility to breast or ovarian cancer. Moreover, a negative test result does not mean a zero risk; the risk then becomes that of the population risk. The American Society of Clinical Oncology (ASCO) offered recommendations for indications for genetic testing for cancer susceptibility in 1996 that they updated in 2003. They have recommended that genetic counseling and testing be offered when:

"1) the person has personal or family history features suggestive of a genetic cancer susceptibility condition; 2) the genetic test can be adequately interpreted; and 3) the test results will aid in diagnosis or influence the medical or surgical management of the patient or family members at hereditrary risk of cancer" (p. 2398).

They go on to say that genetic testing should be done with pre- and post-test counseling that includes possible risks and benefits of early detection and prevention strategies. Because of the rapid evolution of knowledge and testing in regard to genetic testing for susceptibility to cancer and variations and limitations in models, they do not set numerical thresholds for recommending genetic risk assessment but state that "evaluation by a health care professional experienced in cancer genetics be relied on in making interpretations of pedigree information and determinations of the appropriateness of genetic testing" (p. 2398). As part of this they recommend that "practitioners recognize indications for genetic cancer predisposition testing, where testing is part of established or evolving standards of care for risk assessment and management." They go on to say that this "includes families with features of well-defined hereditary syndromes and individuals with very early onset disease or specific rare tumors suggestive of possible genetic hereditary predisposition" (pp. 2398–2399). Examples of the first group would include FAP and von Hippel-Lindau disease. Skolnick (1996), from a commercial company, speaks for wide availability of testing and Collins (1996), speaking for the National Action Plan on Breast Cancer, supports a variety of principles including that individuals should "have complete discretion over the decision to have genetic testing." ASCO (2003) also recommends better regulatory oversight and quality assurance for laboratories involved in genetic testing, and believes that the "health care provider's obligations (if any) to at-risk relatives are best fulfilled by communication of familial risk to the person undergoing testing, emphasizing the importance of sharing this information with family members so that they may also benefit" (p. 2403). They state that case law is not yet developed in regard to the "duty to warn," and that there are differences when the relatives are also patients of the health care provider. What is the obligation of a person to notify their relatives who may be at risk? It has also been found that clients have said they would notify relatives and then have selectively done this, so that some relatives have been informed and others have not received the information (Costalas et al., 2003). To some extent this may depend on their comfort level with those relatives. Offit et al. (2004) review some of the related issues and cite three cases that resulted in lawsuits because of the physician's failure to warn family members about their possible risk of genetic disease.

Various criteria have been used to establish the diagnosis of HNPCC, which was discussed above. In the original Amsterdam criteria, now seen as very stringent by some, the following were included: the presence of histologically verified colorectal cancer in at least three relatives (including a first-degree relative of the other two), cases that span at least two successive generations, with the diagnosis of at least one of the colorectal cancers before 50 years of age, and the elimination of known polyposis syndromes to make the diagnosis. In the more liberal Bethesda criteria, clinical diagnostic criteria include: the Amsterdam criteria, persons with two types of HNPCC-related cancers, persons with colon cancer and a first degree relative with colon cancer and/or HNPCC-associated extracolonic cancer and/or adenoma with the cancer at <45 years of age and adenoma at <40 years of age; persons with colon or endometrial cancer <45 years; persons with right-sided colon cancer with a histologic undifferentiated pattern at <45 years of age; persons with signet-ring-cell type colon cancer at <45 years; and persons with colonic adenomas before age 40 years (Chung & Rustgi, 2003). Family history still remains an important means of identifying those with HNPCC.

Other authors also recommend various conditions before gene testing for cancer, such as a psychological assessment including emotional stability, psychiatric history, and motivations for testing. Others believe that these sorts of conditions increase the tension between the individual right to choose to have testing or not and external groups who are examining various ethical issues. In any case, a number of commercial companies are directly marketing testing to physicians and to patients.

In a study by Lynch and associates (1995), interviews after *BRCA1* testing revealed that 71% of the high-risk women reported depression as compared with 12% of those at low risk; however, 71% of the high and 87% of the low-risk women reported a sense of relief. High-risk women did report more sleep disturbance, anger, and emotional lability than the others. In a study by Lerman et al. (1997), there were no differences in intention to have *BRCA1* mutation testing between those who had education only and those who had education and counseling. When children who were at risk for FAP because of a sibling with this condition were

tested and followed over 23 to 55 months, most did not suffer clinically significant psychological distress but some showed clinically significant anxiety symptoms, leading to the conclusion that all siblings whether positive or negative should have long-term psychological support available (Codori et al., 2003).

How interested are persons in being tested for cancer gene mutations? In one study of 130 women with family histories of breast cancer, 72% indicated that they would opt to be tested immediately (Kash, 1995), and in another study 75% were interested (Lerman, Daly, Masny, & Balshem, 1994). In individuals with colon cancer, another study found that 83% with family histories were interested in the test (Croyle & Lerman, 1993). In one study, women may have not sought breast cancer risk assessment because of concern about future insurance discrimination (Armstrong et al., 2003), but many of those who were found to have a *BRCA1* or *BRCA2* mutation and who could increase their insurance coverage did so. Patenaude, Basili, Fairclough, and Li (1996) found that about half of mothers of pediatric oncology patients would test themselves and their healthy children for genetic cancer predisposition even in the absence of medical benefits. Most would consider their minor children's wishes, and would tell them of the results. Clinical observations suggest that fewer persons actually avail themselves of testing than say they would. A concern surrounding genetic testing for cancer is whether or not health professionals can correctly interpret and explain the results. In one study by Giardiello et al. (1997), only 18.6% of patients received genetic counseling before testing for FAP. In 31.6% of the cases, the results were not interpreted correctly. Health professionals ordering genetic testing must be prepared to offer genetic counseling. If qualified, they may do this personally or by referral. The need for accurate and appropriate pre- and post-test genetic counseling and for the education of health care practitioners has been addressed by ASCO (2003). However, a study of genetic counseling for HNPCC indicated that some clients believed that only one session was needed for pre-test counseling, and in one case stated that patients felt "If I test positive I have to carry on with my screening and if I test negative I can stop" (Brain, Soldan, Sampson, & Gray, 2003). One of the most difficult aspects of testing for *BRCA1* and *BRCA2* mutations in one study was the long wait for the results of the testing (Di Prospero, 2001). Another relevant aspect is that Botkin (2003) found that only 73% of those were tested and found to carry a *BRCA1* or *2* mutation informed their usual health care provider of those results.

Ethical Issues Surrounding Presymptomatic and Predictive Genetic Testing for Cancer

The ethical dilemmas seen in genetic testing for cancer have commonalities with other types of medical testing, genetic testing and screening, prenatal diagnosis, and presymptomatic testing such as for Huntington disease (see chapter 11), and they will not be repeated here. One of the differences lies in the nature of cancer—the varying surveillance and treatment options and the varying outcome possibilities. Issues such as privacy, confidentiality, insurability (although disclosure of a negative test could be to the individual's benefit), possible employment discrimination, stigmatization, possible interference with family relationships, and the impact on marital and reproductive decisions are discussed in chapters 11 and 12. There have been fears that women who are at risk will abandon surveillance methods such as mammograms after a few negative ones, being lulled by false security. Another aspect has centered around access for high-risk women who cannot pay for testing, and testing for those who can pay, but may be deemed at low risk. The latter may be comparable to those who seek prenatal diagnosis because of anxiety, and many consider this to be a legitimate reason. The testing of children in genetically-at-risk families for cancer has been controversial. In some cases, the benefits to be derived are clearer than in others and the family's own beliefs and experiences are important. This is discussed in chapter 10. For example, a child who does not have an *APC* mutation in FAP families would be spared annual colon examinations that might be started at 11 years of age or earlier. Other concerns center around the child's ability to understand the procedure, the implications of what may be found, and the capability to give informed assent. In one study (Codori et al., 1996) of testing for FAP in 41 children, 19 were germline mutation positive. In the short-term, depression and anxiety scores were within normal limits. In keeping with these issues, there is expected to be a demand for prenatal diagnosis for germline mutations in cancer families where there is a transmission risk, presenting another set of issues revolving around pregnancy termination.

Prevention and Surveillance

Once a person is determined to be at risk by virtue of possessing a gene mutation known to be implicated in cancer development, a program of surveillance and of therapeutic preventive interventions can be implemented. For example, the recommendations for women with *BRCA1* or *BRCA2* mutations would include more than the usual recommended monthly breast self-examination. These women would be advised to have an annual mammogram and breast examination by an experienced practitioner beginning by age 25 years. There is some controversy regarding mammography for several reasons, such as radiation exposure sensitivity in those with a gene mutation such as AT heterozygotes. For ovarian cancer surveillance, women should have transvaginal ultrasound and a pelvic examination every 6 to 12 months, and a blood test for cell surface glycoprotein markers in the serum such as CA125 every 6 to 12 months for early ovarian cancer detection beginning at age 25 years, especially for *BRCA1* gene mutation carriers especially. For women with *BRCA1* and *BRCA2* mutations, there is a choice for a prophylactic mastectomy and/or oophrectomy with or without hysterectomy at about age 35 years or older In some studies, prophylactic oophrectomy was preferred to mastectomy. However, these measures are not proven to reduce the risk of cancer development as tissue may remain behind that could become malignant, and they still might develop one of the other associated cancers for which detection is not being pursued as aggressively. In a study by Rebbeck et al. (2004), it was found that bilateral prophylactic mastectomy reduced the risk of breast cancer in women with *BRCA1* or *BRCA2* mutations by about 90%. Olopade and Artoli (2004) found that prophylactic salpingo-oophrectomy in women with *BRCA1* or *BRCA2* mutations reduced the risk of ovarian cancer by about 96% and breast cancer risk by 53%.

Some centers are investigating the use of chemoprevention through such agents as tamoxifen and raloxifene to prevent breast cancer. Aromatase inhibitors such as anastrazole are of interest currently in preventing breast cancer development. Birth control pills may decrease the risk of ovarian cancer. Women with breast cancer gene mutations may want to avoid perimenopausal exogenous estrogen and ingest a low fat diet. Men and women should also have a rectal examination every year and a fecal occult blood test by age 40 years and over, and colonoscopy every 3 to 5 years. Males should have a prostate exam yearly, and a prostate specific antigen test every year after 50 years of age. The Gilda Radner Familial Ovarian Cancer Registry provides information to women with or at risk from ovarian cancer. Another approach is through reducing hormonal influence by use of gonadotropin-releasing hormone inhibitors, though this is still experimental. Men with *BRCA2* mutations should be alert for any breast mass or change.

Persons who are at risk for colorectal cancer by virtue of being a first-degree relative of a person with FAP, or for Gardner syndrome, should have a flexible sigmoidoscopy at 10–12 years of age or earlier if indicated by family history. If no polyps are detected then this should be repeated every 1–3 years (if a germline mutation is present). For HNPCC, it is recommended that colonoscopy be done at about 20–30 years of age, or 5 years earlier than the age at which the index patient was diagnosed. It is recommended that those at higher risk should have full colonoscopy to the cecum every 1 to 3 years. Women should be screened for ovarian cancer, by transvaginal ovarian ultrasonography and CA-125 and annual surveillance for endometrial cancer by endometrial aspirate beginning at age 25–30 years. Eventually, testing may be done on DNA of cells shed in feces. In terms of general health promotion, at-risk patients might also practice dietary modification such as low-fat, high-fiber diet and pharmacologic measures such as nonsteroidal anti-inflammatory drugs that might modify risk but are unproven. Some patients may elect to have prophylactic subtotal colectomy. Data on hysterectomy and bilateral salpingo-oophrectomy are lacking; this option is available preferably by 35 to 40 years of age. Diet modifications (low-fat, high-fiber, fruits and vegetables), and lifestyle modifications (exercise, not smoking) are suggested but are not proven to prevent cancer development. The psychological issues that accompany prophylactic surgery may have some similarities to those observed following mastectomy, hysterectomy, or colectomy for non-familial cancers, and these issues are discussed in detail in other texts.

GENETIC APPROACHES TO CANCER THERAPY

Genetic knowledge has contributed to approaches to the treatment of many diseases including cancer, its complications and metastasis. Some approaches center around gene therapy, whereas others exploit knowledge about the pathogenetic mechanisms underlying the disease or about individual susceptibility to certain drugs. Understanding the disease at the molecular level allows that research to be translated into clinical management. Use of the drugs, azathioprine, thioguanine, and 6-mercaptopurine for leukemia is discussed in chapter 18. Irinotecan (Camptosar) is an agent used to treat metastatic colorectal cancer by stopping cancer cell growth through inhibition of cell division. Among its adverse effects are neutropenia, with potentially fatal outcomes which may occur in up to one-third of patients treated. An enzyme, UDP glucuronosyltransferase 1A1 (UGT1A1), is involved in catabolizing the active metabolite in irinotecan. More than 30 variant alleles have been identified, including a dinucleotide repeat that influences gene expression. Persons (about 10% of the population) with the homozygous *UGT1A1*28 genotype (also called the 7/7 genotype) have lower functional enzyme activity. These people have a more than nine-fold greater risk of developing grade 4 neutropenia than do those with the normal 6/6 genotype or the heterozygous genotype when receiving the standard dose of irinotecan. Thus another regimen can be selected for these people until it is known if there is a safe but effective dose they can be given. An example that is slightly different involves patients with non-small cell lung cancer. Most of these patients do not respond clinically to gefitinib (Iressa) an agent that inhibits tyrosine kinase, which plays a role in cancer metastasis. In a subgroup (about 10–15%) of these patients, their tumors have a somatic mutation in the epidermal growth factor receptor *(EGFR)* gene, which allows a clinical response to gefitinib. This mutation can be screened for in the tumors of patients with this type of lung cancer, allowing tailored therapy. The first drug to be clinically used to inhibit tyrosine kinase activity was imatinib (Gleevec/Glivec) in Philadelphia chromosome positive (Ph+) CML (discussed earlier). In these cases, the *BCR-ABL* fusion gene results in activated BCR-ABL tyrosine kinase which is inhibited by imatinib. Imatinib is being used in newly diagnosed Ph+ adults with CML, and in pediatric patients in the chronic phase whose disease has recurred after initial treatment, thus exploiting what is known about the chromosomal translocation and its fusion gene and products. Imatinib is also proving useful in inhibiting other tyrosine kinases such as in the inhibition of gastrointestinal stromal tumors (GISTs) which over express KIT receptor tyrosine kinase.

BIBLIOGRAPHY

Allan, J. M., Smith, A. G., Wheatley, K., Hills, R. K., Travis, L. B., Hill, D. A., et al. (2004).Genetic variation in XPD predicts treatment outcome and risk of acute myeloid leukemia following chemotherapy. *Blood.*

American Society of Clinical Oncology. (2003). American Society of Clinical Oncology policy statement update: Genetic testing for cancer susceptibility. *Journal of Clinical Oncolgy, 21,* 2397–2406.

American Society of Clinical Oncology. (1996). Statement of the American Society of Clinical Oncology: Genetic testing for cancer susceptibility. *Journal of Clinical Oncology, 14,* 1730–1736.

American College of Medical Genetics. (1996, Summer). Statement on population screening for BRCA-1 mutation in Ashkenazi Jewish women. *College Newsletter, 7,* 9.

Armstrong, K., Weber, B., Fitzgerald, G., Hershey, J. C., Pauly, M. V., Lemaire, J., et al. (2003). Life insurance and breast cancer risk assessment: Adverse selection, genetic testing decisions, and discrimination. *American Journal of Medical Genetics, 120A,* 359–364.

Baglioni, S., & Genuardi, M. (2004). Simple and complex genetics of colorectal cancer susceptibility. *American Journal of Medical Genetics, Part C (Seminars in Medical Genetics), 129C,* 35–43.

Balmain, A., Gray, J., & Ponder, B. (2003). The genetics and genomics of cancer. *Nature Genetics Supplement, 33,* 238–244.

Bataille, V. (2003). Genetic epidemiology of melanoma. *European Journal of Cancer, 39,* 1341–1347.

Bénard, J., Douc-Rasy, S., Ahomadegbe, J-C. (2003). TP53 family members and human cancers. *Human Mutation, 21,* 182–191.

Berry, D. A., Parmigiani, G., Sanchez, J., Schildkraut, J., & Winer, E. (1997). Probability of carrying a mutation of breast-ovarian cancer gene BRCA1 based on family history, *Journal of the National Cancer Institute, 89,* 227–238.

Blackledge, G., & Averbuch, S. (2004). Gefitinib ('Iressa', ZD1839) and new epidermal growth factor receptor inhibitors. *British Journal of Cancer, 90,* 566–572.

Blazer, K. R., Macdonald, D. J., Ricker, C., Sand, S., Uman, G. C., & Weitzel, J. N. (2005). Outcomes from intensive training in genetic cancer risk counseling for clinicians. *Genetics in Medicine, 7,* 40–47.

Boland, C. R., & Meltzer, S. J. (2002). Cancer of the colon and gastrointestinal tract. In D. L. Rimoin, J. M. Connor, R. E. Pyeritz, & B. R. Korf (Eds.), *Emery and Rimoin's principles and practice of medical genetics* (4th ed., pp. 1824–1859). New York: Churchill Livingstone.

Botkin, J. R., Smith, K. R., Croyle, R. T., Baty, B. J., Wylie, J. E., Dutson, D., et al. (2003). Genetic testing for a *BRCA1* mutation: Prophylactic surgery and screening behavior in women 2 years post testing. *American Journal of Medical Genetics, 118A,* 201–209.

Bouchard, L., Blancquaert, I., Eisinger, F., Foulkes, W. D., Evans, G., Sobol, H., et al. (2004). Prevention and genetic testing for breast cancer: Variations in medical decisions. *Social Science & Medicine, 58,* 1085–1096.

Brain, K., Soldan, J., Sampson, J., & Gray, J. (2003). Genetic counselling protocols for hereditary non-polyposis colorectal cancer: A survey of UK regional genetic centres. *Clinical Genetics, 63,* 198–204.

Cardenas, K., & Frisch, K. (2003). Comprehensive breast cancer screening. *Postgraduate Medicine, 113*(2), 34–46.

Carling, T. (2005). Multiple endocrine neoplasia syndrome: Genetic basis for clinical management. *Current Opinion in Oncology, 17,* 7–12.

Cass, I., Baldwin, R. L., Varkey, T., Moslehi, R., Narod, S. A., & Karlan, B. (2003). Improved survival in women with BRCA-associated ovarian carcinoma. *Cancer, 97*, 2187–2195.

Chapman, P.D., Church, W., Burn, J., & Gunn, A. (1989). Congenital hypertrophy of retinal pigment epithelium: A sign of familial adenomatous polyposis. *British Medical Journal, 298*, 353–354.

Chung, D. C., & Rustgi, A. K. (2003). The hereditary nonpolyposis colorectal cancer syndrome: Genetics and clinical implications. *Annals of Internal Medicine, 138*, 560–570.

Codori, A-M., Zawacki, K. L., Petersen, G. M., Mighoretti, D. L., Bacon, J. A., & Trimbath, J. D. (2003). Genetic testing for hereditary colorectal cancer in children: Long-term psychological effects. *American Journal of Medical Genetics, 116A*, 117–128.

Codori, A-M., Petersen, G. M., Boyd, P. A., Brandt, J., & Giardiello, F. M. (1996). Genetic testing for cancer in children. Short-term psychological effect. *Archives of Pediatric and Adolescent Medicine, 150*, 1131–1138.

Collins, F. (1996). Commenatary on the ASCO statement on genetic testing for cancer susceptibility. *Journal of Clinical Oncology, 14*, 1738–1740.

Costalas, J. W., Itzen, M., Malick, J., Babb, J. S., Bove, B., Godwin, A. K., et al. (2003). Communication of BRCA1 and BRCA2 results to at-risk relatives: A cancer risk assessment program's experience. *American Journal of Medical Genetics Part C, Seminars in Medical Genetics, 119C*, 11–18.

Croyle, R. T., & Lerman, C. (1993). Interest in genetic testing for colon cancer susceptibility: Cognitive and emotional correlates. *Preventive Medicine, 22*, 284–292.

D'Andrea, A. D., & Grompe, M. (2003). The Fanconi anaemia/BRCA pathway. *Nature Reviews Cancer, 3*, 23–34.

de la Hoya, M., Fernández, J. M., Tosar, A., Godino, J., Sánchez de Abajo, A., Vidart, J. A., et al. (2003). Association between BRCA1 mutations and ratio of female to male births in offspring of families with breast cancer, ovarian cancer, or both. *Journal of the American Medical Association, 290*, 929–931.

de la Hoya, M., Meijers-Heijboer, H., Fernandez, J. M., Diez, O., Osorio, Alonso, C., et al. (2005). Mutant BRCA1 alleles transmission: Different approaches and different biases. *International Journal of Cancer, 113*, 166–167.

DeMarzo, A. M., Nelson, W. G., Isaacs, W. B., & Epstein, J. I. (2003). Pathological and molecular aspects of prostate cancer. *Lancet, 361*, 955–964.

Deutsch, E., Marriorella, L., Eschwege, P., Bourhis, J., Soria, J. C., & Abdulkarim, B. (2004). Environmental, genetic, and molecular features of prostate cancer. *Lancet Oncology, 5*, 303–313.

Di Prospero, L. S., Seminsky, M., Honeyford, J., Doan, B., Franssen, E., Meschino, W., et al. (2001). Psychosocial issues following a positive result of genetic testing for BRCA1 and BRCA2 mutations: Findings from a focus group and a needs-assessment survey. *Canadian Medical Association Journal, 164*, 1005–1009.

Dome, J. S., & Coppes, M. J. (2002). Recent advances in Wilms tumor genetics. *Current Opinion I in Pediatrics, 14*, 5–11.

Donaldson, S. S., & Hancock, S. L. (1996). Second cancers after Hodgkin's disease in childhood. *New England Journal of Medicine, 334*, 792–794.

Duker, N. J. (2002). Chromosome breakage syndromes and cancer. *American Journal of Medical Genetics (Seminars in Medical Genetics), 115*, 125–129.

Edwards, S. M., & Eeles, R. A. (2004). Unravelling the genetics of prostate cancer. *American Journal of Medical Genetics, Part C (Seminars in Medical Genetics), 129C*, 65–73.

Edwards, S. M., Kote-Jarai, Z., Meitz, J., Hamoudi, R., Hope, Q., Osin, P., et al. (2003). Two percent of men with early-onset prostate cancer harbor germline mutations in the BRCA2 gene. *American Journal of Human Genetics, 72*, 1–12.

Eng, C., & Iglehart, D. (2004). Decision aids from genetics to treatment of breast cancer.

Fanos, J. H. (1997). Developmental tasks of childhood and adolescence: Implications for genetic testing. *American Journal of Medical Genetics, 71*, 22–28.

Friedman, J. M. (1997). Genetics and epidemiology, congenital anomalies and cancer. *American Journal of Human Genetics, 60*, 469–473.

Garber, J. E., & Offit, K. (2005). Hereditary cancer predisposition syndromes. *Journal of Clinical Oncology, 23*, 276–292.

Giardiello, F. M., Brensinger, J. D., Petersen, G. M., Luce, M. C., Hylind, L. M., Bacon, J. A., et al. (1997). The use and interpretation of commercial

APC gene testing for familial adenomatous polyposis. *New England Journal of Medicine, 336,* 823–827.

Goodman, F. R. (2003). Congenital abnormalities of body patterning: Embryology revisited. *Lancet, 362,* 651–662.

Green, D. M., Whitton, J. A., Stovall, M., Mertens, A. C., Donaldson, S. S., Ruymann, F. B., et al. (2003). Pregnancy outcome of partners of male survivors of childhood cancer: A report from the Childhood Cancer Survivor Study. *Journal of Clinical Oncology, 21,* 716–721.

Grisendi, S., & Pandolfi, P. P. (2005). *NPM* mutations in acute myelogenous leukemia. *New England Journal of Medicine, 352,* 291–292.

Grönberg, H. (2003). Prostate cancer epidemiology. *Lancet, 361,* 859–864.

Groupe Français de Cytogénétique Hématologique. (1996). Cytogenetic abnormalities in adult acute lymphoblastic leukemia: Correlations with hematologic findings and outcome. A collaborative study of the Groupe Française de Cytogénétique Hématologique. *Blood, 87,* 3135–3142.

Gurbuxani, S., Vyas, P., & Crispino, J. D. (2004). Recent insights into the mechanisms of myeloid leukemogenesis in Down syndrome. *Blood, 103,* 399–406.

Hadley, D. W., Jenkins, J. F., Dimond, E., de Carvalho, M., Kirsch, I., & Palmer, C. G. S. (2004). Colon cancer screening practices after genetic counseling and testing for hereditary nonpolyposis colorectal cancer. *Journal of Clinical Oncology, 22,* 39–44.

Hampel, H., Sweet, K., Westman, J. A., Offit, K., & Eng, C. (2004). Referral for cancer genetics consultation: A review and compilation of risk assessment criteria. *Journal of Medical Genetics, 41,* 81–91.

Hansen, C. B., Wadge, L. M., Lowstuter, K., Boucher, K., & Leachman, S. A. (2004). Clinical germline genetic testing for melanoma. *Lancet Oncology, 5,* 314–319.

Harper, P. S. (1998). *Practical genetic counseling* (5th ed.). Oxford: Butterworth Heinemann.

Hayward, N. K. (2003). Genetics of melanoma predisposition. *Oncogene, 22,* 3053–3062.

Hemminki, K., Rawal, R., & Bermejo, J. L. (2005). Prostate cancer screening, changing age-specific incidence trends and implications on familial risk. *International Journal of Cancer, 113,* 312–315.

Herrinton, L. J., Zhao, W., & Husson, G. (2003). Management of cryptorchism and risk of testicular cancer. *American Journal of Epidemiology, 157,* 602–605.

Huang, E., Cheng, S. H., Dressman, H., Pittman, J., Tsou, M. H., Horng, C. F., et al. (2003). Gene expression predictors of breast cancer outcomes. *Lancet, 361,* 1590–1596.

Innocenti, F., Undevia, S. V., Iyer, L., Chen, P. X., Das, S., Kocherinsky, M., et al. (2004). Genetic variants in the *UDP-glucuronosyltransferase 1A1* gene predict the risk of severe neutropenia of Irinotecan. *Journal of Clinical Oncology, 22,* 1382–1388.

Kalapurakal, J. A., Dome, J. S., Perlman, E. J., Malogolowkin, M., Hasse, G. M., Grundy, P., et al. (2004). Management of Wilms' tumor: Current practice and future goals. *Lancet Oncology, 5,* 37–46.

Kash, K. M. (1995). Psychosocial and ethical implications of defining genetic risk for cancers. *Annals of the New York Academy of Sciences, 768,* 41–52.

Kern, S. E. (1998). Advances from genetic clues in pancreatic cancer. *Current Opinion in Oncology, 10,* 74–80.

Knudson, A. G., Jr. (1971). Mutation and cancer: Statistical study of retinoblastoma. *Proceedings of the National Academy of Sciences USA, 68,* 820–823.

Knudson, A. G. (2002). Cancer genetics. *American Journal of Medical Genetics, 111,* 96–102.

Kobzev, Y. N., & Rowley, J. D. (2002). Leukemias, lymphomas, and other related disorders. In D. L. Rimoin, J. M. Connor, R. E. Pyeritz, & B. R. Korf (Eds.), *Emery and Rimoin's principles and practice of medical genetics* (4th ed., pp. 1971–1995). New York: Churchill Livingstone.

Kriege, M., Brekelmans, C. T. M., Boetes, C., Bresnard, P. E., Zonderland, H. M., Obdeijn, I. M., Manoliu, R. A., et al. (2004). Efficacy of MRI and mammography for breast-cancer screening in women with a familial or genetic predisposition. *New England Journal of Medicine, 351,* 427–437.

Kurzrock, R., Kantarjian, H. M., Druker, B. J., & Talpaz, M. (2003). Philadelphia chromosome-positive leukemias: From basic mechanisms to molecular therapeutics. *Annals of Internal Medicine, 138,* 819–830.

Lalloo, F., Cochrane, S., Bulman, B., Varley, J., Elles, R., Howell, A., & Evans, D. G. R. (1998). An evaluation of common breast cancer gene mutations in a population of Ashkenazi Jews. *Journal of Medical Genetics, 35,* 10–12.

Lalloo, F., Varley, J., Ellis, D., Moran, A., O'Dair, L., Pharoah, P., et al. (2003). Prediction of pathogenic mutations in patients with early-onset breast cancer by family history. *Lancet, 361,* 1101–1102.

Lerman, C., Biesecker, B., Benkendorf, J. L., Kerner, J., Gomez-Caminero, A., Hughes, C., et al. (1997). Controlled trial of pretest education approaches to enhance informed decision-making for BRCA1 gene testing. *Journal of the National Cancer Institute, 89,* 148–157.

Lerman, C., Daly, M., Masny, A., & Balshem, A. (1994). Attitudes about genetic testing for breast-ovarian cancer susceptibility. *Journal of Clinical Oncology, 12,* 843–850.

Li, F. P., & Fraumeni, J. F., Jr. (1969). Rhabdomyosarcoma in children: Epidemiologic study and identification of a familial cancer syndrome. *Journal of the National Cancer Institute, 43,* 1365–1373.

Li, J., Yen, C., Liaw, D., Podsypanina, K., Bose, S., Wang, S. I., et al. (1997). PTEN, a putative protein tyrosine phosphatase gene mutated in human brain, breast and prostate cancer. *Science, 275,* 1943–1947.

Li, L., Li, X., Francke, U., & Cohen, S. N. (1997). The TSG101 tumor susceptibility gene is located in chromosome 11 band p15 and is mutated in human breast cancer. *Cell, 88,* 143–154.

Liede, A., Karlan, B. Y., & Narod, S. A. (2004). Cancer risks for male carriers of germline mutations in BRCA1 or BRCA2: A review of the literature. *Journal of Clinical Oncology, 22,* 735–742.

Lonser, R. R., Glenn, G. M., Walther, M., Chew, E. Y., Libutti, S. K., Linehan, W. M., et al. (2003). von Hippel-Lindau disease. *Lancet, 361,* 2059–2067.

Lucassen, A., & Parker, M. (2004). Confidentiality and serious harm in genetics—preserving the confidentiality of one patient and preventing harm to relatives. *European Journal of Human Genetics, 12,* 93–97.

Lynch, H. T., & de la Chapelle, A. (2003). Hereditary colorectal cancer. *New England Journal of Medicine, 348,* 919–932.

Lynch, H. T., Smyrk, T., Lynch, J., Fitzgibbons, R., Jr., Lanspa, S., & McGinn, T. (1995). Update on the differential diagnosis, surveillance and management of hereditary non-polyposis colorectal cancer. *European Journal of Cancer, 31A,* 1039–1046.

Lynch, H. T., Snyder, C. L., Lynch, J. F., Riley, B. D., & Rubinstein, W. S. (2003). Hereditary breast-ovarian cancer at the bedside: Role of the medical oncologist. *Journal of Clinical Oncology, 21,* 740–753.

Lynch, T. J., Bell, D. W., Sordella, R., Gurubhagavatula, S., Okimoto, R. A., Brannigan, B. W., et al. (2004). Activating mutations in the epidermal growth factor receptor underlying responsiveness of non-small-cell lung cancer to gefitinib. *New England Journal of Medicine, 350,* 2129–2139.

Magnaldo, T. (2004). Xeroderma pigmentosum: From genetics to hopes and realities of cutaneous gene therapy. *Expert Opinion on Biological Therapy, 4,* 169–179.

Malone, K. L., Daling, J. R., Thompson, J. D., O'Brien, C. A., Francisco, L. V., & Ostrander, E. A. (1998). BRCA1 mutations and breast cancer in the general population. *Journal of the American Medical Association, 279,* 922-929.

Maraschio, P., Spadoni, E., Tanzarella, C., Antoccia, A., di Masi, A., Maghnie, M., et al. (2003). Genetic heterogeneity for a Nijmegen breakage-like syndrome. *Clinical Genetics, 63,* 283–290.

Marsh, S., & McLeod, H. L. (2004). Cancer pharmacogenetics. *British Journal of Cancer, 90,* 8–11.

McConkie-Rosell, A., & Spiridigliozzi, G. A. (2004). "Family matters": A conceptual framework for genetic testing in children. *Journal of Genetic Counseling, 13,* 9–29.

Merg, A., & Howe, J. R. (2004). Genetic conditions associated with intestinal juvenile polyps. *American Journal of Medical Genetics, Part C (Seminars in Medical Genetics, 129C,* 44–55.

Miesfeldt, S., Cohn, W. F., Jones, S. M., Ropka, M. E., & Weinstein, J. C. (2003). Breast cancer survivors' attitudes about communication of breast cancer risk to their children. *American Journal of Medical Genetics, Part C (Seminars in Medical Genetics), 119C,* 45–50.

Miki, Y., Swensen, J., Shattuck-Eidens, D., Futreal, A. P., Harshman, K., Tavtigian, S., et al. (1994). A strong candidate for the breast and ovarian cancer susceptibility gene *BRCA1*. *Science, 266*, 66–71.

Monzon, J., Liu, L., Brill, H., Goldstein, A. M., Tucker, M. A., From, L., et al. (1998). *CDKN2A* mutations in multiple primary melanomas. *New England Journal of Medicine, 338*, 879–887.

Mouchawar, J., Goins, K. V., Somkin, C., Puleo, E., Alford, S. H., Geiger, A. M., Taplin, S., et al. (2003). Guidelines for breast and ovarian cancer genetic counseling referral: Adoption and implementation in HMOs. *Genetics in Medicine, 5*, 444–450.

Murphree, A. L., & Clark, R. D. (2002). Retinoblastoma. In D. L. Rimoin, J. M. Connor, R. E. Pyeritz, & B. R. Korf (Eds.), *Emery and Rimoin's principles and practice of medical genetics* (4th ed., pp. 3604–3635). New York: Churchill Livingstone.

Nadal, E., & Olavarria, E. (2004). Imatinib mesylate (Gleevec/Glivec) a molecular-targeted therapy for chronic myeloid leukaemia and other malignancies. *International Journal of Clinical Practice, 58*, 511–516.

Narod, S. A., Hawkins, M. M., Robertson, C. M., & Stiller, C. A. (1997). Congenital anomalies and childhood cancer in Great Britain. *American Journal of Human Genetics, 60*, 474–485.

National Advisory Council for Human Genome Research. (1994). Statement on use of DNA testing for presymptomatic identification of cancer risk. *Journal of the American Medical Association, 271*, 785.

Nelson, W. G., De Marzo, A. M., & Isaacs, W. B. (2003). Prostate cancer. *New England Journal of Medicine, 349*, 366–381.

Newman, B., Butler, L. M., Millikan, R. C., Moorman, P. G., & King, M-C. (1998). Frequency of breast cancer attributable to *BRCA1* in a population-based series of American women. *Journal of the American Medical Association, 279*, 915–921.

Nieder, A. M., Taneja, S. S., Zeegers, M. P. A., & Ostrer, H. (2003). Genetic counseling for prostate cancer risk. *Clinical Genetics, 63*, 169–176.

Norgauer, J., Idzko, M., Panther, E., Hellstern, O., & Herouy, Y. (2003). Xeroderma pigmentosum. *European Journal of Dermatology, 13*, 4–9.

Offit, K., Groeger, E., Turner, S., Wadsworth, E. A., & Weriser, M. A. (2004). The "duty to warn" a patient's family members about hereditary disease risks. *Journal of the American Medical Association, 292*, 1469–1473.

Olopade, O. I., & Artoli, G. (2004). Efficacy of risk-reducing salpingo-oophrectomy in women with *BRCA-1* and *BRCA-2* mutations. *Breast Journal, 10*(Suppl. 1), S5–S9.

Olopade, O. I., Fackenthal, J. D., Dunston, G., Tainsky, M. A., Collins, F., & Whittfield-Broome, C. (2003). Breast cancer genetics in African Americans. *Cancer, 97*(Suppl. 1), 236–245.

Patenaude, A. F., Basili, L., Fairclough, D. L., & Li, F. P. (1996). Attitudes of 47 mothers of pediatric oncology patients toward genetic testing for cancer predisposition. *Journal of Clinical Oncology, 14*, 415–421.

Peltomaki, P. (2003). Role of DNA mismatch repair defects in the pathogenesis of human cancer. *Journal of Clinical Oncology, 21*, 1174–1179.

Petros, W. P., & Evans, W. E. (2004). Pharmacogenomics in cancer therapy: Is host genome variability important? *Trends in Pharmacological Sciences, 25*, 457–464.

Polsky, D., & Cordon-Cardo, C. (2003). Oncogenes in melanoma. *Oncogene, 22*, 3087–3091.

Rebbeck, T. R., Friebel, T., Lynch, H. T., Neuhausen, S. L., Van't Veer, L., Garber, J. E., et al. (2004). Bilateral prophylactic mastectomy reduces breast cancer risk in BRCA1 and BRCA2 mutation carriers: The PROSE Study Group. *Journal of Clinical Oncology, 22*, 1055-1062.

Richard, S., Graff, J., Lindau, J., & Resche, F. (2004). Von Hippel-Lindau disease. *Lancet, 363*, 1231–1234.

Ross, D. M., & Hughes, T. P. (2004). Cancer treatment with kinase inhibitors: What have we learned from imatinib? *British Journal of Cancer, 90*, 12–19.

Rowley, P. T. (2005). Inherited susceptibility to colorectal cancer. *Annual Review of Medicine, 56*, 539–554.

Ruteshouser, E. C., & Huff, V. (2004). Familial Wilms tumor. *American Journal of Medical Genetics, Part C (Seminars in Medical Genetics), 129C*, 29–34.

Skolnick, M. (1996). Commentary on the ASCO statement on genetic testing for cancer susceptibility. *Journal of Clinical Oncology, 14*, 1737–1738.

Sobol, H., Birnbaum, D., & Eisinger, F. (1994). Evidence for a third breast-cancer susceptibility gene. *Lancet, 344*, 1151–1152.

Speice, J., McDaniel, S. H., Rowley, P. T., & Loader, S. (2002). Family issues in a psychoeducation group for women with a *BRCA* mutation. *Clinical Genetics, 62,* 121–127.

Stary, A., & Sarasin, A. (2002). The genetics of the hereditary xeroderma pigmentosum syndrome. *Biochimie, 84,* 49–60.

Staudt, L. M. (2003). Molecular diagnosis of the hematologic cancers. *New England Journal of Medicine, 348,* 1777–1785.

Stratton, J. F., Gayther, S. A., Russell, P., Dearden, J., Gore, M., Blake, P., et al. (1997). Contribution of BRCA1 mutations to ovarian cancer. *New England Journal of Medicine, 336,* 1125–1130.

Strong, L. C. (2003). General keynote: Hereditary cancer: Lessons from Li-Fraumeni syndrome. *Gynecologic Oncology, 88,* S4–S7.

Struewing, J. P., Abeliovitch, D., Peretz, T., Avishai, N., Kaback, M. M., Collins, F., et al. (1995). The carrier frequency of the BRCA1 185delAG mutation is approximately 1 per cent in ashkenazi Jewish individuals. *Nature Genetics, 11,* 198–200.

Swift, M., Morrell, D. Cromartie, E., Chamberlain, A. R., Skolnick, M. H., & Bishop, D. T. (1986). The incidence and gene frequency of ataxia telangiectasia in the United States. *American Journal of Human Genetics, 39,* 573–583.

Swift, M., Reitnauer, P. J., Morrell, D., Chase, C. L. (1987). Breast and other cancers in families with ataxia telangiectasia. *New England Journal of Medicine, 316,* 1289–1294.

Thull, D. L., & Vogel, V. G. (2004). Recognition and management of hereditary breast cancer syndromes. *The Oncologist, 9,* 13–24.

Tischkowitz, M. D., & Hodgson, S. V. (2003). Fanconi anaemia. *Journal of Medical Genetics, 40,* 1–10.

Tobias, E. S., & Black, D. M. (2002). The molecular biology of cancer. In D. L. Rimoin, J. M. Connor, R. E. Pyeritz, & B. R. Korf (Eds.), *Emery and Rimoin's principles and practice of medical genetics* (4th ed., pp. 514–570). New York: Churchill Livingstone.

Vasen, H. F. A., Mecklin, J. P., Meera Khan, P., & Lynch, H. T. (1991). The international collaborative group on hereditary non-polyposis colorectal cancer. *Diseases of the Colon and Rectum, 34,* 424–425.

Vasen, H. F., Watson, P., Mecklin, J. P., & Lynch, H. T. (1999). New clinical criteria for hereditary nonpolyposis colorectal cancer (HNPCC, Lynch syndrome) proposed by the International Collaborative group on HNPCC. *Gastroenterology, 116,* 1453–1456.

Veersteeg, R. (1997). Aberrant methylation in cancer. *American Journal of Human Genetics, 60,* 751–754.

Velculescu, V., & El-Deiry, W. S. (1996). Biological and clinical importance of the *p53* tumor suppressor gene. *Clinical Chemistry, 42,* 858–868.

Venkitaraman, A. R. (2003). A growing network of cancer-susceptibility genes. *New England Journal of Medicine, 348,* 1917–1919.

Visco, F. M. (1996). Commentary on the ASCO statement on genetic testing for cancer susceptibility. *Journal of Clinical Oncology, 14,* 1737.

Vogel, F., & Motulsky, A. G. (1997). *Human genetics: Problems and approaches* (3rd ed.). Berlin: Springer-Verlag.

Vogelstein, B., & Kinzler, K. W. (Eds.). (2002). *The genetic basis of human cancer.* New York: McGraw Hill.

Watts, J. A., Morley, M., Burdick, J. T., Fiori, J. L., Ewens, W. J., Spielman, R. S., et al. (2002). Gene expression in heterozygous carriers of ataxia telangiectasia. *American Journal of Human Genetics, 71,* 791–800.

Wooster, R., Bignell, G., Lancaster, J., Swift, S., Seal, S., Mangion, J., et al. (1995). Identification of the breast cancer susceptibility gene BRCA2. *Nature, 378,* 789–792.

Wooster, R., & Weber, B. L. (2003). Breast and ovarian cancer. *New England Journal of Medicine, 348,* 2339–2447.

24

Diabetes Mellitus

istorically speaking, diabetes mellitus (DM) has been referred to both as "a geneticist's nightmare" and as the "graveyard of the geneticist's reputation." Although it has been observed for centuries that DM runs in families, the basic genetic defect(s) for most types remains unidentified. DM is not a single disease but "a group of metabolic diseases characterized by hyperglycemia resulting from defects in insulin secretion, insulin action, or both" (American Diabetes Association, 2004, p. S5). Research into DM has been hampered by the reasons common to the common disorders (see chapter 16). In 1997, DM was reclassified after many years to reflect new knowledge, and this was later further revised. The 2004 version of this revised classification is shown in Table 24.1. The two major types, type 1 (formerly called insulin-dependent diabetes mellitus or IDDM) and type 2 (formerly called noninsulin-dependent diabetes mellitus or NIDDM), are quite different both in genetic and in clinical aspects. Impaired glucose tolerance (IGT) and impaired fasting glucose (IFT) are terms used to describe the state between normal and diabetic. They are considered risk factors for future diabetes and not clinical diseases. In addition, the diagnostic criteria for diabetes mellitus have been revised, and a fasting plasma glucose concentration of <100 mg/dl is now defined as the upper limit of "normal" resulting in more individuals being classified as diabetic. Gestational diabetes, one of the classifications, is discussed in chapter 13.

DM is an important cause of morbidity, mortality, and health care costs. In the United States, in 2002, the Centers for Disease Control and Prevention (2004) estimated that the prevalence of diagnosed cases of DM was about 13.0 million, whereas another 5.2 million were believed to be undiagnosed.

Additionally, DM results in complications such as cardiovascular disease, hypertension, blindness, kidney disease, and nerve damage. DM is more frequent in certain ethnic and racial groups. The highest known prevalence is in the Pima Native Americans in Arizona (35–50%) and the Naruans (a Pacific Island group). In such populations, type 2 DM may result from a single major gene rather than multiple ones. Among the U.S. population at age 65 years, the prevalence is 33% in Hispanics, 25% in Blacks, and 17% in Whites.

Evidence for genetic contribution to DM comes from twin studies, sibling studies, migration studies, population studies, genetic and molecular techniques such as linkage analysis, DNA techniques including mapping and genome scans, the identification of genetic markers and variations, and the association with certain HLA types (see chapter 19). The propensity to develop diabetes-related complications such as nephropathy, cardiovascular disease, neuropathy, and retinopathy is also believed to have a genetic component, and susceptibility information may lead to new ways to prevent and treat such complications. Genetic heterogeneity may still exist within classifications, as discussed later in this chapter. The scope of the potential for heterogeneity becomes obvious when one considers the various possibilities for impaired glucose metabolism to occur. The regulation of glucose and of insulin is extremely complex, depending mostly on insulin secretion from pancreatic beta cells, glucagon secretion from alpha cells, and insulin action to promote glucose uptake. Many genes synthesize proteins, hormones, and enzymes that influence the production, secretion, transport, binding, cell entry, and eventual biological action and regulation of a normal insulin molecule. At any phase an alteration of the molecule in

TABLE 24.1   Classification of Diabetes Mellitus

I. Type 1 diabetes
   A. Immune mediated
   B. Idiopathic

II. Type 2 diabetes

III. Other specific types of diabetes mellitus
   A. Genetic defects of β-cell function (example: MODY2)
   B. Genetic defects in insulin action (example: type A insulin resistance)
   C. Diseases of the exocrine pancreas (example: cystic fibrosis)
   D. Endocrinopathies (example: hyperthyroidism)
   E. Drug- or chemical-induced (example: pentamidine)
   F. Infections (example: congenital rubella)
   G. Uncommon forms of immune-mediated diabetes (example: "stiff-man" syndrome)
   H. Other genetic syndromes sometimes associated with diabetes (example: Down syndrome)

IV. Gestational diabetes mellitus

Adapted from the American Diabetes Association (2004). Report of the Expert Committee on the diagnosis and classification of diabetes mellitus. *Diabetes Care, 27*(S11), S8.

question, an inadequate amount of an essential substrate, a decrease in the rate of synthesis, a defective energy system, defective cell membrane receptors, glucose transporter defects, receptor signal defects, defects in ion channels, or lipid metabolism, mediation of insulin uptake, defective or inadequate amounts of enzymes needed for a reaction, or defective transport could occur. Other influencing factors could include the presence of diabetes mellitus susceptibility genes, defective regulation or altered levels of hormones such as glucagon, cortisol, growth hormones, catecholamines, unknown factors connected with obesity, production of insulin antagonists, defects in intracellular glucose metabolism, antibodies against the insulin receptors, and a variety of impaired post-receptor events.

The apparent low frequency of type 2 DM (T2DM) in primitive societies as opposed to its high frequency in civilized societies, as well as the high incidence of T2DM that occurs in a few generations when a formerly isolated hunting society becomes "civilized" has led geneticists to speculate that DM might have had a selective advantage. Neel (1976) postulated that DM represented a "thrifty genotype" allowing the individual to respond rapidly to food intake and by sustaining hyperglycemia when food was scarce, and this idea remained popular. The change in physical activity and the increased incidence of obesity as a component may also influence the high prevalence of T2DM in certain groups. Nutritional status may also play a role as those who experience in utero malnutrition may have interference with proper pancreatic development.

Although genetic disorders that have impaired glucose metabolism as a component are comparatively rare when considering all known causes of diabetes mellitus, they are important because they underscore the fact that known gene mutations at different sites can all result in the same endpoint. This is true regardless of the pathogenetic mechanism involved, whether it is insulin deficiency due to pancreatic degeneration or due to hyperglycemia resulting from production of an abnormal proinsulin molecule. There are more than 60 genetic disorders that have glucose intolerance, DM, or hyperglycemia as components, with a variety of inheritance patterns. These include such diverse disorders as leprechaunism (an autosomal recessive disorder characterized by elfin facies, mental retardation, and insulin-resistant DM), Mendenhall syndrome (an autosomal recessive disorder characterized by insulin-resistant DM), pineal hyperplasia (skin problems, hirsutism, and phallic enlargement), disorders affecting the pancreas such as cystic fibrosis or hemochromatosis (see chapter 3), as well as disorders of the adrenal and pituitary glands.

Many drugs and chemicals are also known to promote glucose intolerance and frank DM. The extent of their ability to cause damage may be influenced by the genotype of the person exposed to the agent, as well as to external factors. Genetic factors may also play a role in the susceptibility for development of certain complications of DM such as diabetic retinopathy and nephropathy.

TYPE 1 DIABETES MELLITUS

Type 1 DM (T1DM) comprising 5% to 10% of all DM, has two subtypes, immune-mediated diabetes and idiopathic diabetes. Few persons with T1DM fit into the idiopathic category, which has a strong inherited component, is frequent in persons of African or Asian origin, has no HLA association, and does not appear to result from autoimmunity. The immune-mediated category results from autoimmune destruction of the pancreatic beta cells, which leads to the absolute extinguishing of insulin secretion. Exogenous insulin is therefore eventually necessary for control. Consequences of the pancreatic beta cell destruction may include increased insulin sensitivity, reduced insulin secretion, hyperglycemia, and insulin deficiency. The destruction may result in the presence of one or more of the following markers: circulating islet cell autoantibodies (ICA), autoantibodies to insulin (IAAs), autoantibodies to glutamic acid decarboxylase, and autoantibodies to tryrosine phosphatases IA-2 and IA-2β. T1DM usually, but not invariably, has its onset before the age of 40 years (considered before 30 by some) with a peak between 5 and 15 years of age, and often another less defined peak at age 20–35 years. It was formerly referred to as juvenile diabetes, although now it is evident that about one-half of the cases are recognized above 20 years of age. Obesity is rarely present. It is the second most common childhood illness in developed countries.

T1DM is considered to be multifactorial in that both genetic and environmental factors are necessary for expression (see chapter 4). The genetic component is generally considered to be polygenic, in which many genes each contribute a susceptibility effect. Some believe that one or a few major genes rather than many minor genes determine this susceptibility. Data from twin studies show a concordance rate of 30% to 50% in monozygotic twins with lower rates in dizygotic twins and sibs. It is not believed that this discordance is caused by an inadequate length of follow-up time, but rather that both genetic and environmental factors play a role in T1DM.

To date, several chromosomal areas have a well-established association with T1DM. These are the HLA region which is the major histocompatibility complex in humans (see chapter 19) on chromosome 6 (6p21) in the histocompatibility region, and the insulin gene region on chromosome 11 (11p15); the putative genes are called *IDDM1* and *IDDM2* respectively. It is estimated that *IDDM1* contributes 40% to 60% and *IDDM2* contributes about 10% to the familial inheritance of T1DM. The insulin gene region includes a region of variable number of tandem repeats (VNTR) that flank the insulin gene. The VNTR region is believed to have a role in modulating insulin gene expression. The variations in number, presence, location, and sequence of elements within this area are associated with susceptibility to T1DM. There are many other possible candidates for T1DM susceptibility loci on chromosome 15, other areas of chromosome 11, and 6, 2, 7, and others which have been designated with putative *IDDM* numbers. The *IDDM12* locus on chromosome 2q33 contains the cytotoxic T-lymphocyte-associated 4 *(CTLA4)* gene in which variants may be associated with T1DM development. Various epigenetic mechanisms, parent-of-origin effects, and gene expression regulation such as alternative splicing may play roles in T1DM development.

A search for an association between HLA and T1DM was reasonable because of previously determined associations between HLA and other diseases sharing chronicity, unknown etiology, and autoimmune components as features. HLA is fully discussed in chapter 19. Within the HLA region, more than 90% of white persons with T1DM express the serologically determined HLA DR3 (DQA1*0501 and DQB10201) and/or DR4 (DQA1*0301 and DRQB1*0302) with the highest risk being for those who are heterozygous for DR3/DR4. But these antigens are also present in persons who do not develop T1DM. Thus, possession of these antigens alone is not sufficient to cause T1DM. Alleles distinguished by molecular means suggest that combinations of DQA1 and DQB1 alleles, especially *DQA1*0501-*

DQB1*0201/DQA1*0301-DQB1*0302, confer even higher susceptibility in all ethnic groups. Various combinations confer varying degrees of susceptibility in different ethnic and racial groups. Of particular interest is the finding that some combinations of HLA alleles appear to be protective in regard to T1DM, particularly *DQB1*0602*. As is the case with other disorders associated with particular HLA types, not all persons with the susceptible HLA type develop diabetes. HLA DR3 or DR4 are present in about 90% of persons with T1DM.

The nature of the nongenetic or environmental contribution to T1DM is believed to be most important in early childhood, and perhaps even in utero. Some of these putative modifiers or triggers are the early introduction of artificial milk (cow's milk) and solid foods to infants under 3 months, viral infections (especially rubella, mumps, and Coxsackie viruses), toxic exposures, maternal-fetal blood group incompatibility, and conditions that increase stress on the beta cells such as a cold climate, puberty, pregnancy, and rapid growth or low vitamin D intake. In those infected with congenital rubella, those with HLA DR3/4 were more likely to develop T1DM than those with other HLA haplotypes. Besides the use of standard methods of insulin replacement therapy, other therapies are being developed including cloning technology and stem cell therapy. For example, DNA or the nucleus from somatic cells from a patient could be used to be transferred into an embryonal stem cell for expansion into a beta cell lineage for insulin replacement. Other methods for transferring cells or genes have been suggested. Islet cell transplantation has also been used.

TYPE 2 DIABETES MELLITUS

T2DM is defined as ranging from predominately insulin resistance with relative insulin deficiency to a predominately insulin secretory defect with insulin resistance (American Diabetes Association, 2004). T2DM was formerly referred to as adult-onset diabetes, as it usually begins after age 40 years. In contrast to T1DM, T2DM is associated with a strong genetic predisposition or may have multiple causes. The number of adults with T2DM has risen rapidly and has been called an epidemic since the number of cases in adults increased by 49% between 1991 and 2000.

It is genetically heterogenous. A few rare single-gene defects that affect small subgroups of those with T2DM have been identified, such as the maturity onset diabetes of the young (MODY) defects and defects in genes encoding glucokinase, insulin, the insulin receptor, and in the mitochondria. In the majority of affected persons, it is considered to be polygenic/multifactorial—caused by a number of genes and influenced by other factors such as obesity and exercise. Some genes may be primary and others may be related—for example those that predispose to obesity. In T2DM there are two essential defects in insulin secretion and action that lead to hyperglycemia (and eventually its complications): the deficient secretion of insulin in response to glucose and the decrease in the ability of insulin to promote glucose uptake in the peripheral tissues (insulin resistance). It is believed that in some cases, insulin resistance may precede and initiate T2DM but persons with insulin resistance do not necessarily develop T2DM. Insulin resistance and obesity are related. Intracellular triglycerides accumulate in muscle and liver occurs in T2DM, adding to insulin resistance. This may predate the clinical development of T2DM by years. In some cases, T2DM susceptibility genes may be population specific. Although various candidate genes for susceptibility have been identified in specific populations, many fewer are replicated and corroborated by others. The HNF-1-α gene mutation known to be responsible for some cases of MODY, discussed below, has also been shown to contribute to the high incidence of T2DM in the Oji-Cree indiginous population in Ontario, Canada. The calpain-10 gene mutation, which encodes a protein-splitting enzyme, appears to be linked to T2DM in certain Mexican-American populations in families and in certain African-American populations. Other gene mutations of current interest are variations (especially the Pro12Ala polymorphism) in the peroxisome proliferator-activated receptor-γ *(PPAR-γ)* gene, which encodes a nuclear receptor, insulin receptor genes that transmit signals to cells, and the *APM1* gene which encodes adiponectin and is involved with fat-induced metabolic syndrome modulating insulin sensitivity. Rare mutations in *PPAR-γ* have been found to cosegregate with T2DM, hypertension, and insulin resistance in a small number of families with autosomal dominant inheritance. It is interesting that the drug class, thiazolidinediones which improves insulin sensitivity and include the agents Actos and Avandia, act in part by stimulating *PPAR-γ* activity. The peroxisome proliferator-activated receptor-γ coactivator 1 (PGC-1) is a transcriptional regulator of genes involved in mitochondrial biogenesis and fat oxidation. A polymorphism of PGC-1 (Gly482Ser) has been linked to an increased T2DM risk in certain Danish populations and altered insulin secretion and lipid oxidation in Pima Indians. Gene expression of PGC-1α has been found to be reduced in overweight people with T2DM, overweight Mexican-American patients with T2DM, and a population of overweight persons who had a family history of diabetes.

In early twin studies 90% to 100% of identical twin pairs were concordant for T2DM, with lower concordance in dizygotic twins and sibs. Because these twin studies were largely concerned with persons in the middle to older age group who had been living apart for a number of years, any environmental factor would have to have exerted its influence in the early years of life when they shared a common environment. These high concordance rates were present even when differences in body weight were present, thus suggesting that the powerful genetic component acts independently of an obesity factor. Another factor that can influence the degree of concordance is the laboratory tests used to determine concordance. It has been suggested that blood glucose values are a much less sensitive indicator than evaluation for impairment of the insulin response or other parameters. Changes that precede T2DM, such as subtle changes in fasting glucose and insulin levels, appear to be evident in children and young adults, suggesting opportunities for early intervention.

GENETIC DEFECTS OF B-CELL FUNCTION

This category includes the following

- Maturity onset diabetes of the young (MODY) (discussed below),
- Mitochondrial DNA mutations,
- Others such as the inability to convert proinsulin to insulin or the production of mutant insulin molecules with impaired receptor

binding. Each of these is inherited in an autosomal dominant (AD) pattern with relatively mild impaired glucose metabolism.

MODY consists of several types of AD single-gene conditions with high penetrance in which DM develops due to a primary defect in insulin secretion, at a young age (usually before age 25 years, and often in the first decade of life) but in which insulin is not usually required. It is considered by some to be a subtype of T2DM, and some feel that the term MODY should not be used but rather autosomal dominant T2DM. At least six gene mutations can result in MODY. The major one is mutations in the hepatocyte nuclear factor *(HNF-1α)* (a transcription factor) on chromosome 12q24, known as MODY3. Others are MODY1 (due to mutations in *HNF-4α*); MODY2 (due to mutations in the gene encoding for glucokinase on chromosome 7p which is also a common form of MODY); MODY4 (due to mutations in the insulin promotor factor-1 (*IPF1* gene): MODY5 (due to mutations in the *HNF-1β* gene on chromosome 17, and MODY6 (due to mutations in the neurogenic differentiation factor-1 *(NeuroD1)* gene. These vary widely in the clinical spectrum and *HNF-1β* mutations have been associated with urogenital malformations in addition to T2DM (Bellané-Chantelot et al., 2004). Another type of AD T2DM results from mutation in the sulfonylurea receptor 1 *(SUR1)* gene and causes hyperinsulinism in infancy as well as a loss of insulin secretory capacity in early adulthood. Obviously genetic counseling is different for those in this category and it is important to have a correct diagnosis.

Observations of persons with DM who had an affected parent revealed that they more frequently had affected mothers than affected fathers, and DM is frequently associated with certain mitochondrial diseases. This suggested that mtDNA mutations (see chapters 4 and 6) might play a role in DM. The first identified association of a specific point mutation in the mtDNA (A3243G, an A to G mutation in mtDNA at position 3243 in the tRNA) with deafness and diabetes is known as MIDD (maternally inherited diabetes and deafness). Since then, other point mutations and deletions in mitochondrial genes have been described in connection with diabetes mellitus.

GENETIC DEFECTS IN INSULIN ACTION

These tend to be rare in frequency and include abnormalities associated with mutations of structure or function of the insulin receptor. These include a variety of syndromes including leprechaunism (an autosomal recessive disorder with characteristic elfin facies, mental retardation, insulin resistance, and early death) and Rabson-Mendenhall syndrome (an autosomal recessive disorder with skin, hair, nail, and teeth abnormalities, insulin resistant DM, and pineal gland hyperplasia). Petersen et al. (2004) in studying a sample of young, lean insulin-resistant offspring of parents with T2DM have suggested that an inherited defect in mitochondrial oxidative phosphorylation leading to reduction of muscle mitochondrial content. This might cause dysregulation of intramyocellular fatty acid metabolism and lipid accumulation, and thus insulin resistance. These data are said to provide a link between defects in beta cell function and muscle that are seen in T2DM (Taylor, 2004).

GENETIC COUNSELING IN DIABETES MELLITUS

The problems in providing accurate genetic counseling in DM can be seen from the preceding discussion. In the past, genetic counseling for DM was based on empirically derived risk data, but today more accurate determinations can be made. Note that the older terminology is used here in places because that is how risks were determined before the reclassification. These risk estimates depend on the evaluation of many individual factors. Histories should contain much more precise information than they did formerly. Nurses should collect the following information: height; weight; age; date of birth; race; ethnic origin; the presence or absence of obesity; type and degree of obesity according to a standard measure; whether any metabolic insults such as infection or trauma were associated with onset; for females, a pregnancy history including weight of infants and age of DM onset; degree of control if diabetic; presence of any disorders with an autoimmune component within the family; any exposure to drugs or chemicals linked with hyperglycemia; and the results of

relevant laboratory tests such as HLA haplotyping for patients who are seeking information relating to T1DM, but not in T2DM where it is not valuable. Diagnosis should be obtained for the individual themselves, and for both the immediate and extended family. The family history may reveal the presence of a specific inheritance mechanism for that family. In addition, other syndromes with DM as a component should be ruled out before attempting counseling. Nutritional status and usual lifestyle habits, especially in regard to physical activity, are useful in implementing appropriate health counseling.

Individuals with impaired glucose tolerance (IGT) and impaired fasting glucose (IFG) have a high potential for developing DM. This is not meant to be diagnostic, and individuals should not be clinically classified as prediabetic because they may face job discrimination or increased health costs. It may be useful in identifying individuals who can benefit from genetic counseling and from health counseling regarding factors that can modify the risk of overt diabetes, such as weight control.

Those individuals at the highest risk for T1DM are as follows:

- Individuals positive for islet cell autoantibodies (ICA)
- Monozygotic twin of person with T1DM
- HLA-identical sibling of person with T1DM
- Sibling sharing one HLA haplotype with person who had T1DM
- Other siblings
- Offspring of parent with T1DM
- Persons with an HLA haplotype conferring susceptibility for T1DM.

Those individuals at the highest risk for T2DM are as follows:

- Monozygotic twin of person with T2DM
- First-degree relative of person with T2DM (sibling, parent, offspring)
- Obese person
- Mother of newborn weighing more than 4.5 kg (9.9 lb)
- Member of racial or ethnic group with a high prevalence of T2DM, such as certain Native Americans, Nauru islanders, Welsh, etc. (A

full listing can be found in the WHO Expert Committee Report on Diabetes Mellitus, 1994.)

- Members of families in which a specific known mutation causing susceptibility or overt disease is segregating.

Genetic counseling will then be based on the number of individuals in the family with diabetes mellitus; the type of DM; the age of onset; the severity; the type of inheritance within the family, if any; the degree of relationship of the person seeking advice to those with diabetes mellitus; the results of HLA haplotyping, if available; the presence of known mutations in other diabetes susceptibility genes, if any; other risk factors; and the results of the findings collected in the history.

Empirical genetic risk data for the relatives of those with T1DM have been estimated by Taylor (1995) as follows: monozygotic twin, 30–50%; dizygotic twin, 15%; HLA-identical sibling, 3–6%; sibling sharing one HLA haplotype, 4–9%; HLA non-identical sibling is estimated at the population frequency, 1%; children, 3–5%. Garner (1995) estimates that the child of a woman with T1DM has a risk of 1–3% of developing T1DM but a risk of 6.1% if it is the father who has T1DM and a 20% risk if both parents are affected. For eventual development of T2DM, Lubin, Lin, Vadheim, and Rotter (1990) give a risk of 10–15% for clinical T2DM and 20–30% for impaired glucose tolerance in first-degree relatives. A general population estimate risk for T1DM is 1 in 500 and 1% to 5% for T2DM. More tailored estimates are made depending on factors noted above and depending on the number and relationship of affected relatives. In T1DM, risk estimates for those with various ICAs and HLA combinations are available and are used to determine risk in specific families.

Prevention of DM is an area of focus. Screening cord blood for HLA types has been suggested with the aim of prevention, for example by removing cow's milk from the infant diet. This is also a potential strategy for infants with a first-degree relative with T1DM. Eventual autoantigen vaccination has been suggested. Administering free-radical scavengers such as nicotinamide to prevent beta cell destruction has been suggested early in life to prevent T1DM, and relatives of T1DM patients with ICA will be enrolled in a trial to test this.

Other trials test the ability of IV or oral insulin in T1DM high-risk relatives with IDA to prevent or delay diabetes by allowing beta cells to rest and encouraging the development of antigen tolerance, which also might be accomplished by oral antigen administration. Immunomodulation and immuno-suppressive therapies have also been suggested. For T2DM, low-fat diets, prevention of obesity, and appropriate exercise are prevention techniques. Exercise has been shown to actually increase the number of insulin receptor sites in muscle tissue. Those who have first-degree relatives with T2DM can have periodic glucose tolerance testing and screening for risk factors associated with cardiovascular disease such as hypertension and hyperlipidemia. For the woman with glucose intolerance during pregnancy, WHO suggests the possibility of insulin treatment during pregnancy, and after delivery, the prevention of obesity and physical exercise programs.

BIBLIOGRAPHY

Åkerblom, H. K., Vaarala, O., Hyöty, H., Ilonen, J., & Knip, M. (2002). Environmental factors in the etiology of type 1 diabetes. *American Journal of Medical Genetics Seminars in Medical Genetics, 115,* 18–29.

American Academy of Pediatrics. Work Group on Cow's Milk Protein and Diabetes. (1994). Infant feeding practices and their possible relationship to the etiology of diabetes mellitus. *Pediatrics, 94,* 752–754.

American Diabetes Association. (2004). Report of the Expert Committee on the Diagnosis and Classification of Diabetes Mellitus. *Diabetes Care, 26*(Suppl. 1), S5–S20.

Anderson, D. C., Jr. (2005). Pharmacologic prevention or delay of type 2 diabetes mellitus. *Annals of Pharmacotherapy, 39,* 102–109.

Bakris, G. L. (2003). The evolution of treatment guidelines for diabetic nephropathy. *Postgraduate Medicine, 113,* 35–40, 43–44, 50.

Barnett, A. H., Eff, C., Leslie, R. D. G., & Pyke, D. A. (1981). Diabetes in identical twins: A study of 200 pairs. *Diabetologia, 20,* 87–93.

Bellanné-Chantelot, C., Chauveau, D., Gautier, J. F., Dubois-Laforgue, D., Clauin, S., Beaufils, S., et al. (2004). Clinical spectrum associated with hepatocyte nuclear factor-1β mutations. *Annals of Internal Medicine, 140,* 510–517.

Bottino, R., Lemarchand, P., Trucco, M., & Giannoukakis, N. (2003). Gene- and cell-based therapeutics for type 1 diabetes mellitus. *Gene Therapy, 10,* 875–889.

Bowden, D. W. (2002). Genetics of diabetes complications. *Current Diabetes Reports, 2,* 191–200.

Centers for Disease Control and Prevention. (2004, May 18). National Diabetes Fact Sheet.

Diamond, J. (2003). The double puzzle of diabetes. *Nature, 423,* 599–602.

Frank, R. N. (2004). Diabetic retinopathy. *New England Journal of Medicine, 350,* 48–58.

Garner, P. (1995). Type 1 diabetes mellitus and pregnancy. *Lancet, 346,* 157–161.

Gerling, I. C., Soloman, S. S., & Bryer-Ash, M. (2003). Genomes, transcriptomes, and proteomes. *Archives of Internal Medicine, 163,* 190–198.

Glaser, B. (2003). Dominant *SUR1* mutation causing autosomal dominant type 2 diabetes. *Lancet, 361,* 272–273.

Guillausseau, P. J., Dubois-Laforgue, D., Massin, P., Laloi-Michelin, M., Bellanne-Chantelot, C., Gin, H., et al. (2004). Heterogeneity of diabetes phenotype in patients with 3243 bp mutation of mitochondrial DNA (Maternally Inherited Diabetes and Deafness or MIDD). *Diabetes and Metabolism, 30,* 181–186.

Harper, P. S. (1998). *Practical genetic counseling* (5th ed.). Oxford, England: Butterworth Heinemann.

Ilonen, J., Sjöroos, M., Knip, M., Veijola, R., Simell, O., Åkerblom, H. K., et al. (2002). Estimation of genetic risk for type 1 diabetes. *American Journal of Medical Genetics (Seminars in Medical Genetics), 115,* 30–36.

Kostraba, J. N., Cruickshanks, K. J., Lawler-Heavner, J., Jobim, L. F., Rewers, M. J., & Gay, E. C. (1993). Early exposure to cow's milk and solid foods in infancy, genetic predisposition and risk of IDDM. *Diabetes, 42,* 288–295.

Laron, Z. (2002). Interplay between heredity and environment in the recent explosion of type 1 childhood diabetes mellitus. *American Journal of Medical Genetics (Seminars in Medical Genetics), 115,* 4–7.

Leslie, R. D. G., & Elliott, R. B. (1994). Early environmental events as a cause of IDDM. Evidence and implications. *Diabetes, 43,* 843–850.

Maassen, J. A. (2002). Mitochondrial diabetes: Pathophysiology, clinical presentation, and genetic analysis. *American Journal of Medical Genetics (Seminars in Medical Genetics), 115,* 66–70.

McCarthy, M. I., & Froguel, P. (2002). Genetic approaches to the molecular understanding of type 2 diabetes. *American Journal of Physiology, Endocrinology, and Metabolism, 283,* E217–E225.

Moustakas, A. K., & Papadopoulos, G. K. (2002). Molecular properties of HLA-DQ alleles conferring susceptibility to or protection from insulin-dependent diabetes mellitus: Keys to the fate of islet β-cells. *American Journal of Medical Genetics (Seminars in Medical Genetics, 115,* 37–47.

Neel, J. V. (1976). Diabetes mellitus-a geneticist's nightmare. In W. Creutzfeldt, J. J. K6bberling, & J. V. Neel (Eds,), *The genetics of diabetes mellitus.* Berlin: Springer-Verlag.

Petersen, K. F., Dufour, S., Befroy, D., Garcia, R., & Shulman, G. (2004). Impaired mitochondrial activity in the insulin-resistant offspring of patients with type 2 diabetes. *New England Journal of Medicine, 350,* 644-671.

Porte, D., Jr., Sherwin, R. S., & Baron, A. (Eds.). (2003). *Ellenberg & Rifkin's diabetes mellitus.* New York: McGraw-Hill, Medical Publishing Division.

Pugliese, A. (2004). Genetics of type 1 diabetes. *Endocrinology and Metabolism Clinics of North America, 33,* 1–16.

Riley, M. D., Blizzard, C. L., McCarty, D. J., Senator, G. B., Dwyer, T., & Zimmet, P. (1997). Parental history of diabetes in an insulin-treated diabetes registry. *Diabetic Medicine, 14,* 35–41.

Seidel, D., & Ziegler, A-G. (1996). Prediction of type 1 diabetes. *Hormone Research, 45*(Suppl. 1), 36–39.

Siebold, C., Hansen, B. E., Wyer, J. R., Harlos, K., Esnouf, R. E., Svejgaard, A., et al. (2004). Crystal structure of HLA-DQ0602 that protects against type 1 diabetes and confers strong susceptibility to narcolepsy. *Proceedings of the National Academy of Sciences, 101,* 1999–2004.

Skolnick, A. A. (1997). First type I diabetes prevention trials. *Journal of the American Medical Association, 277,* 1101–1102.

Taylor, R. (2004). Causation of type 2 diabetes—the Gordian knot unravels. *New England Journal of Medicine, 350,* 639–641.

Taylor, S. I. (1995). Diabetes mellitus. In C. R. Scriver, A. L. Beaudet, W. S. Sly, & D. Valle (Eds.), *The metabolic and molecular bases of inherited disease* (7th ed., pp. 843–896). New York: McGraw-Hill.

Timsit, J., Bellanne-Chantelot, C., Dubois-Laforgue, D., & Velho, G. (2005). Diagnosis and management of maturity onset diabetes of the young. *Treatment in Endocrinology, 4,* 9–18.

Verge, C. F., & Eisenbarth, G. S. (1996). Strategies for preventing type 1 diabetes mellitus. *Western Journal of Medicine, 164,* 249–255.

Warpeha, K. M., & Chakravarthy, U. (2003). Molecular genetics of microvascular disease in diabetic retinopathy. *Eye, 17,* 305–311.

World Health Organization. (1994). *Prevention of diabetes mellitus.* WHO Technical Report Series 844. Geneva, Switzerland: WHO.

25

Mental Illness and Behavior

The brain is the most complex organ, and thousands of genes are involved in some way with brain function. In addition to the large number of neurons and nerve cell connections, cell-to-cell communication occurs through at least 50 known neurotransmitters. About 30% of the known genetic diseases involve nervous system defects. The genetics of cognitive abilities, mental functioning, social attitudes, psychological interests, psychiatric disorders, learning disorders, behavior, addiction, mood, and personality traits have long been of interest to geneticists, but this interest has been complicated by the complexity of brain function as well as the social, ethical, legal, and political implications of research in this area. The contribution of genetic factors to the major types of mental illnesses such as schizophrenia, and the mood or affective disorders (including major depressive disorders and bipolar disease) has long been investigated as have contributions to behavioral, learning, and emotional conditions such as panic disorder, dyslexia, criminal behavior, attention-deficit disorder, personality characteristics such as shyness, risk taking, IQ, and other parameters. Theories regarding the etiology of major mental illnesses and certain behaviors have ranged from that of a single major gene to multiple genes to environmental derangement to a combination of genetic and environmental causes.

The observation that these disorders tend to run in families is claimed as support for all of these theories. Biological families tend to share their genes, cultural heritage, and living environment which includes similar exposure to pathogens, diet, stressors, toxins, dynamic family interactions, patterns of behavior, and other parameters. There has been increasing support for investigation into the contribution of genetic factors in mental illness and behavior. For example, a major workshop on schizophrenia recommended that major efforts be concentrated on looking for predisposing genes. Disorders known to be due to a single gene error (e.g., Lesch-Nyhan syndrome) or to a chromosomal aberration (e.g., Klinefelter syndrome) can have effects manifested in terms of behavior. Many of the genetic disorders can be modified by their external environment, so that behavioral effects may or may not be apparent (e.g., phenylketonuria). In multifactorial disorders, a model for the interaction of genes and environment is already present. It is realistic to expect that genetic factors are at least in part responsible for the etiology of the major psychoses, with the question being to what extent. It is also likely that in some relatively rare families the abnormal phenotype such as schizophrenia may be determined by a single gene error, whereas in others a different gene(s) may confer a susceptibility that depends on certain environmental conditions, triggers, or another gene variation(s) for expression.

The initial establishment of the broad categories of classical schizophrenia and affective, bipolar, or manic-depressive illness was largely based on descriptive symptoms. These categories have been further subdivided over time, but they still represent somewhat heterogenous subtypes that may, as in diabetes mellitus, represent more than one disease and etiology with different inheritance mechanisms. Previously, varying differences in nomenclature and in what was included in "schizophrenia" over the years has made genetic study and interpretation difficult. The major evidence for the role of genetic factors in schizophrenia and the mood disorders originally came from family studies, twin studies, adoption studies, and biochemical analyses. More recently, genetic modeling, linkage, whole genome scans, and other molecular genetic techniques are being used to understand the genetic contribution. Most of the early studies and techniques suffered from methodological problems (see chapter 16) but nearly all of them documented some type of genetic component. At this time, however, the exact nature of the genetic contribution to the major mental disorders remains unknown.

SCHIZOPHRENIA

According to the American Psychiatric Association's *Diagnostic and Statistical Manual* (DSM IV-TR, 2000), schizophrenia is a psychotic disorder that "lasts for at least 6 months, and includes 1 month of active phase symptoms (i.e., two (or more) of the following: delusions, hallucinations, disorganized speech, grossly disorganized or catatonic behavior, negative symptoms)" (p. 273). The worldwide prevalence is about 1%. Subtypes include paranoid, disorganized, catatonic, undifferentiated, and residual. In addition, schizoaffective disorder is a disturbance in which symptoms of schizophrenia and a mood disorder occur together. Harrison and Owen (2003) consider that schizophrenia has a heritability of about 80% but unequivocable single genes have not yet been identified. Major issues in studies include whether pure schizophrenia has been analyzed or whether the clinical spectrum of schizophrenic disorders has been included. At least 40 family and twin studies have been conducted. The essence of these reviews indicates that these studies have consistently found a higher prevalence of the respective illness among relatives. Those studies that have compared the concordance of monozygotic (MZ) twins for schizophrenia with that of dizygotic (DZ) twins have found in all cases that the concordance rate for MZ twins is higher than for DZ twins, although the exact rates have varied from study to study, giving support for a heritability component. Overall concordance rates have varied from 35% to 92% in MZ twins and from 7% to 26% for DZ twins, with an overall pooled rate of 45.6% for MZ and 13.7% for DZ. High concordance rates appear to be associated with severity of the illness. The age of the onset of illness shows greater association between

twins than would be expected by chance. In both groups, twins who have lived apart generally show similar concordance rates to those who have been raised in the same environment.

General conclusions from adoption studies (see chapter 16) reveal that those children born of schizophrenic parents developed schizophrenia at significantly higher rates than did adoptees born of normal parents. Biologic relatives of those adoptees who developed schizophrenia had higher rates of schizophrenia and suicide than did the adoptive relatives and the biologic and adoptive relatives of adoptees who did not become schizophrenic. Those adoptees born of normal parents but raised by schizophrenic adoptive parents did not show an increase in schizophrenia. In order to rule out the intrauterine environment or early interaction with a schizophrenic mother, some researchers studied paternal half-siblings. These half-siblings had the same biologic schizophrenic father, but a different biologic mother. The increased incidence of schizophrenia found was interpreted as ruling out early maternal influences.

More recent studies have looked at the candidate gene approach or linkage, often focusing on those genes or markers having pharmacologic, immunological, and biochemical associations. Based on these, some of those explored have been the gene for catecholamine methyltransferase, which metabolizes the neurotransmitters dopamine, epinephrine, and norepinephrine, as well as both receptors and transmitters for these and for GABA (gamma-aminobutyric acid), serotonin, and monoamine oxidase. Other promising candidate genes for susceptibility include neuregulin (*NRG1*), dysbindin (*DTNBP1*), G72, RGS4 (the regulator of G-protein signalling-4), proline dehydrogenase (*PRODH*), ZDHHC8 (encoding a transmembrane palmitoyltransferase on chromosome 22q11.2, a chromosomal area implicated in DiGeorge syndrome and increased risks for certain neuropsychiatric phenotypes), and catechol-O-methyltransferease (*COMT*). Many of these are located in chromosomal areas that are linked to schizophrenia, as discussed below. Molecular and mapping techniques have been used. Newer strategies such as microarray technology to examine gene expression appear promising. At present, the most promising information appears to be an association and/or linkage for schizophrenia with the following chromosomal sites: 1q21-22, 6p22-24, 6q21-22, 8p21,10p11-15, 13q32, and 22q11-13. A subtype of schizophrenia, periodic catatonia, was also found to be associated with chromosome 15q14. In the case of chromosome 22, chromosomal micro-deletions in chromosome 22q11.21-q11.23 may increase susceptibility. A known genetic syndrome, velocardiofacial syndrome (an autosomal recessive disorder with cardiac anomalies, learning disabilities, and cleft palate), which is associated with small deletions in chromosome 22q11, includes about 10% who develop psychiatric disorders such as chronic paranoid schizophrenia. Karayiorgou et al. (1995) found a microdeletion of the 22q11 region in 2 of 100 schizophrenic patients. A candidate for a susceptibility gene on 22q12-13 is the A2a adenosine receptor, one of the receptors mediating central nervous system effects of adenosine, which showed linkage to schizophrenia in some persons. There has also been the possibility for a vulnerability locus for schizophrenia located on chromosome 6p, which was first described in the Irish Study of High-Density Schizophrenia Families (Kendler et al., 1997) and was also implicated by others such as Straub et al. (2002). This was not confirmed by others such as Daniels et al. (1997), however. Another area of investigation for etiology is unstable tandem repeat expansion (chapters 4 and 20). In at least some cases, anticipation (the appearance of more severe disease progressively earlier in successive generations) and a parent-of-origin effect has been noticed in schizophrenia, giving credence to the possible involvement of unstable tandem repeat nucleotide expansion in etiology. A theory that has had a resurgence of interest is that of events that disrupt neurodevelopmental and thus result in schizophrenia, such as Rh incompatibility and severe nutritional deficiencies. Advanced paternal age has also been associated with a higher risk for adult schizophrenia, perhaps due to de novo paternal mutations. Despite evidence for some yet unknown genetic basis for schizophrenia, environmental disturbances appear to be needed for ultimate expression. It is very likely that there will be multiple susceptibility genes eventually identified which act in conjunction with other genetic configurations, epigenetic processes, and enviornmental factors to result in the phenotype of schizophrenia.

MOOD DISORDERS

The mood disorders (MD), formerly described as affective disorders, may consist of depressive disorders, bipolar disorders, and mood disorders secondary to a general medical condition or substance-induced. They may affect at least 1% of the population. Those who are depressed may have a high risk of suicide. In many of the classic family, twin, and adoptive studies, results were reported in terms of unipolar illness (UP) or bipolar illness (BP). It has been proposed that there may be three distinct BP subgroups defined by age of onset with an early, middle, and late (over age 50 years) onset that might vary etiologically. In BP patients, first-degree relatives had a higher incidence of affective illness than those of UP patients, but both were higher than in the general population. If the index patient has BP disease, the risks to relatives are higher than if the index patient has UP disease (see chapter 4 for a review of multifactorial inheritance). Schlesser and Altshuler (1983) state that 80% to 90% of patients with BP disorders have a family history of an affective disorder, and 50% of UP patients have a family history of a UP disorder, with few having any BP disease. They believe that a family history of BP disorders is important in diagnosis of an individual with depression. There are more female relatives affected than male relatives. This may represent a sex-influenced gene or a sex-related liability threshold as seen in congenital hip disease. Twin studies over time reveal the potential of a hereditary component, and have been reported at about 70% for MZ twins and 20% for DZ twins. Concordance in MZ twins increases with the severity of the proband's illness.

Some adoption studies have been reported for the affective disorders. These basically found that there was an excess of all psychopathology in the biologic parents of the MD adoptees as compared to their adoptive parents. This incidence has been reported as similar to that of the biologic parents of MD persons who were not adopted. The most important finding of the adoption studies is that the incidence of mental illness paralleled that of the biologic relatives of the adoptee rather than that of the adoptive relatives.

Although various biochemical and immunological studies have been investigated, linkage and molecular studies have been the most recent approaches. These have focused on susceptibility regions on chromosomes and on certain biochemical polymorphisms. The latter have included disturbances in dopaminergic and noradrenergic transmitter systems, serotonin 2A receptor *(HTR2A)* gene polymorphisms, gamma-aminobutyric acid (GABA), and the glutaminergic pathways. Gene expression arrays offer new ways to look for associated differences in gene expression. Past reports of linkages in regard to chromosomes have been in conjunction with the X chromosome and chromosomes 11 and 21 but have been difficult to substantiate. X chromosome associations were suggested by an observed excess of females in mood disorders. Various studies have had contradictory findings, and a gene on the X chromosome may represent at least one susceptibility gene. The most significant linkage associations with chromosomal areas for bipolar disorder currently are as follows: 4p15-16, 9p22, 10q11, 11p, 12q23, 13q32, 14q, 18p11.2, 18q12, 18q22, 21q22, 22q11-12. The expansion of unstable tandem repeats has also been suggested as an etiology. Epigenetic mechanisms such as genomic imprinting have been postulated as having a role in the etiology of bipolar disorders. In one family, Darier disease (a genetic skin disorder) has been shown to be associated with bipolar illness.

BEHAVIOR AND GENETICS

The field of behavioral genetics is a very complex and interesting one. It is reasonable to suppose that there are genetic influences on parameters such as behavior as one considers the genetic influence on structural determination and patterning of anatomical configurations, or of the regulation of neurotransmitters, for example. Many of the investigations have been carried out in animal models because of problems in studying human populations, which has been difficult because of the belief that finding a genetic component to a behavioral trait means that the trait is immutable. Rather, such traits can be molded and are indeed shaped by environmental influences. Often understanding the genetics can lead to treatment advances. For example, persons with some types of dyslexia have responded to particular educational approaches that improve outcome. Grigorenko et al. (1997) have presented an interesting study of distinct reading phenotypes, each apparently linked to different chromosomal regions. Mutation in a gene, *FOXP2*, located on chromosome 7, which encodes a transcription factor, leads to a rare speech and language disorder. More often, multiple genes are believed to be involved, with environmental influences as well. Genome-wide scans have identified regions on chromosomes 2, 13, 16, and 19 which may influence speech and language disorders.

In one large family, a defect in the gene for monoamine oxidase A (MAOA) leading to deficiency resulted in an X-linked recessive mild mental retardation and a pattern of aggressive, impulsive, and violent behavior including arson and exhibitionism, and has been named Brunner syndrome. An animal model has also shown the association between deletion of the gene encoding MAOA and aggression in males. In animals, there are many examples of behavioral genetics. For example, ants can manipulate gene expression in developing juveniles so that some larvae that would have become docile workers are stimulated to become aggressive soldiers in response to a threat. A gene that controls social interactions has been found in mice. Dogs maintain specific behavioral traits within breeds. For example, a border collie will maintain eye contact with humans. If put at birth with a type of dog that doesn't, the border collie will continue this trait, and likewise if another breed is put with border collies at birth, they will not develop the eye-contact behavior. The eye-contact behavior is an example of how a genetically determined trait may influence environment. People will respond differently to those who look directly at them as opposed to those who avoid eye contact, thus resulting in different interactions and experiences that shape development. Persons with certain genotypes might create high-stress environments, thus increasing the probability of mental illness. Bouchard (1997) reports that high-sensation seekers might select similar-minded friends and seek dangerous experiences, but those who are novelty seekers might also seek creative careers (Hobert, 2003). A polymorphism in the dopamine D4 receptor gene that is related to novelty-seeking has been reported. There has been considerable opposition to genetic study of some traits such as aggression, intelligence, criminality, personality, sexual orientation, and others. In one well-publicized incident, a conference on genes and criminality was postponed for a considerable time period because of political involvement. However, there has been a recent resurgence in the influence of genes in virtually every realm of behavior including social attitudes, psychological interests, and even such traits as divorce (by virtue of biochemical and personality systems) and religiousness. For example, Bouchard & McGue, p. 31, (2003) quote Dawkins as saying that a "gene for developing the kind of brain that is predisposed to religion when exposed to a religious culture" could be possible. Genes are involved in creating neurons, brain development, and neural connections and transmitters. Religious feelings can be elicited in the brains of non-religious people by cranial stimulation. A recent twin study found that the heritability of cognition in elderly twins was 62%. Other disabilities such as alcoholism, panic disorder, and dyslexia appear to have substantial genetic components. Discussion of these is beyond this text, however. Although it seems likely that many traits have some type of genetic component, how heredity and environment build on each other in complex ways is not understood. Understanding of some of these aspects will make a real contribution to how we approach public policy issues.

Autism is a pervasive developmental disorder that usually has its onset before 3 years of age. It is characterized by impairments in reciprocal social interaction and communication and preferred repetetive, stereotyped behaviors and may include developmental delay, dysmorphic features, and epilepsy; it is more frequent in males. Several closely related disorders such as Asperger syndrome and disintegrative disorder are said to comprise autism spectrum disorders. There are no biological markers for diagnosis. While observations suggest genetic effects, genome-wide linkage and candidate-gene studies have shown some preliminary suggestions of the involvement of areas on chromosomes 2, 7, 13, and 15q11-13. Various gene variations have been implicated in autism including the *RELN* gene, which codes for a protein that guides neuronal migration. As in other disorders, epigenetic and environmental factors appear to play a role although these have not been identified.

ALCOHOLISM, SMOKING, AND ADDICTION

Not everyone who uses recreational drugs, including nicotine from smoking, meet criteria for substance abuse disorder. Thus, while variation in drug metabolism, neuronal physiology, and other biological factors are recognized as important, other factors in development and from the environment play a role. A complete discussion of these complex conditions is not possible here. Alcoholism has been investigated in twin studies and adoption studies, and these have provided evidence of a genetic component. As discussed in chapter 16, complex disorders are difficult to study, and in alcohol dependence, endpoints and definitions have varied—for example, tolerance, acute intoxication, withdrawal symptoms, amount of alcohol consumed, and episodic vs. steady consumption. Chief areas of interest have been variations in the gene for the mitochondrial aldehyde dehydrogenase *(ADLH2)*, which converts an intermediate product of ethanol metabolism, acetaldehyde, to acetic acid. A mutation known as *ALDH2*2/*2*, and to a certain extent, the heterozygote, *ALDH2*1/*2*, result in elevated blood levels of acetaldehyde after ingesting alcohol leading to a flushing reaction. Few with this genotype become alcohol dependent. In another example, the gene encoding the enzyme alcohol dehydrogenase (ADH) converts alcohol to acetaldehyde, and variations in its subunits also affect alcohol dependence risk in various ethnic groups. Other genes of interest have been the dopamine D2 receptor gene, serotonin variations and variations in the μ-opioid receptor gene, especially the single nucleotide polymorphism, A118G. A large, long-term study is being done known as the Collaborative Study of the Genetics of Alcoholism.

Smoking behavior is thought to have both genetic and environmental components. Evidence for genetic components come from twin studies and from variability in nicotine metabolism. The environmental and social influences are also known to be important, especially in the initiation of smoking. A group of enzymes (see chapter 18) known as cytochrome P-450 (CYP) metabolize nicotine to cotinine. Variations in the gene *(CYP2D6)* allow people to be poor, extensive, or ultrarapid metabolizers. People who metabolize nicotine more slowly appear less likely to become dependent while those who are ultrarapid metabolizers may smoke more heavily to maintain their blood nicotine levels. Thus, while people may begin smoking for various reasons, becoming dependent may be related, in part, to metabolism. Polymorphisms of dopamine receptor genes as well as genes encoding the opioid, cannabinoid, and glutamine receptors, also may influence dependence on various drugs. Many of these genes will interact with each other, influencing effects, as well as with the environment. Different gene variations may determine susceptibility to dependence on different drugs.

GENETIC COUNSELING

Awareness of the familial nature of psychiatric disorders among the public has been heightened by the media. Thus, the demand for genetic counseling among relatives of a person with mental illness has increased and nurses may be asked about its availability. Because of our incomplete understanding of the nature and extent of the genetic contribution in these disorders, counseling is based on empirically derived risk figures, or on what has been observed in large studies. The risk figures depend on the number of relatives affected, the severity and age of onset of the disorder in question in the proband, and what the risk entails (e.g., is the risk being given just for one type of schizophrenia or is the entire schizoid spectrum included). In the mood disorders, the sex of the proband and of the family member at risk is also important. In all cases counselees should be advised that the risk can be increased if they marry a relative or someone who has the illness in question, or a close family history of it. Counselees should also understand that risk estimates are empiric and may need to be adjusted to their specific situation. Therefore, if an empiric lifetime risk for developing schizophrenia is cited in the literature, and if a client is 30 years of age or older and free of the disorder, then his/her personal risk is likely to be only 50% that of what it was at birth.

Counselees should also understand that the prevalence of mental illness in the population is about 1.0%. Relatives of those with scihizophrenia are at higher risk. For example, Gottesman (1994) lists the risk to parents, siblings, and children of schizophrenics respectively as 6%, 9% and 13%, and 46% for children of two schizophrenic parents. Commonly cited risk figures for first-degree relatives if the proband has UP disease is about 7% but may be higher in females. Those for first-degree relatives of probands with BP disease may range from 13 to 14% to as high as 25%. In DZ twins it may be 20% ranging up to 70% in MZ twins, and 50% if both parents are affected, according to Harper (1993). These figures should only be used by a qualified geneticist in conjunction with complete diagnostic and family information, as previously discussed. It is possible that the further elucidation of biochemical and genetic markers may allow more precise counseling. Information on genetic counseling in mental illness for consumers may be found in the references by Aschen and Nurberger (1998).

NURSES AND RISK REDUCTION

For any client at risk, nurses may be able to intervene by maximizing positive environmental factors, providing or helping clients to find a supportive atmosphere, and providing access to ongoing counseling or development programs. Techniques for the reduction of stress and promotion of positive family interactions may also help to ameliorate effects due to genetic factors.

SUMMARY

Behavioral genomics is an area of intense interest and renewed research now using molecular methodologies and complex data analysis made possible by technological advances such as the study of gene expression through microarrays. Currently it is believed that the contribution of single-gene mutations to overall behavioral genetics is relatively rare, although such contributions are illuminating because they illustrate that abnormal behaviors can result from single-gene mutations. It is more widely believed that, in the vast majority of cases, multiple genes contribute to behaviors and that these are influenced by both environmental factors and by genes that may not appear to be directly connected with behaviors.

However, when subgroups of psychiatric disorders, such as bipolar disorder, are examined such as by early age of onset, there may be a greater contribution of single mutant genes such as is found in diabetes mellitus. Genetic analysis of various behavioral phenotypes including personality, learning disabilities, psychiatric disorders, and others are still sensitive research areas because of ethical, social, and legal concerns. For example, what would be the implications of genetic testing for behavioral and personality traits if such were available? For example, should the results be made available to school principals and teachers if a child is found to be genetically predisposed to a trait such as shyness or hyperactivity? What are the implications of enhancement of personality traits or intelligence? For a detailed discussion of these issues see chapter 11 and the Nuffield Council on Genetics and Behaviour (2002). Nonetheless it is expected that this area will grow in the future.

BIBLIOGRAPHY

Acosta, M. T., Arcos-Burgos, M., & Muenke, M. (2004). Attention deficit/hyperactivity disorder (ADHD): Complex phenotype, simple genotype? *Genetics in Medicine, 6,* 1–15.

Acosta, M. T., & Pearl, P. L. (2003). The neurobiology of autism: New pieces of the puzzle. *Current Neurological and Neuroscience Reports, 3,* 149–156.

American Psychiatric Association. (2000). *Diagnostic and statistical manual of mental disorders: DSM-IV-TR 2000* (4th ed.). Washington, DC: American Psychiatric Publishing.

Appelbaum, P. S. (2005). Law and psychiatry: Behavioral genetics and the punishment of crime. *Psychiatric Services, 56,* 25–27.

Aschen, S. R., & Nurberger, J. I., Jr. (1998). *Mood disorders and genetic risks.* Indianapolis: Institute of Psychiatric Research, Indiana University Medical Center.

Aschen, S. R., & Nurberger, J. I., Jr. (1998). *Schizophrenia and genetic risks.* Indianapolis: Institute of Psychiatric Research, Indiana University Medical Center.

Baker, C. (2004). *Behavioral genetics.* Washington, DC: American Association for the Advancement of Science.

Batra, V., Patkar, A. A., Berrettini, W. H., Weinstein, S. P., & Leone, L. T. (2003). The genetic determinants of smoking. *Chest, 123,* 1730–1739.

Baud, P. (2005). Personality traits as intermediary phenotypes in suicidal behavior: Genetic issues. *American Journal of Medical Genetics, Part C (Seminars in Medical Genetics), 133C,* 34–42.

Belmaker, R. H. (2004). Bipolar disorder. *New England Journal of Medicine, 351,* 476–486.

Berrettini, W. (2004). Bipolar disorder and schizophrenia: Convergent molecular data. *Neuromolecular Medicine, 5,* 109–117.

Blum, K., & Noble, E. P. (Eds.) (1997). *Handbook of psychiatric genetics.* Boca Raton, FL: CRC Press.

Bouchard, T. J., Jr. (1994). Genes, environment, and personality. *Science, 264,* 1700–1701.

Bouchard, T. J., Jr. (1997). Experience producing drive theory: How genes drive experience and shape personality. *Acta Paediatrica (Suppl.), 422,* 60–64.

Bouchard, T. J., Jr., & McGue, M. (2003). Genetic and environmental influences on human psychological differences. *Journal of Neurobiology, 54,* 4–45.

Bunney, W. E., Bunney, B. G., Vawter, M. P., Tomita, H., Li, J., Evans, S. J., et al. (2003). Microarray technology: A review of new strategies to discover candidate vulnerability genes in psychiatric disorders. *American Journal of Psychiatry, 160,* 657–666.

Chao, J., & Nestler, E. J. (2004). Molecular neurobiology of drug addiction. *Annual Review of Medicine, 55,* 113–132.

Christians, J. K., & Keightley, P. D. (2005). Behavioural genetics: Finding genes that cause complex trait variation. *Current Biology, 15,* R19–R21.

Conneally, P. M. (2003). The complexity of complex diseases. *American Journal of Human Genetics, 72,* 228–232.

Crimes against genetics. (1995). *Nature Genetics, 11,* 223-224.

Daniels, J. K., Spurlock, G., Williams, N. M., Cardno, A. G., Jones, L. A., Murphy, K. C., et al. (1997). Linkage study of chromosome 6p in sibpairs with schizophrenia. *American Journal of Medical Genetics, 74,* 319–324.

De Lilla, E. (Ed.). (2003). *Behavior genetic principles: Development, personality and psychopathology.* Washington, DC: American Psychological Association.

El-Saadi, O., Pedersen, C. B., McNeil, T. F., Saha, S., Welham, J., O'Callaghan, E., et al. (2004. Paternal and maternal age as risk factors for psychosis: Findings from Denmark, Sweden and Australia. *Schizophrenia Research, 67*, 227–236.

Faraone, S. V., Glatt, S. J., & Tsuang, M. T. (2003). The genetics of pediatric-onset bipolar disorder. *Biological Psychiatry, 53*, 970–977.

Faraone, S. V., & Tsuang, M. T. (2003). Heterogeneity and the genetics of bipolar disorder. *American Journal of Medical Genetics, Part C (Seminars in Medical Genetics), 123C*, 1–9.

Fisher, S. E., Lai, C. S., & Monaco, A. P. (2003). Deciphering the genetic basis of speech and language disorders. *Annual Review of Neuroscience, 26*, 57–80.

Fromme, K., de Wit, H., Hutchison, K. E., Ray, L., Corbin, W. R., Cook, T. A., et al. (2004). Biological and behavioral markers of alcohol sensitivity. *Alcoholism: Clinical and Experimental Research, 28*, 247–256.

Gottesman, I. I. (1994). Complications to the complex inheritance of schizophrenia. *Clinical Genetics, 46*, 116–123.

Grigorenko, E. L., Wood, F. B., Meyer, M. S., Hart, L. A., Speed, W. C., Shuster, A., et al. (1997). Susceptibility loci for distinct components of developmental dyslexia on chromosomes 6 and 15. *American Journal of Human Genetics, 60*, 27–39.

Hamann, S., & Canli, T. (2004). Individual differences in emotion processing. *Current Opinion in Neurobiology, 14*, 233–238.

Hampton, T. (2004). Genes harbor clues to addiction, recovery. *Journal of the American Medical Association, 292*, 321–322.

Harper, P. S. (1993). *Genetic counselling* (4th ed.). Oxford, England: Butterworth-Heinemann.

Harrison, P. J., & Owen, M. J. (2003). Genes for schizophrenia? Recent findings and their pathophysiological implications. *Lancet, 361*, 417–419.

Harrison, P. J., & Weinberger, D. R. (2005). Schizophrenia genes, gene expression, and neuropathology: On the matter of their convergence. *Molecular Psychiatry, 10*, 40–68.

Hobert, O. (2003). Introduction: Behavioral genetics—the third century. *Journal of Neurobiology, 54*, 1–3.

Inoue, K., & Lupski, J. R. (2003). Genetics and genomics of behavioral and psychiatric disorders. *Current Opinion in Genetics & Development, 13*, 303–309.

Karayiorgou, M., Morris, M. A., Morrow, B., Shprintzen, R. J., Goldberg, R., Borrow, J., et al. (1995). Schizophrenia susceptibility associated with interstitial deletions on chromosome 22q11. *Proceedings of the National Academy of Sciences USA, 92*, 7212–7216.

Kelsoe, J. R. (2003). Arguments for the genetic basis of the bipolar spectrum. *Journal of Affective Disorders, 73*, 183–197.

Kendler, K. S., Karkowski-Shulman, L., O'Neill, F. A., Straub, R. E., MacLean, C. J., & Walsh, D. (1997). Resemblance of psychotic symptoms and syndromes in affected sibling pairs from the Irish Study of High-Density Schizophrenia Families: Evidence for possible etiologic heterogeneity. *American Journal of Psychiatry, 154*, 191–198.

Kreek, M. J., Nielsen, D. A., & LaForge, K. S. (2004). Genes associated with addiction: Alcoholism, opiate, and cocaine addiction. *Neuromuscular Medicine, 5*, 85–108.

Lai, C. S., Gerrelli, D., Monaco, A. P., Fisher, S. E., & Copp, A. J. (2003). *FOXP2* expression during brain development coincides with adult sites of pathology in a severe speech and language disorder. *Brain, 126*(Pt. 11), 2455–2462.

Lewis, C. M., Levinson, D. F., Wise, L. H., DeLisi, L. E., Straub, R. E., Hovatta, I., et al. (2003). Genome scan meta-analysis of schizophrenia and bipolar disorder, part II: Schizophrenia. *American Journal of Human Genetics, 73*, 34–48.

Malafosse, A. (2005). Genetics of suicidal behavior. *American Journal of Medical Genetics, Part C (Seminars in Medical Genetics), 133C*, 1–2.

McDonald, C., & Murphy, K. C. (2003). The new genetics of schizophrenia. *Psychiatric Clinics of North America, 26*, 41–63.

Middleton, F. A., Pato, Mjj. T., Gentile, K. L., Morley, C. P., Zhao, X., & Eisener, A. F. (2004). Genomewide linkage analysis of bipolar disorder by use of a high-density single-nucleotide-polymorphism (SNP) genotyping assay: A comparison with microsatellite marker assays and finding of significant linkage to chromosome 6q22. *American Journal of Human Genetics, 74*, 886–897.

Muesser, K. T., & McGurk, S. R. (2004). Schizophrenia. *Lancet, 363*, 2063–2072.

Mukai, J., Liu, H., Burt, R. A., Swor, D. E., Lai, W-S.,

Karayiorgou, M., et al. (2004). Evidence that the gene encoding ZDHHC8 contributes to the risk of schizophrenia. *Nature Genetics, 36,* 725–731.

Nestler, E. J. (2004). Historical review: Molecular and cellular mechanisms of opiate and cocaine addiction. *Trends in Pharmacological Sciences, 25,* 210–218.

Newbury, D. F., & Monaco, A. P. (2002). Molecular genetics of speech and language disorders. *Current Opinion in Pediatrics, 14,* 696–701.

Noble, E. P. (2003). D2 dopamine receptor gene in psychiatric and neurologic disorders and its phenotypes. *American Journal of Medical Genetics, Part B (Neuropsychiatric Genetics), 116B,* 103–125.

Nuffield Council on Bioethics. (2002). *Genetics and human behaviour: The ethical context.* London: Nuffield Council on Bioethics.

Owen, M. J., Williams, N. M., & O'Donovan, M. C. (2004). The molecular genetics of schizophrenia: New findings promise new insights. *Molecular Psychiatry, 9,* 14–27.

Parens, E. (2004). Genetic differences and human identities: On why talking about behavioral genetics is important and difficult. *Hastings Center Report, 34,* S4–S35.

Pennisi, E. (2005). Genetics. A genomic view of animal behavior. *Science, 307,* 30–32.

Perkins, D. O., Jeffries, C., & Sullivan, P. (2005). Expanding the 'central dogma': The regulatory role of nonprotein coding genes and implications for the genetic liability to schizophrenia. *Molecular Psychiatry, 10,* 69–78.

Petronis, A. (2003). Epigenetics and bipolar disorder: New opportunities and challenges. *American Journal of Medical Genetics, Part C (Seminars in Medical Genetics), 123C,* 65–75.

Plomin, R., DeFries, J. C., Craig, I. W., & McGuffin, P. (Eds.). (2002). *Behavioral genetics in the postgenomic era.* Washington, DC: American Psychological Association.

Pulver, A. E., McGrath, J. A., Liang, K-Y., Lasseter, V., Nestadt, G., & Wolyniec, P. S. (2004). An indirect test of the new mutation hypothesis associating advanced paternal age with the etiology of schizophrenia. *American Journal of Medical*

Genetics, Part B (Neuropsychiatric Genetics), 124B, 6–9.

Ranade, S. S., Mansour, H., Wood, J., Chowdari, K. V., Brar, L. K., Kupfer, D. J., et al. (2003). Linkage and association between serotonin 2A receptor gene polymorphisms and bipolar I disorder. *American Journal of Medical Genetics, 121B,* 28–34.

Rice, C., Schendel, D., Cunniff, C., & Doernberg, N. (2004). Public health monitoring of developmental disabilities with a focus on the autism spectrum disorders. *American Journal of Medical Genetics, Part C (Seminars in Medical Genetics), 125C,* 22–27.

Schlesser, M. A., & Altshuler, K. Z. (1983). The genetics of affective disorder: Data, theory, and clinical applications. *Hospital and Community Psychiatry, 34,* 415–422.

Segurado, R., Detera-Wadleigh, S. D., Levinson, D. F., Lewis, C. M., Gill, M., Nurnberger, J. I., Jr., et al. (2003). Genome scan meta-analysis of schizophrenia and bipolar disorder, part III: Bipolar disorder. *American Journal of Human Genetics, 73,* 49–62.

Shirts, B. H., & Nimgaonkar, V. (2004). The genes for schizophrenia: Finally a breakthrough? *Current Psychiatry Reports, 6,* 303–312.

Sklar, P. (2002). Linkage analysis in psychiatric disorders: The emerging picture. *Annual Review of Genomics and Human Genetics, 3,* 371–413.

Straub, R. E., MacLean, C. J., Ma, Y., Webb, B. T., Myakishez, M. V., Harris-Kerr, C., Wormley, B., et al. (2002). Genome-wide scans of three independent sets of 90 Irish multiplex schizophrenia families and follow-up of selected regions in all families provides evidence for multiple susceptibility genes. *Molecular Psychiatry, 7,* 542–559.

Sung, Y. J., Dawson, G., Munson, J., Estes, A., Schellenberg, G. D., & Wijsman, E. M. (2005). Genetic investigation of quantitative traits related to autism: Use of multivariate polygenic models with ascertainment adjustment. *American Journal of Human Genetics, 76,* 68–81.

Szatmari, P. (2003). The causes of autism spectrum disorders. *British Medical Journal, 326,* 173–174.

26

Heart Disease

Coronary heart disease is the leading cause of death in most industrialized countries. In the United States cardiovascular disease is responsible for nearly one million deaths per year. Like the other common disorders, early heart disease is more likely to have a strong genetic component than heart disease that develops in middle age or later. Among this early-onset group, disorders caused by mutations in single genes are particularly significant. It is possible for many gene mutations to have coronary involvement as an indirect end result, including those affecting conditions that contribute to cardiac risk factors such as obesity, diabetes mellitus, hypertension, and even susceptibility to organisms that cause related inflammation such as *Chlamydia*. As examples of the broad range of possibilities, malfunctions in many genes could also contribute to heart disease including those that control arterial diameter, reactivity, and branching angles; affect platelet adhesiveness, thrombosis, and fibrinolysis; and regulate endothelial and smooth-muscle function. Hypertension plays a role in heart disease and its regulation and its influence on both the heart and the kidney are complex. A few rare single-gene mutations causing hypertension in humans have been identified, such as Liddle syndrome (an AD disorder from mutation in the beta or gamma subunit of the gene encoding the renal epithelial sodium channel), but the genetic influence in essential hypertension has not been fully elucidated and will not be considered in this chapter. Besides congenital heart disease (discussed in chapter 7), the major categories of heart disease that are caused by or heavily influenced by genetics are the cardiomyopathies, disorders of rhythm, and disease due to hyperlipidemia and atherosclerosis. Each of these will be discussed below. Coronary diseases may also occur as part of the picture of some relatively rare inherited biochemical and neuromuscular disorders (see Table 26.1) and may result from teratogenesis caused by drugs taken in pregnancy, such as lithium, or due to infection in pregnancy, such as rubella.

CORONARY HEART DISEASE AND HYPERLIPIDEMIA

Numerous conditions have been identified as risk factors for coronary artery disease. The major ones include elevated total or low-density lipoprotein cholesterol (LDL-C); decreased high-density lipoprotein cholesterol (HDL-C); family history of myocardial infarction or sudden death in male or female parents or sibs before 55 years and 65 years respectively; male gender aged 45 or above, female gender aged 55 or above; diabetes mellitus; obesity; cigarette smoking; and hypertension. Other factors that affect lipoproteins include high-fat diets, stress, sedentary lifestyle, liver disease, renal disease, certain medications, and excessive alcohol intake. The association among hyperlipidemia, the process of atherosclerosis, and coronary artery disease (CAD) is generally accepted. Genetically determined defects and deficiencies of lipoprotein components alone or in combination, and their transport and metabolism, have been related to the risk for the development of CAD. Both established and emerging cardiovascular risk factors are known. Examples of established ones are family history, cigarette smoking, obesity, elevated LDL-C, and low HDL-C. Examples of emerging ones are small dense LDL levels, metabolic syndrome, and homocysteine levels. Categories of single-gene

494

TABLE 26.1   Selected Genetic Disorders Associated with Cardiac Disease

Genetic disorder	Transmission	Comments
Duchenne muscular dystrophy	XR	Caused by mutation in dystrophin gene. Hypotonia, cardiac muscle failure in about 15%. Respiratory failure. Death usual in adolescence. See chapter 6.
Kearns-Sayre syndrome	mitochondrial	Myopathy, small stature, ophthalmoplegia, pigment degeneration of retina, ataxia, cardiomyophathy, and heart block.
Myotonic dystrophy	AD	Neuromuscular disorder due to unstable trinucleotide repeat expansion. Cataracts, hypogonadism, muscle wasting and weakness, heart block, conduction disturbances, mitral valve prolapse.
Hemochromatosis	AR	Symptoms from iron deposits. Cirrhosis of liver, diabetes mellitus, hepatocellular carcinoma, cardiomyopathy, and skin pigmentation are seen.
Mucopolysaccharidosis IH (Hurler syndrome)	AR	Deficiency of alpha-L-iduronidase. Coarse faces, short stature, hearing loss, valvular heart disease, enlarged tongue, kyphosis, enlarged abdomen. See chapter 6.
Fabry disease	XR	Also known as diffuse angiokeratoma. Skin lesions, autonomic problems, abdominal pain attacks, renal failure, corneal changes, coronary hypertrophy.
Glycogen storage disease II (Pompe disease)	AR	Muscle hypertrophic cardiomyopathy, respiratory insufficiency. In infantile form death is usual in first year. Due to acid alpha glucosidase deficiency.
Ehlers-Danlos syndrome, type IV	AD	A connective-tissue disorder involving collagen mutation with hyperelastic and fragile skin, easy bruisability, joint hypermobility. Mitral valve prolapse, and spontaneous arterial rupture can occur.
Marfan syndrome	AD	A disorder of fibrillin. Includes increased height, chest deformities, arachnodactyly, ectopia lentis and other ocular findings, thoracic lordosis, dilation of the aortic root, mitral valve prolapse possible. See chapter 6.

AD = autosomal dominant, AR = autosomal recessive, XR = X-linked recessive.

disorders causing hyperlipidemias and thus CAD include defects in the apolipoproteins (apo) (example: apo B deficiency leading to classic abetalipoproteinemia), receptor defects (LDL receptor disorder leading to familial hypercholesterolemia), enzyme defects (lipoprotein lipase deficiency), defects in transfer proteins (e.g., cholesteryl ester transfer protein deficiency), and others.

Some characteristics have been noted for genetic susceptibility for CAD that would then allow stratification into familial average, moderate, and high risk categories (see Scheuner, 2003, for details). Based on the risk category, early detection and prevention approaches could be designed. Genetic susceptibility characteristics according to Scheuner (2003, p. 273), include:

- Early onset of CAD (<55 years of age for men and <65 years of age for women
- Involvement of multiple vessels with atherosclerosis
- Angiographic severity
- Two or more close relatives with CAD
- Female relatives with CAD
- Presence of related disorders in close relatives, such as diabetes or hypertension
- Presence of multiple established/emerging CAD risk factors in affected family members such as diabetes, hypertension, insulin resistance, or the prothrombin G20210A mutation and others
- Absence of established risk factors in family members with CAD, such as hypertension or smoking.

Aside from those with single-gene defects, hyperlipidemia as such is not a single disorder, but it exists as various types, each with its own causes, manifestations, and profiles. In the general population, plasma lipid levels are modulated by the interaction of environmental factors within the boundaries set by genetic determinants, environmental factors such as diet acting upon the person with a single-gene disorder affecting lipoprotein, and gene-gene interactions. Blood lipid levels are a continuous curve in the general population and are influenced by age and sex. Usually levels of LDL above the 90th to 95th percentile are considered abnormal. This may be higher in Western countries than in others because of the background of the high lipid content of Western diets. The early identification of those individuals at greatest risk for premature coronary disease would allow the application of measures designed to prevent or minimize morbidity. Recognition of the important role of hyperlipidemia in atherogenesis has led to the strategy of lowering cholesterol in the plasma to reduce the availability of lipoproteins and reduce the accumulation of cholesterol in the arteries. High concentrations of LDL cholesterol and total plasma cholesterol are highly associated with coronary heart disease, as are low levels of HDL. Lipid metabolism is beyond the scope of this chapter. After considering the lipoproteins and apolipoproteins the most important genetic disorders resulting in CAD will be discussed. Others are listed in Table 26.2.

Lipoproteins and Apolipoproteins

Because of their solubility properties, dietary lipids such as cholesterol and triglycerides are transported in the blood mainly in the form of complex macromolecules called lipoproteins. These molecules often consist of a core of nonpolar lipids, a surface layer of polar lipids, and apoproteins (apo). Each class of lipoprotein contains triglycerides (esters of glycerol and long chain fatty acids), cholesteryl esters (esters of cholesterol and long chain fatty acids), free cholesterol, apoproteins, and phospholipids combined in different proportions. The more hydrophobic first two are usually in the core of the molecule and the latter three are at the periphery. Each component in the system has some control, as do other factors such as hormones, cho-

lesterol intake, and metabolic alterations. The components, enzymes and cell surface receptors are involved in the regulation of lipid levels. The major apo functions include (a) serving as mediators of lipoprotein binding to their receptors sites, (b) involvement in biosynthesis and organization of lipoproteins, (c) initiate uptake of lipoproteins by cells, and (d) as structural components of lipoproteins in plasma.

Familial Hypercholesterolemia

Familial hypercholesterolemia (FH, hyperlipoproteinemia, type IIa) is an autosomal dominant (AD) disorder due to mutations (more than 230 are known) in the LDL receptor on chromosome 19p. FH was the first genetic disorder shown to cause myocardial infarction (MI). Goldstein and Brown received a Nobel Prize in 1986 for their work on understanding this disorder. Because it is an AD disorder, heterozygotes and homozygotes are both affected. In the United States, the prevalence of heterozygotes and homozygotes is 1 in 500 and 1 in 1,000,000 respectively, making it a very common genetic disorder. Humphries, Gaton, and Nicholls (1997) estimated that in the United Kingdom, an average health center of 8,000 is likely to have four to five families with FH who are enrolled. Among survivors of MIs, the frequency of heterozygotes has been estimated at 1:20. The result of the gene mutations in FH is reduced numbers of receptors or defective ones, depending on which mutant allele is present. This results in the decreased ability or inability of LDL-C to bind to its cell surface receptors. LDL-C therefore cannot enter the cell to be degraded in adequate amounts. LDL-C accumulates in the plasma and is deposited in abnormal sites such as the arteries (causing atheromas and atherosclerosis) and the tendons (causing xanthomas). In heterozygotes, LDL-C levels are about 3 times normal, in the homozygote they may be 6–10 times normal.

The heterozygote is exposed to the effects of premature and accelerated atherosclerosis even in early childhood. Many clinicians hesitate to institute vigorous therapy at an early age because myelination of the central nervous system is not complete until about 6 years of age, and LDL-C is important in the delivery of lipids to the tissues. For male heterozygotes, the typical age of onset of

TABLE 26.2 Selected Genetic Lipid Disorders

Name	Inheritance pattern	Prevalence	Predisposition to coronary disease	Remarks
Tangier disease	AR	Very rare	Yes	Orange tonsils a feature, peripheral neuropathy, hypersplenism, early CAD. Deficiency or absence of HDL, accumulation of cholesterol esters in tonsils, liver, spleen, bone marrow, cornea, skin, and peripheral nerves. Low plasma cholesterol and apo A. Normal or elevated triglycerides.
Familial hypercholesterolemia (FH) IIa	AD	Heterozygote 1:500; homozygote 1:1,000,000	Yes, severe	LDL receptor deficiency or defect (see text).
Familial hypertriglyceridemia	AD	1:100–1:500	Yes, mild	May not be expressed until person is in his/her 20s or 30s; 5% of survivors of myocardial infarction had disorder; basic defect unknown; VLDL, triglycerides, and occasionally chylomicrons are elevated; episodes of abdominal pain with or without pancreatitis are frequent; eruptive xanthomas can occur; often hypertension, diabetes mellitus, insulin resistance, hyperuricemia are present.
Familial combined hyperlipidemia	AD	1:100	Yes, moderate	May cause 10% of all premature coronary artery disease. Found in 11–20% of survivors of myocardial infarction under 60 years of age; lipoprotein phenotype varies; one third have hypercholesterolemia, one-third have hypertriglyceridemia, one-third have a combination of both; basic defect unknown.
Apo E deficiency	AR	1:5,000	Yes	Familial dysbetalipoproteinemia. Accumulation of LDL in plasma, apolipoprotein ε3 deficient, or structurally altered in 1% of population but not all with alteration show hyperlipidemia; xanthomas seen in palmar creases, tuberous xanthomas in buttocks, elbows and knees; both premature coronary and peripheral vascular disease are common; obesity, hyperuricemia, glucose intolerance are frequently present.

(continued)

TABLE 26.2   Selected Genetic Lipid Disorders (*Continued*)

Name	Inheritance pattern	Prevalence	Predisposition to coronary disease	Remarks
Familial lipoprotein deficiency	AR	1:100,000	Not usual	Increased triglycerides and chylomicrons, lipoprotein lipase deficiency, abdominal pain with or without pancreatitis; hepatosplenomegaly from foam cell deposition; eruptive xanthoma on trunk, tonsils, palate; ophthalmologic examination shows pale retina and increased light reflex (lipemia retinalis); anorexia malaise, abdominal pain follows fat intake.
Apolipoprotein deficiency	AR	1:1,000,000	Sometimes	Lack of Apo C-II as C-II cofactor for lipoprotein lipase results in a similar picture as with familial lipoprotein deficiency, except elevated VLDL.
Lecithin cholesterol acyltransferase (LCAT) deficiency	AR	1:1,000,000	Yes	Enzyme deficiency; increased free cholesterol and lecithin in plasma; triglycerides may be elevated; may detect in childhood due to corneal opacities; can develop anemia, renal disease; foam cells in marrow. HDL abnormalities, renal lesions and failure can occur; LDL abnormal; low-fat diet and symptomatic treatment. One subtype is fish eye disease characterized by corneal opacities; increased VLDL & LDL with HDL abnormalities.
Familial defective apolipoprotein B-100	AD	Heterozygote 1:500–700		See text.

coronary heart disease is 40 years of age, and by 60 years, 85% will have had a MI as compared to 15% for males without the mutant gene. For females, the typical age of onset is 55 years of age, and by 60 years, 50% will have a MI as compared with a 10% risk in unaffected females. Both the heterozygote and homozygote may also have peripheral or cerebral vascular disease. LDL-derived cholesteryl esters are deposited in the soft tissue of the eyelids, cornea (arcus cornae), tendons, elbows, ankles, and knees. Tendon xanthomas of the dorsum of the hand and Achilles tendon may be very painful and are very characteristic. They are not usually seen in the heterozygote before 20 years of age. The finding of such xanthomas on physical examination should alert the practitioner to the need to determine the cause.

The homozygote is much more severely affected. By 4 years of age, most patients will have developed planar yellow-orange xanthomas at the knees, buttocks, elbows, and hands, especially between the thumb and the index finger, as well as tendon xanthomas. MI, angina pectoris, and even sudden death usually occur in the homozygote between 5 and 20 years of age. MIs have been reported as early as 18 months. Cholesterol is also deposited on the heart valves resulting in congestive heart failure. Arcus cornae is frequently present. Death is usual between 5 and 20 years of age. Few live past 30 years. Variability in clinical manifestations may be seen. In the homozygote, therapeutic intervention is particularly aggressive. The statins are a mainstay of therapy but different LDL receptor mutation genotypes can result in varying responses to therapy. The efficacy and safety of specific statins in children and heterozygotes is being studied. Failure of drug therapy to reduce plasma cholesterol levels may indicate the need for surgical procedures such as ileal bypass to prevent the absorption of bile salts or portacaval shunt. Plasma exchange may be also done at intervals. Liver transplantation has also been used. For both the heterozygote and homozygote, diet therapy alone will not lower lipid levels to the normal range, but may be used as adjunctive therapy. The most promising approach is that of gene therapy, and trials have been conducted.

Gene testing and screening by molecular methods for the defective gene are possible. The practicality for generalized screening, such as in newborns, is limited at this time because there does not yet appear to be a small number of mutations that are responsible for the defect in the vast majority of affected persons, nor is there a testing technique that will detect enough mutations to be useful and meet screening test criteria. Such screening, as well as being premature, is somewhat controversial, especially for infants and children. Targeted screening is being done, however, particularly within at-risk families. Relatives may benefit from lifestyle modifications, closer monitoring, or more aggressive lipid lowering therapy depending on the specific mutation, family pattern of disease development (FH tends to have similar patterns within families) and their lipid levels, and other parameters. In a study of those screened for FH in a family screening program, participants correctly perceived they had a higher risk for MI than those without FH, and those with the highest risk used medications more (van Maarle, Stouthard, & Bonsel, 2003). Again, whether or not to test children is controversial. Some, such as Humphries et al. (1997), believe FH meets criteria for genetic testing in children, while others do not because the effect of lipid-lowering therapy is not proven and large randomized studies of the physical and psychosocial impact have not been addressed. A study by Andersen, Jensen, Juul, and Faergeman (1997) revealed that 84% of heterozygotes screened favored family screening, and of those who were screened 13% reported diminished well-being, 37% reported fear of coronary heart disease, and 44% expressed anxiety. Rosenthal, Knaver-Black, Stahl, Catalanotto, and Sprecher (1993) found that anxiety was associated with diagnosis of FH in children, and that families with the best social integration network coped best with the diagnosis and management. Umans-Eckenhausen, Defesche, van Dam, and Kastelein (2003) studied participants in a general screening program for FH in the Netherlands and found that those who were detected and put on medication had significantly reduced their LDL-C levels but needed additional education over time to meet treatment goals.

Familial Defective Apolipoprotein B-100 and Other Contributors to AD Hypercholesterolemia

Familial defective apolipoprotein B-100 (FDB) has been recognized relatively recently. In the heterozygous state the prevalence is estimated at 1:500 to

1:700. Few homozygotes have been reported. In heterozygotes symptoms include tendon xanthomas, arcus lipoides, atherosclerosis, and coronary artery disease. It results from a mutation in apo B, resulting in hypercholesterolemia. LDL receptors are normal but LDL-C accumulates in the blood. In one series, 60% of patients older than 51 years of age had coronary artery disease (CAD) and about 50% of males had CAD by age 50. Inheritance is autosomal dominant. Another type of autosomal dominant hypercholesterolemia, known as FH3, has been found to be due to mutations in the *PCSK9* gene (which encodes neural apoptosis regulated convertase, an enzyme involved in cholesterol homeostasis).

Other Disorders

Among other emerging lipid risk factors are small dense LDL, low HDL-C levels, increased triglyceride levels, and elevated lipoprotein (a). Lipoprotein (a) [Lp(a)] is a cholesterol-rich lipoprotein that is attached to apo B and is associated with LDL. There is a high level of variability of Lp(a) levels that is polymorphic, and there are more than 30 different alleles identified. High Lp(a) levels are associated with coronary heart disease but the way in which this occurs is not well understood, and there may not be a cause-and-effect relationship. About 30% of persons with premature heart disease have Lp(a) levels above the 95th percentile. High density lipoprotein (HDL) levels are inversely associated with coronary heart disease regardless of LDL cholesterol levels. Low levels may be due to single-gene variants, some of which are rare, and a number of candidate genes are under investigation. About half of the variance of HDL levels is attributable to genetic factors.

A specific genotype of APOE, ε4 is associated with elevated LDL levels and the development of CAD. This may account for 4% to 6% of all MIs, and in Korea, those with this allele had a 3-year recurrence rate for ischemic cerebrovascular disease of 53% vs. 16% for persons without this allele. Other conditions that may be related to the development of CAD and increased MI risk are high homocysteine levels, discussed later, factors involved in the thrombosis or hemostasis such as factor V Leiden variants, elevated plasminogen activator inhibitor-1, the G20210A prothrombin gene variant, inflammatory markers such as C-reactive protein, the metabolic syndrome which is comprised of a constellation of factors such as dyslipidemia, abdominal obesity, hypertension, insulin resistance, and others.

Nursing Pointers in Hyperlipidemia and Coronary Disease

The relationship among dietary intake of lipids, various genetic parameters, various risk factors, and plasma levels of various lipid components is a complicated one. Because the consumption of a high cholesterol or lipid-rich diet in persons with an underlying gene abnormality may exacerbate hyperlipidemia, a major therapeutic effort requires lowering dietary fat or cholesterol; however, people handle exogenous lipids in different ways. In some individuals, reduction of dietary lipid intake may not decrease the body's endogenous production of excess lipids or cholesterol. Furthermore, persons may respond differently to the removal of cholesterol from the plasma—they may either increase its excretion from the body (desirable) or deposit it in tissues or arteries (undesirable). Despite recent recommendations for the ideal American diet, some researchers believe that sweeping indiscriminate changes in lipid content may have unknown long-term consequences; however, it is generally agreed that lowering the intake of dietary fat is desirable for persons with hyperlipidemia as a primary or adjunct measure.

The following are some nursing points related to genetic factors in hyperlipidemia and coronary disease:

- Be alert for a genetic component in young persons with hyperlipidemia and CAD, particularly those with MIs who may first be noticed in the coronary care unit.
- Ascertain the family history for lipid-related problems and sudden deaths of persons who have been diagnosed with coronary disease, especially if early onset.
- Be aware of those who have the highest risk for cardiovascular disease based on assessment of genetic risk factors as discussed earlier.
- Close blood relatives of persons having a coronary disorder at an early age may need to be referred for plasma lipid analysis and other testing such as DNA analysis.

- Be alert for the signs and symptoms of hyperlipidemias—xanthomas, abdominal pain of unexplained origin, fatty food intolerance, and so on, and refer such individuals for appropriate evaluation. Be especially alert for these signs in younger persons and children.
- Realize that some symptoms associated with hyperlipidemia, such as xanthomas and arcus cornae, can occur in persons with normal lipid levels.
- Encourage the reduction of secondary risk factors in persons with hyperlipidemia such as cigarette smoking, sedentary life-style, obesity, excess alcohol consumption, stress, and high carbohydrate diet, and also encourage these in their blood relatives.
- Use or develop specific programs for risk reduction that are based on the person's culture, own health belief system, and individual motivational factors in order to maximize success, and that take into account the degree of risk (average, moderate, or high) that they may have based on familial and genetic risk factors as well as lifestyle factors.
- Before a person begins therapy for hyperlipidemia, check to see that secondary disorders (e.g., diabetes mellitus) or contributing factors (e.g., oral contraceptives) have been ascertained, substituted for, or corrected, if possible.
- Optimal health for the particular individual should be a basic goal.
- Treatment of hyperlipidemia will usually involve long-term measures.
- Recognize that the ongoing use of medications that are unpleasant to take, or which have unpleasant side effects, may result in the client's failure to adhere to the treatment plan; techniques for ways to minimize any unpleasantness should be shared and periodically reviewed with the client and family; the compliance literature should be used for ideas on ways to maximize the client's adherence.
- Assess the client's current food and alcohol intake and medication use.
- Recognize that not all persons who adhere to a low-cholesterol, low-fat diet can lower their plasma lipids by dietary means alone.
- For those who are on a lifelong dietary regimen, be able to refer them to a variety of cookbooks and hints for the use of food substitutes.

CARDIOMYOPATHIES

Cardiomyopathies are diseases of the heart muscle that may be primary or secondary and are classified into four categories: hypertrophic, dilated, restrictive, and unclassified cardiomyopathy, and some also use right ventricular cardiomyopathy as another category. They may be part of other inherited disorders such as glycogen storage disease II. The cardiomyopathies are believed to be responsible for about 2% of sudden deaths. Counseling issues are discussed in Yu et al. (1998).

Hypertrophic Cardiomyopathy

The prevalence of hypertrophic cardiomyopathy (HCM) in the general population is about 1:500 and is more common in Iceland. Most cases identified to date are familial although sporadic cases do occur. The mode of transmission is autosomal dominant. Genetic heterogeneity is prevalent, and the pattern of phenotypic expression may be influenced by other modifying genes and environmental factors. HCM results from mutations in genes that encode cardiac sarcomere proteins that are essential for heart muscle contraction. The most prominent of these are mutations in: (a) the β-myosin heavy chain gene on chromosome 14q *(CMH1)*, (b) the cardiac troponin T gene on chromosome 1q *(CMH2)*, (c) the α-tropomyosin gene on 15q *(CMH3)*, and (d) genes encoding cardiac myosin binding protein C on chromosome 11q *(CMH4)*. There are others that are less common including genes that encode: the regulatory and essential myosin light chains, cardiac troponin I, titin, α-tropomyosin, α-actin, and α-myosin heavy chain. Intragenic heterogeneity also exists—at least 150 mutations can occur within these genes. Certain mutations are more frequently associated with varying outcomes, and genotype-phenotype correlations are of great interest. For example, in families with the Arg403Gln (substitution of arginine for glutamine at position 403) mutation of myosin, 50% have died before 45 years of age, whereas the Val606Met, Gly256Glu, and Leu908Val β-myosin heavy chain gene mutations are relatively benign. Persons with troponin T mutations have a poor prognosis despite mild hypertrophy. The mutations Arg453Cys and Arg719Trp are associated with severe hypertrophy as well. Late-onset HCM is associated with mutations in the gene encoding cardiac myosin-binding protein C. This delayed expression, coupled with a favorable prognosis, may mean that the heritable component can be overlooked. Therefore, clinicians should be alert for the possibility of these gene mutations in HCM occurring in middle-aged or elderly patients so that clinical and/or genetic screening can be offered to their families. In families with known HCM, clinical screening may need to be continued throughout adulthood.

HCM is characterized by left ventricular hypertrophy and is the most common cause of sudden death in children and adolescents, especially in athletes. Sometimes sudden death is the initial presentation, and until then the person has been asymptomatic. There are varying degrees of clinical severity including a slow relatively benign course. The most common initial complaints in the 50% who present with symptoms include chest pain, dyspnea, mild exercise intolerance, and syncope. Atrial fibrillation may develop in about 10% to 25%. In affected individuals without symptoms detection usually occurs during a routine physical exam or electrocardiogram (ECG). However, further exploration such as a transthoracic echo Doppler examination, studies to detect ventricular function, and so on is necessary. Outcomes vary and include sudden death, heart failure with congestive features, and atrial fibrillation and its consequences. Treatment depends on manifestations and may include beta blockers, verapamil, disopyramide to reduce left ventricular contractility, or methoxamine to increase peripheral vascular resistance. Other therapy may be given such as amiodarone for atrial fibrillation. Dual-chamber pacing may be used but is controversial. Both surgical and non-surgical approaches are used for septal reduction. An automatic implantable cardioverter defibrillator may be needed to prevent sudden death. Molecular techniques can be used for gene testing and will identify about 60% to 70% of HCM. Presymptomatic testing is possible. If a family member has been diagnosed with HCM as a result of sudden death, screening of children or adolescents is warranted so that preventative measures may be taken. The nurse should be alert to this when taking family histories. In families with multiple affected members, adolescents, even if symptom-free, may be wise to avoid strenuous athletics. Modifier genes are thought to affect the severity such as the extent of hypertrophy and are a subject of interest as pharmacological targets. A potential modifier gene is that encoding the angiotensin-1 converting enzyme 1 (ACE-1).

Dilated Cardiomyopathy

Dilated cardiomyopathy (DCM) occurs with a prevalence of 36.5 per 100,000 and is a chronic heart muscle condition characterized by dilatation and impaired contractility of the left or both ventricles. It may result from familial or genetic causes or from viral, toxic, or metabolic agents, alcohol use, immune dysfunction, or idiopathic causes. Men are more frequently affected. There is a long presymptomatic phase in which the person has no symptoms and the disorder remains unrecognized. Nearly 30% of relatives of persons with DCM have ECG abnormalities. The typical age of onset is 20 to 50 years. The most frequent presentation is end-stage heart failure manifested by exercise intolerance, exertional dyspnea, and chest pain. Sometimes the enlarged heart or ECG abnormalities are detected during a routine examination. Conduction abnormalities may be frequent. Impaired systolic contraction may lead to ventricular dilatation, congestive heart failure, and sudden death. The heart is increased in weight. Mendelian inheritance is seen in about 25% of cases. Inheritance is most commonly autosomal dominant but autosomal recessive, mitochondrial mutation, and X-linked recessive inheritance have been described. Gene mutations identified to date include those in cardiac actin (15q14), desmin (2q35), lamin A and C, and δ-sarcoglycan genes (5q33-34), and loci have been linked to the AD form including *CMD1D* (chromosome 1q32), *CMD1G* (2q31), and *CMD1B* (9q13-22) as well as yet unidentified locations on other chromosomes. In some cases DCM is associated with other features such as sensorineural hearing loss (6q23-24). DCM frequently accompanies both Duchenne and Becker muscular dystrophy. Mutations in the dystrophon gene have been identified in X-linked dilated cardiomyopathy. Other candidate genes are those encoding transcription factors that control the expression of cardiac myocyte genes such as leucine-zipper factor, and members of zinc finger protein families. Treatment includes weight control, restricted sodium intake, ACE inhibitors, digitalis, and diuretics, anti-coagulants, beta blockers and other medications depending on symptoms and need. Implantable cardioverter defibrillators may be useful. DCM is the major indication for heart transplant at present.

Other Cardiomyopathies

Restrictive cardiomyopathy is rare in developed countries, and is inherited rarely as a primary disorder. It is characterized by impaired ventricular filling and progressive left- and right- sided heart failure. Various genetic and acquired causes are known. One gene mutation known is that of cardiac troponin I. Arrhythmogenic right ventricular cardiomyopathy (ARVC), also known as arrhythmogenic right ventricular dysplasia (ARVD), is more recently recognized. Both structural and functional right ventricular abnormalities are seen. Presentation, especially in apparently healthy young athletes, can be sudden death. Sometimes presentation occurs as right ventricular arrhythmias especially with left branch block patterns. In most families with primary genetic causation it appears to have autosomal dominant inheritance. Several loci have been mapped. A full description may be found in Online Mendelian Inheritance in Man (2005). The causative gene mutation in ARVD8 is desmoplakin, and in ARVD2 it is the ryanodine receptor 2 gene.

ARRHYTHMIAS

Primary disorders of the cardiac electrical system resulting from genetic abnormalities include primary rhythm disturbances and those associated with other genetic disorders, such as myonic muscular dystrophy and familial structural cardiac disorders including cardiomyopathy which was discussed previously. Specific syndrome examples and their mode of inheritance include familial ventricular tachycardia (AD), familial absence of sinus rhythm (AD), familial atrioventricular block (AD), mitral valve prolapse (AD), Becker muscular dystrophy (XR), and others. A gene for familial atrial fibrillation has been identified and mapped to chromosome 11p15.5 associated with a mutation in the KCNQ1 gene showing autosomal dominant inheritance in one large family. Certain gene

variations may also increase the risk of drug-related arrhythmias, and are thus significant for treatment choices. The actual prevalence of dysrhythmias due to genetic causes is underestimated.

The most well-described arrhythmia is the long QT syndrome (LQT). LQT is a cardiac arrhythmia showing a prolonged QT interval on ECG. It can present with syncope, ventricular fibrillation, and sudden death. Unexplained cases of near-drowning have revealed families with inherited LQT, and women with hereditary LQT are at risk for untoward cardiac events in the postpartum period which may be prevented prophylactically by using β-adrenergic blockers. LQT is both genetically and phenotypically heterozygous. The genetically transmitted form is caused by mutations in genes encoding ion channels. Mutations in genes of at least 7 loci are implicated in LQT, and three forms are well delineated. These are mutations in potassium channel genes, KCNQ1 or KVLQT1 (LQT1) (described below), HERG or KCNH2 (LQT2 on chromosome 7q), and in the sodium channel gene SCN5A (LQT3). Others include KCNE1 (MinK, LQT5), and KCNE2 (MiRP1, LQT6) while a single mutation in ANKB is responsible for LQT4. Inheritance may be autosomal dominant or, more rarely, autosomal recessive, or the result of non-genetic causes. The autosomal recessive form of LQT1 is known as the Jervell and Lange-Nielsen syndrome and is associated with congenital sensory deafness as well. LQT has been reported in up to 1% of children with congenital deafness and so ECG screening should be done in children with congenital deafness. The AD type of LQT1 has been called the Romano-Ward syndrome. Mutation in the potassium channel gene KCNQ1 may cause both of these as well as play a role in normal hearing. LQT consists of recurrent syncope with abnormal myocardial repolarization; sudden death occurs from ventricular arrhythmias. Occasionally an affected person presents with seizures. Persons with the gene may be asymptomatic when detected. On ECG, prolongation of the QT interval is seen. Genetic testing can identify those with a mutation in one of the genes known to cause LQT5. In addition, untoward events tend to be gene-specific: persons with LQT1 tend to experience cardiac events during exercise; those with LQT2 with arousal-type emotions such as hearing a sudden loud noise; and those with LQT3 without arousal often occurring during sleep. Families and individuals of Asian or Pacific Rim ethnicity may be particularly susceptible to these events. Treatment varies but may include β-adrenergic blockers even if asymptomatic, and mutation-specific therapies are beginning to be examined. Education about preventive medication should include the information that certain drugs can precipitate torsades de pointes. These include cardiac and non-cardiac drugs. Examples of drugs include chlorpromazine, pentamidine, and procainamide. The University of Arizona Center for Education and Research on Therapeutics maintains a list of drugs that can do this. Web sites for patient information may be found in Appendix B. Atrial fibrillation in a parent appears to be a risk factor for atrial fibrillation in offspring. In one report, 30% of offspring in an arrhythmia clinic had affected parents (Fox et al., 2004).

HOMOCYSTEINE AND CARDIOVASCULAR DISEASE

Homocysteine is an amino acid. Elevated homocysteine is considered to be an independent risk factor for coronary artery disease, stroke, and vascular disease. Elevated plasma levels have also been regarded as a predictor of mortality in patients with CAD. This elevation can occur by various mechanisms. These include mutations in the gene for methylenetetrahydrofolate reductase, methionine synthase deficiency, defects in cobalamin metabolism and transport, and by nongenetic causes that interfere with enzymes or with needed cofactors such as folate, cobalamin, and pyridoxine. Classic homocystinuria is a rare autosomal recessive disorder caused by deficiency of cystathionine β-synthetase that includes premature atherosclerosis and recurrent thrombosis. More commonly, persons who were homozygous for certain mutations in the gene coding for methylenetetrahydrofolate reductase, which is involved in the remethylation of homocysteine to methionine, showed elevated levels of homocysteine in those with low folate levels. Those with high folate levels did not show increased homocysteine. Folic acid can be used to lower plasma homocysteine levels and doses as low as 200 μg per day appear effective. Fortification programs such as in flour or baked goods may be a preventative approach to lower

plasma homocysteine in the general population. Natural folate intake is influenced by bioavailability and separate supplementation by adherence. Vitamins B_6 and B_{12} are also useful. Because of the belief that elevated homocysteine levels are risk factors, it has been proposed as a disorder suitable for widespread screening. Elevated homocysteine has also been found to be a risk factor for subsequent stroke after an initial acute event. Hyperhomocysteinemia is also associated with an increased risk of restenosis in patients who have had coronary interventions with stents.

OTHER CONDITIONS

In addition to those discussed, other conditions with a genetic component may also result in heart disease. For example, there is a type of hereditary cardiomyopathy resulting from amyloid deposition that may lead to sudden death. This type results from a variant in transthyretin (a serum carrier protein) and is particularly common among Blacks. Elderly Black patients with heart disease of undetermined etiology should be tested for transthyretin amyloidosis. Alterations in the renin/angiotensin system may be related to heart disease. A particular genotype of the angiotensin-converting enzyme (ACE) gene, DD, has been associated with a susceptibility to both myocardial infarction and CAD, probably because of aberrant blood-pressure regulation. The use of ACE inhibitors may be useful in prevention. Gene mutation in a member of the myocyte enhancer factor 2 transcription factors (MEF2A) has been implicated in CAD as a rare autosomal dominant form in one large family, and is being studied for a larger susceptibility role. Whole genome scans have identified loci linked to premature CAD on chromosome 2q21.1-22, 16p13.3, and Xq23-26 while a linkage to MI was found on chromosome 14q11.2-12 and 2q36-q37.3 in specific population groups. It remains to be seen if these are replicated in other studies and populations. Postmenopausal women with certain genetic variations in the estrogen receptor α (ESR1) gene appeared in one study to be at increased risk for ischemic heart disease and MI (Schuit et al., 2004).

Although beyond the scope of this chapter, the efficacy and adverse effects of some drugs to treat cardiac conditions appear to be related to certain genetic variations. For example, those men with hypercholesterolemia who had the ACE genotype, DD, did not benefit from statin therapy (Maitland-van der Zee et al., 2004). Persons who were heterozygous for a genetic variation in the HMG-CoA reductase gene did not respond as well as the homozygotes to pravastatin therapy to lower cholesterol levels (Chasman et al., 2004). This, along with gene and stem cell therapy to treat cardiac diseases, is an area of intense study.

SUMMARY

Heart disease continues to exact great degrees of morbidity and mortality. Coronary artery disease is associated with a number of lipid and nonlipid risk factors, some of which are modifiable and some, such as age or family history, are not. Risk of certain types of heart disease may be determined by analyzing known risk factors for any individual. Genetic risk assessment including an appropriate family history is possible based on a variety of susceptibility and familial factors discussed above followed by the options of genetic testing and counseling, prenatal diagnosis and reproductive and life planning. Genotype-phenotype correlations are providing new information about the long-term prognosis and best plan of care. Gene therapy aimed at modulation of gene expression, and the application of pharmacogenomics to determine, for example, the most effective drug and the one that will cause the least side effects for a given individual, are allowing great progress in heart diseases.

BIBLIOGRAPHY

Abifadel, M., Varret, M., Rabés, J-P., Allard, D., Ouguerram, K., Devillers, M., et al. (2003). Mutations in *PCSK9* cause autosomal dominant hypercholesterolemia. *Nature Genetics, 34,* 154–156.

Ackerman, M. J., & Porter, C. J. (1998). Identification of a family with inherited long QT syndrome after a pediatric near-drowning. *Pediatrics, 101,* 306–307.

Ackerman, M. J., Tester, D. J., Jones, G. S., Will, M. L., Burrow, C. R., & Curran, M. E. (2003). Ethnic differences in cardiac potassium channel variants: Implications for genetic susceptibility to sudden cardiac death and genetic testing for congenital long QT syndrome. *Mayo Clinic Proceedings, 78,* 1479–1487.

Al-Khatib, S. M., LaPointe, N. M. A., Kramer, J. M., & Califf, R. M. (2003). What clinicians should know about the QT interval. *Journal of the American Medical Association, 289,* 2120–2127.

Andersen, L. K., Jensen, H. K., Juul, S., & Faergeman, O. (1997). Patients' attitudes toward detection of heterozygous familial hypercholesterolemia. *Archives of Internal Medicine, 157,* 553–560.

Baig, M. K., Goldman, J. H., Caforio, A. L., Coonar, A. S., Keeling, P. J., & McKenna, W. J. (1998). Familial dilated cardiomyopathy: Cardiac abnormalities are common in asymptomatic relatives and may represent early disease. *Journal of the American College of Cardiology, 31,* 195–201.

Boysen, G., Brander, T., Christensen, H., Gideon, R., & Truelsen, T. (2003). Homocysteine and risk of recurrent stroke. *Stroke, 34,* 1258–1261.

Burke, L. E. (2003). Primary prevention in patients with a strong family history of coronary heart disease. *Journal of Cardiovascular Nursing, 18,* 139–143.

Chasman, D. I., Posada, D., Subrahmanyan, L., Cook, N. R., Stanton, V. P., Jr., & Ridker, P. M. (2004). Pharmacogenetic study of statin therapy and cholesterol reduction. *Journal of the American Medical Association, 291,* 2821–2827.

Chien, K. R. (2003). Genotype, phenotype: Upstairs, downstairs in the family of cardiomyopathies. *Journal of Clinical Investigation, 111,* 175–178.

Darbar, D., Herron, K. J., Ballew, J. D., Jahangir, A., Gersh, B. J., Shen, W-K., et al. (2003). Familial atrial fibrillation is a genetically heterogeneous disorder. *Journal of the American College of Cardiology, 41,* 2185–2192.

Durrington, P. (2003). Dyslipidaemia. *Lancet, 362,* 717–731.

Finsterer, J., & Stollberger, C. (2003). The heart in human dystrophinopathies. *Cardiology, 99,* 1–19.

Fox, C. S., Parise, H., D'Agostino, R. B., Lloyd-Jones, D. M., Vasan, R. S., Wang, T. J. (2004). Parental atrial fibrillation as a risk factor for atrial fibrillation in offspring. *Journal of the American Medical Association, 291,* 2851–2855.

Gotto, A. M. (2005). Efficacy and safety of statin therapy in children with familial hypercholesterolemia: A randomized controlled trial. *Journal of Pediatrics, 146,* 144–145.

Greene, O., & Durrington, P. (2004). Clinical management of children and young adults with heterozygous familial hypercholesterolaemia in the UK. *Journal of the Royal Society of Medicine, 97,* 226–229.

Hackam, D. G., & Anand, S. S. (2003). Emerging risk factors for atherosclerotic vascular disease. *Journal of the American Medical Association, 290,* 932–940.

Hajjar, R. J., Huq, F., Matsui, T., & Rosenzweig, A. (2003). Genetic editing of dysfunctional myocardium. *Medical Clinics of North America, 87,* 553–567.

Hughes, S. E. (2005). New insights into the pathology of inherited cardiomyopathy. *Heart, 91,* 251–264.

Humphries, S. E., Galton, D., & Nicholls, P. (1997). Genetic testing for familial hypercholesterolaemia: Practical and ethical issues. *Quarterly Journal of Medicine, 90,* 169–181.

Jacobson, D. R., Pastore, R. D., Yaghoubian, R., Kane, I., Gallo, G., Buck, F. S., et al. (1997). Variant-sequence transthretin (isoleucine 122) in late-onset cardiac amyloidosis in black Americans. *New England Journal of Medicine, 336,* 466–473.

Jansen, A. C. M., van Wissen, S., Defesche J. C., & Kastelein, J. J. P. (2003). Phenotypic variability in familial hypercholesterolaemia: An update. *Current Opinion in Lipidology, 13,* 165–171.

Kim, J. S., Han, S. R., Chung, S. W., Kim, B. S., Lee, K. S., Kim, Y. I., et al. (2003). The apolipoprotein E epsilon4 haplotype is an important predictor for recurrence in ischemic cerebrovascular disease. *Journal of Neurological Science, 206,* 31–37.

Kojoglanian, S. A., Jorgensen, M. B., Wode-Tsadik, G., Burchette, R. J., & Aharonian, V. J. (2003). Restenosis in intervened coronaries with hyperhomocysteinemia (RICH). *American Heart Journal, 146,* 1077-1081.

Lashley, F. R. (1999). Genetic testing, screening, and counseling issues in cardiovascular disease. *Journal of Cardiovascular Nursing, 13,* 110–126.

Linton, M. F., & Fazio, S. (2003). A practical approach to risk assessment to prevent coronary artery disease and its complications. *American Journal of Cardiology, 92*(Suppl.), 19i–26i.

Maitland-van der Zee, A. H., Klungel, O. H., Stricker, B. H., Veenstra, D. L., Kastelein, J. J., Hofman A., et al. (2004). Pharmacoeconomic evaluation of testing for angiotensin-converting enzyme genotype before starting beta-hydroxy-beta-methylglutaryl coenzyme A reductase inhibitor therapy in men. *Pharmacogenetics, 14,* 53–60.

Malinow, M. R., Duell, P. B., Hess, D. L., Anderson, P. H., Kruger, W. D., Phillipson, B. E., et. al. (1998). Reduction of plasma homocyst(e)ine levels by breakfast cereal fortified with folic acid in patients with coronary heart disease. *New England Journal of Medicine, 338,* 1009–1115.

Marian, A. J. (2002). Modifier genes for hypertrophic cardiomyopathy. *Current Opinion in Cardiology, 17,* 242–252.

Maron, B. J. (2003). Sudden death in young athletes. *New England Journal of Medicine, 349,* 1064–1075.

McKenna, W. J., Spirito, P., Desnos, M., Dubourg, O., & Komajda, M. (1997). Experience from clinical genetics in hypertrophic cardiomyopathy: Proposal for new diagnostic criteria in adult members of affected families. *Heart, 77,* 130–132.

Mestroni, L. (2003). Genomic medicine and atrial fibrillation. *Journal of the American College of Cardiology, 41,* 2193–2196.

Meyer, J. S., Mehdirad, A., Salem, B. I., Jamry, W. A., Kulikowska, A., & Kulikowski, P. (2003). Sudden arrhythmia death syndrome: Importance of the long QT syndrome. *American Family Physician, 68,* 483–488.

Miller, M., Rhyne, J., Hamlette, S., Birnbaum, J., & Rodriguez, A. (2003). Genetics of HDL regulation in humans. *Current Opinion in Lipidology, 14,* 273–279.

Moolman, J. C., Corfield, V. A., Posen, B., Ngumbela, K., Seidman, C., Brink, P. A., & Watkins, H. (1997). Sudden death due to troponin T mutations. *Journal of the American College of Cardiology, 29,* 549–555.

Moss, A. J. (2003). Long QT syndrome. *Journal of the American Medical Association, 289,* 2041–2044.

Nabel, E. G. (2003). Cardiovascular disease. *New England Journal of Medicine, 349,* 60–72.

Neyroud, N., Tesson, F., Denjoy, I., Leibovici, M., Donger, C., Barhanin, J., et al. (1997). A novel mutation in the potassium channel gene

KVLQT1 causes the Jervell and Lange-Nielsen cardioauditory syndrome. *Nature Genetics, 15,* 186–189.

Nishimura, R. A., & Holmes, D. R., Jr. (2004). Hypertrophic obstructive cardiomyopathy. *New England Journal of Medicine, 350,* 1320–1327.

Omenn, G. S., Beresford, S. A. A., & Motulsky, A. G. (1998). Preventing coronary disease. *Circulation, 97,* 421–424.

Olson, E. N. (2004). A decade of discoveries in cardiac biology. *Nature Medicine, 10,* 467–47x.

Online Mendelian Inheritance in Man, OMIM (TM). (2005). Center for Medical Genetics, Johns Hopkins University (Baltimore, MD) and National Center for Biotechnology Information, Library of Medicine (Bethesda, MD). Retrieved from http://www.ncbi.nlm.nih.gov/omim/

Priori, S. G., Schwartz, P. J., Napolitano, C., Bloise, R., Ronchetti, E., Grillo, M., et al. (2003). Risk stratification in the long-QT syndrome. *New England Journal of Medicine, 348,* 1866–1874.

Pyeritz, R. E. (2001). Genetics and cardiovascular disease. In E. Braunwald, D. P. Zipes, & P. Libby (Eds.), *Heart disease. A textbook of cardiovascular medicine* (6th ed., pp. 1977-2018). Philadelphia: W.B. Saunders.

Roberts, R., & Brugada, R. (2003). Genetics and arrhythmias. *Annual Review of Medicine, 54,* 257–267.

Rosenthal, S. L., Knauer-Black, S., Stahl, M. P., Catalanotto, T. J., & Sprecher, D. L. (1993). The psychological functioning of children with hypercholesterolemia and their families. *Clinical Pediatrics, 32,* 135–141.

Scheuner, M. T. (2003). Genetic evaluation for coronary artery disease. *Genetics in Medicine, 5,* 269–285.

Schuit, S. C. E., Oei, H-H., S., Witteman, J. C. M., Geurts van Kessel, C. H., van Meurs, J. B. J., Nijhuis, R. L., et al. (2004). Estrogen receptor α gene polymorphisms and risk of myocardial infarction. *Journal of the American Medical Association, 291,* 2969–2977.

Song, Y., Stampfer, M. J., & Liu, S. (2004). Meta-analysis: Apolipoprotein E genotypes and risk for coronary heart disease. *Annals of Internal Medicine, 141,* 137–147.

Staessen, J. A., Wang, J., Bianchi, G., & Birkenhäger, W. H. (2003). Essential hypertension. *Lancet, 361,* 1629–1641.

Sturm, A. C. (2004). Cardiovascular genetics: Are we there yet? *Journal of Medical Genetics, 41,* 321–323.

Tester, D. J., McCormack, J., & Ackerman, M. J. (2004). Prenatal molecular genetic diagnosis of congenital long QT syndrome by strategic genotyping. *American Journal of Cardiology, 93,* 788–791.

Topol, E. J. (Ed.). (2002). *Textbook of cardiovascular medicine* (2nd ed.). Philadelphia: Lippincott-Raven.

Towbin, J. A. (2002). Familial dysrhythmias and conduction disorders. In D. L. Rimoin, J. M. Connor, R. E. Pyeritz, & B. R. Korf (Eds.), *Emery and Rimoin's principles and practice of medical genetics* (4th ed., pp. 1417–1474). New York: Churchill Livingstone.

Turner, S. T., & Boerwinkle, E. (2003). Genetics of blood pressure, hypertensive complications, and antihypertensive drug responses. *Pharmacogenomics, 4,* 53–65.

Umans-Eckenhausen, M. A., Defesche, J. C., van Dam, M. J., & Kastelein, J. J. (2003). Long-term compliance with lipid-lowering medication after genetic screening for familial hypercholesterolemia. *Archives of Internal Medicine, 163,* 65–68.

Van Maarle, M. C., Stouthard, M. E., & Bonsel, G. J. (2003). Risk perception of participants in family-based genetic screening program on familial hypercholesterolemia. *American Journal of Medical Genetics, 116A,* 136–143.

Vosberg, H-P., & McKenna, W. J. (2002). Cardiomyopathies. In D. L. Rimoin, J. M. Connor, R. E. Pyeritz, & B. R. Korf (Eds.), *Emery and Rimoin's principles and practice of medical genetics* (4th ed., pp. 1342–1416). New York: Churchill Livingstone.

Worman, H., & Courvalin, J-C., (2004). How do mutations in lamins A and C cause disease? *Journal of Clinical Investigation, 113,* 349–351.

Yu, B., French, J. A., Jeremy, R. W., French, P., McTaggart, D. R., Nicholson, M. R., et al. (1998). Counselling issues in familial hypertrophic cardiomyopathy. *Journal of Medical Genetics, 35,* 183–188.

V

In Closing

27

Genes and Future Generations

Human genetics, perhaps more than any other science, has influenced and been influenced or manipulated by social, economic, political, and religious forces. The practical application of developments in genetics as seen in genetic testing, screening, counseling, prenatal diagnosis, advanced therapeutic management, and the exercise of such reproductive options as gamete donation, in vitro fertilization, embryo implantation, contraception, sterilization, gender selection, abortion, and adoption, affect both individuals and society, raising important questions of rights and responsibilities that impact on both present and future generations. Is the "brave new world" now? James Watson once said that our fate used to be thought of as being in the stars; now it is in our genes. The results of the research under the auspices of the Human Genome Project have emphasized the influence of genetics. Moral, social, and ethical problems posed by human genetics have been discussed throughout this book, most specifically in chapters 10, 11, and 12. The work of the Human Genome Project as discussed in chapter 1 has brought to the forefront many of these issues. Early in the Project its significant impact on society was recognized, and therefore ethical, legal, and social implications were made an integral part of the Project. This chapter concentrates on problems concerning cloning, transgenic plants, assisted reproductive technologies, eugenics, the effects of genetic practices on the gene pool (the collection of genes in a population) in present and future generations, the rights of the individual vs. society, genetic discrimination (defined by Natowicz, Alper, & Alper (1992) as "discrimination against an individual or against members of that individual's family solely because of real or perceived differences from the 'normal' genome in the genetic constitution of that individual" p. 466), and the implications of the "new genetics." While issues of gene patents and ownership have become important to industry, they are beyond the scope of this chapter.

CLONING

One of genetics' recent reported advances was announced in February, 1997, when the cloning of a lamb (Dolly) from an adult sheep cell caused considerable stir. At one university, human embryos were cloned from embryonic cells and grown to the 32-cell stage, at which point they could have been implanted in a woman's uterus although they were not. Much discussion and speculation arose from the story, however, and the question is, "Will Mary follow Dolly?" Since that time, other animals have been cloned, such as cows and mules. Even a report of the birth of a cloned infant was made in 2002, by the religious cult the Raëlians, but this was not substantiated. Cloned human cells are being used, however, for the production of embryonic stem cells which are used for bone marrow transplantation and for therapies for damaged cells and tissues. The embryo is sacrificed during harvesting of these cells. The stem cell controversy has become increasingly political, particularly in the United States.

Probably a clone would not be identical to its origin as an adult due to the environmental impact and shaping that occurs with every person. For example, if Beethoven had been raised in the Amazon basin would his same talent have emerged and been recognized? Cloning, however, raises many issues and questions. Some have been tackled in books, movies, and other media, such as *The Boys From Brazil* by Ira Levin in which multiple boys were cloned from Hitler. Other implications have to do with the possibility of raising cloned humans for spare body parts, for replacing a person with extraordinary talent or characteristics either "good" or "evil," or for many other reasons. Could a person be cloned without his or her knowledge or permission? What decisions should be made if any? Who will make them? Who will enforce them and how? As Rabbi Moses Tendler said, "In science, the one rule is that what *can* be done *will* be done" (Woodward, 1997, p. 60).

GENETICALLY ALTERED AND TRANSGENIC PLANTS

Genetically altered plants has been a source of controversy although humans have improved crops and domesticated animals by selective breeding for many years. Some of the ways to improve farm crops include making plants resistant to disease and predators, making plants resistant to weed killers, improving crop production, increasing the nutritional value, altering features such as color, taste, resistance to spoilage and freezing, and so on. While the National Research Council stated that it was not aware of unsafe conditions brought on by genetically altered plants, the ecological impact and the impact of gene modification on the environment, the possibility of horizontal gene transfer, and other aspects are being examined (Kaiser, 2000). For example, soybeans were modified with a Brazil nut gene, in one instance. These were given to people who were allergic to the nut, who showed allergic reactions; thus such modification could expose consumers to hidden allergies. There are also political and economic ramifications.

ASSISTED REPRODUCTIVE TECHNIQUES

It was in July, 1978, that the first "test tube" baby, Louise Joy Brown, was born in the United Kingdom using in vitro fertilization, and in 1992, the first birth using intracytoplasmic sperm injection occurred. It is now estimated that assisted reproductive procedures are used in 1 in 150 births in the United States. The use of assisted reproductive technology (ART), including in vitro fertilization (IVF) and embryo transfer, embryo donation, intracytoplasmic sperm injection (ICSI), and other approaches including the cryopreservation of both reproductive cells and embryos, has vastly benefitted infertile couples but has created a variety of questions and ethical issues. Many experimental techniques are being used in order to find the most effective and safest approaches that minimize multiple pregnancies and unwanted side effects. In spite of these successes, questions have been raised that focus on the health and development outcomes of children born after ART, and of ethical issues that have emerged from this technology. Among the problems in examining health and development of children born using ART are that the procedure is generally done in a population in which at least one parent is infertile, and the effects of parental age, parity, the cause of the infertility, whether hormonal or other therapy is used to maintain pregnancy, the maturity of sperm used, and delayed fertilization of the oocyte are all factors that may influence results. In addition, it is difficult to assemble a large enough sample size, standardize definitions and assessments particularly as to the time period that assessment of a birth defect, for example, is recorded since some become obvious later in life. There is also the question of whether or not the cellular stress that occurs during manipulation can modify fetal and placental gene expression, and whether epigenetic modification of gene expression might occur. Further, in ICSI, most natural selection mechanisms are bypassed, there is the risk of mechanical injury to the spindle, there is a delay in DNA replication of the paternal genome, the introduction of sperm components into the egg, culture media entry into the egg during injection, changes in certain oscillations and kinetics, compromised mitochondrial function, and preferential localization of the sex chromosomes in the sperm head. Cytoplasmic transfer has been used from donor oocytes to rejuvenate recipient oocytes from women who have had repeated IVF failures, but this procedure raises concerns about mitochondrial disease and the effects of the transfer of mRNA and other cytoplasmic elements.

ICSI has become commonly used in as many as 80% of all ART procedures. In regard to ICSI, in which a single spermatozoon is injected into the oocyte cytoplasm, lower birthweights have been observed. There is also an increase in multiple pregnancies, which in and of themselves can lead to complications. In one study by Hansen, Kurinczuk, Bower, and Webb (2002), ICSI has been associated with a higher number of major birth defects than among naturally conceived children, especially in regard to chromosomal defects including those of the sex chromosomes. Those conceived using IVF had a greater number of cardiovascular and urogenital defects, particularly hypospadias. This study adjusted for maternal age, parity, infant sex, singletons, sibling correlation, and classification issues. Other studies have noted an increase in chromosomal abnormalities in IVF. In other studies, there have been suggestions of neurodevelopmental delays in early childhood but these have not been confirmed. Niemitz and Feinberg (2004) suggest that ART may be associated with the development of Beckwith-Wiedemann syndrome, Angelman syndrome and retinoblastoma as well as other epigenetic defects in offspring and call for further research in the area. Preimplantation genetic screening is often done in conjunction with ART and is discussed in chapter 12.

A variety of social, legal, and ethical issues are engendered by ART. These have to do with the creation of multiple embryos for ART, and their potential selection for characteristics or sex not related to a genetic disorder; the possibility of the use of unused embryos who are under 14 days post conception, and of those between 14 and 18 days, for research purposes; induction of twins; the use of eggs, sperm, or embryos for research when the donor has not given explicit consent; induction of twins through division of embryos; creation of embryos for research purposes; constructing embryonic cell lines from unused embryos; and selective reduction of multifetal pregnancies after ART. In some of these issues of informed consent and the right to keep and store cells and tissues for later research and other purposes are of concern. The American Society for Reproductive Medicine has devoted much of the September 2004 (volume 82, supplement 1) issue of *Fertility and Sterility* to issues connected with ART including issues relating to gamete donors and recipients. Issues have also been created by mistakes during IVF that in

one case involved implantation of the "wrong embryo," and in another, a White woman's eggs were fertilized by mixed sperm due to a poorly sterilized pipette so that she gave birth to one Black and one White twin. Such instances have led to looking at what determines who is a parent and what determines parental rights and duties by various authors such as Fuscaldo (2003), Spriggs (2003), and Murray and Kaebnick (2003). Another issue has been the potential for ART children to seek their donor parent(s) in much the same way people who are adopted have done, and issues of disclosure and confidentiality for gamete donors have been raised.

The Ethics Committee of the American Society for Reproductive Medicine (ASRM) (2004) have issued a statement on disclosure to offspring of their conception by gamete donation. Their opinions include the following:

1. ART programs and sperm banks should discuss issues of offspring disclosure with both gamete donors and recipients before attempting pregnancy.
2. All prospective recipients and donors should receive counseling about the implications of donation and disclosure for the recipients, donors, and children.
3. All gamete donors should undergo a complete medical history, physical examination, family genetic history, and laboratory screen following ASRM guidelines.
4. ART programs and sperm banks should retain medical and genetic donor information in a secure location, and consider how to preserve these in the case of closure or retirement.
5. Gamete donors should be encouraged to inform the program or sperm bank of information that might have genetic implications for offspring.
6. The level of desired disclosure (anonymous, known or identified, identifiable later) should be clearly addressed in counseling, informed consent, and consent forms for both donors and recipients.
7. Nonidentifying medical and genetic information regarding the donor should be provided to recipients when they are choosing a donor.

8. Programs and sperm banks should consider how to accommodate the different disclosure options preferred by donors and recipients.
9. After successful anonymous donation, the following should apply:
   a. The original agreements should be honored unless the donor and recipients agree to disclose more or less than originally agreed upon or the donor and adult child agree to additional disclosure.
   b. Donors and recipients need to be aware that the program or sperm bank could be compelled to disclose or protect the donor's identity by court order or future legislation.
   c. Programs or sperm banks should expect inquiries about donors from the offspring and should consider developing a written policy to respond to these issues (p. 530).

Recent trends have favored disclosure to offspring, and there is a trend in telling children earlier in order that they can absorb this information over time although it depends on the readiness of the child. The Ethics Committee of ASRM (2004) supports disclosure while recognizing that this personal decision should be made by the parents. Considerations for disclosure include that: (1) people have a fundamental right to know their biological origins and that not telling the child about their biological origins violates that child's autonomy; (2) openness may be important in development of identity; (3) open and honest communication is important; (4) disclosure may have a positive effect on the parent-child relationship; (5) prevents the child from accidentally discovering information about their origin; (6) avoids secrets in families which can create dynamics between those who know and those who don't as well as cause confusion; (7) can provide information about potential health problems; and (8) can protect against inadvertent consanguinity. Considerations against disclosure include: (1) that telling the child can subject them to psychological turmoil; (2) may create barriers between the child and the non-biological parent; and (3) allows parents to retain privacy about their infertility which may be especially important in some cultural groups (pp. 528–529).

Genetic risks associated with embryo donation where the recipient couple makes no direct genetic contribution to the child are still to be fully developed but some guidelines have been suggested (Eydoux et al., 2004).

EUGENICS, THE EUGENICS MOVEMENT, AND GENETIC ENHANCEMENT

Eugenics refers to the improvement of a species through genetic manipulation. Positive eugenics seeks to accomplish this by increasing the frequency of traits considered desirable through encouraging selective mating and reproduction of those possessing such traits (the "fit"). Negative eugenics seeks to reduce the frequency of traits considered undesirable by preventing the reproduction of those persons possessing such traits (the "unfit"). Although plant and animal breeders have long practiced eugenics to improve crops and livestock, in humans, active advocacy of formal programs began in the latter part of the 19th century. In America a Eugenics Record Office was established in Cold Spring Harbor, New York, in 1910.

One of their major goals was the preservation of the "racial welfare" of the United States, through the application of positive and negative eugenics by encouraging the propagation of those whom they considered to be fit and by preventing the propagation of those they considered unfit. Those whom they considered fit were individuals who were healthy, intelligent, of high moral character, of Anglo-Saxon or Nordic extraction, affluent, Protestant, and of the upper or upper-middle class. In fact, these characteristics were generally synonymous with those possessed by the eugenicists themselves. Although many proponents of eugenics were sincere in their intent to strengthen the human race and alleviate suffering, the movement was also a refuge for bigots, racists, and male supremists who came to dominate it. Genetics was used in an attempt to biologically justify the perceived inferiority of blacks, Jews, southern and eastern Europeans, as well as the Irish because they were Catholics. The activities and influence of the eugenicists ranged from sponsoring blue-ribbon baby contests at county and state fairs to issues with a far more serious impact, such as the eugenic sterilization laws, and the Immigration Restriction Act of 1924 (the Johnson Act). The latter restricted immigration to 2% of the number of each nationality listed in the 1890 census, a year that was well before the mass immigration of persons from southern and eastern Europe. This situation existed until the passage of the Celler Act of 1965. In Germany, the Nazis, with the assistance of scientists, used the concept of racial hygiene to sterilize people such as the mentally retarded, and annihilate others such as the Jews and gypsy people in attempts to "protect" the German people from those they considered unclean or "genetically diseased."

Compulsory sterilization was seen as a way to prevent the propagation of the "unfit," a term that in its various interpretations included the mentally retarded, the insane, alcoholics, orphans, paupers, derelicts, epileptics, diseased and degenerate persons, and even chicken thieves. Campaigns for eugenic sterilization laws were launched, although some enthusiasts were already performing sterilizations in state institutions. The first state to institute involuntary sterilization laws was Indiana in 1907. The wording and provisions of the laws varied greatly from state to state and by 1935, more than 30 states had passed such laws. California was most active in their implementation and by 1935 had sterilized about 10,000 persons, whereas in the entire United States about 20,000 sterilizations were performed. While these laws remain on the books in many states, they are rarely invoked. In Oregon, recently, Governor Kitzhaber apologized for past abuses of sterilization, occuring from 1923 to 1981. In addition to the institutionalized mentally retarded, involuntary sterilization abuses extended to those who were Black or poor. It has been suggested that the use of Norplant(r) might allow a type of eugenic control. In the People's Republic of China, those persons with "a genetic disease of a serious nature" and those who are married and of childbearing age who are "considered to be inappropriate for childbearing" are asked to be sterilized or take long-term contraceptive methods (Beardsley, 1997; "Brave new now," 1997). The Minister of Public Health (Chen Mingzhang) in 1994 was quoted as saying that "births of inferior quality are serious among the old revolutionary base, ethnic minorities, the frontier, and economically poor areas" (Dickson, 1994, p. 3). Some have said that prenatal diagnosis with selective pregnancy termination already constitutes eugenics. Others believe these techniques constitute disease prevention instead. The question of preimplantation genetic diagnosis following in vitro fertilization to allow the selection and implantation of an unaffected embryo is generally considered more ethically acceptable than prenatal diagnosis followed by abortion. In the former case, spare embryos are not allowed to further develop, and this is seen by many as a more acceptable choice.

The misuse and misunderstanding of genetic knowledge, coupled with an emerging doctrine of racial superiority, led to disenchantment and denouncement of the movement by many geneticists and citizens. By the 1930s, the visible abuse of genetics and eugenics for totalitarian aims and the flagrant disregard for human rights were so evident in Nazi Germany that not only did the movement die in this country, but the discipline of human genetics itself was left with a tinge of suspicion that permeates many programs even today. Fears of genetic discrimination remain. For example, when it was discovered that a specific gene mutation for colon cancer was most common among Ashkenazi Jews, there were fears raised about discrimination that led to statements issued such as this one by Dr. Francis Collins, "I think it is very unlikely that the total number of genetic aberrations carried around by Jewish individuals is any greater than that of any other group" and "There is no perfect genetic specimen. We are all flawed" (Wade, 1997). However, as gene studies in Ashkenazi Jews continue, many leaders are refusing to participate, fearing vulnerability to discrimination.

As genetic manipulation and selective choice progresses, the question of genetic enhancement has been raised. For example, certain characteristics are known to be associated with success in certain sports. In some instances, physicians have been asked to administer growth hormone not because the given individual is particularly short but in order to produce a taller individual so that they could play basketball, for example. The concept of "gene doping" is defined by the World Anti-Doping Agency as "the non-therapeutic use of genes, genetic elements, and or cells that have the capacity to enhance athletic performance" (Unal & Unal, 2004, p. 358). Examples include the potential for using gene therapy such as using the gene that encodes erythropoetin to increase oxygen transport in the tissues to increase aerobic capacity; or to use the insulin-like growth factor-1 gene to stimulate muscle hypertrophy in specific muscles to enhance performance. Athletes using such methodologies would be subjecting themselves to known and unknown health risks. Various agencies are developing various warnings and standards. Another aspect is genotyping of athletes. It has been noted that certain gene variations might convey certain performance enhancements. For example the R577X polymorphism in the gene that encodes for α-actinin-3 which is responsible for generating muscle force at high velocity appears to produce advantages in performance (Yang et al., 2003). Conceivably using genotying to select athletes early based on possession of identified favorable genetic polymorphisms and discouraging others have serious ethical and societal implications. It could even result in the planning of children who would carry a certain configuration of these polymorphisms to create a potential class of superathletes. As the future ability to perform genetic manipulations, gene therapy, and other direct and indirect genetic technologies looms on the horizon, will we be asked to enhance human abilities and traits? Will embryo manipulation for enhancement and therapy become increasingly common? Will such options only be for those with the financial means to afford them? What kinds of discrimination could result?

EFFECTS OF CURRENT PRACTICES ON THE GENE POOL

The improved medical management of persons with genetic disorders such as phenylketonuria (PKU), hemophilia, retinoblastoma, cystic fibrosis, and others has led to longer life spans with an improved quality of life. Thus, persons with certain genetic disorders who earlier did not live long enough or were too incapacitated to reproduce are now able to do so. In genetic terms this means that the selective forces that formerly acted against the survival and transmission of these mutant genes are now counteracted or relaxed by medical treatment. One of the genetic consequences is that these genes can be transmitted to succeeding generations instead of being lost from the gene pool. Some have expressed concern that the result of genetic and medical advances in testing, screening, prenatal diagnosis, assisted reproductive techniques,

counseling, and treatment will ultimately be to weaken and "pollute" the gene pool of future generations. This line of thought poses certain questions. Among them are the following: Does this generation have a responsibility to prevent the "deterioration" of the gene pool? If so, how great a responsibility? How far into the future does this responsibility extend? Should the well-being of individuals in this generation supersede responsibility to future individuals? Should genetic counselors and geneticists consider the individual rights and wishes of their clients above those of today's society? Should they be considered above concerns for succeeding generations? How much do we value individual freedom and personal privacy? Is it ever proper to subsume such freedoms for the greater good of society? How do we decide what the greater good of society is? What are the actual effects of some practices on the gene pool? Such estimates vary because of differences in the mutation rate, the frequency of the gene in the population, fertility and fitness, marriage and mating practices, and the effect of using alternative reproductive options coupled with prenatal diagnosis and genetic counseling. Assuming full fertility and fitness for an autosomal recessive disorder with a gene frequency of .01, a disease frequency of 1 in 10,000, and a mutation rate of 10^{-4}, the World Health Organization (WHO) estimates that it would be 100 generations before the gene frequency in the population would double and the frequency of the disorder would quadruple. The rarer the autosomal recessive disorder, the more genes would be present in the heterozygote states than in the affected homozygote. For autosomal dominant disorders that would have been genetically lethal without medical therapy, assuming a mutation rate of 5×10^{-5}, and a frequency of the trait of 0.0001, the incidence of the disorder would double in the next generation. Thus, change has greater immediate genetic consequences than does the result of treatment in autosomal recessive disorders. For X-linked recessive disorders, the effects of relaxed selection will not be seen in the first generation, but the incidence of the disease will double in about four generations. The effects of relaxed selection on multifactorial disorders such as pyloric stenosis and congenital heart disease are more difficult to determine because of differences in the extent of the genetic contribution and of the possibility of changes occurring in contributing environmental factors. WHO estimates that the incidence of each of these disorders will increase between 3% and 5% per generation. Thus, it can be expected that an increase in each autosomal recessive disorder will have the least short-term impact on the population.

The gene pool can also be influenced by assortative rather than random nonassortative mating practices. Persons with the same genetic disorders often choose to marry each other, and to take the risk of having natural children. This has been attributed to social proximity, lack of social acceptance by others, lack of opportunity to interact with "normal" individuals, and mutual understanding of problems created by the disorder. Phillips, Newton, and Gosden (1982), in studying couples who were blind from birth, noted that having natural children is one way of demonstrating their own normality in at least one sphere, and showing that they are able to overcome difficulties. In addition, choosing adoption may be difficult as many agencies are unwilling to give a child to disabled couples. The couple may, however, not consider the impact on the natural child of later discovering that his/her parents knowingly chose to have a child who would be affected instead of choosing another reproductive option such as gamete donation, and some believe that knowingly imposing a lifetime burden on an affected child is wrong. In fact, children have been allowed to enter "wrongful life" suits against their parents. For certain disorders the use of genetic testing/screening can identify couples who are both heterozygous carriers for the same deleterious genes. The birth of an affected child could then be prevented if desired, by prenatal diagnosis followed by the selective pregnancy termination of affected fetuses. The actual impact on the gene pool would vary according to the mode of transmission of the genetic disorder in question and the number of children the couple chose to have. Kaback estimates that if all Ashkenazi Jewish couples were screened for Tay Sachs and allowed to have 2 unaffected children, it would take 8,750 years to double the carrier rate in that population. Parents could still contribute single copies of deleterious genes to the next generation by way of heterozygous offspring. Trying to eliminate all fetuses who were heterozygous for deleterious genes would mean eliminating the entire human race because each of us carries single copies of 5 to 7 deleterious genes in the recessive state. The effect of genetic counseling on the gene pool would also depend on the reproductive course chosen by the couple seeking counseling. How directive the counseling is can influence that choice and thus influence effects on succeeding generations (see chapter 10).

INDIVIDUAL RIGHTS vs. THOSE OF OTHERS

The rights of individuals to make reproductive and other decisions are increasingly complicated by outside forces. For example, if a fetus is found to be affected with Down syndrome, the parents may decide to give birth to this child. If insurance companies or society would say that if they knowingly gave birth to this child, no medical or health insurance coverage would apply for the birth or future care, however, how would that influence their decision? The issues of insurance in regard to genetics include life insurance, disability-income insurance, long-term care insurance, critical-illness coverage, and medical-expense insurance, and are well reviewed by Pokorski (1997). In another instance, a Los Angeles TV anchorwoman, Bree Walker Lampley, was criticized on a talk show and elsewhere for deciding to have a child despite the fact that she had ectrodactyly (a hand deformity where some digits are fused, known as "lobster claw"), for which there is a 50% risk of transmission.

In order to provoke thought, some of the questions and problems relating to individual versus societal good and rights are exemplified by the following: Should society allow affected individuals to marry or mate if no prenatal diagnosis is available for the specific condition in question? Should they be prohibited from procreation? What should society do if a couple chooses not to abort an affected fetus? Should such measures be compulsory? Should there be more subtle pressures such as the refusal of society to contribute financially to the care and education of such children? How do these questions apply to women who are eligible for prenatal diagnosis because of advanced maternal age or because of other indications? Should prenatal diagnosis be mandatory for everyone? Should newborn screening be more inclusive such as for adult-onset diseases and presymptomatic disorders? When one member of a couple is at a high risk for inheriting the gene for a disorder such as Huntington disease, should that couple be "allowed" by society to have natural children without having molecular testing for the Huntington disease gene? And if the gene is present, does that person have the right to reproduce if he or she so chooses? Does he or she have a duty not to reproduce? Should society enforce sterilization of the person at risk? Does the right of the person to reproduce always supersede the possible burden to society? Does a person have the right to reproduce no matter what the effects are on his/her direct descendants? Should the right of the individual prevail? Further advances in treatment will continue to reduce the burden of certain disorders. For example, the inborn inability to synthesize a certain vitamin may be compensated for relatively simply by taking a pill once a day. Would this disorder be considered a burden? What about other types of selection? For example, in one survey, a substantial percentage of respondents said they would want to choose a more intelligent or attractive fetus. How large a burden is the correction of a disorder such as pyloric stenosis by surgery? Would it be important enough to limit the reproduction of persons who have had this disorder? Who would make such decisions? On what basis? Should genetic counseling be firmly directive? Should it consider the interests of society or the interests of the individuals seeking counseling? Should the number of children a heterozygous couple is allowed to have be limited by law to reduce the frequency of the gene? What about all of the genotypes not detectable by current screening or diagnostic methods? What about possession of traits apart from the mainstream (including variations) whose meaning is unclear? Other meanings are legal ones: would criminals be able to mount a defense on the basis of their genetic constitution, for example, if they possessed genes with susceptibility to violence or aggression? For example, in a California murder case, a woman was found not guilty because her violence was attributed to her having Huntington disease. Other defenses have been mounted on the basis of genetic constitution (see Andrews, 1997). Should couples who decide to give birth to children with serious genetic conditions be criminally guilty of child abuse, as has

been suggested by some? In a California case, the court stated that a child with a genetic condition could sue the parents for not having prenatal diagnosis and terminating the pregnancy. New techniques are constantly raising new ethical questions. For example, should fetal oocytes be taken from the ovaries of aborted fetuses and used in assisted reproduction? What about posthumous reproduction? What should be done with embryos that have been cryopreserved? What do the terms "mother" and "father" mean?

FUTURE GENERATIONS

Suppose that it was decided that society could now think about instituting a type of eugenics program for the good of future generations. In addition to the problem of the inherent rights of the individual, some of the problems that could be identified at present are as follows: (a) Knowledge about the inheritance of many traits is inadequate. (b) It is not known what genotypes may be needed for humans coping with different environments in the future. (c) It is not known what traits would be most desirable. For example, tallness might be a liability because of crowded conditions, whereas shortness might become highly valued. (d) The consequences of the total elimination of a particular genotype cannot be foreseen. (e) New mutations would probably continue to add new deleterious genes and traits to the population. (f) Not all traits or genes are currently detectable or diagnosable. (g) What traits should be included—would late-onset diseases be detected presymptomatically? If so, perhaps no one would be free of such genetic susceptibility. (h) The development of new treatments for disorders cannot be accurately predicted. (i) Would the political and social ramifications of restricted reproduction compensate for perceived benefits? (j) What would happen if harmful genes that were eliminated were tightly linked to essential ones? (k) Who would make decisions about such programs? (l) How could we reconcile such programs with the value we place on individual freedom in a democratic society? Have we already set foot down a eugenics path by offering testing, screening, prenatal diagnosis with the option of pregnancy termination, and assisted reproductive techniques? These questions and problems are significant. Some have advocated the creation of a eugenics board to decide on traits amenable to and conditions for either a voluntary or compulsory eugenics program. Instead it seems as if efforts should be concentrated on the support of society for a couple and family in making knowledgeable, voluntary decisions in their own best interests, and in the elucidation and elimination of genetic disorders and birth defects.

END NOTES

Advances in genetics have a profound impact on contemporary society as well as future generations. Such advances include predictive susceptibility and other genetic testing and reproductive planning, prenatal diagnosis, assisted reproductive technologies, the potential for genetic manipulation and technology for both therapy and enhancement, the use of cloning, stem cell research and therapy, pharmacogenomic selection for therapy, cloning, use of population data bases such as in Iceland to search for variations, and use of genetic engineering in agriculture. What happens today affects both individuals and the larger society. It is important that we ensure that ethical standards and policies safeguard the rights of individuals as well as enable responsible scientific progress and research.

BIBLIOGRAPHY

Andrews, L. (1997). Body science. *American Bar Association Journal, 83,* 44–49.

Annas, G. J. (2002). Cloning and the U.S. Congress. *New England Journal of Medicine, 346,* 1599–1602.

Bachrach, S. (2004). In the name of public health—Nazi racial hygiene. *New England Journal of Medicine, 351,* 417–420.

Barritt, J., Willadsen, S., Brenner, C., & Cohen, J. (2001). Cytoplasmic transfer in assisted reproduction. *Human Reproduction Update, 7,* 428–435.

Beardsley, T. (1997). China syndrome. *Scientific American, 276*(3), 33–34.

Begley, S. (1997, March 10). Little lamb, who made thee? *Newsweek,* 52–59.

Boyle, K. E., Vlahos, N., & Jarow, J. P. (2004). Assisted reproductive technology in the new millennium: Part I. *Urology, 63,* 2–6.

Brave new now. (1997). *Nature Genetics, 15,* 1–2.

Cameron, C., & Williamson, R. (2003). Is there an ethical difference between preimplantation genetic diagnosis and abortion. *Journal of Medical Ethics, 29,* 90–92.

Chakravarthy, M. V., & Booth, F. W. (2004). Eating, exercise, and "thrifty" genotypes: Connecting the dots toward an evolutionary understanding of modern chronic diseases. *Journal of Applied Physiology, 96* 3–10.

Clayton, E. W. (2003). Ethical, legal and social implications of genomic medicine. *New England Journal of Medicine, 349,* 562–569.

Cranshaw, M. (2002). Lessons from a recent adoption study to identify some of the service needs of, and issues for, donor offspring wanting to know about their donors. *Human Fertility, 5,* 6–12.

Crow, J. F. (2001). The beanbag lives on. *Nature, 409,* 771.

Dresser, R. (2004). Genetic modification of preimplantation embryos: Toward adequate hnuman research policies. *Milbank Quarterly, 82,* 195–214.

Ethics Committee of the American Society for Reproductive Medicine. (2004). Informing offspring of their conception by gamete donation. *Fertility and Sterility, 81,* 527–531.

Evers, K. (2002). European perspectives on therapeutic cloning. *New England Journal of Medicine, 346,* 1579–1582.

Eydoux, P., Thepot, F., Fellmann, F., Francannet, C., Simon-Bouy, B., Jouannet, P., Bresson, J. L., et al. (2004). *Human Reproduction, 19,* 1685–1688.

Fost, N. C. (2004). Conception for donation. *Journal of the American Medical Association, 291,* 2125–2126.

Fuscaldo, G. (2003). What makes a parent? It's not black or white. *Journal of Medical Ethics, 29,* 66–67.

Gogarty, B. (2003). What exactly is an exact copy? And why it matters when trying to ban human reproductive cloning in Australia. *Journal of Medical Ethics, 29,* 84–89.

Goodheart, L. B. (2004). Rethinking mental retardation: Education and eugenics in Connecticut, 1818–1917. *Journal of the History of Medicine and Allied Sciences, 59,* 90–111.

Gurdon, J. B., & Byrne, J. A. (2003). The first half-century of nuclear transplantation. *Proceedings of the National Academy of Sciences,, USA, 100,* 8048–8052.

Hansen, M., Kurinczuk, J. J., Bower, C., & Webb, S. (2002). The risk of major birth defects after intracytoplasmic sperm injection and in vitro fertilization. *New England Journal of Medicine, 346,* 725–730.

Herrera-Estrella, L., Simpson, J., & Martinez-Trujillo, M. (2005). Transgenic plants: An historical perspective. *Methods in Molecular Biology, 286,* 3–32.

Holtzman, N. A., & Rothstein, M. A. (1992). Invited editorial: Eugenics and genetic discrimination. *American Journal of Human Genetics, 50,* 457–459.

Hook, C. C., DiMagno, E. P., & Tefferi, A. (2004). Primer on medical genomics. Part XIII: Ethical and regulatory issues. *Mayo Clinic Proceedings, 79,* 645–650.

Jain, T., Missmer, S. A., & Hornstein, M. D. (2004). Trends in embryo-transfer practice and in outcomes of the use of assisted reproductive technology in the United States. *New England Journal of Medicine, 350,* 1639–1645.

Jonsen, A. R., Durfy, S. J., Burke, W., & Motulsky, A. G. (1996). The advent of the 'unpatients.' *Nature Medicine, 2,* 622–624.

Jorgenson, E., Tang, H., Gadde, M., Province, M., Leppert, M., Kardia, S., Schork, N., et al. (2005). Ethnicity and human genetic linkage maps. *American Journal of Human Genetics, 76,* 276–290.

Josephson, D. (2002). Oregon's governor apologises for forced sterilisations. *British Medical Journal, 325,* 1380.

Kaiser, J. (2000). Transgenic crops report fuels debate. *Science, 288,* 245–247.

Kluger, J. (1997, March 10). Will we follow the sheep? *Time.*

Knoppers, B. M., & Chadwick, R. (2005). Science and society: Human genetic research. Emerging trends in ethics. *Nature Reviews Genetics, 6,* 75–79.

Lo, B., Chou, V., Cedars, M. I., Gates, E., Taylor, R. N., Wagner, R. M., et al. (2003). Consent from donors for embryo and stem cell research. *Science, 301,* 921.

Ludmerer, K. M. (1972). *Genetics and American society.* Baltimore: Johns Hopkins University Press.

Ludwig, M., & Diedrich, K. (2003). Follow-up of children born after assisted reproductive technologies. *Reproductive Biomedicine Online, 5,* 317–322.

Mallia, P., & ten Have, H. (2003). From what should we protect future generations: Germline therapy or genetic screening. *Medical and Health Care Philosophy, 6,* 17–24.

Marteau, T., & Richards, M. (Eds.). (1999). *The troubled helix: Social and psychological implications of the new human genetics.* Cambridge: Cambridge University Press.

Mertus, J., & Heller, S. (1992). Norplant meets the new eugenicists. *Saint Louis University Public Law Review, 11,* 359–383.

Murray, T. H. (2002). Reflections on the ethics of genetic enhancement. *Genetics in Medicine, 4*(Suppl. 6), 27S–32S.

Murray, T. H., & Kaebnick, G. E. (2003). Genetic ties and genetic mixups. *Journal of Medical Ethics, 29,* 68–69.

Natowicz, N. R., Alper, J. R., & Alper, J. S. (1992). Genetic discrimination and the law. *American Journal of Human Genetics, 50,* 465–475.

Niemitz, E. L., & Feinberg, A. P. (2004). Epigenetics and assisted reproductive technology: A call for investigation. *American Journal of Human Genetics, 74,* 599–609.

Ossorio, P., & Duster, T. (2005). Race and genetics: Controversies in biomedical, behavioral and forensic sciences. *American Psychologist, 60,* 115–128.

Patel, D. R., & Greydanus, D. E. (2002). Genes and athletes. *Adolescent Medicine, 13,* 249–255.

Phillips, C. I., Newton, M. S., & Gosden, C. M. (1982). Procreative instinct as a contributory factor to prevalence of hereditary blindness. *Lancet, 1,* 1169–1172.

Pokorski, R. J. (1997). Insurance underwriting in the genetic era. *American Journal of Human Genetics, 60,* 205–216.

Rabino, I. (2003). Gene therapy: Ethical issues. *Theoretical Medicine and Bioethics, 24,* 31–58.

Rakowski, E. (2002). Who should pay for bad genes? *California Law Review, 90,* 1345–1414.

Reilly, P. R., Boshar, M. F., & Holtzman, S. H. (1997). Ethical issues in genetic research: Disclosure and informed consent. *Nature Genetics, 15,* 16–20.

Rothenberg, K., Fuller, B., Rothstein, M., Duster, T., Kahn, M. J. E., Cunningham, R., et al. (1997). Genetic information and the workplace: Legislative approaches and policy challenges. *Science, 275,* 1755–1757.

Sankar, P. (2003). Genetic privacy. *Annual Review of Medicine, 54,* 393–407.

Schatten, G. (2002). Safeguarding ART. *Nature Cell Biology, 4*(S1), s19–s22.

Schieve, L. A., Rasmussen, S. A., Buck, G. M., Schendel, D. E., Reynolds, M. A., & Wright, V. C. (2004). Are children born after assisted reproductive technology at increased risk for adverse health outcomes? *Obstetrics & Gynecology, 103,* 1154–1163.

Schulman, J. D., & Edwards, R. G. (1996). Preimplantation diagnosis is disease control, not eugenics. *Human Reproduction, 11,* 463–464.

Seligmann, J., & Foote, D. (1991, October 28). Whose baby is it, anyway? *Newsweek,* p. 73.

Sharp, R. R., Yudell, M. A., & Wilson, S. H. (2004). Shaping science policy in the age of genomics. *Nature Reviews Genetics, 5,* 1–6.

Silver, R. I., Rodriguez, R., Chang, T. S. K., & Gearhart, J. P. (1999). In vitro fertilization is associated with an increased risk of hypospadias. *Journal of Urology, 161,* 1954–1957.

Spriggs, M. (2003). IVF mixup: White couple have black babies. *Journal of Medical Ethics, 29,* 65.

Stolberg, S. G. (1998, April 22). Concern among Jews is heightened as scientists deepen gene studies. *New York Times (National Edition),* p. A24.

Sutcliffe, A. G., Taylor, B., Saunders, K., Thornton, S., Lieberman, B. A., & Grudzinskas, J. G. (2001). Outcome in the second year of life after in-vitro fertilisation by intracytoplasmic sperm injection: A UK case-control study. *Lancet, 357,* 2080–2084.

Thomas, S. M. (2004). Society and ethics—the genetics of disease. *Current Opinion in Genetics & Development, 14,* 287–291.

Thompson, J. G., Kind, K. L., Roberts, C. T., Robertson, S. A., & Robinson, J. S. (2002). Epigenetic risks related to assisted reproductive technolgies: Short- and long-term consequences for the health of children conceived through assisted reproduction technology: More reason for caution? *Human Reproduction, 17,* 2783–2786.

Unal, M., & Unal, D. O. (2004). Gene doping in sports. *Sports Medicine, 34,* 357–362.

Van Steirteghem, A., Bonduelle, M., Liebaers, I., & Devroey, P. (2002). Children born after assisted reproductive technology. *American Journal of Perinatology, 19,* 59–65.

Weissman, I. L. (2002). Stem cells—scientific, medical , and political issues. *New England Journal of Medicine, 346,* 1576–1579.

Winston, R. M. L., & Hardy, K. (2002). Are we ignoring potential dangers of *in vitro* fertilization and related treatments? *Nature Cell Biology, 4*(S1), s14–s18.

Woods, G. L., White, K. L., Vanderwall, D. K., Li, G-P., Aston, K. I., Bunch, T. D., et al. (2003). A mule cloned from fetal cells by nuclear transfer. *Science, 301,* 1063.

Woodward, K. L. (1997, March 10). Today the sheep . . . *Newsweek,* p.60.

Wright, V. C., Reynolds, M. A., Jeng, G., & Kissin, D. (2004). Assisted reproductive technology surveillance—United States, 2001. *Morbidity and Mortality Weekly Report, 51*(SS-01), 1–20

Yang, N., MacArthur, D. G., Gulbin, J. P., Hahn, A. G., Beggs, A. H., Easteal, S., et al. (2003). ACTN3 genotype is associated with human elite athletic performance. *American Journal of Human Genetics, 73,* 627–6331.

Glossary

All terms in this section refer to their application in humans and human genetics.

aberration (chromosome)—any abnormality of chromosome structure or number

acentric fragment—a chromosome piece without a centromere, due to breakage

acrocentric chromosome—one in which the centromere is near the end of the chromosome

agenesis—imperfect development or absence of an organ, or its failure to form

allele—any one of two or more alternate forms of a gene located at the same locus

allogeneic—members of the same species with different genotype

allograft—graft between members of the same species who have different genotypes, for example, between two humans who are not identical twins

allozymes—enzymes that differ in electrophoretic mobility because of different alleles at a gene locus

amelia—complete congenital absence of one or more limbs

amnion—the innermost membrane of the amniotic sac that surrounds the fetus

amplification—the production of extra copies of genes or a section of DNA

anencephaly—a neural tube defect with partial or complete absence of the cranial vault and a rudimentary brain

aneuploid—any chromosome number that is not an exact multiple of the haploid (N) set, thus, trisomy 18 with 47 chromosomes is an aneuploidy, but triploidy with 69 chromosomes is a polyploidy

anhidrosis—absence of sweating

aniridia—absence of the iris of the eye

anodontia—absence of teeth

anomaly—abnormal variation in form or structure

anotia—absence of pinna of the ear

anticipation—the occurrence of a trait or disorder at an earlier age with each successive generation and/or the increased severity of a disorder with each successive generation

antimongoloid slant—downward slant of palpebral fissures of eye

aplasia—absence of or irregular structure of tissue or organ

apoenzyme—the protein part of a complex (conjugated) holoenzyme

apoptosis—the normal cellular process of programmed cell death

arcus cornae—an opaque ring seen in the cornea that is caused by a deposit of cholesteryl esters

ascertainment—the process of finding individuals or families for inclusion in genetic studies

association—the occurrence of anomalies that

occur together more often than would be expected by chance, but which have not yet been recognized as a syndrome

assortative mating—nonrandom mating practices based on choosing or rejecting mates with certain traits

atresia—absence or closure of a normal opening

autograft—a self graft

autosome(al)—any chromosome that is not a sex chromosome (X or Y); in normal human somatic cells there are 22 pairs (44) of autosomes and 2 sex chromosomes (XX or XY)

Barr body—sex chromatin found at the edge of the cell nucleus in normal females that represents the genetically inactive X chromosome

base pair—two nitrogenous bases bonded together. In DNA, adenine pairs with thymine and cytosine pairs with guanine

base sequence—the order of bases on a chromosome or DNA fragment

Bayes theorem—method of computing the probability of the occurrence of an event, considering prior and conditional probabilities

brachydactyly—abnormally shortened digits

Brushfield spots—speckled areas noted on the iris in a small percentage of normal individuals and in a large percentage of persons with Down syndrome

camptodactyly—flexion contracture or curvature of finger(s), usually the fifth finger

candidate gene—one which may be the site of causation for a given disease

canthus—outer or inner corner of eye where upper and lower lids meet

carrier—a person who is heterozygous, possessing two different alleles of a gene pair (e.g., Aa as opposed to aa or AA)

centromere—the primary constriction of a chromosome where the long and short arms meet

CHARGE association—the nonrandom association of coloboma, heart disease, atresia choanal, retarded growth and/or nervous system anomalies, genital anomalies, and ear anomalies or deafness

chimera—an organism composed of two or more cell lines; the product of the fusion of embryos

chromatid—after replication of a chromosome, two subunits attached by the centromere can be seen; each is called a chromatid, and after separation each becomes a chromosome of a daughter cell

chromatin—the material of which chromosomes are composed; it contains DNA, RNA, histones, and nonhistone proteins

chromosome—microscopic structures in the cell nucleus composed of chromatin that contain genetic information and are constant in number in a species; humans have 46 chromosomes, 22 autosome pairs and 2 sex chromosomes

clinodactyly—crooked finger that is curved inward sideways, usually the fifth digit

clone—a genetically identical cell population derived from a common ancestor; to clone an organism is to make a genetically identical copy of that organism

cloning DNA—manipulation to produce multiple copies of a single gene or groups of genetically identical cells from the same ancestor

codominance—the expression of each of a pair of alleles when present in the heterozygous state

codon—triplet bases in nucleic acids specifying placement of a specific amino acid in a polypeptide chain

coenzyme—an organic molecule that acts as a cofactor (e.g, vitamin B_{12})

cofactor—the nonprotein component of a conjugated enzyme that is required for activity; it can be organic or inorganic; if organic, often called coenzyme

coloboma—defect in, or absence of, tissue, usually in the iris of the eye; usually seen as a gap

complementary DNA (cDNA)—DNA that is synthesized from an mRNA template. Usually used as a probe in physical mapping

complementation—ability of cells with different gene mutations to cross-correct in cell culture

compound heterozygote—presence of two different alleles of a given gene, one on each allele on each chromosome

concordance—the presence of a certain trait in two individuals, usually twins

congenital—present at birth; a congenital trait may or may not be caused by genetic factors

consanguineous—related by descent from a common ancestor, usually in preceding few generations; blood relatives

consultand—the person whose genotype is of primary importance to the genetic counseling problem at hand; in practice, often used synonymously with counselee

contig—groups of clones representing overlapping regions in the genome. Used to create a contig map

contiguous gene syndrome—name given to disorders arising from small chromosome deletions or duplications of adjacent but functionally unrelated genes

CpG islands—stretches of DNA rich in cytosine and guanine base pairs

crossing over—the physical event or exchange that gives rise to recombinant chromatids

crossovers—chromatid with genetic material from each homologous chromosome

deformation—anomaly resulting from mechanical forces causing constraint on the fetus

deletion—loss of all or part of a chromosome

deoxyribonucleic acid—the primary genetic material in humans consisting of nitrogenous bases, a sugar group, and phosphate combined into a double helix

diploid—the number of chromosomes normally present in somatic cells. In humans, this is 46, and is sometimes symbolized as $2N$

discordance—when two members of a twin pair do not exhibit the same trait

dizygotic—twins originating from two different fertilized eggs; fraternal twins

DNA—deoxyribonucleic acid

DNA fingerprint—a person's unique pattern in regard to a selected section or total DNA

DNA hybridization—the process of the joining of two complementary DNA strands to form a double stranded molecule

DNA probe—a selected fragment of DNA that is labelled, often with a radioactive isotope, and through molecular hybridization, is used to find very similar or complementary regions of DNA in a sample

dominant—a trait that is expressed when one copy of the gene determining it is present

drumstick—the sex chromatin of polymorphonuclear leukocytes that is contained in a nuclear protrusion resembling a drumstick

dyshistogenesis—result from aberrant development of a specific tissue type

dysplasia—developmental abnormality of a tissue; an example is a nevus

empiric risk—one that is based on observed data, not theoretical models *epigenetics*—alterations in a gene that do not involve the DNA sequence

epimutations—abnormal changes in epigenetic alterations

epistasis—the prevention of the expression of one gene by another gene at a different locus

eugenics—improvement of a species by genetic manipulations

euploidy—having a complete correct chromosome set

exons—structural gene sequences retained in messenger RNA, and eventually translated into amino acids

expressivity—variation in the degree to which a trait is manifested; clinical severity

familial—the occurrence of more than one case of an anomaly in a family; a trait that appears with a higher frequency in close relatives than in the general population; it is not synonymous with hereditary

fitness—ability of a person with a certain genotype to reproduce and pass his/her genes to the next generation

flanking region—DNA on either side of a particular locus

forme fruste—minimal manifestation or mild form of a disorder

gamete—mature reproductive cells containing the haploid number of chromosomes (sperm or ovum)

gastroschisis—a congenital abdominal wall defect characterized by antenatal evisceration of the intestine through a small opening

gene—the functional unit of heredity; a sequence of nucleotides along the DNA of a chromosome that codes for a functional product such as RNA or a polypeptide

gene mapping—assignment of genes to specific sites on specific chromosomes

gene pool—all of the genes in a specific breeding population at a certain time

genetic code—nucleotide base sequence in DNA or RNA coding for specific amino acids

genetic constitution—a person's genetic make-up; used for either one gene pair or all

genetic load—the recessive deleterious genes concealed in the heterozygous state within a population

genocopy—the production of the same phenotypic appearance by different genes

genome—the total genetic complement of an individual genotype—a person's genetic constitution at one locus or in total

genomic imprinting—differences in gene expression depending on whether the gene in question is inherited from the individual's mother or father

genomics—the study of the genome including gene sequencing, mapping, and function

hallux—big toe

hamartoma—an overgrowth of tissue normally present but in abnormal proportion and distribution; it is not malignant

haploid—the number of chromosomes present in the gamete; in humans this is 23, and can be symbolized as N

haploinsufficiency—the condition wherein one copy of a specific gene is not enough for normal development or function if one copy of that gene has been inactivated or deleted

haplotype—the set of alloantigens produced by the closely linked HLA complex genes located on chromosome 6

hemizygous—the condition in which only one

copy of a gene pair is present, and so its effect is expressed (e.g., the genes on the X chromosome of the male as there is no counterpart present)

heterogeneity—in genetic usage, the production of the same phenotype by different genetic mutations—in clinical usage, differences within the same disorder

heteromorphism—morphologic chromosome polymorphism or variant

heterozygous—state in which the two alleles of a gene pair are different (e.g., Aa as opposed to aa or AA)

HLA complex—the major histocompatibility region on chromosome 6

holandric—a trait controlled by genes on the Y chromosome; Y-linked inheritance

holoenzyme—a conjugated or complex enzyme consisting of an apoenzyme and cofactor

homologous chromosomes—chromosomes that are members of the same pair and normally have the same number and arrangement of genes

homozygous—state in which both alleles of a given gene pair are identical (e.g., AA or aa as opposed to Aa)

hydrocephalus—abnormal accumulation of fluid in cranium, usually in ventricles or subarachnoid space, leading to an enlarged head and pressure on the brain

hyperlipidemia—increased blood lipid levels

hyperlipoproteinemia—elevation of blood lipoproteins

hypertrichosis—excessive hair growth

inborn errors of metabolism—inherited biochemical disorders caused by single-gene mutations affecting enzymes involved in metabolic pathways

in vivo—in the living organism

in vitro—in the test tube or laboratory

introns—intervening gene sequences in messenger RNA that are "cut out" and are not translated into amino acids

inversion—a chromosome aberration in which a segment has become reversed due to breakage, 180° rotation, and reunion

ion channel—essentially a protein tunnel that crosses the cell membrane and changes conformation as it opens and closes in response to various signals. Ion channels exist for such ions as calcium, chloride, potassium, and sodium.

isochromosome—chromosome composed of either two long or two short arms due to abnormal separation during division

karyotype—the arrangement of chromosome pairs by number according to centromere position and length

Kayser-Fleischer ring—pigmented brownish gold ring resulting from copper deposition in the cornea and seen in Wilson disease

library—a collection of cloned DNA probes

linked genes—genes located on the same chromosome within 50 map units of each other; they do not assort independently, and the closer they are to each other the more frequently they are transmitted together

locus—the place on a chromosome where a gene resides

Lyon hypothesis—in the normal female (46,XX), one of the two X chromosomes is randomly inactivated and appears in somatic cells as sex chromatin

macroglossia—an unusually large tongue

macrosomia—growth excess of prenatal onset associated with several genetic disorders and seen in infants of diabetic mothers *malformation*—morphologic defect of an organ resulting from an intrinsically abnormal developmental process

meiosis—reduction division of diploid germ cells resulting in haploid gametes

meiotic drive—mechanism resulting in unequal, nonrandom, or preferential assortment of chromosomes into gametes during meiosis

meningocele—bulging of meninges without involvement of the spinal cord

metabolome—the complement of all metabolites in the genome

metacentric chromosome—one in which the centromere is in the center of the chromosome

methylation—attachment of a methyl group to cytosine in DNA

microcephaly—small head circumference, usually defined as below the third percentile for age, height, and weight; associated with mental retardation in most cases

micrognathia—undersized jaws, especially the mandible

microstomia—unusually small mouth

microtia—unusually small external ear

minute—a very small chromosome fragment

missense mutation—one in which the nucleotide alteration results in the placement of a different amino acid in the polypeptide chain than the one that was originally specified

mitosis—somatic cell division that normally results in no change from the usual diploid number of chromosomes

monosomy—missing one of a chromosome pair in normally diploid cells ($2N$-1 = 45); a person with Turner syndrome (45, X) has a chromosome number of 45 instead of 46 and is monosomic for the X chromosome

monozygotic—twins originating from one fertilized egg; identical twins

mosaic—presence in the same individual of two or more cell lines that differ in chromosome or gene number or structure but are derived from a single zygote

multifactorial—determined by the interaction of several genes with environmental factors

multiple alleles—the occurrence of more than two alternate forms of a gene that can occupy the same locus, although only one can be present on each chromosome at a time

multiplexing—using several pooled samples simultaneously in analysis

MURCS association—nonrandom association of Mullerian duct aplasia, renal aplasia, and cervicothoracic somite dysplasia

mutagen—any agent that causes mutation or increases the mutation rate above the usual background rate existing

mutation—a heritable alteration in the genetic material

myelomeningocele—spina bifida with cord and membranes protruding

nondisjunction—the failure of two homologous chromosomes or of sister chromatids to separate in meiosis appropriately during cell division, resulting in abnormal chromosome numbers in gametes or cells

nuchal translucency—a thickening of the fetal neck seen on ultrasound examinination in the first trimester. Called cystic hygroma, and nuchal fold when seen in the later trimesters

nucleotide—a nucleic acid "building block" comprised of a nitrogenous base, a five carbon sugar, and a phosphate group

oligonucleotide—a short segment of nucleotides

omphalocele—congenital abdominal wall defect, commonly known as umbilical hernia

p—in cytogenetics, refers to the short arms of a chromosome; in population genetics, it stands for the gene frequency of the dominant allele

PCR—polymerase chain reaction

penetrance—fraction of individuals known to carry the gene for a trait who manifest the condition; a trait with 90% penetrance will not be manifested by 10% of the persons possessing the gene

pedigree—essentially a diagrammatic representation of the family history

phenocopy—a phenotype that mimics one that is genetically determined but is actually due to non-genetic causes

philtrum—vertical groove between upper lip and nose

phocomelia—a type of limb defect in which proximal parts of extremities are missing so that a hand might be directly attached to the shoulder or attached by a single irregular bone

pleiotropy—the production of multiple phenotype effects by a single gene

polydactyly—presence of extra (supernumerary) digits

polygenic—a phenotypic trait whose expression is controlled by several genes at different loci, each having an additive effect

polymerase chain reaction—a technique to amplify a sequence of DNA and/or detect a specific DNA sequence in a sample

polymorphism—a genetic variation with two or more alleles that is maintained in a population so that the frequency of the most common one is not more than 0.99, and the frequency of one of the uncommon ones is maintained at at least 0.01

polypeptide—chain of amino acids formed during protein synthesis; may be a complete protein molecule or combined with other polypeptides to form one

polyploidy—a cell or individual having more than two haploid sets in an exact multiple; examples are triploidy, tetraploidy, etc.

proband—the index patient; the person who brings the family to the attention of the geneticist

probe—see DNA probe

promotor—DNA site where the enzyme, RNA polymerase, binds to initiate transcription

propositus—essentially the same as proband

proteome—the complete set of all proteins in the genome

q—in cytogenetics, refers to the long arms of a chromosome; in population genetics, it stands for the gene frequency of the recessive allele

recessive—when the effect of a gene is expressed phenotypically only when two copies are present, as in the homozygous recessive state (aa)

recombinant DNA—hybrid produced by combining DNA pieces from different sources

recombination—reassortment of genes to form new nonparental types

restriction enzymes—enzymes that recognize a specific base sequence in DNA and cut the DNA everywhere that the sequence occurs

restriction fragment length polymorphism—variation in a restriction enzyme recognition site in the fragments of DNA that have been cut by a restriction enzyme

RFLP—restriction fragment length polymorphism

sentinel phenotype—disorders followed to monitor populations for genetic damage as an early warning system; usually refers to sporadic disorders that follow an autosomal dominant mode of inheritance

sequence—a pattern of multiple anomalies derived from a single prior anomaly; order of nucleotide bases in DNA or RNA

sequencing—a method to determine the order of bases in DNA or RNA

sex chromatin—the inactive X chromosome

sex chromosome—the X or the Y chromosome

sex influenced—an autosomally inherited trait whose degree of phenotypic expression is controlled by the sex of the individual

sex limited—an autosomally inherited trait that is only manifested in one sex

shagreen patch—raised, thickened skin plaque commonly seen in tuberous sclerosis

short tandem repeats—see STR

sibs (siblings)—brothers and sisters from the same natural parents

sister chromatids—identical chromatids of the same duplicated chromosome before cell division

spina bifida—neural tube defect of the spinal column through which the cord or the membranes can protrude

sporadic—an isolated occurrence of a trait in a family

STRs—short tandem repeats. The STRs usually comprise pairs such as CG of 2 bases (although 3 to 5 pairs have been noted) that are repeated a few to many times.

structural gene—one that determines the amino acid sequence of the polypeptide chain

submetacentric chromosome—one in which the centromere is between the metacentric and acrocentric position

syndactyly—webbing or fusion of adjacent fingers or toes

syndrome—recognizable pattern of multiple anomalies, presumed to have the same etiology

syntenic—genes on the same chromosome that are more than 50 map units apart

tandem repeats—multiple copies of the same base sequence in a segment of DNA

teratogen—an agent acting on the embryo or fetus prenatally, altering morphology or subsequent function; causes teratogenesis

teratogenesis—exogenous induction of structural, functional, or developmental abnormalities caused by agents acting during embryonic or fetal development

tetraploid—cell or person with four copies of each chromosome, having a chromosome number of $4N = 96$

TORCH—abbreviation for the following organisms: *t*oxoplasmosis, *r*ubella, *c*ytomegalovirus, and *h*erpes simplex

transcription—the process by which complementary mRNA is synthesized from a DNA template

transcriptome—the complete set of RNA in the genome

translation—the process whereby the amino acids in a given polypeptide are synthesized from the mRNA template

translocation—transfer of all or part of a chromosome to another chromosome

transposable element—segment of DNA that can move from place to place in the genome; a jumping gene

triploid—cell or person with three copies of each chromosome, having a chromosome number of $3N = 69$

trisomy—the presence of one extra chromosome in an otherwise diploid chromosome complement ($2N + 1 = 47$); the most common autosomal trisomy is trisomy 21, or Down syndrome

uniparental disomy—both chromosomal homologues are inherited from the same parent instead of inheriting one copy of each chromosome pair from the mother and the father

VACTERL association—the nonrandom finding of *v*ertebral, *a*nal, *c*ardiac, *t*racheoesophageal, *r*enal, and *l*imb anomalies

variable number of tandem repeats—see VNTRs

VATER association—a nonrandom association of vertebral defects, anal atresia, tracheoesophageal fistula, and radial or renal anomalies

VNTRs—variable number of tandem repeats. Short sequences of base pairs in DNA (such as CAG) that are repeated in order a varying number of times

wild type—the form of a gene or characteristic usually found in nature and thus usually considered the "normal" one. It is usually the most common as well

X-linked—located on the X chromosome

xenobiotics—foreign drugs and chemicals not normally found in the body

Y-linked—located on the Y chromosome

zygote—the diploid ($2N$) cell formed by fusion of a haploid egg and a haploid sperm during fertilization that develops into the embryo

Appendices

The following appendices were up-to-date as of January 2005. When an organization that serves many rare disorders is listed, the reader is referred to the listing under the major disorders it serves. Some genetic disorders may feature a general impairment such as visual impairment as one feature. Therefore, help may be found for some clients in more than one category listed below. For most clients, listings under advocacy, disabilities, self-help aids, genetic disorders (general), should also be consulted. State agencies such as public health, maternal–child health, division of crippled children's services and genetic disease sections and the appropriate institute at the National Institutes of Health should be considered as resources. Some organizations listed below serve individuals with disorders that have a genetic component, but which are not wholly genetic, so listing disorders below does not imply etiology. This list does not constitute an endorsement of any organization. These lists are not intended to be exhaustive. The author welcomes any additions or corrections to this list.

Appendix A

Useful Genetic Web Sites for Professional Information

American Board of Genetic Counseling
http://www.abgc.net

American Board of Medical Genetics
http://www.faseb.org/genetics/abmg/abmgmenu.htm

American College of Medical Genetics
http://www.acmg.net

American Society of Human Genetics
http://www.faseb.org/genetics/ashg/ashgmenu.htm

Association of Professors of Human and Medical Genetics
http://www.faseb.org/genetics/aphmg/aphmg1.htm

Biosis
http://www.biosis.org

Center for Disease Control and Prevention Office of Genomics and Disease Prevention
http://www.cdc.gov/genomics/

Genetic Alliance
http://www.geneticalliance.org

The Genetics Education Center at the University of Kansas Medical Center
http://www.kumc.edu/gec

Genetics Education Partnership
http://genetics-education-partnership.mbt.washington.edu

Genetic Science Learning Center
http://gslc.genetics.utah.edu

HumGen
http://www.humgen.umontreal.ca/en/

International Society of Nurses in Genetics
http://www.isong.org

National Coalition for Health Professional Education in Genetics
http://www.nchpeg.org

National Human Genome Research Institute, National Institutes of Health
http://www.nhgri.nih.gov/

National Organization of Rare Disorders (NORD)
http://www.rarediseases.org

National Society of Genetic Counselors
http://www.nsgc.org

Online Mendelian Inheritance in Man (OMIM) National Center for Biotechnology Information
http://www.ncbi.nlm.nih.gov/omim

Appendix B

Organizations and Groups with Web Sites that Provide Information, Products, and Services for Genetic Conditions

GROUPS PROVIDING A LARGE AMOUNT OF GENETIC SUPPORT GROUP INFORMATION

Canadian Directory of Genetic Support Groups
http://www.lhsc.on.ca/programs/medgenet/

Canadian Organization for Rare Disorders
http://www.cord.ca

Center for Jewish Genetic Diseases
Mt. Sinai School of Medicine
http://www.mssm.edu/jewish_genetic

Directory of Online Genetic Support Groups
http://www.mostgene.org/support/index.html

Easter Seal Society National Headquarters
http://www.easter-seals.org

European Organisation for Rare Diseases
http://www.euroordis.org

Family Village
http://www.familyvillage.wisc.edu/index.html

Genetic Alliance
http://www.geneticalliance.org

The Genetics Education Center at the University of Kansas Medical Center
http://www.kumc.cdu/gec

Heredity Disease Foundation
http://www.hdfoundation.org

March of Dimes Birth Defects Foundation
http://www.modimes.org

Maternal and Child Health Bureau
Health Resources and Services Administration
http://mchb.hrsa.gov

National Center on Birth Defects and Developmental Disabilities
Centers for Disease Control and Prevention
http://www.cdc.gov/ncbddd

National Coalition of Health Professionals in Genetics (NCHPEG)
http://www.nchpeg.org

National Organization for Rare Disorders, Inc.
http://www.rarediseases.org

Office of Rare Diseases
National Institutes of Health
http://rarediseases.info.nih.gov/

GROUPS PROVIDING SUPPORT INFORMATION ON SPECIFIC GENETIC DISORDERS

Aarskog Syndrome
Aarskog Syndrome Parent Support Group
http://www.familyvillage.wisc.edu/lib_aars.htm

Achondroplasia—See Short Stature

Acid Maltase Deficiency—See Muscular Dystrophy, Glycogen Storage Diseases, Liver Diseases

Acoustic Neuroma—Also see Neurofibromatosis
Acoustic Neuroma Association
http://anausa.org

Adrenal Disorders—Also see Ambiguous Genitalia, Growth Problems
    National Adrenal Diseases Foundation *
    http://www.medhelp.org/www/nadf
    * Includes Addison disease, congenital adrenal hyperplasia, Cushing syndrome, and adrenal hyperplasia.

Adrenoleukodystrophy and Adrenomyeloneuropathy
    United Leukodystrophy Foundation, Inc.
    http://www.ulf.org

Agammaglobulinemia—See Immune Deficiency Diseases

Alagille Syndrome—Also see liver disease
    Alagille Syndrome Alliance
    http://www.alagille.org

Albinism
    National Organization for Albinism and
        Hypopigmentation
    http://www.albinism.org/

Alcohol and Drug Abuse Including Fetal Alcohol Syndrome
    Al-Anon/Alateen
    http://www.al-anon.alateen.org

    Alcoholics Anonymous
    http://www.aa.org
    National Organization on Fetal Alcohol
        Syndrome
    http://www.nofas.org

    SAMHSA's National Clearinghouse for Alcohol
        and Drug Information
    http://ncadi.samhsa.gov

Alpha-1-Antitrypsin Deficiency—Also see Liver Diseases
    Alpha-1 Association
    http://www.alpha1.org/

Alzheimer Disease
    Administration on Aging
    Department of Health and Human Services
    http://www.aoa.gov

    Alzheimer's Association, Inc.
    http://www.alz.org/

    Alzheimer's Disease Education and Referral Center
    http://www.alzheimers.org

National Institute on Aging
National Institutes of Health
http://www.nia.nih.gov

Ambiguous Genitalia
    Ambiguous Genitalia Support Network
    http://www.geneticalliance.org/Resources

    Intersex Society of North America) *
    http://www.isna.org
    * Includes ambiguous genitalia, hermaphroditism, congenital adrenal hyperplasia, Klinefelter syndrome, and hypospadias.

Amputees—Also see Disabilities
    Amputee Coalition of America
    http://www.amputee-coalition.org

    Amputee Information Network
    http://amp-info.net

    National Amputee Foundation, Inc.
    http://www.nationalamputation.org

Amyotrophic Lateral Sclerosis—Also see Muscular Dystrophy
    ALS Association
    http://www.alsa.org

    Les Turner Amyotrophic Lateral Sclerosis
        Foundation, Ltd.
    http://wwwlesturnerals.org

Anderson Disease—See Glycogen Storage Disease

Angelman Syndrome
    Angelman Syndrome Foundation, Inc.
    http://www.angelman.org

Angioedema—See Hereditary Angioedema, Immune Disorders

Ankylosing Spondylitis—Also see Arthritis
    Spondylitis Association of America *
    http://www.spondylitis.org
    * Includes ankylosing spondylitis, Reiter's syndrome, psoriatic arthritis, and arthritis associated with inflammatory bowel disease.

Anophthalmia
    International Children's Anophthalmia Network
    http://www.ioi.com/ican

Apert Syndrome—Also see Craniofacial Anomalies
    Aperts Syndrome Pen Pals
    http://www.familyvillage.wisc.edu/lib_aprt.htm

Argininosuccinic Aciduria—See Organic Acidemias

Arnold-Chiari—Also see Hydrocephalus
American Syringomyelia Alliance Project Inc. *
http://www.asap4sm.com
* Includes syringomyelia and Chiari I and II.

World Arnold-Chiari Malformation
Association
http://www.pressenter.com/~wacma/

Arrhythmias—Also see Heart Defects/Disease,
Cardiac Arrhythmias Reseach and Education
Foundation
QTsyndrome.ch Group
http://www.qtsyndrome.ch

Sudden Arrhythmia Death Syndromes Foundation
http://www.sads.org

Arthritis
American Juvenile Arthritis Organization
http://www.arthritis.org/communities/juve-
nile_arthritis/about_ajao.asp

Arthritis Foundation
http://www.arthritis.org

The Arthritis Society (Canada)
http://www.arthritis.ca/

National Institute of Arthritis and
Musculoskeletal and Skin Diseases
National Institutes of Health
http://www.niams.nih.gov

Arthrogryposis Multiplex Congenita—Also see
Muscular Dystrophy
AVENUES, National Support Group for
Arthrogryposis Multiplex Congenita
http://www.sonnet.com/avenues

Ataxia—Also see Friedreich Ataxia, Muscular
Dystrophy
National Ataxia Foundation *
http://www.ataxia.org
* Includes ataxia telangiectasia, Charcot-Marie-
Tooth disease, hereditary tremor, hereditary
spastic paraplegia.

Ataxia Telangiectasia (Louis Bar Disease)—Also
see Ataxia, Tay Sachs disease
A-T Children's Project
http://www.med.jhu.edu/ataxia/

Autism
Autism Network International
http://ani.autistics.org

Autism Society of America
http://www.autism-society.org/

Cure Autism Now (CAN)
http://www.canfoundation.org/

Barth Syndrome
Barth Syndrome Foundation
http://www.barthsyndrome.org

Batten Disease (Batten Vogt Syndrome)—Also see
Tay-Sachs Disease
Batten's Disease Support and Research Association
http://www.bdsra.org

Beta-Glucuronidase Deficiency—See
Mucopolysaccharidoses, Tay-Sachs Disease

Biedl-Bardet syndrome—See Laurence Moon
Syndrome

Bilary Atresia—See Liver Disease

Biotinidase Deficiency—See Metabolic Disorders

Birth Defects, General—Also see Disabilities,
Genetic Diseases
Birth Defect Research for Children
http://www.birthdefects.org

Center for Jewish Genetic Diseases, Inc.
http://www.mssm.edu/jewish_genetics

Easter Seals
http://www.easter-seals.org

March of Dimes Birth Defects Foundation
http://www.modimes.org

National Center for Birth Defects and
Developmental Disabilities
Centers for Disease Control and Prevention
http://www.cdc.gov/ncbddd

Blindness—See Visual Impairment

Bloom Syndrome
Center for Jewish Genetic Diseases, Inc.
http://www.mssm.edu/jewish_genetics

Bone Diseases—Also see Osteogenesis Imperfecta,
Paget Disease, Osteoporosis
Osteoporosis and Related Bone Diseases—
National Resource Center

National Institutes of Health
http://www.osteo.org/

Breast Cancer—Also see Cancer
National Breast Cancer Coalition
http://www.natlbcc.org

Susan G. Komen Breast Cancer Foundation
http://www.komen.org

Breast-Feeding
La Leche League International
http://www.lalecheleague.org

Burke Syndrome—See Shwachman Syndrome

Byler Disease—See Liver Disease

Canavan disease—See Tay-Sachs Disease

Cancer—also see specific type
American Cancer Society, Inc.
http://www.cancer.org

Candlelighters Childhood Cancer Foundation
http://www.candlelighters.org

Kidscope
http://www.kidscope.org

National Cancer Institute, National Institutes
   of Health
http://www.nci.nih.gov

National Childhood Cancer Foundation
http://www.nccf.org/

Starlight Children's Foundation
http://www.starlight.org

Cardiac Arrhythmias/Disease—See Heart
Defects/Disease

Carnitine Deficiency—Also see Muscular
Dystrophy
FOD Communication Network
http://www.fodsupport.org

Cartilage Hair Hypoplasia—See Short Stature

Celiac Disease—See Gluten Intolerance

Central Core Disease—See Muscular Dystrophy
Cerebral Palsy
Easter Seals
http://www.easter-seals.org

UCP United Cerebral Palsy
http://www.ucp.org/

Charcot-Marie-Tooth Disease—Also see
Muscular Dystrophy, Ataxia
Charcot-Marie-Tooth Association
http://www.charcot-marie-tooth.org

CHARGE Syndrome
CHARGE Family Support Group (UK)
http://www.widerworld.co.uk/charge/index.htm

CHARGE Syndrome Foundation
http://www.chargesyndrome.org

Chromosome Abnormalities—Also see specific
disorder (e.g., Down, Klinefelter, Turner,
Cri-du-Chat, etc.), Genetic Diseases, Mental
Retardation, Disabilities (General).
11q Net (UK)
http://web.ukonline.co.uk/c.jones/11q/con-
   tents.htm

4p-Support Group
http://www.4p-supportgroup.org

The CHARGE Family Support Group
http://www.widerworld.co.uk/charge/index.htm

Chromosome 22 Central
http://www.nt.net/~a815/chr22.htm

Chromosome Deletion Outreach, Inc. *
http://www.chromodisorder.org
* Includes chromosome deletions, chromosome
   duplications, translocations, and inversions.

Chromosome 18 Registry & Research
   Society
http://www/chromosome18.org

Chromosome and Genetic Links
http://www.trisomyonline.org/chromlinks.htm

Cri-du-Chat Syndrome Support Group
http://www.personal.u-net.com/~cridchat

IDEAS: IsoDicentric 15 Exchange Advocacy
   & Support
http://www.idic15.org
* Includes inverted duplication of chromosome
   15, supernumerary marker chromosomes,
   duplication of chromosome 15, and
   chromosomal anomalies.

Parents and Researchers Interested in
   Smith-Magenis Syndrome *
http://www.prisms.org
* Also includes deletion 17p11.2

SOFT (UK)
http://www.soft.org.uk

Support Organization for Trisomy (SOFT) 18,
    13 and Related Disorders
http://www.trisomy.org

Trisomy 9 International Parent Support
http://www.multilim.com.au/~softwa/9tips.htm

Unique, Rare Chromosome Disorder Support
    Group
http://www.rarechromo.org

Wolf Hirschhorn Support Group UK
http://www.whs.webk.co.uk

Cleft Lip/Palate—Also see Craniofacial
Anomalies

Children's Craniofacial Association
http://www.ccakids.com

Cleft Palate Foundation
http://www.cleftline.org

Prescription Parents, Inc.
http://www.samizdat.com/pp1.html

Smiles
http://www.cleft.org

Wide Smiles
http://www.widesmiles.org/

Cockayne Syndrome
Share and Care Cockayne Syndrome Network
http://www.cockayne-syndrome.org

Coffin-Lowry Syndrome
Coffin-Lowry Syndrome Foundation
http://www.clsf.info

Colorectal cancer—Also see Cancer
Familial Gastrointestinal Registry (Canada)
http://www.mtsinai.on.cafamilialgicancer/

Communicative Disorders—Also see Hearing
Impairment
National Center for Stuttering
http://www.stuttering.com

Sensory Access Foundation
http://www.sensoryaccess.com

Sertoma International
http://sertoma.org/

Trace Center (communication devices and
    research)
University of Wisconsin
http://www.tracecenter.org/

Congenital Adrenal Hyperplasia—See Adrenal
Disorders, Ambiguous Genitalia, Growth
Disorders

Congenital Heart Disease—See Heart Disease

Conjoined Twins
Conjoined Twins International
http://www.conjoinedtwinsint.com

Cooley Anemia—See Thalassemia

Cornelia De Lange Syndrome
Cornelia de Lange Syndrome Foundation, Inc.
http://www.cdlsusa.org

Craniofacial Anomalies—Also see Cleft Lip/Palate
About Face, U.S.A.*
http://www.aboutfaceusa.org
* Includes facial anomalies, cleft lip/palate,
    Crouzon syndrome, Apert syndrome,
    Treacher-Collins syndrome, hemangioma,
    and cystic hygroma.

Children's Craniofacial Association
http://www.ccakids.com

Craniofacial Foundation of America
http://www.erlanger.org/craniofacial/found1.html

Let's Face It, Inc.
http://www.faceit.org

The National Craniofacial Association
http://www.faces-cranio.org

National Foundation for Facial Reconstruction
http://www.nffr.org

Cri-du-Chat—Also see Chromosome
Disorders
The 5p- Society (Cri-du-Chat Syndrome)
http://www.fivepminus.org

Crohn Disease—Also see Inflammatory Bowel
Disease, Gastrointestinal Disease
Crohn's and Colitis Foundation of America
http://www.ccfc.org

Crohn's and Colitis Foundation of Canada
http://www.ccfc.ca

National Institute of Diabetes, Digestive and
Kidney Diseases
National Institutes of Health
http://www.niddk.nih.gov

Cutis Laxa—See Ehlers-Danlos

Cystic Fibrosis
Cystic Fibrosis Foundation
http://www.cff.org

Cystic Fibrosis Trust
England, United Kingdom
http://www.cftrust.org.uk

National Institute of Diabetes and Digestive and
Kidney Diseases
National Institutes of Health
http://www.niddk.nih.gov

Dandy-Walker Syndrome
Dandy-Walker Syndrome Network
http://www.familyvillage.wisc.edu/lib_dandy.htm

Darier Disease—See Ichthyosis, Skin Disease

de Lange syndrome—See Cornelia de Lange
Syndrome

Deaf-Blind—Also see Hearing Impairment, Usher
Syndrome, Visual Impairment
American Association of the Deaf-Blind
http://www.aadb.org

The National Information Clearinghouse on
Children who are Deaf-Blind (DB-LINK)
http://www.tr.wou.edu.dblink/

Deaf—See Hearing Impairment

Death, Neonatal and Infant—Also see Sudden
Infant Death Syndrome
A.M.E.N.D. (Aiding a Mother and Father
Experiencing Neonatal Death)
http://www.amendinc.com

Born Angels Pregnancy Loss Support
http://www.bornangels.com

Center for Loss in Multiple Birth (CLIMB, Inc.)
http://www.climb-support.org

Compassionate Friends (TCF)
http://www.compassionatefriends.org

A Heartbreaking Choice
http://www.aheartbreakingchoice.com

SHARE
Pregnancy and Infant Loss Support, Inc.
http://www.nationalshareoffice.com

Stork Net
http://www.storknet.com/cubbies/pil/

Dental Care
National Foundation of Dentistry for the
Handicapped
http://www.nfdh.org

Depression
Depression and Bipolar Support Alliance

Depression and Related Affective Disorders
Association
http://www.drada.org

http://www.ndmda.org

National Institute of Mental Health
National Institutes of Health
http://www.nimh.nih.gov

Diabetes Mellitus
American Diabetes Association
http://www.diabetes.org

Canadian Diabetes Association
http://www.diabetes.ca/

Juvenile Diabetes Research Foundation
International
http://www.jdfcure.org

National Institute of Diabetes and Digestive and
Kidney Diseases
National Institutes of Health
http://www.niddk.nih.gov

Diethylstilbesterol (DES)
DES Action, USA
http://www.desaction.org

National Women's Health Network
http://www.womenshealthnetwork.org

National Women's Health Resource Center
http://www.4woman.gov

Di George Syndrome—Also see Immune
Deficiency Diseases, Chromosome
Abnormalities
VCFS Educational Foundation *
http://www.vcf

* Includes DiGeorge syndrome, Shprintzen syndrome, velocardiofacial syndrome, and 22q11.2 deletions.

Disabilities, General—Also see Mental Retardation

ADA & IT Technical Assistance Centers
http://www.adata.org

Administration on Developmental Disabilities
http://www.acf.dhhs.gov/programs/add

Association of University Centers on Disabilities
http://www.aucd.org

Council for Exceptional Children
http://www.cec.sped.org

Disability Connections
http://www.disabilityconnections.org

DisabilityInfo.gov
http://www.disabilityinfo.gov

Disability Rights Center
http://www.drcme.org

Exceptional Parent Magazine
http://www.eparent.com

Family Resource Center on Disabilities
http://www.frcd.org

Friends Health Connection
http://www.friendshealthconnection.org

Information Center for Individuals with Disabilities
http://www.disability.net

Maternal and Child Health Bureau
Health Resources and Services Administration
http://mchb.hrsa.gov

Medic Alert Foundation International
http://www.medicalert.org

Mobility International USA
http://www.miusa.org

National Association of the Physically Handicapped, Inc.
http://www.naph.net

National Center for Education in Maternal and Child Health
http://www.ncemch.org

National Dissemination Center for Children with Disabilities
http://www.nichcy.org

National Clearinghouse on Disability and Exchange
http://www.miusa.org/ncde/

National Council on Independent Living
http://www.ncil.org

National Easter Seal Society
http://www.easter-seals.org

National Organization on Disability
http://www.nod.org

National Parent to Parent Support and Information System, Inc.
http://www.nppsis.org

Parents Helping Parents*
http://www.php.com
* General disabilities, children with special needs, tuberous sclerosis.

Social Security Administration
Office of Communications
http://www.ssa.gov

Down Syndrome—Also see Chromosome Abnormalities

Association for Children with Down Syndrome
http://www.acds.org

Canadian Down Syndrome Society
http://www.cdss.ca

Caring, Inc.
http://www.caringinc.org

Down Syndrome Research Foundation (Canada)
http://www.dsrf.org

Down's Syndrome Association (UK)
http://www.downs-syndrome.org.uk
National Down Syndrome Congress
http://www.ndsccenter.org

National Down Syndrome Society
http://www.ndss.org

Dubowitz Syndrome

Dubowitz Syndrome Parent Support Network
http://www.dubowitz.org

Dwarfism—See Short Stature

Dysautonomia (Riley-Day Syndrome)
Center for Jewish Genetic Diseases
http://www.mssm.edu/jewish_genetics/

Dysautonomia Foundation, Inc.
http://www.familialdysautonomia.org

Dysautonomia Treatment and Evaluation Center
http://www.med.nyu.edu

Dyslexia—See Learning Disabilities

Dystonia (Torsion Dystonia)—Also see Jewish
Genetic Diseases
Center for Jewish Genetic Diseases
http://www.mssm.edu/jewish_genetics/

Dystonia Medical Research Foundation
http:/www.dystonia-foundation.org

Ectodermal Dysplasia
Ectodermal Dysplasia Society
http://www.ectodermaldysplasia.org

National Foundation for Ectodermal Dysplasias
http://www.ednf.org

Edwards Syndrome—See Trisomy 18/13, and
Chromosome Abnormalities

Ehlers-Danlos Syndrome
Ehlers-Danlos National Foundation
http://www.ednf.org

Environmental Mutagens
Centers for Disease Control and Prevention
(CDC)
http://www.cdc.gov

Clinical Teratology Web
Teratogen Information System (TERIS)
http://depts.washington.edu/~terisweb/

The Environmental Health Clearinghouse
National Institute of Environmental Health
Sciences
http://infoventures.com/e-hlth

National Library of Medicine
http://www.nlm.nih.gov/

Epidermolysis Bullosa
(Dystrophic) Epidermolysis Bullosa Research
Association of America
http://www.debra.org

Epilepsy
Epilepsy Canada
http://www.epilepsy.ca

Epilepsy Foundation
http://www.epilepsy foundation.org

Epilepsy Information Service
http://www.wfubmc.edu/neuro/epilepsy/infor-
mation.htm

Fabry Disease—See Tay-Sachs Disease

Fanconi Anemia
Fanconi Anemia Research Fund, Inc.
http://www.fanconi.org

Farber syndrome—See Tay-Sachs disease

Fetal Alcohol Syndrome—See Alcohol Abuse

Fibrodysplasia
International Fibrodysplasia Ossificans Progressiva
www.ifopa.org

Fragile X Syndrome— Also see Chromosome
Abnormalities
FRAXA Research Foundation, Inc.
http://www.fraxa.org

National Fragile X Foundation
http://www.nfxf.org/

Freeman-Sheldon Syndrome
Freeman-Sheldon Parent Support Group *
http://www.spsg.org
* Includes Whistling Face Syndrome and
craniocarpotarsal dysplasia.

Friedreich Ataxia—See Ataxia, Muscular Dystrophy

Fucosidosis—See Tay-Sachs Disease

Galactosemia—Also see Liver Disease
Parents of Galactosemic Children
http://www.galactosemia.org

Gardner syndrome—See Colorectal Cancer,
Polyposis

Gaucher Disease—Also see Tay-Sachs Disease,
Jewish Genetic Diseases
Center for Jewish Genetic Diseases
http://www.mssm.edu/jewish_genetics/

National Gaucher Foundation
http://www.gaucherdisease.org

Genetic Disorders, General—Also see Disabilities, Birth Defects

Canadian Organization for Rare Disorders
http://www.cord.ca

Center for Jewish Genetic Diseases
http://www.mssm.edu/jewish_genetics/

Genetic Alliance
http://www.geneticalliance.org

Heredity Disease Foundation
http://www.hdfoundation.org

Maternal and Child Health Bureau
Health Resources and Services Administration
http://mchb.hrsa.gov

Med Help International
http://www.medhelp.org

MUMS National Parent-to-Parent Network
http://www.netnet.net/mums/

National Health Information Center
Department of Health and Human Services
http://www.health.gov/nhic

National Organization for Rare Disorders, Inc.
http://www.rarediseases.org

Office of Rare Diseases
National Institutes of Health
http://rarediseases.info.nih.gov/

Gluten Intolerance

Celiac Sprue Association USA, Inc. (CSA/USA)
http://www.csacceliacs.org

Gluten Intolerance Group of North America
(GIG)
http://www.gluten.net

National Digestive Diseases Information
Clearinghouse
http://digestive.niddk.nih.gov

Glycogen Storage Disorders—See Liver Diseases
The Association for Glycogen Storage Disease *
http://www.agsdus.org
* Glycogen storage disease, acid maltase deficiency, Anderson disease, amlopectinosis.

Goldenhar Syndrome

Goldenhar Syndrome Support Network
http://www.goldenhar syndrome.org

Granulomatous Disease—Also see Immune Dysfunction

Chronic Granulomatous Disease Association
http://home.socal.rr.com/cgda

Growth Problems—Also see Short Stature, Tall Stature, specific disorder

Human Growth Foundation (HGF)
http://www.hgfound.org

MAGIC Foundation *
http://www.magicfoundation.org
* Includes growth disorders, growth hormone deficiency, McCune Albright syndrome, congenital adrenal hyperplasia, precocious puberty, growth retardation in Down syndrome.

Handicapped—See Disabilities

Hearing Impairment

Alexander Graham Bell Association for the Deaf
http://www.agbell.org

American Society for Deaf Children
http://www.deafchildren.org

Better Hearing Institute
http://www.betterhearing.org

Canadian Hearing Society
http://www.chs.ca/

Deafness Research Foundation
http://www.drf.org

International Hearing Society
http://www.ihsinfo.org

Laurent Clerc Deaf Education Center
http://clerccenter.gallaudet.edu/InfoToGo

National Association for the Deaf
http://www.nad.org

National Institute on Deafness and Other Communication Disorders Information
National Institutes of Health
http://www.nidcd.nih.gov/health

Self Help for Hard of Hearing People, Inc.
http://www.shhh.org

Heart Defects/Diseases

American Heart Association, Inc.
http://www.americanheart.org/

Cardiac Arrhythmias Research and Education
Foundation
http://www.longqt.org

Congenital Heart Anomalies-Support,
Education, and Resources (CHASER, Inc.)
http://www.csun.edu/~hcmth011

Congenital Heart Information Network
http://www.tchin.org

National Heart, Lung, and Blood Institute
National Institutes of Health
http://www.nhlbi.nih.gov

QTsyndrome.ch Group
http://www.qtsyndrome.ch.

Sudden Arrhythmia Death Syndrome Foundation
http://www.sads.org

Hemangiomas—See Vascular Birthmarks

Hemochromatosis—Also see Iron Overload
Canadian Hemochromatosis Society
http://www.cdnhemochromatosis.ca

Hemochromatosis Foundation, Inc.
http://www.hemochromatosis.org

Iron Overload Diseases Association
http://www.ironoverload.org

Hemophilia
National Hemophilia Foundation *
http://www.hemophilia.org/
* Includes von Willebrand disease, and other
clotting disorders.

World Federation of Hemophilia
http://www.wfh.org/
Hereditary Angioedema—Also see Immune
Disorders
U.S. Hereditary Angioedema Association
http://www.hereditaryangioedema.com

Hereditary Exostoses, Multiple
Multiple Hereditary Exostoses Family Support
Group
http://www.radix.net/~hogue/mhe.htm

Hereditary Hemorrhagic Telangiectasia
Hereditary Hemorrhagic Telangiectasia
Foundation International, Inc. *
http://www.hht.org
* Also includes Osler-Weber-Rendu syndrome.

Hermansky-Pudlak Syndrome—See Albinism

Hirschsprung Disease
International Foundation for Functional
Gastrointestinal Disorders
http://www.aboutkidsgi.org

National Institute of Diabetes, Digestive and
Kidney Diseases
National Institutes of Health
http://www.niddk.nih.gov

Homocystinuria—See Metabolic Disorders

Hunter Disease—See Mucopolysachharide
Disorders, Tay-Sachs Disease

Huntington Disease
Heredity Disease Foundation
http://www.hdfoundation.org

Huntington's Disease Society of America
http://www.hdsa.org

Huntington Society of Canada
http://www.hsc-ca.org

Hurler Disease—See Mucopolysaccharidoses,
Tay-Sachs Disease

Hydrocephalus—Also see Arnold-Chiari
Association for Spina Bifida and Hydrocephalus
http://www.asbah.org

Hydrocephalus Association
http://www.hydroassoc.org

National Hydrocephalus Foundation
http://www.nhfonline.org

Hypercholesterolemia—Also see Heart Disease
Inherited High Cholesterol Foundation
http://cholesterol.med.utah.edu/medped

I-cell Disease—See Mucolipidoses

Ichthyosis—Also see Skin Disease
Foundation for Ichthyosis and Related Skin Types *
http://www.scalyskin.org
* Includes skin disorders, ichthyosis, Darier
disease, Rud syndrome, Sjogren-Larsson
syndrome, erythrokeratodermas, peeling skin
syndrome, acquired ichthyosis, bullous
ichthyosis (epidermolytic hyperkeratosis),
Chanarin-Dorfman syndrome, child
syndrome (unilateral CIE), epiderma nevus

syndrome, progressiva symmetrica, Harlequin fetus, ichthyosis linearis circumflexa, ichthyosis vulgaris, keratitis-ichthyosis deafness (KID) syndrome, lammellar ichthyosis/congenital ichthyosiform erythroderma.

National Registry for Ichthyosis and Related Disorders
http://depts.washington.edu/ichreg/ichthyosis.registry

Immune Disorders
The Immune Deficiency Foundation
http://www.primaryimmune.org

National Jewish Center for Immunology and Respiratory Medicine
http://www.njc.org

U.S. Hereditary Angioedema Association
http://www.hereditaryangioedema.com

Incest
Clearinghouse on Child Abuse and Neglect Information
http://nccanch.acf.hhs.gov

Survivors of Incest Anonymous
http://www.siawso.org

Incontinentia Pigmenti
Incontinentia Pigmenti International Foundation
http://imgen.bcm.tmc.edu/IPIF

Infertility
Resolve, The National Infertility Association
http://www.resolve.org/

International Council on Infertility Information Dissemination
http://www.inciid.org

Inflammatory Bowel Disease—Also see Crohn's Disease
National Digestive Diseases Education Information Clearinghouse
National Institutes of Health
http://www.niddk.nih.gov

Iron Overload Diseases—Also see Hemochromatosis, Thalassemia
Iron Overload Diseases Association, Inc.
http://www.ironoverload.org

Isovaleric Acidemia—See Organic Acidemias

Joseph Disease
International Joseph Diseases Foundation, Inc.
http://69.10.163.110/bastiana

Joubert Syndrome
Joubert Syndrome Foundation
http://www.joubertfoundation.com

Kearn-Sayre—See Mitochondrial Diseases

Kidney Diseases
American Association of Kidney Patients
http://www.aakp.org/

National Institute of Diabetes and Digestive and Kidney Diseases
National Institutes of Health
http://www.niddk.nih.gov/

National Kidney Foundation
http://www.kidney.org/

Klinefelter Syndrome—Also see Chromosome Abnormalities
Klinefelter Syndrome and Associates, Inc.
http://www.genetic.org/ks

Klinefelter Syndrome Support Group
http://klinefeltersyndrome.org

Klippel-Trenaunay Syndrome
Klippel-Trenaunay Support Group
http://www.k-t.org

Krabbe Disease—See Tay-Sachs Disease

Kugelberg-Welander Disease—See Muscular Dystrophy

Lactic Acidosis
Congenital Lactic Acidosis Support Group
http://www.Kumc.edu/gec/support/lactic_a.html

Laurence Moon Syndrome—Also see Retinitis Pigmentosa, Vision Problems
Foundation Fighting Blindness
http://www.blindness.org/laurence-moon-bardet-biedel-syndrome.asp

Laurence Moon Bardet Biedl Syndrome Network
http://mlmorris.com/lmbbs

Learning Disabilities
Council for Learning Disabilities
http://www.cldinternational.org

Learning Disabilities Association of America
http://www.Ldanatl.org

Learning Disabilities Association of Canada
http://www.ldac-taac.ca

National Attention Deficit Disorder Association
http://www.add.org

NLDline (nonverbal learning disorders)
http://www.nldline.com

The Orton Dyslexia Society
http://www.selu.edu/Academics/Education/
   TEC/orton.htm

Recording for the Blind and Dyslexic
http://www.rfbd.org

Leigh Disease—Also see Mitochondrial Disorders
National Leigh's Disease Foundation
http://www.kumc.edu/gec/support/leigh_di.html

Leukemia—Also see Cancer
Leukemia & Lymphoma Society of America, Inc.
http://www.leukemia.org/

National Children's Leukemia Foundation
http://www.leukemiafoundation.org

Leukodystrophy—See Adrenoleukodystrophy

Lissencephaly
Lissencephaly Network, Inc.
http://www.lissencephaly.org

Liver Diseases
American Liver Foundation
http://www.liverfoundation.org

Biliary Atresia and Liver Transplant Network *
http://www.transweb.org/people/recips/resource
   s/support/oldbilitree.html
* Also includes Alagille syndrome, alpha-1-
   anti-trypsin, Byler's disease, galactosemia,
   glycogen storage diseases, tyrosinemia,
   Wilson disease, and acid maltase
   deficiency.

Long QT Syndrome
Cardiac Arrhythmias Research and Education
   Foundation
http://www.longqt.org

QTsyndrome.ch Group
http://www.qtsyndrome.ch

Sudden Arrhythmia Death Syndromes Foundation
http://www.sads.org

Lowe Syndrome (Oculocerebrorenal Disease)
Lowe Syndrome Association
http://www.lowesyndrome.org

Lupus Erythematosus—Also see Arthritis
Lupus Foundation of America, Inc.
http://www.lupus.org

Lymphangioleiomyomatosis
LAM Foundation
http://lam.uc.edu

Lymphoma—Also see Cancer
The Leukemia & Lymphoma Society of
   America, Inc.
http://www.leukemia.org/

Lymphedema
National Lymphedema Network
http://www.lymphnet.org

Machado-Joseph Disease—See Joseph Disease

Macular Diseases—Also see Visual Impairment
Association for Macular Diseases
http://www.macula.org

Macular Degeneration International
http://www.maculardegeneration.org

Maffucci Disease—See Ollier disease

Malignant Hyperthermia—Also see Muscular
Dystrophy
Malignant Hyperthermia Association of the
   United States
http://www.mhaus.org

Mannosidosis—See Tay-Sachs Disease

Maple Syrup Urine Disease—Also see Metabolic
Diseases
Maple Syrup Urine Disease Family Support Group
http://www.msud-support.org

Marfan Syndrome—Also see Tall Stature
National Marfan Foundation
http://www.marfan.org

Canadian Marfan Association
http://www.marfan.ca

Marfan Association (United Kingdom)
http://www.marfan.org.uk

Maroteaux-Lamy Disease—See Tay-Sachs Disease, Mucopolysaccharide Disorders

McArdle Disease—See Muscular Dystrophy

McCune Albright Syndrome—See Growth Problems

Medium Chain Acyl-CoEnzyme A Dehydrogenase (MCAD) Deficiency—Also see Mitochondrial Disease
    Fatty Oxidation Disorders (FOD) Family Support Group
    http://www.fodsupport.org

    Save Babies Through Screening
    http://www.savebabies.org/

MELAS—See Mitochondrial Diseases

Menke Disease
    Corporation for Menke's Disease
    http://www.familyvillage.wisc.edu/lib_menk.htm

    National Institute of Neurological Disorders and Stroke
    National Institutes of Health
    http://www.ninds.nih.gov

Mental Retardation—Also see Disabilities, General; specific disorders
    American Association on Mental Retardation
    http://www.aamr.org/

    The Arc of the United States (formerly Association for Retarded Citizens of the United States)
    http://TheArc.org/

    President's Committee for People with Intellectual Disabilities
    http://www.acf.hhs.gov/programs/pcpid

Mental Retardation/Mental Illness
    National Organization of the Dually Diagnosed
    http://www.thenadd.org

MERFF—See Mitochondrial Disorders

Metabolic Disorders—Also see specific disorder
    The Association for Neuro-Metabolic Diseases *
    http://www.kumc.edu/gcc/support/metaboli.html
    * Includes biotinidase deficiency, methylenetetrahydrofolatereductase deficiency, phenylketonuria, maple syrup urine disease, propionic acidemia, galactosemia, and more.

Children Living With Inherited Metabolic Disease (United Kingdom)
http://www.climb.org.uk

Fatty Oxidation Disorders Family Support Group *
http://www.fodsupport.org
* Includes MCAD, LCHAD, LCAD, SCAD, GAII, CPT.

National Institute of Diabetes, Digestive & Kidney Diseases
National Institutes of Health
http://www.niddk.nih.gov

National Urea Cycle Disorders Foundation
http://www.nucdf.org

Organic Acidemia Asssociation, Inc.
http://www.oaanews.org

Oxalosis and Hyperoxaluria Foundation
http://www.ohf.org

Purine Research Society
http://www2.dgsys.com /~purine

Save Babies Through Screening
http://www.savebabies.org/

Metachromatic Leukodystrophy—See Tay-Sachs Disease

Methylenetetrahydrofolate Reductase Deficiency—See Metabolic Disorders

Methylmalonic Acidemia—See Organic Acidemias

Microphthalmia—See Anophthalmia

Miller Syndrome
    Foundation for Nager & Miller Syndromes *
    http://www.nagerormillersynd.com

Miscarriages—See Death, Neonatal and Infant

Mitochondrial Diseases
    The Children's Mitochondrial Disease Network *
    http://www.emdn.mitonet.co.uk
    * Includes Leigh disease, Kearns-Sayre syndrome, Pearson marrow-pancreas syndrome, MELAS (mitochondrial encephalomyopathy/lactic acidosis and strokelike episodes), MERRF (myoclonic epilepsy/ragged red fibers), NARP (neurogenic weakness, ataxia, retinitis pigmentosa).

United Mitochondrial Disease Foundation *
http://www.umdf.org
* Includes Alpers disease (progressive infantile poliodystrophy)

Moebius Syndrome
Moebius Syndrome Foundation
http://www.ciaccess.com/moebius/homepage.html

Morquio Disease—See Tay-Sachs Disease

Mucolipidoses—Also see Tay-Sachs Disease
ML4 Foundation
http://www.Ml4.org

National MPS Society, Inc. *
http://www.mpssociety.org
* Includes mucopolysaccharidosis, mucolipidosis, Hunter syndrome, Hurler syndrome, Maroteaux-Lamy syndrome, Sanfilippo syndrome, and Scheie syndrome.

Mucopolysaccharide Disorders—Also see Tay-Sachs Disease
National MPS Society, Inc.
http://www.mpssociety.org

Multiple Births
International Twins Association
http://www.intltwins.org

Mothers of Supertwins (MOST)
http://www.MOSTonline.org

Multiple Births Foundation (UK)
http://www.multiplebirths.org.uk

National Organization of Mothers of Twins Clubs, Inc.
http://www.ntmotc.org

Twins Clubs (UK)
http://www.twinsclubs.co.uk

The Twins Foundation
http://www.twinsfoundation.com

Twins and Multiple Births Association
http://www.tamba.org.uk

Multiple Sclerosis
International MS Support Foundation
http://www.imssf.org/ms/

Multiple Sclerosis Society of Canada
http://www.mssociety.ca

National Multiple Sclerosis Society
http://www.nmss.org/

Muscular Dystrophy
FacioScapuloHumeral Muscular Dystrophy Society, Inc. *
http://www.fshsociety.org
* Includes muscular dystrophy, facioscapulo- humeral muscular dystrophy, Landoozy- Dejerine facioscapulohumeral muscular dystrophy.

Families of Spinal Muscular Atrophy *
http://www.fsma.org
* Includes spinal muscular atrophy, Werd nig-Hoffman disease, Oppenheim's disease, Kugelberg-Welander disease, Aran-Duchenne type.

Muscular Dystrophy Association *
http://www.mdausa.org/
* Includes many muscle diseases such as Becker, Duchenne, congenital, facioscapulohumeral, limb-girdle   muscular dystrophy, myotonic dystrophy; amyotophic lateral sclerosis; Werd- nig-Hoffmann, Kugelberg-Welander, Char- cot-Marie-Tooth diseases; Friedreich ataxia; myasthenia gravis; McArdle, Pompe, Cori diseases; phosphofructokinase deficiency; carnitine palmityltransferase deficiency; malignant hyperthermia; arthrogryposis; miscellaneous myopathies.

Muscular Dystrophy Association of Canada
http://www.mdac.ca

Parent Project Muscular Dystrophy
http://www.parentprojectmd.org

Myasthenia Gravis—Also see Muscular Dystrophy
Myasthenia Gravis Foundation of America, Inc.
http://www.myasthenia.org

Myelin Disorders
Organization for Myelin Disorders Research and Support *
http://www.familyvillage.wisc.edu/lib.myel.htm
* Also includes hypomyelination, delayed myelination, dysmyelination, periventricular leukomylasia, macroencephaly, microencephaly.

Myoclonus
Myoclonus Research Foundation
http://www.myoclonus.com

Worldwide Education for Movement Disorders
http://www.wemove.org/myo

Myotonia Congenita—See Muscular Dystrophy

Myotubular Myopathy
Centronuclear and Myotubular Myopathy (UK)
http://tonilouise.tripod.com

Myotubular Myopathy Resource Group *
http://www.mtmrg.org
* Includes centronuclear myopathy.

Nager Syndrome
Foundation for Nager & Miller Syndromes*
http://www.nagerormillersynd.com

Nail-Patella Syndrome
Nail-Patella Syndrome Worldwide
http://www.nailpatella.org

Narcolepsy
Narcolepsy Network, Inc.
http://www.narcolepsynetwork.org

Narcolepsy & Sleep Disorders: An International
Newsletter
http://www.narcolepsy.com

National Institute of Neurological Disorders and
Stroke
National Institutes of Health
http://www.ninds.nih.gov

National Sleep Foundation
http://www.sleepfoundation.org

Neural Tube Defects—See Hydrocephalus, Spina
Bifida

Neurofibromatosis
National Neurofibromatosis Foundation, Inc.
http://www.nf.org/

Neurofibromatosis, Inc.
http://www.nfinc.org

Neurological Disorders—Also see specific disorder
National Institute of Neurological Disorders and
Stroke
National Institutes of Health
http://www.ninds.nih.gov

Nevoid Basal Cell Carcinoma Syndrome—Also
see Cancer
BCCNS Life Support Network
http://www.bccns.org

Niemann-Pick Disease—Also see Tay-Sachs Disease
Center for Jewish Genetic Diseases
http://www.mssm.edu/jewish_genetics/

National Niemann-Pick Disease Foundation, Inc.
http://www.nnpdf.org

Noonan Syndrome
Noonan Syndrome Support Group, Inc.
http://www.noonansyndrome.org

Ollier Disease
American Association of Multiple
Enchondroma Disease *
http://www.aamed.net
* Also includes multiple cartilaginous enchon-
dromatosis, Ollier osteochondromatosis,
Maffucci syndrome.

Oppenheim Disease—See Muscular Dystrophy

OptizG/BBB, Opitz G and Related Syndromes
The Opitz G/BBB Family Network
http://www.opitznet.org

Organic Acidemias—Also see Metabolic Diseases
Organic Acidemia Association *
http://www.oaanews.org
* Includes organic aciduria, isovaleric acidemia,
methylmalonic acidemia, proprionic
acidemia, acidemia, and errors of amino acide
fatty acid metabolism.

Osler Weber Rendu Syndrome—See Hereditary
Hemorrhagic Telangiectasia

Osteogenesis Imperfecta—Also see Bone Diseases
The Osteogenesis Imperfecta Foundation, Inc.
http://www.oif.org

Osteoporosis
National Osteoporosis Foundation
http://www.nof.org/

Osteoporosis and Related Bone Diseases—
National Research Center,
NIH
http://www.osteo.org/

Ovarian Cancer—Also see Cancer
Gilda Radner Familial Ovarian Cancer Registry
http://www.ovariancancer.com

Oxalosis—Also see Kidney Diseases
Oxalosis and Hyperoxaluria Foundation *
http://www.ohf.org

* Also includes primary hyperoxaluria (PH), hyperoxaluria, oxaluria, calcium-oxalate kidney stones.

Paget Disease (of the Bone)
The Paget Foundation
http://www.paget.org

Pallister-Hall Syndrome
Pallister-Hall Foundation (Aust.)
http://www.pallisterhall.com

Pallister-Killian Syndrome
Pallister-Killian Syndrome Support Group
http://www.pk-syndrome.org

Parkinson Disease
The American Parkinson Disease Association, Inc.
http://www.apdaparkinson.org

National Parkinson Foundation, Inc.
http://www.parkinson.org/

Parkinson's Action Network
http://www.parkinsonsaction.org

Parkinson's Disease Foundation
http://www.pdf.org

http://www.umanitoba.ca

Parkinson's Disease Information
http://www.parkinsons.org

Patau Syndrome—See Trisomy 18/13, Chromosome Abnormalities

Peutz-Jeghers Syndrome—See Polyposis

Phenylketonuria (PKU)—Also see Metabolic Disorders
Children's PKU Network (CPN)
http://www.pkunetwork.org

National Coalition for PKU & Allied Disorders
http://www.pku-allieddisorders.org

National PKU News
http://www.pkunews.org

Pierre Robin Syndrome—See Stickler Syndrome

Pigment Disorders—See specific disorder such as Albinism, Vitiligo

Polycystic Kidney Disease—Also see Kidney Disease
National Institute of Diabetes, Digestive & Kidney Diseases

National Institutes of Health
http://www.niddk.nih.gov

Polycystic Kidney Research Foundation
http://www.pkdcure.org

Polyposis
Familial Gastrointestinal Cancer Registry (Canada)
http://www.mtsinai.on.ca/familialgicancer

Porphyria—Also see Iron Overload
American Porphyria Foundation
http://www.enterprise.net/apf

Prader-Willi Syndrome
Prader-Willi Syndrome Association (UK)
http://www.pwsa-uk.demon.co.uk/

Prader-Willi Syndrome Association (USA)
http://www.pwsausa.org

Progeria
Progeria Research Foundation, Inc. *
http://www.progeriaresearch.org
* Includes progeria, Cockayne syndrome, Werner syndrome.

Propionic Acidemia—See Organic Acidemias, Metabolic Diseases

Prune Belly Syndrome
Prune Belly Syndrome Network *
http://www.prunebelly.org
* Also includes Eagle Barrett syndrome.

Pseudoxanthoma Elasticum
National Association for Pseudoxanthoma Elasticum, Inc.
http://www.pxenape.org

PXE International, Inc. (PXE)
http://www.pxe.org

Rare Disorders—See Genetic Disorders, General

Recreation and Leisure
Canadian Wheelchair Basketball Association
http://www.cwba.ca

Cooperative Wilderness Handicapped Outdoor Group (CWHOG)
Idaho State University
http://www.isu.edu/cwhog/

Disabled Sports, USA
http://www.dsusa.org

HSA International (Handicapped Scuba
Association)
http://www.hsascuba.com

National Disability Sports Alliance
http://www.ndsaonline.org

North American Riding for the Handicapped
Association, Inc.
http://www.narha.org

Special Equestrian Riding Therapy, Inc.
http://www.sert.org/main.html

Special Olympics International
http://www.specialolympics.org/

WheelchairSports USA
http://www.wsusa.org

Wilderness on Wheels
http://www.wildernessonwheels.org

Refsum Disease—See Tay-Sachs Disease

Rehabilitation
National Clearinghouse of Rehabilitation
Training Materials
http://www.nchrtm.okstate.edu

National Rehabilitation Association
http://www.nationalrehab.org

National Rehabilitation Information Center
http://www.naric.com/

Rehabilitation International
http://www.rehab-international.org

Resources for Rehabilitation
http://www.rfr.org

Reiter Syndrome—See Ankylosing Spondylitis,
Arthritis

Renal Disorders—See Kidney Disorders, specific
disease

Respite
National Respite Network
http://www.archrespite.org

Retinitis Pigmentosa—Also see Visual Impairment
Foundation Fighting Blindness
http://www.blindness.org

Laurence Moon Bardet Biedl Syndrome Network
http://www.mlmorris.com/lmbbs/

RP International
http://www.rpinternational.org

Rett Syndrome
International Rett Syndrome Association, Inc.
http://www.rettsyndrome.org

Rubinstein-Taybi Syndrome
Rubinstein-Taybi Parent Group
http://www.rubinstein-taybi.org

Russell-Silver Syndrome
The Magic Foundation *
http://www.magicfoundation.org
* Also includes Silver syndrome, Russell
syndrome, Silver-Russell syndrome.

Sandhoff Disease—See Tay-Sachs Disease

Sanfillippo Disease—See Tay-Sachs Disease,
Mucopolysaccharide Disorders

Scheie Disease—See Mucopolysaccharide Disorders

Scleroderma
Scleroderma Foundation
http://www.scleroderma.org

Scoliosis
National Scoliosis Foundation
http://www.scoliosis.org

Scoliosis Association, Inc.
http://www.scoliosis-assoc.org

Scoliosis Research Society
http://www.srs.org

Scoliosis Treatment Advanced Recovery System
(STARS)
http://www.scoliosis.com/

Self-Help Clearinghouses
American Self-Help Group Clearinghouse
http://www.mentalhelp.net/selfhelp

National Self-Help Clearinghouse
http://www.selfhelpweb.org

Sexuality
Sexuality Information and Education Council
of the U.S.
http://www.siecus.org

Short Stature—Also see Growth Problems
Human Growth Foundation
http://www.hgfound.org

Little People of America, Inc.
http://www.lpaonline.org

The MAGIC Foundation for Children's
Growth
http://www.magicfoundation.org

Short Persons Support
http://www.shortsupport.org

Shprintzen Syndrome—See Chromosome
Abnormalities

Shwachman Syndrome
Shwachman-Diamond Syndrome International *
http://www.shwachman-diamond.org
* Also includes Shwachman-Diamond, Burke's
syndrome, Shwachman-Vodian.

Shy-Drager Syndrome
Shy-Drager Syndrome Support Group
http://www.shy-drager.com

Siblings
Siblings for Significant Change
http://wwwmed.umich.edu/1libr/yourchild/spec
need.htm

Sibling Support Project
http://www.thearc.org/siblingsupport

Sickle Cell Disease
American Sickle Cell Anemia Association
http://www.ascaa.org

National Heart, Lung, and Blood Institute
National Institutes of Health
http://www.nhlbi.nih.gov

Sickle Cell Disease Association of America, Inc.
http://www.sicklecelldisease.org

Silver-Russell Syndrome—See Russell-Silver
Syndrome

Sjögren Syndrome
National Sjögren's Syndrome Association
http://www.sjogrenssyndrome.org

Sjogren's Syndrome Foundation, Inc.
http://www.sjogrens.com

Skeletal Dysplasias
Greenberg Center for Skeletal Dysplasias
http://www.hopkinsmedicine.org/greenbergcen-
ter/Greenbrg.htm

Skin Disorders—Also see specific disorder
Foundation for Ichthyosis and Related Skin Types
http://www.scalyskin.org

Smith-Magenis Syndrome—See also Chromo-
some Abnormalities
Parents and Researchers Interested in
Smith-Magenis Syndrome *
http://www.prisms.org
* Also includes deletion 17p11.2

Sotos Syndrome
Sotos Syndrome Support Association
http://www.well.com/user/sssa

Sotos Syndrome Support Group of Canada
http://www.sssac.com

Spina Bifida
Association for Spina Bifida and Hydrocephalus
(UK)
http://www.asbah.org

Spina Bifida Association of America
http://www.sbaa.org

Spina Bifida and Hydrocephalus Association
of Canada
http://www.sbhac.ca

Hydrocephalus Support Group, Inc.
http://www.hydrocephaly.com

Spinal Muscular Atrophy
Families of Spinal Muscular Atrophy
http://www.fsma.org

Sprue—See Gluten Intolerance

Stickler Syndrome
Stickler Involved People *
http://www.sticklers.org
* Includes Stickler syndrome, hereditary
progressive arthro-opthalmopathy,
Pierre Robin syndrome.

Sturge-Weber Syndrome—Also see Vascular
Malformations
Sturge-Weber Foundation
http://www.sturge-weber.com

Sudden Infant Death Syndrome—Also see Death,
Neonatal, and Infant
First Candle/SIDS Alliance, Inc.
http://www.sidsalliance.org

National SIDS/Infant Death Resource Center
http://www.sidscenter.org

Syringomyelia
American Syringomyelia Alliance Project, Inc.
http://www.asap4sm.com

Tall Stature—Also see Growth Problems
Tall Clubs International
http://www.tall.org

Tangier Disease—See Tay-Sachs Disease

Tay-Sachs Disease
Center for Jewish Genetic Diseases
http://www.mssm.edu/jewish_genetics/

National Tay-Sachs & Allied Diseases
   Association, Inc. *
http://www.ntsad.org
* Includes the following disorders: Batten,
   Canavan, Fabry, Farber, fucosidosis, Gaucher,
   Krabbe, Landing, mannosidosis, metachro-
   matic leukodystrophy, mucolipidoses
   I-IV (sialidosis, I-cell disease, etc.),
   mucopolysaccharidoses (Hunter, Hurler,
   Scheie, Maroteaux-Lamy, Morquio,
   Sanfillippo, Sly or betaglucuronidase
   deficiency), Niemann-Pick, Pompe,
   Refsum, Tangier, Tay-Sachs, Wolman
   disease, and others.

Thalassemia—Also see Iron Overload
AHEPA-American Hellenic Educational
   Progressive Association *
http://www.ahepa.org
* Thalassemia minor, thalassemia major,
   thalassemia intermedia, beta-thalassemia,
   Cooley's anemia.

Cooley's Anemia Foundation, Inc.
http://www.cooleysanemia.org

Thrombocytopenia Absent Radius (TAR) Syndrome
Thrombocytopenia Absent Radius Syndrome
   Association
http://www.kumc.edu/gec/support/tarsynd.html

Thyroid Disorders
American Foundation of Thyroid Patients
http://www.thyroidfoundation.org

National Graves' Disease Foundation
http://www.ngdf.org

Thyroid Foundation of America
http://www.tsh.org

Torsion Dystonia—See Dystonia

Tourette Syndrome
Tourette Syndrome Association, Inc.
http://www.tsa-usa.org

National Institute of Neurological Disorders
   and Stroke
National Institutes of Health
http://www.ninds.nih.gov

Travel
AccessAbility Travel
http://www.access-ability.org/travel.html

Handicapped Travel Club
http://www.handicappedtravelclub.com

Mobility International
http://www.miusa.org

Society for Accessible Travel and Hospitality
http://www.sath.org

Travel Outlet, Inc.
http://www.traveloutlet.org

Travelin' Talk
http://www.travelintalk.net

Treacher Collins Syndrome
Treacher Collins Foundation
http://www.treachercollinsfnd.org

Tremor, familial
Coping With Essential Tremor
http://www.essentialtremor.org

Triple X Syndrome—See also Chromosome
Disorders
Triplo-X Syndrome
http://www.triplo-x.org

Trisomy 9—See Chromosome Disorders

Trisomy 18/13—See also Chromosome
Disorders
Chromosome 18 Registry and Research
   Society
http://www.chromosome18.org

Support Organization for Trisomy (SOFT) 18,
   13, and Related Disorders
http://www.trisomy.org

Tuberous Sclerosis
Tuberous Sclerosis Alliance.
http://www.tsalliance.org

Turner Syndrome—Also see Short Stature,
Chromosome Disorders
Turner's Syndrome Society of Canada
http://www.turnersyndrome.ca

Turner Syndrome Society of the United States
http://www.turner-syndrome-us.org/

Turner Syndrome Support Society
http://www.tss.org.uk

Twins—See Multiple Births

Tyrosinosis—See Liver Disease

Tyrosinemia—See Liver Disease, Metabolic
Disorders

Ulcerative Colitis—See Inflammatory Bowel
Disease

Urea Cycle Disorders—Also see Organic
Acidemias, Metabolic Disorders
National Urea Cycle Disorders Foundation
http://www.nucdf.org

Usher Syndrome—See Deaf-Blind, Hearing
Impairment, Retinitis Pigmentosa, Visual Impairment

Vascular Birthmarks and Malformations—Also
see Sturge-Weber Syndrome, Von Hippel-Lindau
Syndrome
Vascular Birthmarks Foundation *
http://www.birthmark.org
* Includes vascular malformations, port wine
stain, Klippel-Trenaunay syndrome, hereditary hemorrhagic telangiectasia, Sturge Weber
syndrome, arteriovenous malformations, Von
Hippel-Lindau syndrome, lymphangiomas.

VATER Syndrome and Association
TEF VATER National Support Network
http://www.tefvater.org

Velo-Cardio Facial Syndrome
Velo-Cardio Facial Syndrome Educational
Foundation
http://www.vcfsef.org

Vision Impairment—Also see Disabilities
American Council of the Blind
http://www.acb.org/

American Foundation for the Blind
http://www.afb.org

Association for Education and Rehabilitation of
the Blind and Visually Impaired
http://www.aerbvi.org

Blind Children's Center
http://www.blindcntr.org

Braille Institute
http://www.brailleinstitute.org

Canadian National Institute for the Blind
http://www.cnib.ca

Carroll Center for the Blind, Inc.
http://www.carroll.org

Center for the Partially Sighted
http://65.18.208.35

Choice Magazine Listening
http://www.choicemagazinelistening.org

Descriptive Video Service
http://main.wgbh.org/wgbh/access

Foundation Fighting Blindness
http://www.blindness.org/

Guide Dogs for the Blind, Inc.
http://www.guidedogs.com

Guide Dog Foundation for the Blind
http://www.guidedog.org

Guiding Eyes for the Blind
http://www.guiding-eyes.org

Jewish Guild for the Blind
http://www.jgb.org

Leader Dogs for the Blind
http://www.leaderdog.org

Library of Congress-Persons with Disabilities
http://www.loc.gov/access

National Association for Parents of the Visually
Impaired
http://www.spedex.com/napvi

National Association for the Visually Handicapped
http://www.navh.org

National Braille Association, Inc.
http://www.nationalbraille.org

National Federation of the Blind
http://www.nfb.org

Recording for the Blind and Dyslexic
http://www.rfbd.org

The Seeing Eye, Inc.
http://www.seeingeye.org

Vision Council of America
http://www.visionsite.org

Vitiligo
National Vitiligo Foundation, Inc.
http://www.nvfi.org

Von Hippel-Lindau Syndrome—Also see
Sturge Weber Syndrome, Vascular Malformations,
Cancer
VHL Family Alliance
http://www.vhl.org

Von Willebrand Disease—See Hemophilia

Werdnig-Hoffman Disease—See Muscular
Dystrophy

Werner Syndrome—See Progeria

Williams Syndrome
Williams Syndrome Association
http://www.williams-syndrome.org

Wilson Disease—Also see Liver Diseases
Wilson's Disease Association
http://www.wilsonsdisease.org

Wolf-Hirschhorn Disease—Also see Chromosome
Abnormalities
4p-Support Group
http://www.4p-supportgroup.org

Wolf Hirschhorn Support Group UK
http://www.whs.webk.co.uk

Wolman Disease—See Tay-Sachs Disease

Xeroderma Pigmentosum
Share and Care Cockayne Syndrome Network
http://www.cockayne-syndrome.org

Xeroderma Pigmentosum Society, Inc.
http://www.xps.org

Index

Springer Publishing Company

Guidelines for Nurse Practitioners in Gynecologic Settings

8th Edition

Joellen W. Hawkins, RNC, PhD, FAAN
Diane M. Roberto-Nichols, BS, APRN-C
J. Lynn Stanley-Haney, MA, APRN-C

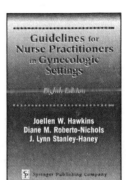

This extensively revised and updated edition is designed to be used as a guide for nursing management of the common gynecological conditions of women, for use in community-based or ambulatory settings.

Contents:

Part I: Clinical Guidelines
- Methods of Family Planning
- Infertility
- Vaginal Discharge, Vaginitis, and STDs
- Miscellaneous Gynecological Aberrations
- Breast Conditions
- Cervical Aberrations
- Menstrual Disorders
- Postabortion Care
- Abuse, Battering, Violence, and Sexual Assault
- Sexual Dysfunction
- Peri- and Postmenopause
- Smoking Cessation
- Loss of Integrity of Pelvic Floor Structures
- Genitourinary Tract, Urinary Tract Infection
- Preconception Care

- Weight Management
- Complementary Therapies
- Emotional/Mental Health Issues Appropriate for Assessment and Treatment in a Women's Health Care Setting

Part II: Appendixes
- Patient Education Handouts
- Health History Forms
- Gynecological Annual Exam Form
- Informed Consent Forms
- Danger Assessment
- Self Assessment of AIDS (HIV) Risk
- Vulvar Self Examination
- Women and Heart Disease: Risk Factor Assessment
- General Women's Health Web Sites
- Body Mass Index Table

2004   424pp   0-8261-1626-4   softcover

11 West 42nd Street, New York, NY 10036-8002 • Fax: 212-941-7842
Order Toll-Free: 877-687-7476 • Order On-line: www.springerpub.com

Springer Publishing Company

From the Springer Series on Advanced Practice Nursing...

Nurse Practitioners
Evolution of Advanced Practice
4th Edition

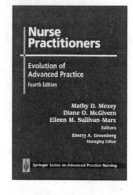

Mathy D. Mezey, EdD, RN, FAAN
Diane O. McGivern, RN, PhD, FAAN
Eileen M. Sullivan-Marx, PhD, CRNP, FAAN
Editors
Sherry A. Greenberg, MSN, RN, BC Managing Editor

"Nothing could be more propitious to herald in the 21st century than this Fourth Edition...It chronicles the depth and breadth of advanced practice nursing historically, clinically, professionally, organizationally, legally and politically...A vital descriptive link in the illustrious, if torturous, history of advanced practice nursing."
—from the Foreword by **Loretta C. Ford,** RN, EdD, PNP, FAAN, FAANP
Co-Founder with Pediatrician Henry Silver
of the Pediatric Nurse Practitioner Role (1965)

This comprehensive textbook provides a broad and balanced picture of this important part of professional nursing, and is a valuable resource for students in advanced practice nursing programs as well as new advanced practice graduates.

Partial Contents:
Part I: Perspectives: History, Education, Philosophy, and Research
• Philosophical and Historical Basis of Advanced Nursing Roles • Primary Care as an Academic Discipline
Part II: The Practice Arena: Many Voices, Many Roles • Nurse-Midwifery and Primary Health Care for Women • Pediatric Nurse Practitioner and Pediatrician: Collaborative Practice • Adolescent Family Practice
Part III: A Range of Settings for Care • Nurse Practitioners in the School-Based Health Care Environment • Primary Care in the Home: The Nurse Practitioner's Role • Caring for Residents in Public Housing-Based Nursing Centers
Part IV: Payment, Policy, and Politics • Systems of Payment for Advanced Practice Licensure, Certification and Credentialing • Workforce Policy Perspectives on Advanced Practice Nursing

2003   514pp   0-8261-7772-7   hardcover

11 West 42nd Street, New York, NY 10036-8002 • Fax: 212-941-7842
Order Toll-Free: 877-687-7476 • Order On-line: www.springerpub.com